Diagnostic and Treatment Methods for Ulcerative Colitis and Colitis-Associated Cancer

Ashok Kumar Pandurangan
B. S. Abdur Rahman Crescent Institute of Science and Technology, India

A volume in the Advances in Medical Diagnosis, Treatment, and Care (AMDTC) Book Series

IGI Global
PUBLISHER of TIMELY KNOWLEDGE

Published in the United States of America by
IGI Global
Medical Information Science Reference (an imprint of IGI Global)
701 E. Chocolate Avenue
Hershey PA, USA 17033
Tel: 717-533-8845
Fax: 717-533-8661
E-mail: cust@igi-global.com
Web site: http://www.igi-global.com

Library of Congress Cataloging-in-Publication Data

Names: Pandurangan, Ashok Kumar, 1982- editor.
Title: Diagnostic and treatment methods for ulcerative colitis and colitis-associated cancer / Ashok Kumar Pandurangan, editor.
Description: Hershey, PA : Medical Information Science Reference, [2020] | Includes bibliographical references and index. | Summary: "This book provides innovative insights that describe the fundamental understanding of UC and CAC and the molecular mechanisms behind the etiology as well as modern diagnostic methods that are employed in UC and CAC. Current prevention and therapeutic strategies practiced in the pre-clinical level are also discussed"-- Provided by publisher.
Identifiers: LCCN 2019057171 (print) | LCCN 2019057172 (ebook) | ISBN 9781799835806 (h/c) | ISBN 9781799835813 (eISBN)
Subjects: MESH: Colitis, Ulcerative--diagnosis | Colitis, Ulcerative--therapy | Colitis, Ulcerative--complications | Colonic Neoplasms--diagnosis | Colonic Neoplasms--therapy
Classification: LCC RC862.C63 (print) | LCC RC862.C63 (ebook) | NLM WI 522 | DDC 616.3/4473--dc23
LC record available at https://lccn.loc.gov/2019057171
LC ebook record available at https://lccn.loc.gov/2019057172

This book is published in the IGI Global book series Advances in Medical Diagnosis, Treatment, and Care (AMDTC) (ISSN: 2475-6628; eISSN: 2475-6636)

British Cataloguing in Publication Data
A Cataloguing in Publication record for this book is available from the British Library.

All work contributed to this book is new, previously-unpublished material.
The views expressed in this book are those of the authors, but not necessarily of the publisher.

For electronic access to this publication, please contact: eresources@igi-global.com.

Advances in Medical Diagnosis, Treatment, and Care (AMDTC) Book Series

ISSN:2475-6628
EISSN:2475-6636

MISSION

Advancements in medicine have prolonged the life expectancy of individuals all over the world. Once life-threatening conditions have become significantly easier to treat and even cure in many cases. Continued research in the medical field will further improve the quality of life, longevity, and wellbeing of individuals.

The **Advances in Medical Diagnosis, Treatment, and Care (AMDTC)** book series seeks to highlight publications on innovative treatment methodologies, diagnosis tools and techniques, and best practices for patient care. Comprised of comprehensive resources aimed to assist professionals in the medical field apply the latest innovations in the identification and management of medical conditions as well as patient care and interaction, the books within the AMDTC series are relevant to the research and practical needs of medical practitioners, researchers, students, and hospital administrators.

COVERAGE

- Chronic Conditions
- Medical Testing
- Cancer Treatment
- Internal Medicine
- Disease Management
- Alternative Medicine
- Disease Prevention
- Diagnostic Medicine
- Patient-Centered Care
- Critical Care

IGI Global is currently accepting manuscripts for publication within this series. To submit a proposal for a volume in this series, please contact our Acquisition Editors at Acquisitions@igi-global.com or visit: http://www.igi-global.com/publish/.

The Advances in Medical Diagnosis, Treatment, and Care (AMDTC) Book Series (ISSN 2475-6628) is published by IGI Global, 701 E. Chocolate Avenue, Hershey, PA 17033-1240, USA, www.igi-global.com. This series is composed of titles available for purchase individually; each title is edited to be contextually exclusive from any other title within the series. For pricing and ordering information please visit http://www.igi-global.com/book-series/advances-medical-diagnosis-treatment-care/129618. Postmaster: Send all address changes to above address.

Titles in this Series

For a list of additional titles in this series, please visit: http://www.igi-global.com/book-series

Exploring the Efficacy and Beneficence of Complementary and Alternative Medicinal Products in Disease herapy
Etetor Roland Eshiet (Sustainable Energy Environmental and Educational Development (SEEED), USA)
Medical Information Science Reference • © 2021 • 315pp • H/C (ISBN: 9781799841203) • US $295.00

Climate Change and Its Impact on Fertility
Khursheed Ahmad Wani (Goverment Degree College, Bijbehara, India) and Nibedita Naha (ICMR, National Institute of Occupational Health, Ahmedabad, India)
Medical Information Science Reference • © 2021 • 416pp • H/C (ISBN: 9781799844808) • US $265.00

Treating Endocrine and Metabolic Disorders With Herbal Medicines
Arif Hussain (Manipal Academy of Higher Education, UAE) and Shalini Behl (Manipal Academy of Higher Education, UAE)
Medical Information Science Reference • © 2021 • 489pp • H/C (ISBN: 9781799848080) • US $295.00

Handbook of Research on Advancements in Cancer Therapeutics
Sumit Kumar (National Institute of Pathology, New Delhi, India) Moshahid Alam Rizvi (Jamia Millia Islamia, India) and Saurabh Verma (National Institute of Pathology, India)
Medical Information Science Reference • © 2021 • 913pp • H/C (ISBN: 9781799865308) • US $465.00

Cases on Medical Nutrition Therapy for Gastrointestinal Disorders
Elham Abbas Aljaaly (King Abdulaziz University, Saudi Arabia) Nahlaa Abdelwahab Khalifa (King Abdulaziz University, Saudi Arabia) Rouba Khalil Naaman (King Abdulaziz University, Saudi Arabia) and Manar Abduljalil Bakhsh (King Abdulaziz University, Saudi Arabia)
Medical Information Science Reference • © 2021 • 254pp • H/C (ISBN: 9781799838029) • US $245.00

IGI Global
PUBLISHER of TIMELY KNOWLEDGE

701 East Chocolate Avenue, Hershey, PA 17033, USA
Tel: 717-533-8845 x100 • Fax: 717-533-8661
E-Mail: cust@igi-global.com • www.igi-global.com

Editorial Advisory Board

Table of Contents

Detailed Table of Contents

Daniela Ribeiro, LAQV-REQUIMTE, Laboratório de Química Aplicada, Departamento de Ciências Químicas, Faculdade de Farmácia, Universidade do Porto, Portugal
Marisa Freitas, LAQV-REQUIMTE, Laboratório de Química Aplicada, Departamento de Ciências Químicas, Faculdade de Farmácia, Universidade do Porto, Portugal
José Miguel P. Ferreira de Oliveira, LAQV-REQUIMTE, Laboratório de Química Aplicada, Departamento de Ciências Químicas, Faculdade de Farmácia, Universidade do Porto, Portugal
M. Luisa Corvo, Faculdade de Farmácia, Instituto de Investigação do Medicamento (iMed.ULisboa), Universidade de Lisboa, Portugal
Félix Dias Carvalho, UCIBIO-REQUIMTE, Laboratório de Toxicologia, Departamento de Ciências Biológicas, Faculdade de Farmácia, Universidade do Porto, Portugal
Eduarda Fernandes, LAQV-REQUIMTE, Laboratório de Química Aplicada, Departamento de Ciências Químicas, Faculdade de Farmácia, Universidade do Porto, Portugal

Inflammatory bowel disease (IBD) is a physically incapacitating disorder that significantly disturbs patients' quality of life. IBD is classified into two main pathophysiological forms, ulcerative colitis and Crohn's disease. Literature studies indicate that chronic colitis may contribute to the development of up to 25% of all diagnosed colorectal tumors. The complexity and development of IBD onset is intermediated by a variety of inflammatory mediators and pathways that are intrinsically linked and are summarized in this chapter. This complexity resulted in the development of various in vivo models to surpass the enormous challenges in the finding of new drugs for IBD treatment. These models are mostly based on rodents and on three types of inflammatory activation: chemical induction, transfer of naïve CD4+ T cells, and generation of engineered mouse strains, with specific target gene manipulations. The most broadly described models in literature are here presented and discussed.

Mohamed Adil, Saveetha Institute of Medical and Technical Sciences, India
Anandraj K. Vaithy.k, Mahatma Gandhi Medical College and Research Institute, India
Ashok Kumar Pandurangan, B. S. Abdur Rahman Crescent Institute of Science and Technology, India
Mohammad Waseem, B. S. Abdur Rahman Crescent Institute of Science and Technology, India
Neesar Ahmed, B. S. Abdur Rahman Crescent Institute of Science and Technology, India

Chronic inflammation in the large intestinal epithelial to rectum is a major risk for malignancies. The pathogenesis of colitis associated cancer is distinct with perilous molecular mechanism. The inflammation leads to damage of cells resulting in symptomatic conditions including cancer. This suggest the relationship between certain cancer due to its associated factors such as environment, genetics, and chronic inflammation leading to cancer. Colorectal cancer (CRC) has also been acknowledged as bowel, rectal, or colon cancer. The most common types of adenocarcinomas are associated with colorectal cancer. The lymphomas, carcinoids, sarcoma, and gastrointestinal tumors are also associated with CRC. Most disorders with chronic inflammation and exposure of immunosuppressant have an increased risk with the development of cancer leading towards the treatment of cancer by various therapies like radiation therapy, chemotherapy, hormonal therapy, further into immunotherapy, and targeted therapy. The prognosis of CRC has always been controversial.

Inflammatory bowel disease (IBD) is characterized by sustained inflammatory processes in the gastrointestinal tract. One of the most threatening risks for IBD patients is the development of colorectal cancer, resulting from the chronic inflammatory state. Current IBD treatment presents limitations in safety and efficacy. As such, it is of paramount importance to find novel therapeutic strategies. The antioxidant and anti-inflammatory properties of flavonoids are widely recognized. Flavonoids currently found in our daily diet are likely to yield biological actions at the gastrointestinal level, suggesting a potential protective effect in IBD. However, the number of studies concerning the effects of flavonoids on intestinal inflammation is limited. This chapter intends to summarize the known effects of flavonoids in the different phases of IBD inflammatory pathways, covering all the concerning available in vivo studies.

Ulcerative colitis (UC) is a serious health problem around the world. Inflammatory bowel disease (IBD) is comprised of both Crohn's disease (CD) and UC. IBD is a clinical condition referred as inflammation in the colon. So far there is no proper medication available to treat IBD. On the other hand, untreated UC can be developed as colitis associated cancer. Natural agents are diverse molecules possess many beneficial effects. Many researchers have proven that natural agents can be better option to treat UC. Natural agents such as chrysin, chelidonic acid, euphol, fish oil, diallyl trisulfide, embelin, isatin, and rutin were already reported to have anti-colitic activity. In this chapter, the authors documented the natural agents that were used as treatment for UC.

Ulcerative colitis is a chronic inflammation of the inner part of the colonic mucosa. It is a type of inflammatory bowel disease which is idiopathic in nature. It is multifactorial, debilitating disorder which may cause life threatening complications. Given to the architecture of colon, conventional medicines have limitation in treating the disease. Thus, the need for alternative methods of drug delivery is important. Nanoparticle is one of the preferred drug delivery system owing to its unique properties. Nanoparticles resist undesired and premature degradation of the drugs, increases bioavailability, and target specificity. Different nanoparticle-based drug delivery systems like metallic, liposome, silica, or polymeric nanoparticles have been designed to administer therapeutic agents through oral route to treat ulcerative colitis. Natural compounds and active components isolated from the plant extracts and other bioactive agents are also delivered by nanoparticle. In the current chapter, nanoparticle-mediated drug and phytochemicals delivery to treat ulcerative colitis are discussed.

Inflammatory bowel disease (IBD) is a psychosomatic disorder characterized by chronic inflammation of the gastrointestinal tract. Metabolism of an individual affected with IBD is equated to imbalance of jatharagni (digestive fire) which results in atijeernam (hyper digestive disorder), ajeernam (hypo digestive disorder), or kutajeernam (erroneous digestive disorder). Yoga stabilizes jatharagni that helps energy transformation of 1) food substances into nutritious substance, 2) nutritious substance into tissues. It improves anabolic and catabolic processes which help absorption of energy. Yogic cleansing techniques promote elimination of ama (toxic products) and kleda (waste products). Yoga therapy along with herbal medicine and lifestyle modification helps develop balanced state of doshas in individuals with IBD. Yoga practice has a healing effect on mind and body, reduces stress, increases emotional and physical self-awareness, and improves the ability to manage physical symptoms.

Colitis-associated cancers are a metastatic form of inflammatory bowel disease considered a vital health associated risk factor causing the death of approximately five lacs people every year throughout the world. There are trillions of bacteria that are associated with our gut as a part of our healthy microbiome. The microbiota plays a plethora of important role in determining the normal physiological processes of the cells and, subsequently, the body. The imbalance in microbiome diversity (dysbiosis) due to abnormal dietary habitats, hectic lifestyle, and other factors thus alters the normal physiological processes of the body, thereby causing several chronic diseases. Therefore, it is essential to maintain the homeostasis between the host and their gut microbiome. So, based on the facts mentioned above, this chapter is entirely devoted to providing an overview of colitis-associated cancer and their relation with the dysbiosis of a healthy microbiome. Moreover, the mechanism involved in the development of colorectal cancer and its preventive insights has also been addressed.

Ulcerative colitis or Crohn's illness patients are in danger of colon cancer due to chronic inflammation, resulting from the reaction of the immune system to bacterial disease caused by genetic alterations in the colonic mucosa. Somatic cells gain genomic changes, such as TP53 that regulates MUC2 production and APC alterations linked with β-catenin and MUC1 contribution in the slight proliferation of cells. Mathematical modeling describes developmental modifications and uses the phrases to link parameter to curves of age-dependent incidence of epidemiological cancer. By using the long-lasting investigation of IBD patients to gather the genomic estimations for increasingly exact computations of IBD-explicit developmental parameters as initiation, birth, and death. Colon cancer genetic trajectory follows the structure of the composition of functions that leads to malignancies. Models of population level can be utilized to consolidate epidemiological information and in this manner describe malignant growth advancement in a population with IBD.

Colorectal cancer the third-leading cause of cancer mortality Worldwide; it's a well characterised model at molecular level among various cancera. Chronic ulcerative colitis is one of the causes of colorectal cancer. Recent cancer research focuses on tumor-initiating cells which are the cause of tumor initiation, invasions, drug-resistant, recurrence, and metastasis. Emerging research findings support the presence of colon cancer stem cells in sporadic colorectal cancer and in colitis-associated colorectal cancer. Colitis-associated cancer cells exhibit increased colon cancer stem cell marker expression along with activated developmental signaling pathways. Also, emerging reports exhibit that inhibition stem cell markers in chronic ulcerative colitis cells impedes progression of cancer in genetically engineered animal models and primary samples. This chapter deals of colitis-cancer transition, microenvironment of colitis-associated colorectal cancer, and articulates that cancer stem cells are ideal targets for colorectal cancer.

Inflammatory bowel disease (IBD) is comprised of ulcerative colitis (UC) and Crohn's disease (CD) that was recognized by the inflammation in the colon. There are no proper medications are available to control the IBD in patients. NASIDs such as Aspirin, diclofenac, and ibuprofen are widely used to control the inflammation. On the other hand, the untreated prolonged inflammation leads to the development of cancer in the colon termed as colitis-associated cancer or inflammation-driven colon cancer. Oxidative stress and inflammation play key roles in the pathogenesis of colitis-associated cancer. Single dose of azozymethane (AOM) and three cycles of 2% dextran sodium sulfate (DSS) induces colitis-associated cancer (CAC) in mouse. Hence, many natural products were tested in the preclinical model of colitis-associated cancer. Each of these natural agents modulate important signaling pathway to control the colitis-associated cancer (CAC). In this review, the authors tabulated all the natural agents that culminate the colitis-associated cancer in the preclinical models.

Foreword

Ulcerative colitis (UC) and Crohn's disease (CD) is a chronic idiopathic inflammatory bowel disease (IBD) characterized by continuous mucosal inflammation that starts in the rectum and extends proximally. Typical presenting symptoms include bloody diarrhea, abdominal pain, urgency, and tenesmus. The etiology of the disease not fully known. The risk factors include a history of recent infection with Salmonella or Campylobacter, living in Western industrialized nations and at higher latitudes, and a family history of the disease. The incidence peaks in early adulthood, but patients can develop the disorder from early childhood through adulthood. There are no proper medications are available for the treatment of UC. Especially, the non-steroidal anti-inflammatory drugs (NSAIDs) were used to control the inflammation. When UC is untreated that leads to the chronic inflammation further developed as colitis associated cancer (CAC). CAC is totally different from familial based colorectal cancer.

This book has the collection of chapters of different aspects of ulcerative colitis and colitis associated cancer. Daniela Ribeiro et al reported that various inflammatory, transcription signaling pathways that contribute to the development of UC was discussed in Chapter 1. Adil et al., reported that how immuo-profiling and immuno-scoring helps in the detection of biomarkers of UC and CAC. In addition, the advancement of immunotherapy in CAC was discussed in Chapter 2. Marisa Freitas et al., reported that the preclinical evidence on the list of flavonoids showed promising effects on UC in Chapter 3. Syed Nasar Rahaman et al., reported that the diagnostic methods and mechanism of action of some of the natural products against UC was discussed in Chapter 4. Subhamoy Banerjee reported that the novel and modern therapeutic approaches in the treatment of UC in Chapter 5. Soccalingam Artchoudane reported that the types of yoga pose's that help to prevent the IBD diseased such as UC and CD in Chapter 6. Gut microbiome plays a vital role in many disease conditions and also provide valuable information about individual. Priyamvada reported that the role of gut microbiome correlated with the colitis associated cancer was discussed in Chapter 7. Rubeena et al., reported that some of the mathematical approaches in analyzing the data of IBD and CAC such as fuzzy logic methods and etc. was discussed in Chapter 8. Vasudeven reported that cancer stem cells are the main culprit for the re-occurrence of all type of cancers. He discussed that the markers that expressed in CAC and singling that regulated by Cancer stem cells in CAC in Chapter 9. Pandurangan et al., reported that the major signaling pathways that dysregulated in CAC and natural agents that influence these signaling to suppress the CAC was discussed in Chapter 10.

I strongly believe this book will be helpful for the researchers in particular and also for clinicians and graduate (Under and post) students studying in this field. Moreover, it will help the teachers, and healthcare professionals who is interested to know about UC and CAC.

I wish thank Dr. Ashok Kumar Pandurangan and all the authors who contributed chapters for this book for bringing such a nice collection of chapters for the benefit of human beings among the world and I wish the book will have grand success.

Norhaizan Mohd Esa
Department of Nutrition and Dietetics, Faculty of Medicine and Health Sciences, Universiti Putra Malaysia, Serdang, Malaysia

Preface

A common chronic inflammatory disease of the gastrointestinal tract (IBD) is inflammatory bowel disease (IBD). Ulcerative colitis and Crohn's Disease (CD), considered common health conditions, are included in IBD. UC is characterised by erosion, mucosal ulceration, and inflammatory cell invasion, and exhibits clinical symptoms that include weight loss, blood and mucus-accompanied diarrhoea, fever, gastric dysmotility, and colon shortening. Ulcerative colitis pathogenesis is complicated and can include genetic, environmental and immunological influences. A breakdown of the epithelial barrier, accompanied by improper reactions to microbial products and persistent inflammation in genetically susceptible hosts, is suggested to play a key role in this disease.

More than 1 million new cases of colorectal cancer (CRC) are diagnosed around the world every year. The third most prevalent malignancy and fourth most prevalent cause of mortality worldwide is CRC. Chronic inflammation of the intestine and colon results in epithelial injury. Inflammation is induced by locally generated cytokines and the proliferation of crypt cells is stimulated to compensate for epithelial cell loss. The development of CAC can eventually lead to this chronically stimulated condition of the epithelium. The stages of cancer growth between non-inflammatory CRC and CAC, including the formation of aberrant crypt focuses, polyps, adenomas, and carcinomas, are similar. Some distinct pathogenic sequences have, however, been suggested for CAC, including chronic inflammation and injury-dysplasia carcinoma that occurs without well-defined adenoma development. In sporadic CRC and CAC, typical genetic and signalling pathways such as Wnt / β-catenin, K-ras, p53 and transforming growth factor (TGF)-β are altered, although the timing between CRC and CAC may be different for p53 and adenomatous polyposis coli (APC) inactivation and K-Ras activation. In the early stage of CAC, aberrant activation of inflammatory cytokines, transcription factors such as NF-eB and STAT3, was observed.

Azoxymethane (AOM) and dextran sodium sulphate (DSS) are the classic and commonly used models for inducing CAC in rodents. In animal models of CRC, several researchers use AOM, 1,2-dimethylhydrazine (DMH, a precursor of AOM) and/or methyl azoxy methane (MAM) acetate. The spectrum of epithelial lesions caused by AOM parallels that of the different forms of human CRC neoplastic lesions. In addition, the definition in which tumour initiation is accompanied by tumour promotion and development in a sequential manner tends to obey AOM-induced CRC. Specifically, as the precursor lesion and Mucin deficient foci, AOM causes the onset of aberrant crypt foci, followed most frequently by the onset of distal colon adenocarcinoma, and, eventually, by metastasis of mesenteric lymph nodes and liver.

Chronic inflammation in a variety of organs is related to the development of cancer. Chronic inflammatory disorders, such as Barrett oesophagus, chronic gastritis, and chronic pancreatitis, of the gastrointestinal tract confer a predisposition to malignancy. The production of reactive oxygen and nitrogen species that can cause oxidative damage to DNA, proteins, and lipids is one mechanism by which inflammation may contribute to the development of cancer. Increased levels of oxidative damage were observed explicitly at cancer sites in a study of multiple inflammation-associated cancers, including colitis-associated CRC. Continuous exposure to cytokines induces an up-regulation of ROS production based on iNOS and DNA instability that leads to cancer. Hence, Oxidative stress plays a crucial role in the development of CAC from chronic inflammation.

In the intestinal immune system, cytokines are essential signalling molecules and are believed to engage in the disturbance of the so-called natural state of regulated inflammation. They are small peptide proteins generated mainly by immune cells that facilitate cell-to - cell contact, promote the proliferation of antigen-specific effector cells, and mediate autocrine, paracrine, and endocrine local and systemic inflammation. IL-6 is a pleiotropic cytokine that, through its soluble IL-6 receptor (sIL-6R), exerts its pro-inflammatory effects mainly through mediation. Soluble IL-6 (sIL-6R) and IL-6 receptor combinations activate cells that express only gp130 and not IL-6R, a mechanism known as trans-signaling. There has been thorough research of IL-6 signalling by STAT3. In many immunologic reactions during the production of IBD, this pathway plays a central function, and circulating levels of IL-6 and sIL-6R interact with several CD and UC clinical features.

Cytokines are key signaling molecules in the intestinal immune system, and are known to participate in the disruption of the so-called normal state of controlled inflammation. They are small peptide proteins produced mainly by immune cells that enable communication between cells, stimulate the proliferation of antigen specific effector cells, and mediate the local and systemic inflammation in an autocrine, paracrine and endocrine pathways. IL-6 is a pleiotropic cytokine that exerts its pro-inflammatory effects largely by mediated through its soluble IL-6 receptor (sIL-6R). The combination of soluble IL-6 receptor (sIL-6R) and IL-6 stimulates cells that only express gp130 and not IL-6R, a process known as trans-signaling. IL-6 signaling through STAT3 has been extensively studied. This system plays a central role in several immunologic reactions during the development of IBD, and circulating levels of IL-6 and sIL-6R correlate with many clinical features of CD and UC. Blocking of IL-6 trans-signaling causes T-cell apoptosis, indicating that the IL-6-sIL-6R system mediates the resistance of T cells to apoptosis in CD. IL-6 protein and mRNA are also often upregulated in serum and tumor samples of humans and mice suffering from breast, prostate, lung, liver and colon cancer. IL-6 enhances the proliferation of human colon carcinoma cells *in vitro* and interference with IL-6 signaling during late stages of CAC development slows down tumor growth. There are extensive reports are stating the IL-6 and STAT3 are required for survival of intestinal epithelial cells and development of CAC and blocking this will inhibit the tumor formation in CAC.

IL-17A is an important pro-inflammatory cytokine that is secreted by CD 41 T cells that produce IL-17 (IL-17A) and express a specific transcription factor, retinoid-related orphan receptor -γt, have been distinguished from other Th1 and Th2 cells, and termed Th17 cells, while the monocyte/macrophage lineage also produces this cytokine. In mice, IL-17A is furthermore secreted by NKT-like cells as well as cd T cells. The IL-17 receptor A (IL-17RA) is ubiquitously expressed on a variety of cell types and essentially involved in the IL-17A and IL-17F signaling. IL-17 plays a key role in animal models of chronic inflammation and several human chronic inflammatory diseases. IL-17 has been reported to be important in the initiation and/or progression of several inflammatory diseases through the recruitment of neutrophils or other cells in the immune system and amplifies the inflammation. IL-21 is a member of large family of cytokines and is made by a range of activated $CD4^+$ Th cells, including Th1, Th17 and activated natural killer cells. An IL-21 protein level is elevated in the intestinal inflamed patients with CD and patients of UC as compared to normal controls. Excessive evidence supports that, elevated levels of IL-21 in the gut has deleterious consequences for the host. DSS or TNBS-induced wild-type colitis mice produce high level of IL-21; also IL-21-knockout mice are largely protected against disease in both models. IL-21 was highly expressed in human CRC patients and IL-21-deficient mice were resistant to CAC induced with AOM and DSS. IL-21, like IL-6 and IL-17A, is a powerful activator of the transcription factor STAT3, which is a critical modulator of chronic inflammation. Absence of IL-21 reduced STAT3 Activation and reduced the expression of Bcl-xL, a STAT3-induced anti-apoptotic protein in tumor and stromal cells.

The Signal Transducer and Activator Transcription 3 (STAT3) protein is a part of STAT's transcription factor family, which is initially inactive in the cytoplasm. After stimulation with extracellular signals, including cytokines, growth factors, and hormones, Janus kinase (JAKs), which then induces STAT3 phophorylateation with tyrosine residue 705 (Y705), is enabled. Phosphorylated STAT3 proteins dimerate and translocate to the nucleus through their Src-homology 2 (SH2) domains where many of the essential genes involved in cell cycle progressive, proliferative, migratory and invasive growth and survival are regulated. In clinical samples of a broad range of human carcinoma, especially CAC, the constitutive activation of STAT3 is always detected. Importantly, high levels of STAT3 were associated with the invasion of the tumour, metastasis and weaker CAC prognoses. The IL-6 / STAT3 signalling pathway has ample evidence to play an important role for CAC and was therefore considered a primary focus for the treatment of CAC. The book comprised of the following chapter

Chapter 1 emphasize the involvement of various signaling molecules and pathways that contribute to the development of UC and CD. The signaling such as Eicosanoids, Reactive oxygen species, Reactive nitrogen species, adhesion molecules and some of the transcription factors such as NF-κB and Nrf2. The authors discussed how these signaling were dysregulated in UC.

Chapter 2 depicts about the how chronic inflammation will lead to the development of colitis Associated cancer (CAC). In this juncture, the immune cells play a vital role as tumor microenvironment that contribute CAC. In this chapter, authors proposing immuno-profiling and immuno-scoring as potential biomarkers for CAC. This chapter also, highlights the treatment options such as immunotherapy in the form of monoclonal antibodies.

Chapter 3 denotes that the preclinical treatment option such as the flavonoids on IBD. The flavonoids are one kind of natural active ingredients produced by plants and they have many classifications. Flavonoids possess many beneficial effects against variety of diseases. Here authors of this chapter discussed the beneficial flavonoids such as Apigenin, Luteolin, Genistein, catechin, epicatechin, daidzein and hesperidin against IBD and their mechanism of action.

Chapter 4 describes the use of various natural products and their pharmacological properties and also, they possess a significant effect in ameliorating inflammatory bowel disease in animal models. The compilated data suggests that there is a future for new herbal-based therapies in the treatment of ulcerative colitis.

Chapter 5 demonstrates that more than the free drugs, the nanoparticle mediated delivery of both natural products and synthetic compounds. The overview, of how the drugs attached to nanoparticles and their mode of action in treating ulcerative colitis was discussed in detail.

Chapter 6 depicts that Yogic practices have a calming effect on mind and body, reduces stress, and improves emotional and physical self-awareness. Several studies have found that yoga improves quality of life and anxiety in individuals with IBD as well as ulcerative colitis.

Chapter 7 demonstrates the cause and development of IBD and CAC as well as its treatment by modulating the existing microbiome altered during the course of IBD and CAC development.

Chapter 8 describes a number of mathematical models that can be used in the CAC, such as probability models, population-based models, time series models, and statistical models.

Chapter 9 Cancer stem cells are small sub-population of tumor cells, they are immortal tumor-initiating cells, possess self-renewal and pluripotent capacity. Cancer stem cells are the basis for tumor initiation, development, metastasis, recurrence and drug resistance. In this chapter, the author detailed the role of cancer stem cells in the colon cancer and colitis associated cancer along with markers and signaling that is associated to cancer stem cells.

Chapter 10 Natural products the class of molecules which shows many beneficial effects. Natural products can be sub classed into flavonoids, alkaloids, Terpenoids. The authors of this chapter discussed the pre-clinical evidence on how natural products such as Ziziphus jujuba Fruit, Bufalin, Cocoa, Digitoflavone, Astaxanthin and etc. control the CAC. In addition, the authors also discussed the mechanism of action of these natural products.

In a nutshell, this book comprised of versatile chapters that covers all the aspects of ulcerative colitis and colitis associated cancer. Both Ulcerative colitis and colitis associated cancer that need to address at this moment since their aggressiveness. The incidence is increasing day by and the treatment options are limited. This book will provide a clear insight on the various treatment options available that were proven pre-clinically. This information will be beneficial for the clinicians who are interested to develop drugs for bot ulcerative colitis and colitis associated cancer.

Chapter 1
Inflammatory Pathways and In Vivo Studies of Inflammatory Bowel Disease

Daniela Ribeiro
LAQV-REQUIMTE, Laboratório de Química Aplicada, Departamento de Ciências Químicas, Faculdade de Farmácia, Universidade do Porto, Portugal

Marisa Freitas
LAQV-REQUIMTE, Laboratório de Química Aplicada, Departamento de Ciências Químicas, Faculdade de Farmácia, Universidade do Porto, Portugal

José Miguel P. Ferreira de Oliveira
LAQV-REQUIMTE, Laboratório de Química Aplicada, Departamento de Ciências Químicas, Faculdade de Farmácia, Universidade do Porto, Portugal

M. Luisa Corvo
https://orcid.org/0000-0002-6332-3937
Faculdade de Farmácia, Instituto de Investigação do Medicamento (iMed. ULisboa), Universidade de Lisboa, Portugal

Félix Dias Carvalho
https://orcid.org/0000-0003-3858-3494
UCIBIO-REQUIMTE, Laboratório de Toxicologia, Departamento de Ciências Biológicas, Faculdade de Farmácia, Universidade do Porto, Portugal

Eduarda Fernandes
https://orcid.org/0000-0003-3858-3494
LAQV-REQUIMTE, Laboratório de Química Aplicada, Departamento de Ciências Químicas, Faculdade de Farmácia, Universidade do Porto, Portugal

DOI: 10.4018/978-1-7998-3580-6.ch001

ABSTRACT

Inflammatory bowel disease (IBD) is a physically incapacitating disorder that significantly disturbs patients' quality of life. IBD is classified into two main pathophysiological forms, ulcerative colitis and Crohn's disease. Literature studies indicate that chronic colitis may contribute to the development of up to 25% of all diagnosed colorectal tumors. The complexity and development of IBD onset is intermediated by a variety of inflammatory mediators and pathways that are intrinsically linked and are summarized in this chapter. This complexity resulted in the development of various in vivo models to surpass the enormous challenges in the finding of new drugs for IBD treatment. These models are mostly based on rodents and on three types of inflammatory activation: chemical induction, transfer of naïve CD4+ T cells, and generation of engineered mouse strains, with specific target gene manipulations. The most broadly described models in literature are here presented and discussed.

INTRODUCTION

Inflammatory bowel disease (IBD) is a physically incapacitating disorder that significantly disturbs the patients' quality of life (Rohr *et al.*, 2018). IBD diagnosis is based on descriptive characteristics and symptomology, including vomiting, diarrhea, and nausea, particularly when specific food groups are ingested. IBD has two key pathophysiological forms: ulcerative colitis (UC) and Crohn's disease (CD). Both forms present analogous characteristics and symptomology, mainly differing in the anatomical involvement of the gastrointestinal tract (Table 1) (Rohr *et al.*, 2018; Sairenji *et al.*, 2017).

Recently, a systematic analysis for the "Global Burden of Disease Study 2017" reported 6.8 million [95%, uncertainty intervals (UI) 6.4 - 7.3] cases of IBD globally, in 2017. Interestingly, in 1990, the number of individuals with IBD was 3.7 million (95%, UI 3.5 - 3.9), corresponding to an increase of 85.1% (UI 79.5 - 89.9) in global prevalent cases of IBD (1990 - 2017). This study estimates that more than 3 million people in Europe and USA have IBD; with an estimated prevalence exceeding 0.3% in many countries in Europe (Alatab *et al.*, 2020). Particularly, the prevalence of IBD in Europe is high, with up to 2 million people affected by this condition. In the United States, more than 1.6 million inhabitants are affected by IBD, 910,000 with UC and 785,000 with CD. Interestingly, the incidence of IBD has been growing in developing countries of Africa, South America, and in Eastern Europe, demonstrating the relevance of environmental issues in the expansion of chronic inflammatory disorders (Ramos & Papadakis, 2019).

Table 1. Characterization of Crohn's disease and ulcerative colitis based on their site of origin, progression, inflammation, risk factors and symptoms (Rohr et al., 2018)

	Crohn's Disease	Ulcerative Colitis
Site of origin	No particular localization (terminal ileum, most frequently)	Rectum (descending and sigmoid colon)
Progression	Irregular lesions	Proximally contiguous
Inflammation	Transmural	Mucosal and submucosal
Risk factors	Subtypes of pathogenic bacteria; high-fat diets; genetic mutations	Ethnic origin; age; smoking; family history; isotretinoin use
Symptoms	Abdominal pain; cramping or swelling; anaemia; nausea; vomiting, rectal and gastrointetsinal bleeding; malabsorption; persistent or recurrent diarrhoea; stomach ulcers; weight loss; fever; joint pain	Abdominal pain; anaemia; bloody diarrhoea; rectal bleeding; malabsorption; loss of appetite; urgent bowel movements; ulceration; weight loss; fatigue; fever; dehydration; joint pain

In the past two decades, important developments in IBD treatment have occurred. However, the complexity of IBD and the traditional scientific methods have created enormous challenges, and drug research and development still need optimization (Olivera *et al.*, 2019; Weisshof *et al.*, 2018). The scientific community continuously looks for the best, more practical and representative model of human IBD. Despite the most recent advances of human intestinal microphysiological systems (e.g. "Gut-on-a-Chip"), the *in vivo* models are the ones that best fit these aims, and the rodent models are the most used ones (Bang & Lichtenberger, 2016; Kang & Kim, 2016).

This chapter intends to present and discuss the most relevant inflammatory pathways involved in the genesis and development of IBD, and a summary of the *in vivo* rodent models commonly used to study and discover new molecules that modulate these inflammatory pathways.

Inflammatory Pathways in IBD

The precise cause of IBD is still unknown. However, due to the constant research in this field, the pathogenesis of IBD have been associated with environmental factors (*e.g.* food intake, smoking, psychological stress, and drugs), genetic susceptibility of the host (while many individuals carry the risk loci associated to IBD, only a small population develops IBD), immunological anomalies, and intestinal microbiota. Apparently, IBD may result from the combination of these two last factors: an abnormal host immune response to the intestinal microbiota (Guan, 2019).

The gut contains between 1000 to 5000 of different species of microorganism, with 99% coming from the phyla *Actinobacteria*, *Bacteroidetes*, *Firmicutes*, and

Proteobacteria - the gut microbiome. This microbiome is vital for the host metabolism and gastrointestinal development, and differentiation of the local and systemic immune system, and finally for the overall intestinal homeostasis and function. The composition on commensal and pathogenic microorganisms of the gut may be affected by antibiotics, diet, lifestyle, hygiene, among others, resulting in an alteration of their composition and function - dysbiosis. This consequently causes an imbalance in the interaction with the intestinal immune system, contributing to the progress of intestinal inflammation (Guan, 2019; Mentella *et al.*, 2020). Indeed, higher bacterial instability, reduced bacterial diversity and dysregulated gut microbiota have already been reported in IBD patients (compared to heathy controls). Dysbiosis is clearly associated with the inflammatory state of IBD, causing: the dysregulation of T-cell differentiation, the changing of epithelial cell death mechanisms, the induction of oxidative stress, and the disruption of epithelial barrier integrity (Aggeletopoulou *et al.*, 2019).

In the gut, various types of immune cells coexist, namely B and T cells, macrophages, natural killer cells, neutrophils, dendritic cells, eosinophils, and mast cells. These cells are also responsible for a homeostatic state, even under normal conditions, protecting the gut (Ribeiro *et al.*, 2018). Despite the presence of all these types of cells, the most noticeable feature of IBD is immune cell infiltration, comprising a wide recruitment of neutrophils and monocytes, the latter in a smaller degree (Chami *et al.*, 2018). There are other cells involved in IBD, but mostly in resolution of inflammation. This process appears to be essentially dependent on regulatory T cells, and on the recently discovered regulatory lymphoid cells (ILCreg) (Schett & Neurath, 2018). The most relevant T cells in IBD are postulated to be $CD4^+$ T effector lymphocytes, as regulatory T cells, Th17, Th2, and Th1 (Maynard & Weaver, 2009). The crucial role of these cells in the progression and resolution of inflammation are generally linked to their ability to modulate the production of cytokines. These cytokines recruit other immune cells, influence the action of antigen-presenting cells, and consequently modulate the adaptive immune response (Chami *et al.*, 2018; Schett & Neurath, 2018). The immunopathogenesis of IBD is complex and is described as a 3-stage model: a) luminal antigen penetration, b) reduced normal antigenic clearance, and c) compensatory immune response. Generally, it is anticipated that an antigenic stimulus activates gut mucosal immune cells, which in turn release anti- and proinflammatory cytokines. It is believed that IBD results from the dysregulated production of these cytokines (Rohr *et al.*, 2018). However, in IBD, there are also other inflammatory targets that can be modulated, not only cytokines production, as transcription factors and arachidonic acid pathways, tight-junction (TJ) function, reactive oxygen and nitrogen species (ROS/RNS) and adhesion molecules (Ribeiro *et al.*, 2018; Vezza *et al.*, 2016). These mediators and pathways are intrinsically linked, and therefore their modulation results in an extensive crosstalk, as following demonstrated.

Transcription Factors

The most recent pharmacotherapies applied in IBD resort to biologics, i.e., immunotherapies that block downstream signaling pathways, namely those related to the production of cytokines. These pathways include Janus kinases (JAKs), a family of tyrosine kinases [JAK1, 2, 3, and tyrosine kinase 2 (TYK2)]; signal transducer and activator of transcription (STATs) proteins (STAT1, 2, 3, 4, 5A, 5B, and 6), that bind to JAKs (Ramos & Papadakis, 2019); p38 and extracellular signal regulated kinase (ERK)1/2; nuclear factor-κB (NF-κB); and Akt (Chami *et al.*, 2018; Mitchell & Carmody, 2018). Indeed, in the specific inflammatory process of IBD, JAKs mediate the intracellular communication between nuclear signals and cytokine receptors, and between cytokines receptors and intranuclear proteins, namely STATs. STATs, in their turn, bind to JAKs, and upon phosphorylation, STATs dimerize with each other and initiate the intracellular effects of a specific cytokine pathway. In the case of CD pathogenesis, the cytokines interleukin (IL)-12 and -23 are crucial, being responsible for the stimulation of the non-receptor JAK2 and of tyrosine kinase 2 (TYK2) activity, resulting in the phosphorylation of STAT1, 3, 4, and 5. These intranuclear signals are linked to the control of Th1/Th17 cell responses (Ramos & Papadakis, 2019; Teng *et al.*, 2015). The classical mitogen activated protein kinases (MAPK), ERK1/2, and p38 are also crucial intermediaries in the inflammatory cascade (Ribeiro *et al.*, 2018). These MAPKs, upon activation, are responsible for the production of IL-8 in colonic epithelial cells. This chemokine is a powerful neutrophil chemoattractant which indirectly contribute to the hypochlorous acid (HOCl) production and MAPK activation, that ultimately results in cell death. An unregulated production of HOCl activates p38 that subsequently can promote the expression of tumor necrosis factor (TNF), propagating the inflammatory process (Chami *et al.*, 2018). In its turn, TNF strongly activates the redox-sensitive NF-κB, which is an evolutionarily conserved transcription factor responsible for a master regulation of the inflammatory response. In general, NF-κB regulates the expression of hundreds of immune relevant genes, particularly those encoding the proinflammatory cytokines and chemokines (Mitchell & Carmody, 2018). NF-κB is constituted by p65 (RelA), c-Rel, RelB, p50 and p52, where only the initial three straightly activate target genes transcription. In the cytoplasm of resting cells, the NF-κB set of inhibitory proteins, known as IκB family, bind to NF-κB dimers, maintaining this transcription factor inactive. NF-κB can be activated and translocated to the nucleus by a classic pathway or by an alternative pathway. In the classic one, the phosphorylation of IκB is mostly done by IκB kinases (IKK). IKK is a trimeric complex of a regulatory subunit (IKKγ or NF-kB essential modulator or NEMO) and two catalytic subunits (IKKα and IKKβ). IκB phosphorylation leads to its proteasomal degradation, particularly the degradation of IκBα. In the alternative pathway, the NF-κB heterodimers p52/RelB, upon activation of the NF-κB-inducing kinase (NIK) and IKKα, reach the nucleus (Ribeiro *et al.*, 2018). In an inflammatory context, NF-κB activation can be triggered by the overproduction of ROS/RNS. However, this effect is not clear, as it was also recently described that ROS/RNS can both activate and repress NF-κB signaling. Indeed, hydrogen peroxide (H_2O_2) is widely recognized due the activation of NF-κB in endothelial, epithelial and T cells; nevertheless, its underlying molecular mechanisms remain unclear. In its turn, HOCl has been described as a probable inhibitor of NF-κB. NF-κB not only overturns the apoptotic signal induced by TNF; but also raises the production and secretion of TNF, IL-1 and -6, in mucosal macrophages, that together can preserve the inflammatory response (Chami *et al.*, 2018). Along with NF-κB, the activating nuclear erythroid-related factor 2 (Nrf2) pathway is also a critical signaling pathway related to inflammation and oxidation. Nrf2 suppresses the production of cytokines with a proinflammatory action and increases the expression of antioxidant genes (He *et al.*, 2018). Akt is a serine/threonine kinase classified as a crucial IBD mediator and probably correlated to disease prognosis. Upon activation, Akt is responsible for downstream antiapoptotic signaling. Indeed, active Akt increases the active NF-κB, consequently increasing the expression of TNF, IL-1, and -6. In their turn, IL-1 and TNF activate Akt, further spreading the activation of NF-κB and the succeeding inflammatory response (Chami *et al.*, 2018). Akt activity can also be modulated by ROS/RNS (Chami *et al.*, 2018).

The c-Jun NH2-terminal Kinase (JNK) is another sub-group of the MAPKs that play an eminent role in the inflammatory disease state through the targeting of specific proteases and cytokines expression. JNK regulates T cells maturation and activity, and the synthesis of the proinflammatory cytokines, as IL-2, -6 and TNF. The precise mechanism of action of JNK on intestinal inflammation onset is not yet elucidated. Crosstalk has been reported between the JNK pathway and other signaling pathways, namely ERK and p38 MAPK; nevertheless, this crosstalk needs to be further clarified (Roy *et al.*, 2008). JNK transmits signals to the nucleus, resulting in transcription factor activator protein-1 (AP-1) activation. AP-1 is responsible for adaptive modifications, in damaged cells related to the expression of genes encoding for proinflammatory and apoptotic mediators in damaged cells. In this sense, reduction of JNK activation and of AP-1 may reduce colon damage (Zingarelli *et al.*, 2004).

The nuclear human pregnane X receptor (PXR) is considered the main controller of xenobiotic metabolism and is plentifully expressed in the liver and intestine, contributing to maintain the intestinal barrier integrity. In animal studies, intestinal inflammation has been related to PXR loss; and, in UC patients, low levels of PXR have been observed (Dou *et al.*, 2014). Peroxisome proliferator-activated receptor gamma (PPARγ), constitutes a nuclear receptor family and regulates the inflammatory signaling pathways. It acts on kinases and transcription factors [*e.g.* NF-κB, nuclear factor of activated T cell, c-Fos, and c-Jun], inhibiting cytokines and chemokines production, the expression of some adhesion molecules and consequently the decreased proliferation of inflammatory cells (Dubuquoy *et al.*, 2006).

Eicosanoids

In general, the major arachidonic pathways involved in IBD are those that involve cyclooxygenase (COX)-2 and 1-, 5- and 12-lipoxygenase (LOX) (Stenson, 2014). COXs are responsible for the production of prostaglandins (PGs). PGs are considered primary promoters of immune tolerance and epithelial homeostasis. In this sense, any pharmacotherapy with COX-1 and COX-2 inhibitors will probably disturb the homeostasis of the epithelium and reduce immune tolerance, leading to the exacerbation of the clinical course of IBD. On the contrary, in installed IBD, high levels of PGs are produced, amplifying the inflammatory response, consequently promoting Th17 cells activity, vascular permeability and blood flow (Stenson, 2014). These apparently opposing effects raise important issues on the efficacy of strategies for the inhibition of arachidonic acid pathways in IBD treatment. As example, PGE_2 has been described as supporter of immune tolerance, epithelial homeostasis and proinflammatory activity of Th17 cells, finally promoting the resolution of inflammation in the gastrointestinal mucosa (Stenson, 2014). PGD_2 is also associated with inflammation resolution, as it binds to PGD_2 receptors (DP) on neutrophils, blocking their activity, and to DP and chemokine receptor homologous molecule expressed in Th2 lymphocytes (CRTH2), monocytes and erythrocytes (Stenson, 2014). It is also described that the PGD_2 receptor (DP2) and the PGE_2 receptor (EP4) are both over-expressed during experimental colitis. EP4 is not only involved in intestinal homeostasis, but also in IBD progression, since it drives the differentiation of Th1 and proliferation of Th17 cells, which are essential in the exacerbation of the disease. The activation of another PGE_2 receptor, EP2, also exacerbates IBD symptoms by lowering the expression of IL-12 and IL-27 and increasing the expression of IL-23, leading to the differentiation of T-cells into Th17 (Moreno, 2017).

5-LOX and 12-LOX are responsible for the synthesis of leukotrienes (LTs). The 5-LOX pathway leads to the production of LTB_4, among other LTs. LTB_4 is a potent neutrophil chemotactic agent and its levels are markedly increased in UC. It is believed that LTB_4, together with IL-8, is responsible for the neutrophils migration into the mucosa from the blood stream (Stenson, 2014). 12-LOX is responsible for metabolizing arachidonic acid into the unstable intermediate 12-hydroperoxyeicosatetraenoic acid. This intermediate is further metabolized, in epithelial cells, into hepoxilin A3 (HXA3). HXA3 is secreted through the apical membrane of these cells to the intestinal lumen, mediating the migration of neutrophils into the lumen, from the mucosa (Moreno, 2017; Stenson, 2014). These deceptive proinflammatory effects of the metabolites of arachidonic acid lead some authors to conclude that dual inhibitors of COX-2 and 5-LOX might act synergistically, leading to an effective IBD treatment (Ribeiro *et al.*, 2018).

Cytokines

Cytokines (including chemokines) play pivotal roles in the development, maintenance, and, more importantly, in the resolution of IBD, because they are correlated with all the other mediators and pathways. In general, the cytokines that are described as directly related to IBD are: IL-1β, -4, -6, -12, -15, -18, and -23, interferon (IFN)-γ, and TNF, as their levels are clearly increased in UC and CD. IL-6, -15, -18, -23, IFN-γ, and TNF seem to exert their immune triggering roles without the generation of tissue damage. In damaged tissues, IL-1β, -4, -6, and -12 seem to have a positive link with mucosal markers. In particular, IL-1β and -6 are implicated in the regulation of the damage to the mucosa through the enhanced presence of macrophages and neutrophils. This last factor justifies the presence and involvement of the granular enzyme myeloperoxidase (MPO) in IBD pathogenesis (Chami *et al.*, 2018). IL-17, IFN-γ and TNF are another proinflammatory cytokines produced by Th1 and Th17 cells. The latter cytokines are responsible for a self-sustaining amplification cycle, where macrophages, fibroblasts, and endothelial cells are stimulated to produce, IL-1, -6, -8, -12, -18 and TNF (Ramos & Papadakis, 2019). There are other cytokines that have been described as having a pivotal role in resolution of inflammation, the transforming growth factor (TGF)-β, which is produced by T cells and during IBD changed their transcriptional profile acquiring regulatory properties; and IL-10 and -35, produced by Treg cells (Schett & Neurath, 2018). The newly discovered regulatory ILCreg cells, present in the human intestine's *lamina propria*, are also a source of the anti-inflammatory cytokines TGF-β and IL-10, but simultaneously block IFN-γ and IL-17 production. In addition, IL-22, -28 and -36 were also shown to promote resolution of colitis (Schett & Neurath, 2018).

Chemokines are a group of heparin binding cytokines. Chemokines are able to induce the migration of leukocytes and can be virtually expressed and secreted by any stimulated cell type, including epithelial, endothelial, leukocytes, and stromal cells (Trivedi & Adams, 2018). In the gut, distinct patterns of chemokine expression exist according to different intestinal sites. These patterns may serve to compartmentalize leukocyte recruitment, regulating, in this way, regional immunity and the nature of inflammation in disease. As example, in absence of inflammatory process, the chemokine CCL25 is just expressed in small intestine, recruiting T and B cells. Under inflammatory conditions, other chemokines are released, as the IFN-induced CXCL10, that can recruit effector cells expressing the receptor CXCR3 to the small bowel (Trivedi & Adams, 2018). The chemokine CCL25 activates its receptor CCR9 and induces pro-migratory responses, on mucosal vessels: α4β1 integrin to bind vascular cell adhesion molecule (VCAM)-1 and α4β7 integrin to bind mucosal addressin cell adhesion molecule (MAdCAM)-1, leading to the development of cryptopatches. CCL20 is another inflammatory chemokine secreted by the epithelium, that is responsible for the attraction of cells that secrete IL-17 and express CCL20 receptor, CCR6. The secretion of CCL20 is, in its turn, induced by TNF (Trivedi & Adams, 2018).

Monocyte chemoattractant protein (MCP)-1 is another up-regulated chemokine found in mucosal tissues in IBD. However, the precise role of this chemokine or its mechanisms in IBD pathogenesis remain to be determined (Takada *et al.*, 2010).

Reactive Oxygen and Nitrogen Species

Large cohort studies have already identified the infiltration of immune cells, namely neutrophils, as a crucial IBD characteristic. These cells migrate to the tissues via chemotaxis, where they mediate the antimicrobial defense through the production of ROS/RNS, phagocytosis and degranulation of soluble protein antimicrobials (Chami *et al.*, 2018). The unregulated ROS/RNS production leads to alterations in cellular signaling, causing direct damage to the inflamed mucosa, favoring in this way a proinflammatory outcome. This overproduction of ROS/RNS, without an efficient response of the antioxidant defenses, known as oxidative stress, plays a significant role in IBD pathogenesis. It has been well described that, in IBD, the apoptosis process in neutrophils, monocytes and other proinflammatory cells are delayed. In UC, for example, dysregulated neutrophil apoptosis could contribute to the release of granulocyte-macrophage colony-stimulating factor (GM-CSF). This anti-apoptotic cytokine extends the longevity of granulocytes, prolonging ROS/RNS formation and an overall exacerbation of the inflammation-associated mucosal injury (Chami *et al.*, 2018).

Superoxide anion radical ($O_2^{\bullet-}$) is the first ROS produced by neutrophils during the inflammatory process of IBD, being the precursor of other harmful ROS/RNS. $O_2^{\bullet-}$ can be produced through different enzymatic systems, namely xanthine oxidase (XO), nitric oxide synthase (NOS), nicotinamide adenine dinucleotide phosphate (NADPH) oxidase (both contained in phagocytes) or through the mitochondrial electron transport chain. Once formed, $O_2^{\bullet-}$ can be rapidly converted into H_2O_2, either spontaneously or by the action of superoxide dismutase (SOD). The enzymes catalase and/or glutathione peroxidase (GSH-Px) are likewise able to control the levels of H_2O_2, since they can convert it into water. In neutrophils, the majority of H_2O_2 is converted into HOCl, via MPO (Ribeiro *et al.*, 2018). Elevated levels of MPO in IBD are widely reported, and have an interesting close correlation between IL-8 and MPO levels in UC (Chami *et al.*, 2018). HOCl is an oxidizing agent of thiols and thioethers (reacts with sulfur atoms), amines and amides (reacts with nitrogen atoms), affecting in this way cysteine residues in low-molecular weight thiols [*e.g.* glutathione (GSH)] and in proteins. In this sense, HOCl is responsible for the conversion of GSH into its oxidation products glutathione sulfonamide (GSA) and glutathione disulfide (GSSG), dropping the endogenous antioxidant pool and increasing the susceptibly to damage, through oxidative stress, in the surrounding cells and tissues (Chami *et al.*, 2018; Ribeiro *et al.*, 2018). There are three known isoforms in mammals: two constitutive enzymes, expressed in neuronal cells (nNOS) or in endothelial cells (eNOS), and an inducible isoform (iNOS) expressed by immune cells. nNOS and eNOS produce little levels of nitric oxide (•NO) essentially with physiological functions. iNOS produces higher levels of •NO with an immune function. In the intestinal submucosa and mucosa, iNOS is expressed in selected cells and converts the amino acid L-arginine into L-citrulline and •NO. iNOS expression is induced by NF-κB as a response to several stimuli as TNF, IFN-γ, IL-1α, -6, lipopolysaccharide bacterial and viral components. Both upregulation of iNOS and the presence of high levels of •NO occur in experimental and human IBD (Soufli *et al.*, 2016).

Adhesion Molecules

Leukocyte migration is an extremely controlled process, mediated by the expression and/or regulation of several chemoattractant molecules and receptors, and by adhesion molecules from immune and stromal cells. In IBD there are dramatic alterations in the production of chemokines and endothelial adhesion molecules, affecting the type of cells that will be recruited (Panes & Salas, 2018). Leukocyte trafficking to the gut is crucial to the pathophysiological mechanisms of IBD (Katsanos & Papadakis, 2017). Extravasation of leukocytes into the gut mucosa takes place in three stages: rolling, adhesion and migration. Upon damage or infection of a tissue, upregulation of several chemokines production firstly occurs, but also the upregulation of several adhesion molecules, as MAdCAM-1, VCAM-1, and intercellular adhesion molecule (ICAM)-1, (Panes & Salas, 2018). ICAM-1 primary ligands comprise Mac-1 (αMβ2, CD11b/ CD18), β2-integrins, and leukocyte function associated antigen-1 (CD11a/CD18, αLβ2, LFA-1). The adhesion of leukocytes to vascular endothelium and possible transmigration to the mucosa depends on the communication between ICAM-1 on endothelial cells and LFA-1 on leukocytes (Reinisch *et al.*, 2018).

VCAM-1 binds to both α4β1 and α4β7 integrins, but, in humans, its expression is lower compared to ICAM-1 (Thomas & Baumgart, 2012). MAdCAM is typically expressed on high endothelial venules (cell surface) and its ligand, α4β7 integrin, is expressed on lymphocytes. MAdCAM regulates the rolling, adhesion and diapedesis of the lymphocytes expressing α4β7 to the gastrointestinal tract endothelium. In the inflammatory site, IL-1 and TNF are responsible for the increased expression of ICAM-1 and MAdCAM (Katsanos & Papadakis, 2017; Reinisch *et al.*, 2018).

Tight Junctions

CD and UC share common features such as reduction in TJ strands, glandular atrophy, and epithelial breaks. As it is broadly known, the intercellular spaces between cells, which are connected by junctional complexes, are vital in the mucosal barrier regulation. TJ define the border between the basolateral and apical membranes. They are part of a dynamic intestinal barrier that controls the uptake of electrolytes, water and nutrients. TJ are assembled by peripheral membrane proteins [*e.g.* cingulin and zona occludens (ZO)-1, -2, -3] and transmembrane proteins [*e.g.* claudins, occludin, tricellulin, and junctional adhesion molecules (JAMs)] (Landy *et al.*, 2016). Myosin light chain kinase (MLCK) has also emerged as a key regulator of TJ permeability. MLCK1 and MLCK2 transcription appears to be activated similarly by TNF (Cunningham & Turner, 2012). Dysfunction of this barrier, which is characteristic of IBD, occurs upon epithelium damage, namely by ulceration, erosion, and apoptosis (Landy *et al.*, 2016). TJ dysregulation leads to an augmented permeability to large molecules and transport of solutes, instigating leak-flux diarrhea. All these induce an immune response and sustain the inflammatory process (Barmeyer *et al.*, 2017). Interestingly, this increased barrier permeability in CD is essentially related with an unsuccessful antimicrobial response, and in UC essentially disturbs the mucus layer (Holmberg *et al.*, 2018).

In Vivo Studies of IBD

Animal models are the most widely used models in preclinical and translational studies as only the whole animal physiology mimics the best the clinical pathology and the potential effects of novel molecules on humans (Johnson & Greenwood-Van Meerveld, 2017). Still, over the last 50 years, the principles of the 3Rs (replacement, refinement and reduction) have been developed and have been crucial to perform more humane animal research. In general, these principles refer to: replacement, by using alternative in vitro methods for screening purposes; refinement, by housing and treat animals, minimizing their suffering and improving welfare (use of humane endpoints and approval of institutional and national ethical committees); and reduction, by using appropriate experimental design, sample size determination, and statistical analysis.

Several animal species used as models have advantages and limitations (Table 2) that will affect the translation significance of the studies.

Table 2. Animal models potentially used in gastrointestinal (GI) studies: advantages and limitations

Animal models	Advantages	Limitations	References
Zebrafish (*Danio rerio*) larvae	Easy to cultivate and highly fecund; embryos with rapid development and transparent, facilitating observation, manipulation, and drug screening; immune system analogous to humans	Duplicated genes; have no lymph glands and their gut lacks Peyer's patch; T and B lymphocytes maturation sites and subtypes of antibodies are different from mammals; intestinal epithelium lacks crypts; the intestinal microorganisms of mammals do not survive in the gut of zebrafish	(Hanyang *et al.*, 2017)
Rodents (rats, mice, guinea pigs)	Have a very similar GI tract to humans; have an enteric nervous system, like humans; enable the study of large numbers of animals, and genetically modified strains	Lack of emetic reflex; have a marked cecum which impairs the studies on GI transit	(Johnson & Greenwood-Van Meerveld, 2017)
Non-rodents (rabbits, ferrets, and opossums)	Larger animals; enable additional surgical manipulations	Limited availability from accredited sellers; more expensive; additional animal wellbeing conditions	
Cats, dogs, and pigs	Mild to large animals; tolerate recurrent experimental testing	Bigger expense (per animal); additional regulatory oversight; unable chronic surgical manipulations	
Nonhuman primates	Enables spontaneous GI disease, and aging effects	Additional ethical concerns and associated costs	

The search for more practical and representative models of human IBD has led, throughout the past decades, to the refinement of the adequacy of the species used, number of individuals *per* group, and relevant parameters to be investigated. Considering the most prominent features of IBD, it is expected that most *in vivo* studies have been focused on the interrelated aspects of IBD such as inflammation and oxidative stress, immune cell regulation, maintenance and repair of epithelial architecture and alterations in the gut microbiome (Martin *et al.*, 2017; Mizoguchi, 2012).

In IBD experimental animal models, the disease may be developed by exogenous induction with chemical agents or by the selection of mouse and rat lines that spontaneous develop colitis, due to gene deletion or transgene expression (Kolios, 2016). In the first case, the inflammation is limited to the colon, and, according to the chemical inflammatory stimuli, the inflammatory mediators' expression may be affected, because the collected tissue sample may have both inflamed and healthy segments. In the second case, spontaneous colitis is generally developed in adulthood, but the infection route may diverge from the clinical course (Johnson & Greenwood-Van Meerveld, 2017).

Currently, there are, at least, 66 different animal models identified for the study of IBD. However, the majority of the *in vivo* studies of IBD used, are based on rodent models. These models are mostly based on three types of inflammatory activation: chemical induction, transfer of naïve $CD4^+$ T cells and generation of engineered mouse strains, with specific target gene manipulations (Figure 1) (Bang & Lichtenberger, 2016; Mizoguchi, 2012).

Figure 1. Rodent models in IBD. DSS - dextran sulfate sodium, RAG - recombinase activating gene, SCID - severe combined immunodeficiency, TNBS - trinitrobenzene sulfonic acid.

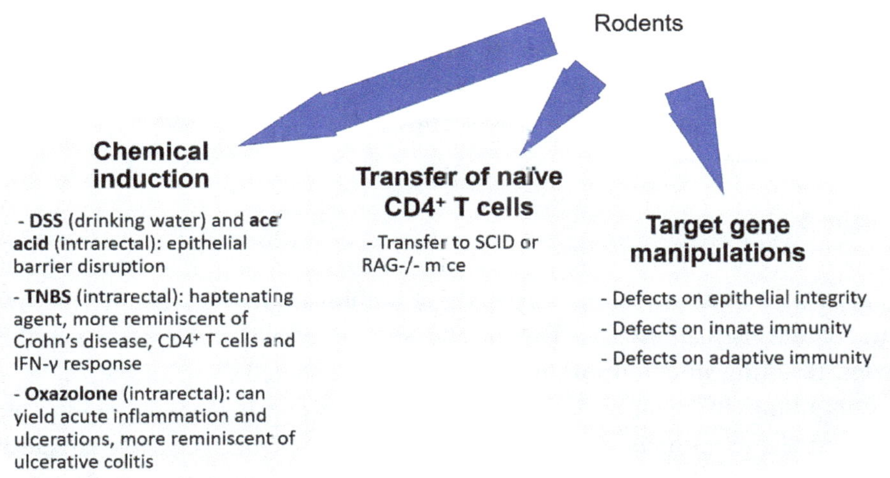

CHEMICAL INDUCTION

Dextran Sulfate Sodium

Dextran sulfate sodium (DSS) is a sulfated polysaccharide, and its mechanism of action regarding IBD is not yet completely understood. DSS seems to chemically disrupt the epithelial barrier of the gut, being toxic to the colonic epithelium, leading to inflammatory response. DSS is typically administered to rodents in the drinking water and, depending on the model (acute or chronical colitis), different concentrations, periods of exposure and cyclic administration can be attempted (Bang & Lichtenberger, 2016). Generally, ingestion of a solution of DSS will result in acute colitis over a week or less. This colitis is limited to the colonic mucosa and will get worse over time; an animal subjected to cycles of DSS will develop chronic colitis (Bramhall *et al.*, 2015; Johnson & Greenwood-Van Meerveld, 2017). The type of lesion is more widespread, which is less reminiscent of human IBD. Moreover, there are other factors that can influence the severity and the susceptibility to DSS, as its manufacturer, its molecular weight, the animal strain (*e.g.* BALB/c and C3HeJ have an augmented susceptibility, when compared to C57BL/6 mice), and the conditions/environment in which the animals are raised in (*e.g.* germ-free or pathogen-free). Despite this, because of its simplicity, reduced cost and decreased experimental time, this model is broadly used (Bramhall *et al.*, 2015; Mizoguchi, 2012). This model is especially suited to the study of epithelial barrier function, and because inflammation is not exclusively dependent on adaptive immunity, it is also adapted to the study of innate immunity processes leading to colon inflammation (Kiesler *et al.*, 2015).

Acetic Acid

In acetic acid-induced colitis, the mode of administration is typically intrarectal (intracolonic instillation). Like DSS, acetic acid also causes damage to the epithelial barrier, resulting in colon inflammation. The protonated form of the acetic acid releases protons in the intracellular space, most likely causing massive acidification, resulting in large epithelial damage. Indeed, acetic acid induces several characteristic features of human ulcerative colitis, as vascular dilation, edema, increased neutrophil infiltration, and submucosal and mucosal necrosis and ulceration. The induced colitis has a fast development, 4 h after acetic acid administration, with a subsequent rapid healing, 7 days after acetic acid administration. Again, the concentration and period of exposure can vary depending on the severity and type of colitis (acute or chronic) (Qin *et al.*, 2011; Randhawa *et al.*, 2014).

Haptenating Agents

2,4,6-Trinitrobenzenesulfonic acid (TNBS) is a haptenating agent that is administered intrarectally and renders self-proteins immunogenic to the host, thereby promoting colitis (Bang & Lichtenberger, 2016). TNBS leads to the development of a transmural diffuse inflammation or local ulcers and necrosis (Johnson & Greenwood-Van Meerveld, 2017) reminiscent of Crohn's disease. The enema consists in a mixture of TNBS and ethanol, and the peak and duration of the inflammatory response vary according to the TNBS/ethanol concentration (Bang & Lichtenberger, 2016). As for the other chemically induced colitis models, the severity of colitis also largely depends on the animal strain used (Bramhall *et al.*, 2015), Balb/c, C3HeJ, and SJL/J are susceptible strains, while DBA/2 and C57BL/6 are very resistant strains (Mizoguchi, 2012). This is a particularly useful model to study immune cell responses and differential cytokine secretion (Bang & Lichtenberger, 2016). TNBS is considered a very relevant model to mimic Crohn's disease due to the involvement of the key susceptibility gene, NOD2. This is considered a time saving and economical model (Mizoguchi, 2012).

Oxazolone (4-ethoxymethylene-2-phenyl-2-oxazolin-5-one), as TNBS, is also a haptenating agent. However, unlike TNBS, its intrarectal administration results in a pattern of colonic inflammation that is more like ulcerative colitis than Crohn's disease (Boismenu & Chen, 2000). The induced colitis is characterized by severe submucosal edema and hemorrhagic inflammation. Another limitation of oxazolone is that, in general, conventional mouse strains are resistant to its colitis induction. In this sense, a pre-sensitization of skin with oxazolone before the intrarectal administration is needed (Mizoguchi, 2012). In comparison to TNBS-induced colitis, oxazolone most easily induces colitis in SJL/J and C57BL/10 mice. Oxazolone weekly administration, in low doses, to BALB/c induces chronic colitis. All in all, this model is particularly valuable because it resembles the morphology and the immunopathogenesis of the human ulcerative colitis (Kiesler *et al.*, 2015).

Transfer OF Naïve $CD4^+$ T Cells

T lymphocytes are crucial in colitis onset, as they mediate the process that comprises the antigen presenting cells and the generation of targeted immune responses to commensal enteric bacteria (Bramhall *et al.*, 2015). Immune cell transfer of naïve $CD4^+$ T cells from a donor to a receptor rodent suffering from severe combined immunodeficiency (SCID) or deficiency in recombinase activating gene ($RAG^{-/-}$) will result in intestinal inflammation. This method is increasingly popular and most suitable for the study of immunoregulation (Boismenu & Chen, 2000). This curious model is based on the fact that mature T-cell population comprises Treg cells that suppress inflammation; on the contrary, naïve T-cell population lacks these cells (Kiesler *et al.*, 2015). On one hand, this model entails a more complex protocol that requires the extraction, isolation, purification and injection of the cells. Moreover, there are several factors that can interfere with the induced colitis, as the number/viability of the transferred T cells, the animal strain, and finally, the presence of B cells in the receptor rodent (Bramhall *et al.*, 2015). On the other hand, Treg cells have a crucial role in this model as it is crucial to understand how the intestinal immune homeostasis is regulated, making this one of the most used models (Kiesler *et al.*, 2015).

Target Gene Manipulations

The use of rodents with target gene modifications enables the study of specific processes that are linked to human IBD (Mizoguchi, 2012). The modifications can change a plethora of processes, from mucin production, IL-10 function, epithelial transport, regulation of innate immune response, NF-κB signaling, epithelial senescence, oxidative stress or overexpression of IL-7, among others (Mizoguchi, 2012). Lee and colleagues (Lee *et al.*, 2020) recently reviewed the possible target genes for immunomodulation in autoimmune diseases, namely IBD. They identified the following target genes or immunomodulation strategy to mimic IBD: cytokines (IL-10, -4, -22, -35, -6), antimicrobial peptides (human defensin-5), endoplasmic-reticulum stress in Crohn's disease (autophagy-related protein 16-like1), and genes easily manipulated in their expression levels in ulcerative colitis (GATA binding protein 3 using homologous DNAzyme, NF-κB using miR-214) (Lee *et al.*, 2020). Mizoguchi and colleagues (Mizoguchi, 2012) also described genetically engineered mice lacking STAT3, XBP1, and IL-2Ra or overexpressing (transgenic) TNFSF15, and IL-7 as capable of developing spontaneous intestinal inflammation (Mizoguchi, 2012).

As example, the gene encoding the anti-inflammatory cytokine IL-10 is identified as a susceptibility gene for the development of both CD and UC. IL-10 or its receptor are knocked out, and these IL-$10^{-/-}$ mice, when housed under normal conditions, develop gut chronic inflammation. Noteworthy, if the mice are kept under germ-free conditions or under antibiotics administration, they do not develop colitis. In this sense, care should be taken when mice are raised under germ-free housing; to develop the disease they will need to be inoculated with specific enteric microbes (*e.g. Helicobacter hepaticus*, *Enterococcus faecalis*) (Bramhall *et al.*, 2015; Kiesler *et al.*, 2015).

Model Disease Evaluation

The evaluation of prophylactic or therapeutic actions of new drugs can be investigated *in vivo* upon determination of various complementary parameters, e.g., macroscopic (ulceration, gross inflammation) and histological (immune cell infiltration, inflammation, ulceration) scores, colon weight/length, disease activity index (DAI - stool consistence and presence of blood), comprising scores for weight loss, stool consistency and the presence of blood in feces (Maxwell *et al.*, 2009).

CONCLUSION

IBD, in its two main pathophysiological forms, UC and CD, have a huge and disquieting prevalence all over the world, with increasing numbers every year. IBD is an extremely complex inflammatory condition that results from the crosstalk of several inflammatory mediators (transcription factors, eicosanoids, cytokines, chemokines, ROS/RNS, adhesion molecules, TJ, among others) and pathways. Currently, multiple animal models allow the study of IBD; however, most of them are based on rodent models, mainly due to their similarities with the human disease and to the relatively simple and moderate costs associated. Each model (chemical induced or genetically engineered) has advantages and limitations, which reinforces the importance of continuous accumulation of data, when looking for new intervention drugs. The use of more than one model may compensate the drawbacks of each other. Finally, there still is a vast body of knowledge that has yet to be gathered from the currently known *in vivo* models and methodologies.

ACKNOWLEDGMENT

This work was supported by UIDB/50006/2020, UIDB/04378/2020, and UID/DTP/04138/2020 with funding from Fundação para a Ciência e Tecnologia / Ministério da Ciência, Tecnologia e Ensino Superior (FCT/MCTES) through national funds and also by the "Programa Operacional Competitividade e Internacionalização" (COMPETE) (POCI-01-0145-FEDER-029248). Daniela Ribeiro and Marisa Freitas acknowledge the financial support from the European Union [FEDER funds through the Operational Competitiveness Program (COMPETE)] (POCI-01-0145-FEDER-029253 and POCI-01-0145-FEDER-029248, respectively). FCT/MCT supported J.M.P. Ferreira de Oliveira (grant number SFRH/BPD/74868/2010) as defined by Decree-Law No. 57/2016, of 29 August, amended by Law No. 57/2017, of 19 July.

REFERENCES

Aggeletopoulou, I., Konstantakis, C., Assimakopoulos, S. F., & Triantos, C. (2019). The role of the gut microbiota in the treatment of inflammatory bowel diseases. *Microbial Pathogenesis*, *137*, 103774. doi:10.1016/j.micpath.2019.103774 PMID:31586663

Alatab, S., Sepanlou, S. G., Ikuta, K., Vahedi, H., Bisignano, C., Safiri, S., Sadeghi, A., Nixon, M. R., Abdoli, A., Abolhassani, H., Alipour, V., Almadi, M. A. H., Almasi-Hashiani, A., Anushiravani, A., Arabloo, J., Atique, S., Awasthi, A., Badawi, A., Baig, A. A. A., ... Naghavi, M. (2020). The global, regional, and national burden of inflammatory bowel disease in 195 countries and territories, 1990-2017: A systematic analysis for the Global Burden of Disease Study 2017. *The Lancet. Gastroenterology & Hepatology*, *5*(1), 17–30. doi:10.1016/S2468-1253(19)30333-4 PMID:31648971

Bang, B., & Lichtenberger, L. M. (2016). Methods of inducing inflammatory bowel disease in mice. *Current Protocols in Pharmacology, 72*(5), 51-42.

Barmeyer, C., Fromm, M., & Schulzke, J. D. (2017). Active and passive involvement of claudins in the pathophysiology of intestinal inflammatory diseases. *Pflügers Archiv*, *469*(1), 15–26. doi:10.100700424-016-1914-6 PMID:27904960

Boismenu, R., & Chen, Y. P. (2000). Insights from mouse models of colitis. *Journal of Leukocyte Biology*, *67*(3), 267–278. doi:10.1002/jlb.67.3.267 PMID:10733087

Bramhall, M., Florez-Vargas, O., Stevens, R., Brass, A., & Cruickshank, S. (2015). Quality of methods reporting in animal models of colitis. *Inflammatory Bowel Diseases*, *21*(6), 1248–1259. doi:10.1097/MIB.0000000000000369 PMID:25989337

Chami, B., Martin, N. J. J., Dennis, J. M., & Witting, P. K. (2018). Myeloperoxidase in the inflamed colon: A novel target for treating inflammatory bowel disease. *Archives of Biochemistry and Biophysics*, *645*, 61–71. doi:10.1016/j.abb.2018.03.012 PMID:29548776

Cunningham, K. E., & Turner, J. R. (2012). Myosin light chain kinase: Pulling the strings of epithelial tight junction function. *Annals of the New York Academy of Sciences*, *1258*(1), 34–42. doi:10.1111/j.1749-6632.2012.06526.x PMID:22731713

Dou, W., Zhang, J., Li, H., Kortagere, S., Sun, K., Ding, L., Ren, G., Wang, Z., & Mani, S. (2014). Plant flavonol isorhamnetin attenuates chemically induced inflammatory bowel disease via a PXR-dependent pathway. *The Journal of Nutritional Biochemistry*, *25*(9), 923–933. doi:10.1016/j.jnutbio.2014.04.006 PMID:24913217

Dubuquoy, L., Rousseaux, C., Thuru, X., Peyrin, L., Romano, O., Chavatte, P., & ... . (2006). PPARg as a new therapeutic in inflammatory bowel diseases. *Gut*, *55*(9), 1341–1349. doi:10.1136/gut.2006.093484 PMID:16905700

Guan, Q. (2019). A Comprehensive Review and Update on the Pathogenesis of Inflammatory Bowel Disease. *Journal of Immunology Research*, *2019*, 7247238. doi:10.1155/2019/7247238 PMID:31886308

Hanyang, L., Xuanzhe, L., Xuyang, C., Yujia, Q., Jiarong, F., Jun, S., & Zhihua, R. (2017). Application of zebrafish models in inflammatory bowel disease. *Frontiers in Immunology*, *8*, 501. doi:10.3389/fimmu.2017.00501 PMID:28515725

He, F., Wu, C., Li, P., Li, N., Zhang, D., Zhu, Q., Ren, W., & Peng, Y. (2018). Functions and signaling pathways of amino acids in intestinal inflammation. *BioMed Research International*, *2018*, 9171905. doi:10.1155/2018/9171905 PMID:29682569

Holmberg, F. E. O., Pedersen, J., Jorgensen, P., Soendergaard, C., Jensen, K. B., & Nielsen, O. H. (2018). Intestinal barrier integrity and inflammatory bowel disease: Stem cell-based approaches to regenerate the barrier. *Journal of Tissue Engineering and Regenerative Medicine*, *12*(4), 923–935. doi:10.1002/term.2506 PMID:28636192

Johnson, A. C., & Greenwood-Van Meerveld, B. (2017). Critical evaluation of animal models of gastrointestinal disorders. *Handbook of Experimental Pharmacology*, *239*, 289–317. doi:10.1007/164_2016_120 PMID:28176046

Kang, T. H., & Kim, H. J. (2016). Farewell to animal testing: Innovations on human intestinal microphysiological systems. *Micromachines*, *7*(7), 107. doi:10.3390/mi7070107 PMID:30404281

Katsanos, K. H., & Papadakis, K. A. (2017). Inflammatory bowel disease: Updates on molecular targets for biologics. *Gut and Liver*, *11*(4), 455–463. doi:10.5009/gnl16308 PMID:28486793

Kiesler, P., Fuss, I. J., & Strober, W. (2015). Experimental models of inflammatory bowel diseases. *Cellular and Molecular Gastroenterology and Hepatology*, *1*(2), 154–170. doi:10.1016/j.jcmgh.2015.01.006 PMID:26000334

Kolios, G. (2016). Animal models of inflammatory bowel disease: How useful are they really? *Current Opinion in Gastroenterology*, *32*(4), 251–257. doi:10.1097/MOG.0000000000000287 PMID:27206158

Landy, J., Ronde, E., English, N., Clark, S. K., Hart, A. L., Knight, S. C., Ciclitira, P. J., & Al-Hassi, H. O. (2016). Tight junctions in inflammatory bowel diseases and inflammatory bowel disease associated colorectal cancer. *World Journal of Gastroenterology*, *22*(11), 3117–3126. doi:10.3748/wjg.v22.i11.3117 PMID:27003989

Lee, K. H., Ahn, B. S., Cha, D., Jang, W. W., Choi, E., Park, S., Park, J. H., Oh, J., Jung, D. E., Park, H., Park, J. H., Suh, Y., Jin, D., Lee, S., Jang, Y.-H., Yoon, T., Park, M.-K., Seong, Y., Pyo, J., ... Kronbichler, A. (2020). Understanding the immunopathogenesis of autoimmune diseases by animal studies using gene modulation: A comprehensive review. *Autoimmunity Reviews*, *19*(3), 102469. doi:10.1016/j.autrev.2020.102469 PMID:31918027

Martin, R., Chain, F., Miquel, S., Motta, J. P., Vergnolle, N., Sokol, H., & Langella, P. (2017). Using murine colitis models to analyze probiotics-host interactions. *FEMS Microbiology Reviews*, *41*(Supp_1), S49–S70. doi:10.1093/femsre/fux035 PMID:28830096

Maxwell, J. R., Brown, W. A., Smith, C. L., Byrne, F. R., & Viney, J. L. (2009). Methods of inducing inflammatory bowel disease in mice. Current Protocols in Pharmacology.

Maynard, C. L., & Weaver, C. T. (2009). Intestinal effector T Cells in health and disease. *Immunity*, *31*(3), 389–400. doi:10.1016/j.immuni.2009.08.012 PMID:19766082

Mentella, M. C., Scaldaferri, F., Pizzoferrato, M., Gasbarrini, A., & Miggiano, G. A. D. (2020). Nutrition, IBD and gut Microbiota: A review. *Nutrients*, *12*(4), 944. doi:10.3390/nu12040944 PMID:32235316

Mitchell, J. P., & Carmody, R. J. (2018). NF-kappa B and the transcriptional control of inflammation. *International Review of Cell and Molecular Biology*, *335*, 41–84. doi:10.1016/bs.ircmb.2017.07.007 PMID:29305014

Mizoguchi, A. (2012). Animal models of inflammatory bowel disease. *Progress in Molecular Biology and Translational Science*, *105*, 263–320. doi:10.1016/B978-0-12-394596-9.00009-3 PMID:22137435

Moreno, J. J. (2017). Eicosanoid receptors: Targets for the treatment of disrupted intestinal epithelial homeostasis. *European Journal of Pharmacology*, *796*, 7–19. doi:10.1016/j.ejphar.2016.12.004 PMID:27940058

Olivera, P., Danese, S., Jay, N., Natoli, G., & Peyrin-Biroulet, L. (2019). Big data in IBD: A look into the future. *Nature Reviews. Gastroenterology & Hepatology*, *16*(5), 312–321. doi:10.103841575-019-0102-5 PMID:30659247

Panes, J., & Salas, A. (2018). Past, present and future of therapeutic interventions targeting leukocyte trafficking in inflammatory bowel disease. *Journal of Crohn's and Colitis*, *12*(suppl_2), S633–S640. doi:10.1093/ecco-jcc/jjy011 PMID:30137311

Qin, H. Y., Wu, J. C., Tong, X. D., Sung, J. J., Xu, H. X., & Bian, Z. X. (2011). Systematic review of animal models of post-infectious/post-inflammatory irritable bowel syndrome. *Journal of Gastroenterology and Hepatology*, *46*(2), 164–174. PMID:20848144

Ramos, G. P., & Papadakis, K. A. (2019). Mechanisms of disease: Inflammatory bowel diseases. *Mayo Clinic Proceedings*, *94*(1), 155–165. doi:10.1016/j.mayocp.2018.09.013 PMID:30611442

Randhawa, P. K., Singh, K., Singh, N., & Jaggi, A. S. (2014). A review on chemical-induced inflammatory bowel disease models in rodents. *The Korean Journal of Physiology & Pharmacology; Official Journal of the Korean Physiological Society and the Korean Society of Pharmacology*, *18*(4), 279–288. doi:10.4196/kjpp.2014.18.4.279 PMID:25177159

Reinisch, W., Hung, K., Hassan-Zahraee, M., & Cataldi, F. (2018). Targeting endothelial ligands: ICAM-1/alicaforsen, MAdCAM-1. *Journal of Crohn's and Colitis*, *12*(suppl_2), S669–S677. doi:10.1093/ecco-jcc/jjy059 PMID:29757363

Ribeiro, D., Proenca, C., Rocha, S., Lima, J. L. F. C., Carvalho, F., Fernandes, E., & Freitas, M. (2018). Immunomodulatory effects of flavonoids in the prophylaxis and treatment of inflammatory bowel diseases: A comprehensive review. *Current Medicinal Chemistry*, *25*(28), 3374–3412. doi:10.2174/0929867325666180214121734 PMID:29446723

Rohr, M., Narasimhulu, C. A., Sharma, D., Doomra, M., Riad, A., Naser, S., & Parthasarathy, S. (2018). Inflammatory diseases of the gut. *Journal of Medicinal Food*, *21*(2), 113–126. doi:10.1089/jmf.2017.0138 PMID:29389238

Roy, P. K., Rashid, F., Bragg, J., Ibdah, J. A., Hepatology, D. G., Medicine, U. M. S., Columbia, Missouri, & States, U. (2008). Role of the JNK signal transduction pathway in inflammatory bowel disease. *World Journal of Gastroenterology*, *14*(2), 200–202. doi:10.3748/wjg.14.200 PMID:18186555

Sairenji, T., Collins, K. L., & Evans, D. V. (2017). An update on inflammatory bowel disease. *Primary Care*, *44*(4), 673–692. doi:10.1016/j.pop.2017.07.010 PMID:29132528

Schett, G., & Neurath, M. F. (2018). Resolution of chronic inflammatory disease: Universal and tissue-specific concepts. *Nature Communications*, *9*(1), 9. doi:10.103841467-018-05800-6 PMID:30111884

Soufli, I., Toumi, R., Rafa, H., & Touil-Boukoffa, C. (2016). Overview of cytokines and nitric oxide involvement in immuno-pathogenesis of inflammatory bowel diseases. *World Journal of Gastrointestinal Pharmacology and Therapeutics*, *7*(3), 353–360. doi:10.4292/wjgpt.v7.i3.353 PMID:27602236

Stenson, W. F. (2014). The universe of arachidonic acid metabolites in inflammatory bowel disease: Can we tell the good from the bad? *Current Opinion in Gastroenterology*, *30*(4), 347–351. doi:10.1097/MOG.0000000000000075 PMID:24837228

Takada, Y., Hisamatsu, T., Kamada, N., Kitazume, M. T., Honda, H., Oshima, Y., Saito, R., Takayama, T., Kobayashi, T., Chinen, H., Mikami, Y., Kanai, T., Okamoto, S., & Hibi, T. (2010). Monocyte chemoattractant protein-1 contributes to gut homeostasis and intestinal inflammation by composition of IL-10-producing regulatory macrophage subset. *Journal of Immunology (Baltimore, Md.: 1950)*, *184*(5), 2671–2676. doi:10.4049/jimmunol.0804012 PMID:20107182

Teng, M. W., Bowman, E. P., McElwee, J. J., Smyth, M. J., Casanova, J. L., Cooper, A. M., & Cua, D. J. (2015). IL-12 and IL-23 cytokines: From discovery to targeted therapies for immune-mediated inflammatory diseases. *Nature Medicine*, *21*(7), 719–729. doi:10.1038/nm.3895 PMID:26121196

Thomas, S., & Baumgart, D. C. (2012). Targeting leukocyte migration and adhesion in Crohn's disease and ulcerative colitis. *Inflammopharmacology*, *20*(1), 1–18. doi:10.100710787-011-0104-6 PMID:22205271

Trivedi, P. J., & Adams, D. H. (2018). Chemokines and chemokine receptors as therapeutic targets in inflammatory bowel disease; pitfalls and promise. *Journal of Crohn's and Colitis*, *12*(12), 1508–1508. doi:10.1093/ecco-jcc/jjy130 PMID:30272117

Vezza, T., Rodriguez-Nogales, A., Algieri, F., Utrilla, M. P., Rodriguez-Cabezas, M. E., & Galvez, J. (2016). Flavonoids in inflammatory bowel disease: A review. *Nutrients*, *8*(4), 211. doi:10.3390/nu8040211 PMID:27070642

Weisshof, R., El Jurdi, K., Zmeter, N., & Rubin, D. T. (2018). Emerging therapies for inflammatory bowel disease. *Advances in Therapy*, *35*(11), 1746–1762. doi:10.100712325-018-0795-9 PMID:30374806

Zingarelli, B., Hake, P. W., Burroughs, T. J., Piraino, G., O'Connor, M., & Denenberg, A. (2004). Activator protein-1 signalling pathway and apoptosis are modulated by poly(ADP-ribose) polymerase-1 in experimental colitis. *Immunology*, *113*(4), 509–517. doi:10.1111/j.1365-2567.2004.01991.x PMID:15554929

Chapter 2
Protagonist of Immuno-Profiling, Immuno-Scoring, and Immunotherapy Towards Colitis-Associated Cancer:
Systematic Review

Mohamed Adil
https://orcid.org/0000-0002-6497-7684
Saveetha Institute of Medical and Technical Sciences, India

Anandraj K. Vaithy.k
Mahatma Gandhi Medical College and Research Institute, India

Ashok Kumar Pandurangan
https://orcid.org/0000-0003-2824-1757
B. S. Abdur Rahman Crescent Institute of Science and Technology, India

Mohammad Waseem
B. S. Abdur Rahman Crescent Institute of Science and Technology, India

Neesar Ahmed
B. S. Abdur Rahman Crescent Institute of Science and Technology, India

DOI: 10.4018/978-1-7998-3580-6.ch002

ABSTRACT

Chronic inflammation in the large intestinal epithelial to rectum is a major risk for malignancies. The pathogenesis of colitis associated cancer is distinct with perilous molecular mechanism. The inflammation leads to damage of cells resulting in symptomatic conditions including cancer. This suggest the relationship between certain cancer due to its associated factors such as environment, genetics, and chronic inflammation leading to cancer. Colorectal cancer (CRC) has also been acknowledged as bowel, rectal, or colon cancer. The most common types of adenocarcinomas are associated with colorectal cancer. The lymphomas, carcinoids, sarcoma, and gastrointestinal tumors are also associated with CRC. Most disorders with chronic inflammation and exposure of immunosuppressant have an increased risk with the development of cancer leading towards the treatment of cancer by various therapies like radiation therapy, chemotherapy, hormonal therapy, further into immunotherapy, and targeted therapy. The prognosis of CRC has always been controversial.

INTRODUCTION

The chronic inflammation in the large intestinal epithelial to rectum is a major risk for the malignancies. The pathogenesis of colitis associated cancer is distinct with perilous molecular mechanism. The inflammation leads to damage of cells resulting in symptomatic conditions including cancer. This suggest the relationship between certain cancer and the ulcerative colitis due to its various factors such as environment, genetics and chronic inflammation leading to cancer. Colorectal cancer (CRC), also acknowledged as bowel cancer, rectal or colon cancer. The most common types of adenocarcinomas are associated with colorectal cancer, the adenocarcinomas form mucus within the cells. The lymphomas, carcinoids, sarcoma and gastrointestinal tumors are also associated with CRC. Genetic mutations also associate in development of cancer forming polyps. The CRC are mostly found with polyp by creating and establishing internal mass of cells on the linings. The inflammatory bowel disease with chronic inflammation also results in the development of gastrointestinal malignancies but the pathogenicity behind the mechanism of formation of malignancies is unknown. Most disorders with chronic inflammation and exposure of immunosuppressant have an increased risk with the development of cancer leading towards the treatment of cancer by various therapies like radiation therapy, chemotherapy, hormonal therapy and further into immunotherapy. About 1.8 million cases of new colorectal cancer and about 881,000 deaths are estimated to occur in 2018 by colorectal cancer. The pathogenesis of colitis associated cancer is distinctive towards sporadic colorectal carcinoma. Moreover patients with CRC have found to develop metastasis during their lifetime. Hence the development of effective treatment is critical and treatment towards modulation of own immune system towards destroying cancers could be a viable treatment for the cancers by using checkpoint inhibitors and other immunotherapy.

The classification of tumor progression by TNM classification established by American joint committee on cancer is the most common classification method for evaluating the malignancies is often inadequate because the cancer patients with the histological same stages of tumors have been found to demonstration various clinical outcomes. The important part of tumor microenvironment and its immune environment has become a pivotal role towards the integral component for immunotherapy for the therapy of cancer. Medical therapies that weaken the immune system with increased inflammatory response have been found with evidences supporting their disease progression with outcome. However immune therapies altering the immune system are also been evidenced to promote the carcinogenesis with chronic inflammation. Diseases such as ulcerative colitis, crohn's disease and other diseases have been evidenced with immune mediated disorders leading with chronic intestinal inflammation supporting towards gastrointestinal malignancy such as colorectal cancer, small bowel adenocarcinoma, gastrointestinal lymphoma, anal cancer, cholangiocarcinoma. The risk of the disease progression and outcome is highly inflammation associated, moreover the mutations by DNA methylation, aneuploidy, adenomatous polyposis coli (APC) gene mutation, activation of *k-ras* oncogene and *COX-2*, mutation in tumor suppressor gene DPC4, loss of *p53* function and other associated factors like transcription factors, DNA mismatch repair and DNA base excision repair, signalling proteins leads into genomic changes. Even though clear reason is unknown oxidative stress is highly involved with ROS produced by the inflammatory cells. Mouse models have also been shown that with inflammation they are genetically prone to develop CRC with bacterial colonization. Adaptive and innate immune responses with these machineries and system are found to be associated with the formation of cancer.

In the immune microenvironment, the oxidative stress and other immune response contribute towards the initiation, promotion and progression of the tumor with unsimplifiable complexity leading towards the tumor microenvironment consisting variety of cells and factors like immune cells like lymphocytes, monocytes, dendritic cells, natural killer cells, epithelial cells, stromal cells, fibroblast, tumor derived exosomes cytokines, chemokines, stem cells and immune infiltrates (Adil, Vallinayagam, Chitra et al, 2019; Ahmed et al., 2014). As many carcinomas are found to arise from chronic inflammation and chronic irritation from the site of infections, the inflammatory cells along with immune cells orchestrate the tumor microenvironment with the stages of carcinoma leading with neoplastic process with proliferation of tumor cells leading with invasion of tumor cells with migration and metastasis (Coussens & Werb, 2002). The relationship between the innate immunity and inflammation with cancer is based widely accepted based upon the cellular and the molecular mechanism but still the process involved is clueless and unclear. Association of soluble factors in the peripheral environment could sculpture the activity of factors trafficked to the tumors microenvironment (Adil, Bommanabonia, Vaithy et al, 2019), the interaction between the signalling of these immune response and the soluble factors play a critical role in inflammation leading towards initiation of colitis associated cancer. Prolonged immunosuppression with antimetabolites have been found with various carcinoma, lymphomas, leukemia and melanomas but the data is limited as they are found to harmonize angiogenesis with immunosuppressive factors influencing favourable microenvironment for the tumor (Olejarz et al., 2020). After the introduction of radiotherapy in 1900's, chemotherapy in 1940's and with the human genome project had brought a noticeable understanding attitude towards the treatment of cancer. Even though with multitude of chemotherapy drugs available still distinct side effects are also included with the package towards treatment of cancer. Immunotherapy uses the body immune system by stimulating immune system towards fighting cancer cells. The treatment with immunotherapy have different approaches towards different type of tumors and its immune system. The major type of immunotherapy include Monoclonal antibodies, immune check point inhibitors and cancer vaccines. Infiltration of factors and cells into the cancer microenvironment retards the evaluation of cancer tissues resulting with improper cancer treatment.

Immunoprofiling in Immunotherapy

As immunotherapy has been successfully progressing as for therapies associating cancer. Immunosuppression or suppressed immune environmental system is where the tumors strategically work towards the escape of immune microenvironment leading to immunosuppression. The main itinerary of immunotherapy is primarily to restore effective immune surveillance and regulate the immune microenvironment. The immunosuppression inhibits rejection of tumor with the help of check point inhibitors, immuno modulating molecules and other immunosuppressive enzymes help in impacting towards the disease prognosis with the survival of the cancer patients (Guerrouahen et al., 2020). With the identification of antitumor immune response help in better clinical outcomes (Papaioannou et al., 2016). The major cancer immunotherapies are based upon active and passive treatments based with the administration of monoclonal antibodies, antibody drug conjugates, cytokine therapy, immune cells based adoptive cell transfer, anti-cancer vaccines, oncolytic viruses and immune checkpoint inhibitors help in enhancing anti-cancer targeted approaches. Most commonly immunotherapy are administered in conjugation with radiotherapy, chemotherapy and targeted gene therapy (Osmani et al., 2018). Immunoprofiling is highly advantageous in predicting prognosis of malignancies thus providing target for immunotherapy. The tumor microenvironment can be simultaneously detected with various immune markers in CRC (Soh et al., 2019). The T cells are associated with development of malignancies and progression of tumors by adaptive immune system, the T cells densities were higher in colitis associated lesion compared with sporadic colorectal cancer (Soh et al., 2019). Cancer at unidentified primary sites constitutes for approximately 3 to 5% of diagnosed cancers have outcome with poor prognosis and metastasis (Haratani et al., 2019). Cancer at unidentified primary sites are mostly heterogeneous and based upon the molecular Immunoprofiling like chemotherapy with gene expression guidance or immunotherapy with gene expression guidance personalized medical therapy are been develop with clinical benefits but their background remains unclear, hence immune checkpoint like CTLA4, PD1, PD-L1 might prove efficient for the treatment of the cancer patients. Explorative studies based on the immune profile of the cancer patients gets retarded because of immune infiltration, hence cell specific immune cells evaluation using RNA sequencing, Intracellular staining by flow cytometry, protein array with barcoded antibodies, nanostring's nCounter analysis system, cytometry by time of flight (CyTOF) and other immune profiling methods provide information of the specific immune cells to immune oncology samples (Lyons et al., 2017). In cancer patients, tumor antigens are mainly responsible for the immune response. With the recognition of the new biomarkers help in diagnosis of cancer and help in targeting for the immunotherapy (Young et al., 2019). Microarrays with antibody secreting probes help in Immunoprofiling by the identification of the tumor antigens of the patients with cancer. With recent advancement in immunoassays and microarrays based antibody profiling has made accordingly with the specificity and sensitivity in selecting anti tumor antibodies (Meeusen et al., 2017). Targeted tumor therapy, anticancer drug discovery and diagnostic biomarkers and antigen specific antibody secreting probes help in immunotherapy applications (Salmaninejad et al., 2016).

Immunotherapy, Combination Therapy and Immunoscore

The tumor microenvironment contribute to the overlay of immune measurement, the cancer initiation and progression is supervised by the host's immune system. Immunological biomarkers determine the prognosis of the disease and help in providing response to the immunotherapy, this concept is coined as immunoscore. The data obtained from the cancer patient's samples provide the prognosis value and disease outcome by augmenting to the TNM classifications. Basically immunoscore is used to quantify the *insitu* infiltration of the T cell by determining the predictive and prognostic value (Galon et al., 2013). The host's immune system also play a critical role in shaping up the tumor microenvironment, pre-existing intratumoral adaptive immunity has been found effective with immune check point inhibitors based immunotherapy. The immunoscore could decipher and provide a sceptical method in describing tumor fitness, forecast and separate patients. Those can be benefitted from the combinational immunotherapies with biomarkers. As there are no immune based classification of the host immune response and the TNM staging affords partial information on disease prognosis on tumor cells and its complex tumor microenvironment and does not give the status of immune system of the tumor (Bruni et al., 2020). The immunoscore provides the quantification based upon lymphocyte population established at the center of tumor and invasive margin. As the T cell infiltration into the tumor is immunoscore any activity or mechanism with tumor immunogenicity will affect the immunoscore category. Other than measuring the T cell infiltration, immunoscore could also help in envisaging markers like CTLA4, PD-1, PD-L1 (Galon et al., 2012). With immunotherapies and combination therapies are being shown with positive impact on the cancers patients, the complexity of tumors and its microenvironment and prognosis of cancer patients can be determined and patients with high risk of tumor recurrence can be improved with the immunoscore (Galon & Bruni, 2019). In CRC, the type of tumor, density and the position of immune cells in the tumor site helped in predicting the disease outcome accurately than the classical TNM staging system leading to the concept and development of the immunoscore (Galon et al., 2007). With the new classification based on the immunoscore, the tumors are defined based on hot immune tumors, altered immunosuppressed immune tumors, altered excluded immune tumors and cold immune tumors (Galon & Bruni, 2019). The immune coordination profiles of hot, altered and cold immune tumors were observed and classified based upon the immune coordination and the escape of tumor (Camus et al., 2009) . CRC can be problematic with advanced stage malignancy and chemotherapy is normally used for the treatment of CRC with metastasis, combinational targeted immunotherapies have been proven to be effective with the CRC patients with promising results (Lichtenstern et al., 2020). The main principle of most cancer immuno therapies is to re-establish effective immunosurveillance, the soluble factors and immune cells regulating the tumor microenvironment are responsible for the immunosuppression and retarding the success rate of immunotherapy (Guerrouahen et al., 2019).

Immune Targeting Therapies

Targeted treatment with drugs targeting towards focusing on the cancer cells by arresting the food for tumor, eliciting the immune system towards the attack of tumor cells, modulating and modifying the proteins in cancer cells, modulating or hindering the signals supporting the progression of cancer and directly targeting cancer cells by inducing poison for them. But their specificity is questionable towards different cancer variations and treatment could alter accordingly. Targeted drugs are mostly found to work differently than chemotherapy drugs, still they can be used with chemotherapy drugs or can be used as standalone. Stivarga (Regorafenib) a kinase inhibitor that blocks many kinase proteins that help cancer cells proliferate to form new blood vessels for helping tumor. This drug is primarily used in advanced colorectal cancer where no other cancer drug works (Aljubran et al., 2019). Regorafenib blocks multiple protein kinases that are highly active in oncogenesis, helping tumor angiogenesis by regulating the tumor microenvironment. Even though chemotherapy and surgery has been the choice for treatment for the patients with colitis associated cancers especially with lesions of metastasis. The targeted therapy has become approachable option for treatment for patients. Cetuximab (anti EGFR) (Jonker et al., 2007) and bevacizumab (anti VEGF) (Rosen et al., 2017) and other check point inhibitors are emerging into the market impeding the tumor microenvironment including immune cells, factors enhancing tumor growth and regulating the proteins supporting tumor growth. Chemotherapy for CRC treatment is the primary treatment but it is associated with limitation in treatment of the CRC. The targeted therapies for CRC has been guaranteed to progress with new methodologies to enhance with the supplementary or replace with existing chemotherapy for CRC. Small molecules such as monoclonal antibodies or therapeutic antibodies work as major performers in targeted therapies. Hence Immunoprofiling could provide helping hand towards the treatment of CRC through targeted therapies.

Landscaping of CRC Targeted Therapy

Immunotherapies are categorized as passive and active cancer immunotherapy. Immune checkpoint inhibitors such as Cetuximab, Bevacizumab, Panitumumab, Ziv-aflibercept, Regorafenib, Ramucirumab, Pembrolizumab, Nivolumab, Ipilimumab, Gefitinib, erlotinib, Fluorouracil (5-FU), Irinotecan, Leucovorin, oxaliplatin, Capecitabine and other monoclonal antibodies have been approved for targeted therapies of CRC (Xie et al., 2020). Mediating pathways and signalling cascades such as Hedgehog, Notch, Wnt (β-catenin), TGF β/SMAD, PI3K/AKT, RAS/RAF, VEGF/VEGFR, EGF/EGFR, HGF/c-MET, IGF/IGF1R, JAK/STAT have been found to contain ideal targets for the targeted therapy (Krishnamurthy & Kurzrock, 2018; Tiwari et al., 2018).Based up on the difficulties in understanding the complex downstream signalling mechanism and its associated difficulties in the specific interactions in the biological system retards the successful interpretation of the specific targets for the CRC. Even though many targets have been identified but most are in preclinical stages of development (Ohhara et al., 2016; Willett et al., 2007). Some targets have been approved and recommended for second line of treatment for the CRC. Chemo combination based humanized monoclonal antibodies have been effective with antitumor effects in CRC (Moore et al., 2016; Schmoll et al., 2012). Murine human chimeric antibodies have been found to have immunogenic reactions, hence humanized antibody such as panitumumab does not trigger antibody dependent cell mediated cytotoxicity with reduced hypersensitivity such as cetuximab in patients with metastatic CRC (Douillard et al., 2014; Douillard et al., 2010). Antibody dependent cell mediated cytotoxicity were not found to have major contrivance with cetuximab and panitumumab, But panitumumab have been found to efficient than cetuximab for treatment of patients with CRC (Price et al., 2014). trametinib, irinotecan, encorafenib, vemurafenib, binimitinib, dabrafenib are recommended for the patients with BRAF mutated metastatic CRC (Kopetz et al., 2019).anti HER2 inhibitors also provide a new hope for the patients with EGFR resistant CRC patients (Sartore-Bianchi et al., 2016) the development of these biological and cytotoxic agents have helped metastatic CRC patients with prolonged survival. These personalized targeted therapy based upon the evidenced have demonstrated clinical remunerations for patients with metastatic CRC patients (Ohhara et al., 2016). Dendritic cell based vaccines, whole tumor cell vaccines, viral vector vaccines are being used widely and clinical trials with adoptive immunotherapy have shown promising results with CRC. Combining immunotherapies, predominantly agents targeting different immune checkpoints could be a promising approach. Preliminary clinical findings indicate that combined targeted therapies and simultaneous blockade of multiple immune checkpoints could promote therapeutic interaction and long-term antitumor immunity to improve clinical outcomes of CRC.

CONCLUSION

Immune escape, a key mechanism in progression and metastasis of cancer aiding with capable of escaping immune surveillance and antitumor immunity. Immunosuppressive cells such as T regulatory cells (Tregs), Myeloid derived suppressive cells (MDSCs), or loss of immunogenicity through down regulation of MHC-1 help in immune escape (Havel et al., 2019; Ishihara & Ishihara, 2019). Anti PD-1/ anti PD-L1, anti CTLA-4 and other checkpoint inhibitors have found to demonstrate promising effect against patients with CRC. Taking into consideration the efficiency of these check point inhibitors could lead with adverse effects. Hence identifying potential biomarker for the patients with CRC has become a vital task. Immunoprofiling, immuno recognition based with T cell infiltration in essential for predicting the drug response with clinical validation for CRC to have valid immunoscore for analysis. Targeting agents in adjuvant and neo adjuvant therapy for

CRC have been advancing resulting in identification of novel targets. Individualized treatments could help in better prognosis of CRC patients.

REFERENCES

Adil, A.A.M., Bommanabonia, A.K., Vaithy, A., Kumar, S., Waseem, M., & Jamal, S. (2019). Differential expression of Helios, Neuropilin-1 and FoxP3 in head and neck squamous cell carcinoma (HNSCC) patients. *Biotech., 9*(5), 178.

Adil, A.A.M., Vallinayagam, L., Chitra, K., Jamal, S., Pandurangan, A.K., & Ahmed, N. (2019). Increased Expression of TGF-β and IFN-γ in Peripheral Blood Mononuclear Cells (PBMCs) Cultured in Conditioned Medium (CM) of K562. *Cell Culture, 38*(2), 173-83.

Ahmed, N., Mohamed Adil, A. A., Lavanya, V., & Jamal, S. (2014). Cancer immunotherapy: Targeting immunosuppressive tumor microenvironment. *Oncobiology and Targets.*, *1*(1), 16–21. doi:10.4103/2395-4469.145382

Aljubran, A., Elshenawy, M. A., Kandil, M., Zahir, M. N., Shaheen, A., Gad, A., Alshaer, O., Alzahrani, A., Eldali, A., & Bazarbashi, S. (2019). Efficacy of Regorafenib in Metastatic Colorectal Cancer: A Multi-institutional Retrospective Study. *Clinical Medicine Insights. Oncology*, *13*, 1179554918825447. doi:10.1177/1179554918825447 PMID:30728734

Axelrad, J. E., Lichtiger, S., & Yajnik, V. (2016). Inflammatory bowel disease and cancer: The role of inflammation, immunosuppression, and cancer treatment. *World Journal of Gastroenterology*, *22*(20), 4794–4801. doi:10.3748/wjg.v22.i20.4794 PMID:27239106

Bray, F., Ferlay, J., Soerjomataram, I., Siegel, R. L., Torre, L. A., & Jemal, A. (2018). Global cancer statistics 2018: GLOBOCAN estimates of incidence and mortality worldwide for 36 cancers in 185 countries. *CA: a Cancer Journal for Clinicians*, *68*(6), 394–424. doi:10.3322/caac.21492 PMID:30207593

Bruni, D., Angell, H. K., & Galon, J. (2020). The immune contexture and Immunoscore in cancer prognosis and therapeutic efficacy. *Nature Reviews. Cancer*, *20*(11), 662–680. doi:10.103841568-020-0285-7 PMID:32753728

Camus, M., Tosolini, M., Mlecnik, B., Pagès, F., Kirilovsky, A., Berger, A., Costes, A., Bindea, G., Charoentong, P., Bruneval, P., Trajanoski, Z., Fridman, W.-H., & Galon, J. (2009). Coordination of intratumoral immune reaction and human colorectal cancer recurrence. *Cancer Research*, *69*(6), 2685–2693. doi:10.1158/0008-5472.CAN-08-2654 PMID:19258510

Colitis-Associated Cancer. (2016). Overview. Springer.

Coussens, L. M., & Werb, Z. (2002). Inflammation and cancer. *Nature*, *420*(6917), 860–867. doi:10.1038/nature01322 PMID:12490959

Douillard, J. Y., Siena, S., Cassidy, J., Tabernero, J., Burkes, R., Barugel, M., Humblet, Y., Bodoky, G., Cunningham, D., Jassem, J., Rivera, F., Kocákova, I., Ruff, P., Błasińska-Morawiec, M., Šmakal, M., Canon, J. L., Rother, M., Oliner, K. S., Tian, Y., ... Sidhu, R. (2014). Final results from PRIME: Randomized phase III study of panitumumab with FOLFOX4 for first-line treatment of metastatic colorectal cancer. *Annals of Oncology: Official Journal of the European Society for Medical Oncology*, *25*(7), 1346–1355. doi:10.1093/annonc/mdu141 PMID:24718886

Douillard, J. Y., Siena, S., Cassidy, J., Tabernero, J., Burkes, R., Barugel, M., Humblet, Y., Bodoky, G., Cunningham, D., Jassem, J., Rivera, F., Kocákova, I., Ruff, P., Błasińska-Morawiec, M., Šmakal, M., Canon, J.-L., Rother, M., Oliner, K. S., Wolf, M., & Gansert, J. (2010). Randomized, phase III trial of panitumumab with infusional fluorouracil, leucovorin, and oxaliplatin (FOLFOX4) versus FOLFOX4 alone as first-line treatment in patients with previously untreated metastatic colorectal cancer: The PRIME study. *Journal of Clinical Oncology*, *28*(31), 4697–4705. doi:10.1200/JCO.2009.27.4860 PMID:20921465

Eaden, J. A., Abrams, K. R., & Mayberry, J. F. (2001). The risk of colorectal cancer in ulcerative colitis: A meta-analysis. *Gut*, *48*(4), 526–535. doi:10.1136/gut.48.4.526 PMID:11247898

Galon, J., Angell, H. K., Bedognetti, D., & Marincola, F. M. (2013). The continuum of cancer immunosurveillance: Prognostic, predictive, and mechanistic signatures. *Immunity*, *39*(1), 11–26. doi:10.1016/j.immuni.2013.07.008 PMID:23890060

Galon, J., & Bruni, D. (2019). Approaches to treat immune hot, altered and cold tumours with combination immunotherapies. *Nature Reviews. Drug Discovery*, *18*(3), 197–218. doi:10.103841573-018-0007-y PMID:30610226

Galon, J., Fridman, W. H., & Pagès, F. (2007). The adaptive immunologic microenvironment in colorectal cancer: A novel perspective. *Cancer Research*, *67*(5), 1883–1886. doi:10.1158/0008-5472.CAN-06-4806 PMID:17332313

Galon, J., Pagès, F., Marincola, F. M., Thurin, M., Trinchieri, G., Fox, B. A., Gajewski, T. F., & Ascierto, P. A. (2012). The immune score as a new possible approach for the classification of cancer. *Journal of Translational Medicine*, *10*(1), 1. doi:10.1186/1479-5876-10-1 PMID:22214470

Guerrouahen, B. S., Maccalli, C., Cugno, C., Rutella, S., & Akporiaye, E. T. (2019). Reverting Immune Suppression to Enhance Cancer Immunotherapy. *Frontiers in Oncology*, *9*, 1554. doi:10.3389/fonc.2019.01554 PMID:32039024

Guerrouahen, B. S., Maccalli, C., Cugno, C., Rutella, S., & Akporiaye, E. T. (2020). Reverting Immune Suppression to Enhance Cancer Immunotherapy. *Frontiers in Oncology*, *9*, 1554. doi:10.3389/fonc.2019.01554 PMID:32039024

Haratani, K., Hayashi, H., Takahama, T., Nakamura, Y., Tomida, S., Yoshida, T., Chiba, Y., Sawada, T., Sakai, K., Fujita, Y., Togashi, Y., Tanizaki, J., Kawakami, H., Ito, A., Nishio, K., & Nakagawa, K. (2019). Clinical and immune profiling for cancer of unknown primary site. *Journal for Immunotherapy of Cancer*, *7*(1), 251. doi:10.118640425-019-0720-z PMID:31519206

Havel, J.J., Chowell, D., & Chan, T.A. (2019). *The evolving landscape of biomarkers for checkpoint inhibitor immunotherapy*. Academic Press.

Ishihara, J., & Ishihara, A. (2019). *Targeted antibody and cytokine cancer immunotherapies through collagen affinity*. Academic Press.

Jonker, D. J., O'Callaghan, C. J., Karapetis, C. S., Zalcberg, J. R., Tu, D., Au, H.-J., Berry, S. R., Krahn, M., Price, T., Simes, R. J., Tebbutt, N. C., van Hazel, G., Wierzbicki, R., Langer, C., & Moore, M. J. (2007). Cetuximab for the Treatment of Colorectal Cancer. *The New England Journal of Medicine*, *357*(20), 2040–2048. doi:10.1056/NEJMoa071834 PMID:18003960

Kopetz, S., Grothey, A., Yaeger, R., Van Cutsem, E., & Desai, J. (2019). Encorafenib, Binimetinib, and Cetuximab in BRAF V600E-Mutated. *Colorectal Cancer*, *381*(17), 1632–1643. PMID:31566309

Krishnamurthy, N., & Kurzrock, R. (2018). Targeting the Wnt/beta-catenin pathway in cancer: Update on effectors and inhibitors. *Cancer Treatment Reviews*, *62*, 50–60. doi:10.1016/j.ctrv.2017.11.002 PMID:29169144

Lichtenstern, C.R., Ngu, R.K., & Shalapour, S. (2020). *Immunotherapy, Inflammation and Colorectal Cancer*. Academic Press.

Lyons, Y.A., Wu, S.Y., Overwijk, W.W., Baggerly, K.A., & Sood, A.K. (2017). Immune cell profiling in cancer: molecular approaches to cell-specific identification. *NPJ Precision Oncology, 1*(1), 26.

Ma, K. W., Cheung, T. T., Leung, B., She, B. W. H., Chok, K. S. H., Chan, A. C. Y., Dai, W. C., & Lo, C. M. (2019). Adjuvant chemotherapy improves oncological outcomes of resectable intrahepatic cholangiocarcinoma: A meta-analysis. *Medicine, 98*(5), e14013. doi:10.1097/MD.0000000000014013 PMID:30702559

Meeusen, E., Lim, E., & Mathivanan, S. (2017). Secreted Tumor Antigens - Immune Biomarkers for Diagnosis and Therapy. *Proteomics, 17*(23-24), 1600442. doi:10.1002/pmic.201600442 PMID:28714192

Moore, M., Gill, S., Asmis, T., Berry, S., Burkes, R., Zbuk, K., Alcindor, T., Jeyakumar, A., Chan, T., Rao, S., Spratlin, J., Tang, P. A., Rothenstein, J., Chan, E., Bendell, J., Kudrik, F., Kauh, J., Tang, S., Gao, L., ... Strevel, E. (2016). Randomized phase II study of modified FOLFOX-6 in combination with ramucirumab or icrucumab as second-line therapy in patients with metastatic colorectal cancer after disease progression on first-line irinotecan-based therapy. *Annals of Oncology: Official Journal of the European Society for Medical Oncology, 27*(12), 2216–2224. doi:10.1093/annonc/mdw412 PMID:27733377

Ohhara, Y., Fukuda, N., Takeuchi, S., Honma, R., Shimizu, Y., Kinoshita, I., & Dosaka-Akita, H. (2016). Role of targeted therapy in metastatic colorectal cancer. *World Journal of Gastrointestinal Oncology, 8*(9), 642–655. doi:10.4251/wjgo.v8.i9.642 PMID:27672422

Olejarz, W., Dominiak, A., Żołnierzak, A., Kubiak-Tomaszewska, G., & Lorenc, T. (2020). Tumor-Derived Exosomes in Immunosuppression and Immunotherapy. *Journal of Immunology Research, 2020*, 6272498. doi:10.1155/2020/6272498 PMID:32537468

Osmani, L., Askin, F., Gabrielson, E., & Li, Q. K. (2018). Current WHO guidelines and the critical role of immunohistochemical markers in the subclassification of non-small cell lung carcinoma (NSCLC): Moving from targeted therapy to immunotherapy. *Seminars in Cancer Biology, 52*, 103–109. doi:10.1016/j.semcancer.2017.11.019 PMID:29183778

Papaioannou, N. E., Beniata, O. V., Vitsos, P., Tsitsilonis, O., & Samara, P. (2016). Harnessing the immune system to improve cancer therapy. *Annals of Translational Medicine, 4*(14), 261. doi:10.21037/atm.2016.04.01 PMID:27563648

Price, T. J., Peeters, M., Kim, T. W., Li, J., Cascinu, S., Ruff, P., Suresh, A. S., Thomas, A., Tjulandin, S., Zhang, K., Murugappan, S., & Sidhu, R. (2014). Panitumumab versus cetuximab in patients with chemotherapy-refractory wild-type KRAS exon 2 metastatic colorectal cancer (ASPECCT): A randomised, multicentre, open-label, non-inferiority phase 3 study. *The Lancet. Oncology*, *15*(6), 569–579. doi:10.1016/S1470-2045(14)70118-4 PMID:24739896

Rosen, L. S., Jacobs, I. A., & Burkes, R. L. (2017). Bevacizumab in Colorectal Cancer: Current Role in Treatment and the Potential of Biosimilars. *Targeted Oncology*, *12*(5), 599–610. doi:10.100711523-017-0518-1 PMID:28801849

Salmaninejad, A., Zamani, M. R., Pourvahedi, M., Golchehre, Z., Hosseini Bereshneh, A., & Rezaei, N. (2016). Cancer/Testis Antigens: Expression, Regulation, Tumor Invasion, and Use in Immunotherapy of Cancers. *Immunological Investigations*, *45*(7), 619–640. doi:10.1080/08820139.2016.1197241 PMID:27603913

Sartore-Bianchi, A., Trusolino, L., Martino, C., Bencardino, K., Lonardi, S., Bergamo, F., Zagonel, V., Leone, F., Depetris, I., Martinelli, E., Troiani, T., Ciardiello, F., Racca, P., Bertotti, A., Siravegna, G., Torri, V., Amatu, A., Ghezzi, S., Marrapese, G., ... Siena, S. (2016). Dual-targeted therapy with trastuzumab and lapatinib in treatment-refractory, KRAS codon 12/13 wild-type, HER2-positive metastatic colorectal cancer (HERACLES): A proof-of-concept, multicentre, open-label, phase 2 trial. *The Lancet. Oncology*, *17*(6), 738–746. doi:10.1016/S1470-2045(16)00150-9 PMID:27108243

Schmoll, H. J., Cunningham, D., Sobrero, A., Karapetis, C. S., Rougier, P., Koski, S. L., Kocakova, I., Bondarenko, I., Bodoky, G., Mainwaring, P., Salazar, R., Barker, P., Mookerjee, B., Robertson, J., & Van Cutsem, E. (2012). Cediranib with mFOLFOX6 versus bevacizumab with mFOLFOX6 as first-line treatment for patients with advanced colorectal cancer: A double-blind, randomized phase III study (HORIZON III). *Journal of Clinical Oncology*, *30*(29), 3588–3595. doi:10.1200/JCO.2012.42.5355 PMID:22965961

Shirwaikar Thomas, A., Schwartz, M., & Quigley, E. (2019). Gastrointestinal lymphoma: The new mimic. *BMJ Open Gastroenterology*, *6*(1), e000320. doi:10.1136/bmjgast-2019-000320 PMID:31645987

Soh, J. S., Jo, S. I., Lee, H., Do, E., Hwang, S. W., Park, S. H., Ye, B. D., Byeon, J.-S., Yang, S.-K., Kim, J. H., Yang, D.-H., Kim, S.-Y., & Myung, S.-J. (2019). Immunoprofiling of Colitis-associated and Sporadic Colorectal Cancer and its Clinical Significance. *Scientific Reports*, *9*(1), 6833. doi:10.103841598-019-42986-1 PMID:31048714

Sokol, H., Beaugerie, L., Maynadié, M., Laharie, D., Dupas, J. L., Flourié, B., Lerebours, E., Peyrin-Biroulet, L., Allez, M., Simon, T., Carrat, F., & Brousse, N. (2012). Excess primary intestinal lymphoproliferative disorders in patients with inflammatory bowel disease. *Inflammatory Bowel Diseases*, *18*(11), 2063–2071. doi:10.1002/ibd.22889 PMID:22271569

Tiwari, A., Saraf, S., Verma, A., Panda, P. K., & Jain, S. K. (2018). Novel targeting approaches and signaling pathways of colorectal cancer: An insight. *World Journal of Gastroenterology*, *24*(39), 4428–4435. doi:10.3748/wjg.v24.i39.4428 PMID:30357011

Ullman, T. A., & Itzkowitz, S. H. (2011). Intestinal inflammation and cancer. *Gastroenterology*, *140*(6), 1807–1816. doi:10.1053/j.gastro.2011.01.057 PMID:21530747

Van Der Kraak, L., Gros, P., & Beauchemin, N. (2015). Colitis-associated colon cancer: Is it in your genes? *World Journal of Gastroenterology*, *21*(41), 11688–11699. doi:10.3748/wjg.v21.i41.11688 PMID:26556996

Willett, C. G., Duda, D. G., Czito, B. G., Bendell, J. C., Clark, J. W., & Jain, R. K. (2007). Targeted therapy in rectal cancer. *Oncology (Williston Park, N.Y.)*, *21*(9), 1055. PMID:17910311

Xie, Y.-H., Chen, Y.-X., & Fang, J.-Y. (2020). Comprehensive review of targeted therapy for colorectal cancer. *Signal Transduction and Targeted Therapy*, *5*(1), 22. doi:10.103841392-020-0116-z PMID:32296018

Young, A. R. D. J., Coulson, R., O'Brien, M., Deb, S., Lopata, A., Behren, A., Mathivanan, S., Lim, E., & Meeusen, E. (2019). Immunoprofiling of Breast Cancer Antigens Using Antibodies Derived from Local Lymph Nodes. *Cancers (Basel)*, *11*(5), 682. doi:10.3390/cancers11050682 PMID:31100936

Chapter 3
Insights on the Potential Preventive and Healing Effects of Flavonoids in Inflammatory Bowel Disease

Marisa Freitas
LAQV-REQUIMTE, Laboratório de Química Aplicada, Departamento de Ciências Químicas, Faculdade de Farmácia, Universidade do Porto, Portugal

José Miguel Pimenta Ferreira de Oliveira
LAQV-REQUIMTE, Laboratório de Química Aplicada, Departamento de Ciências Químicas, Faculdade de Farmácia, Universidade do Porto, Portugal

M. Luísa Corvo
https://orcid.org/0000-0002-6332-3937
Faculdade de Farmácia, Instituto de Investigação do Medicamento (iMed. ULisboa), Universidade de Lisboa, Portugal

Félix Carvalho
https://orcid.org/0000-0003-3858-3494
UCIBIO-REQUIMTE, Laboratório de Toxicologia, Departamento de Ciências Biológicas, Faculdade de Farmácia, Universidade do Porto, Portugal

Eduarda Fernandes
https://orcid.org/0000-0003-3858-3494
LAQV-REQUIMTE, Laboratório de Química Aplicada, Departamento de Ciências Químicas, Faculdade de Farmácia, Universidade do Porto, Portugal

Daniela Ribeiro
LAQV-REQUIMTE, Laboratório de Química Aplicada, Departamento de Ciências Químicas, Faculdade de Farmácia, Universidade do Porto, Portugal

DOI: 10.4018/978-1-7998-3580-6.ch003

ABSTRACT

Inflammatory bowel disease (IBD) is characterized by sustained inflammatory processes in the gastrointestinal tract. One of the most threatening risks for IBD patients is the development of colorectal cancer, resulting from the chronic inflammatory state. Current IBD treatment presents limitations in safety and efficacy. As such, it is of paramount importance to find novel therapeutic strategies. The antioxidant and anti-inflammatory properties of flavonoids are widely recognized. Flavonoids currently found in our daily diet are likely to yield biological actions at the gastrointestinal level, suggesting a potential protective effect in IBD. However, the number of studies concerning the effects of flavonoids on intestinal inflammation is limited. This chapter intends to summarize the known effects of flavonoids in the different phases of IBD inflammatory pathways, covering all the concerning available in vivo studies.

INTRODUCTION

Inflammatory bowel disease (IBD), which includes ulcerative colitis and Crohn's disease, is a general designation for a chronic, non-infectious, and immune-mediated intestinal disease of complex etiology, resulting from the interaction of multiple factors, such as diet, microbiota, environment, and genes (Olivera *et al.*, 2019).

In the past two decades, important developments in IBD treatment have occurred. Nowadays, the generally followed treatment strategy is: a) for mild IBD, upkeep therapies are usually achieved with 5-aminosalicylic acid alone or budesonide; b) for moderate or refractory mild IBD, immunosuppressants (*e.g.* methotrexate, azathioprine, corticosteroids) are commonly used; c) for severe or refractory moderate IBD, biologics such as small molecule inhibitors or immunoglobulins, as anticytokine antibodies, are used [e.g., anti-tumour necrosis factor (TNF) (adalimumab), transcription signaling pathway inhibitors (filgotinib, tofacitinib, etc.), β7 integrin inhibitor (etrolizumab)]; d) finally, surgical resection of the affected bowel is required in severe refractory IBD. Recently, another adopted strategy is based on the manipulation of the interactions between beneficial and pathogenic microorganisms of the gut biota (Flamant & Roblin, 2018; Rohr *et al.*, 2018). However, the complexity of IBD has created enormous challenges, and drug research and development still need optimization (Olivera *et al.*, 2019; Weisshof *et al.*, 2018). Flavonoids are known to modulate the production and expression of several inflammatory mediators (Ribeiro *et al.*, 2015). Thus, studies about their use in the prevention and treatment of chronic inflammatory disorders, as IBD, have been increasing (Ribeiro *et al.*, 2018). This chapter intends to summarize the known properties of flavonoids in the diverse stages of IBD inflammatory pathways, covering all the concerning available *in vivo* studies.

FLAVONOIDS

Flavonoids display a diphenylpropane basic structure. This structure is made of 2 benzene rings (A and B rings) and a third pyran heterocyclic ring (C ring) (Figure 1). Flavonoids are divided in different subclasses according to the substitution pattern and oxidation of the C ring. Within the same subclass, and according to the substitution pattern of the A or B rings, various flavonoids can be identified (Table 1).

Figure 1. General scaffold of flavonoids

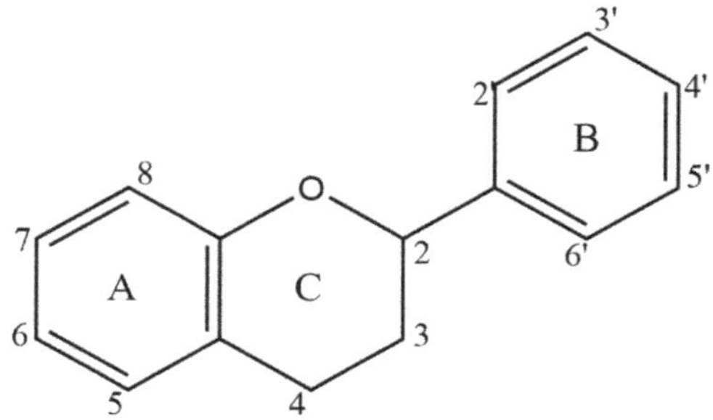

Flavonoids are broadly distributed in nature and are present in the human diet on a daily basis (Table 1). However, they can also be found in commercially available products, namely in dietary supplements (e.g., capsules of resveratrol and quercetin), phytotherapeutic extracts (e.g., green tea extracts), and as isolated products (Ribeiro *et al.*, 2015). In nature, flavonoids occur as methylated derivatives, glycosides and aglycones. Most of them, except flavanols (monomers and proanthocyanidins), occur in plants as *O*-glycosides.

The number of flavonoids ingested, and the levels detected in our body vary according to the diet of each individual, and also to the cooking and food processing methods, among other factors (Shivashankara & Acharya, 2010). In a comprehensive review published in 2004 (Manach & Donovan, 2004), the total ingested values (glycosides expressed as the equivalent dose of aglycone) of diverse flavonoid subclasses were presented. The obtained values varied between 68 and 307 mg for flavonols; 32 and 664 mg for catechins; 23 and 199 mg for flavanones; and 68 and 139 mg for anthocyanidins. The discrepancies among the values within the same flavonoid subclasses may derive from the fact that each study used different types of supplementation, different flavonoid concentrations, administered during different periods of time (Manach & Donovan, 2004). A study performed in 2007 (Mullie *et al.*, 2007) evaluated the daily intake of flavonoids present in food, using a four-day non-consecutive food diary (4DFR) and a semi-quantitative food frequency questionnaire (FFQ), by 300 female subjects. The FFQ included a list of 86 flavonoids and their consumption was registered in a frequency table. The determined daily intake was approximately between 0.6 and 2.7 mg for flavonols; 0.5 and 27.5 mg for flavanones; 0.4 and 2.7 mg for anthocyanidins; and 0.3 and 5.9 for flavones (Mullie *et al.*, 2007). Despite these spread values, all subclasses of flavonoids were daily ingested in mg range.

Table 1. Chemical structure and dietary sources of several subclasses of flavonoids (Ribeiro et al., 2018)

Subclass	Chemical structure	Examples	Dietary sources
Flavone	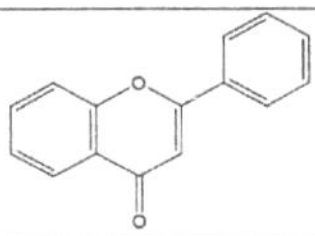	Apigenin, baicalin, chrysin, luteolin	Fruit peel, red pepper, tomato skin
Flavanol	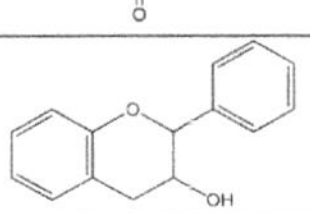	Catechin, epichatechin	Cocoa, fruits, tea
Flavonol	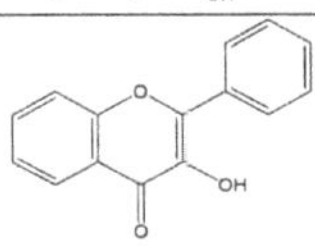	Fisetin, myricetin, quercetin	Berries, onion, red wine
Flavanone	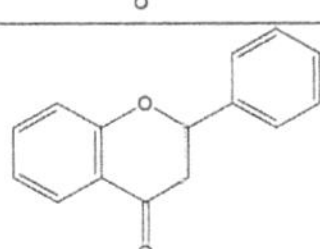	Hesperetin, naringenin	Citrus fruits
Flavanonol	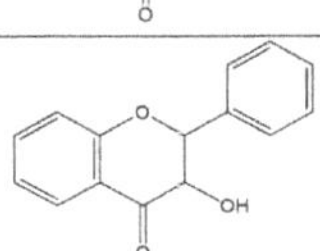	Astilbin, taxifolin	Onion
Isoflavone	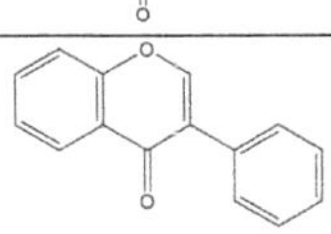	Daidzein, genistein	Leguminous plants
Anthocyanidin	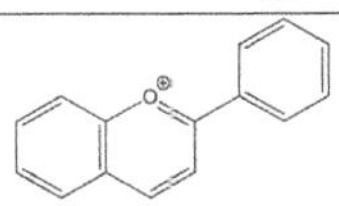	Cyanidin, malvidin	Berries, red wine, vegetables

Absorption and metabolism of flavonoids depend on their molecular lipophilicity, solubility, pKa, size, and configuration. In the intestine, due to the hydrophilicity of flavonoid glycosides, specific active transport mechanisms or hydrolysis of the sugar conjugates are required for intestinal absorption. In the intestinal epithelial cells, flavonoid aglycones can suffer glucuronidation, sulphation, or methylation, which enables the production of other phenolic compounds that enter the bloodstream (Ribeiro *et al.*, 2018). In general, it is difficult to relate plasma levels of flavonoids reported in the diverse studies, mostly due to the population and intake variabilities. Regardless of the ingested amounts, flavonoids are found in human plasma in micromolar concentrations. One of the previously mentioned reviews (Manach & Donovan, 2004) pointed to maximal plasma concentrations between 0.2 and 7.6 μM for flavonols; 0.02 and 5.9 μM for catechins; 0.06 and 5.99 μM for flavanones; and 0.0014 and 0.17 μM for anthocyanidins. More recently, 77 healthy females and males were subjected to a 2-week flavonoid supplementation (329 mg/day of anthocyanins, flavan-3-ols and quercetin mixture). After this period, the average sum of 76 plasma gut-derived phenolics was calculated. The authors found an average of 2.19 μM gut-derived phenolic metabolites (Nieman *et al.*, 2018). In fact, the immunomodulatory effect of flavonoids in IBD may be potentiated by increasing the intestinal concentration of flavonoids (Ribeiro *et al.*, 2018).

IN VIVO STUDIES OF IBD: PROPHYLACTIC EFFECTS OF FLAVONOIDS

In this section, an overview will be presented on the prophylactic potential of different subclasses of flavonoids. In all cases, mice or rats were pre-treated (hours to days) with flavonoids in the order of 1–100 mg/kg and then colitis was induced by acetic acid (3–7.5%), dextran sulfate sodium (DSS) (1–5%) or 2,4,6-trinitrobenzenesulfonic acid (TNBS) (2–12%). In some cases, the treatment with flavonoids also continued after colitis induction. Unless otherwise stated, the parameters presented refer exclusively to the colon, including epithelial and immune cells.

Flavones

Chrysin, 5,7-dihydroxyflavone, is a flavone with low number of chemical substitutions compared to other mentioned flavones. C57BL/6 mice were exposed to DSS, with a pre-treatment with chrysin [25 mg/kg body weight (BW)], for 3 days before DSS exposure. Chrysin led to the amelioration of colon length, decreased phosphorylation of nuclear factor-κB (NF-κB) p65 and kB inhibitor (IκB)-α, increased total IκB-α levels, decreased the transcript and protein levels of inducible nitric oxide synthase (iNOS), cyclooxygenase (COX)-2, monocyte chemoattractant protein (MCP)-1, intercellular adhesion molecule (ICAM)-1, interleukin (IL)-6 and TNF (Dou, Zhang, Zhang, *et al.*, 2013).

Apigenin, 4',5,7-trihydroxyflavone, has been studied at doses of 1–10 mg/kg BW, depending on the rodent model, in different regimes of chemically-induced colitis. Generally, apigenin-induced amelioration of colon length was associated with decreased histological scores, disease activity index (DAI), and damage scores. More importantly, its ingestion by Wistar rats lowered the levels of proinflammatory IL-1β and increased the expression of ICAM-1 and the chemokine CCL2 (Mascaraque *et al.*, 2015). Moreover, in C57BL/6 mice, co-housing with mice treated with apigenin ameliorated the inflammatory state of non-treated animal, through acquired gut microbiota, and this effect was shown to rely on the NLRP6 inflammasome signaling pathway (Radulovic *et al.*, 2018).

Baicalein, 5,6,7-trihydroxyflavone, administered daily (20 mg/kg BW, oral route) to C57BL/6 mice exposed to DSS and to BALB/c mice exposed to TNBS, starting 2 days before colitis induction, reduced histological score, and decreased proinflammatory gene expression and TNF levels (Dou *et al.*, 2012; Luo *et al.*, 2017). In the TNBS model, BALB/c mice pre-treated with baicalein showed decreased macrophage infiltration, lower levels of NF-κB, and reduced iNOS, COX-2, and IL-1β gene expression (Luo *et al.*, 2017).

Luteolin, 3′,4′,5,7-tetrahydroxyflavone, has shown varying effects, depending on the pre-treatment and chemical exposure. In C57BL/6 mice, luteolin in diet (0.5–5%), administered for 3 days before colitis induction, aggravated the disease symptoms induced by DSS, increased proinflammatory NF-κB activity, and enhanced apoptotic caspase 3 activation (Karrasch *et al.*, 2007). Notwithstanding, in another study with C57BL/6CrSlc mice, colon length, histological score, colon infiltration of macrophages, $CD4^+$ T cells, interferon (IFN)-γ^+ cells, and gene expression of IFN-γ were ameliorated by luteolin (5–20 mg/kg BW). However, no effect was observed on COX-2 gene expression (Nishitani *et al.*, 2013).

BALB/c mice were treated with 3′-hydroxy-4',5,7-trimethoxyflavone (FVN625) and 6-hydroxy-5,7-dimethoxyflavone (FVN1087) (25 mg/kg BW), 2, 24 and 48 h before; and 24 h after the induction of colitis by TNBS. These synthetic flavones did not induce a change in colon length/weight, but increased myeloperoxidase (MPO) activity, revealing macrophage infiltration in the gut. Nevertheless, an increase in glutathione (GSH) was found, suggestive of increased antioxidant capacity (Seito *et al.*, 2015).

Baicalin, baicalein 7-*O*-glucuronide, is one of the most studied flavonoids in *in vivo* colitis models. In DSS colitis model in C57BL/6 mice, baicalin pre-treatments (20–100 mg/kg BW) resulted in a decrease of histological score and TNF levels (Dou *et al.*, 2012; Zhu *et al.*, 2016). Mice pre-treated with baicalin and exposed to DSS, showed *lamina propria* mononuclear cells with larger proportion of macrophages associated with tissue repair *versus* proinflammatory macrophages (Zhu *et al.*, 2016).

Diosmin, diosmetin 7-*O*-rutinoside, pre-treatment doses for colitis vary between 2.5-100 mg/kg BW, depending on the study (Crespo *et al.*, 1999; Shalkami *et al.*, 2018). Wistar rats were exposed to TNBS, and Swiss mice to acetic acid. Diosmin reduced damage, malondialdehyde (MDA) content, and (MPO) activity (a marker of neutrophil infiltration), and increased GSH content (Crespo *et al.*, 1999; Shalkami *et al.*, 2018).

Orientin, luteolin 8-C-glucoside, administered to C57BL/6 mice (50, 100 mg/kg BW) 2 days before DSS-induced colitis, ameliorated colon length, decreased histological score, MPO activity and cytokine production. Moreover, it decreased nitric oxide radical (•NO) content, and gene expression of iNOS, COX-2, IL-1β and -6, MCP-1, TNF, p-p65 (phosphorylated NF-κB), and p-IκB-α, suggesting a relation between inflammation and oxidative stress (A. N. Sun *et al.*, 2016).

Dosmalfate is a derivative of diosmin, with improved solubility. In Wistar rats with colitis induced by TNBS, pre-treatment with this derivative (200–800 mg/kg BW) before the induction of colitis (1, 24 and 48 h) and after (24 h), decreased colon weight/volume, macroscopic damage, MPO activity, and TNF levels (Villegas, La Casa, *et al.*, 2003).

Flavanols

The prophylactic role in colitis of epigallocatechin gallate (EGCG) also known as (-)-epigallocatechin-3-*O*-gallate, has been extensively investigated (Chiou *et al.*, 2012; Geagea *et al.*, 2017; Guan *et al.*, 2012; Mochizuki & Hasegawa, 2005, 2010). In DSS models, it was found that EGCG (0.5%), administration 2 weeks before colitis induction in C57BL/6 mice, resulted in no significant improvement in colon length, and no change in leukotriene (LT)B_4 and prostaglandin (PG)E_2 levels (Guan *et al.*, 2012). At lower concentrations, EGCG decreased lymphoid nodule number and inflammation, ameliorated colon length, and decreased serum LTB_4 and PGE_2 levels (Chiou *et al.*, 2012). In TNBS models, EGCG pre-treatment (1–30 mg/kg BW) decreased macroscopic damage and histological score, number of mast cells, gene expression of proinflammatory TNF and IL-6. Moreover, it decreased histamine levels, MPO activity and increased superoxide dismutase (SOD) activity (Geagea *et al.*, 2017; Mochizuki & Hasegawa, 2005, 2010).

Peracetylated epigallocatechin gallate (AcEGCG) is a flavanol derivative of EGCG. AcEGCG pre-treatment (0.017 and 0.085%) 1 week before DSS-induced colitis in ICR mice, ameliorated colon shortening, decreased inflammation, lesions, as well as levels of COX-2, iNOS, NF-κB, and p65 phosphorylation (Chiou *et al.*, 2012).

Flavonols

Fisetin, 3,3',4',7-tetrahydroxyflavone, pre-treatment (10 mg/kg BW) 1 day before and during the induction of colitis in BALB/c mice through DSS, ameliorated colon length, and decreased DAI and the levels of proinflammatory IL-1β, and -6, iNOS, COX-2, TNF, p-IκBα, and NF-κB and also MPO activity (Sahu *et al.*, 2016).

In C57BL/6J mice exposed to DSS, pre-treatment (0.1–0.3%) with kaempferol, 3,4',5,7-tetrahydroxyflavone, 14 days before and during colitis induction, ameliorated colon length, decreased DAI, histological score, MPO activity, LTB_4 levels, and gene expression of PGE_2, COX-2, IL-6, -1β, TNF, and iNOS. Kaempferol presence also increased TFF3 gene expression, a marker of columnar epithelium, suggesting improved epithelial barrier integrity (Park *et al.*, 2012).

The prophylactic effects of morin, 3,2',4',5,7-pentahydroxyflavone, were tested by administration of 5–200 mg/kg BW, at 3 time points before TNBS-induced colitis and 24h later to Wistar rats (Ocete *et al.*, 1998). No significant changes were observed; however, bowel wall thickening and increased LTB_4 levels were found, suggestive of colitis aggravation. Notwithstanding, decreased damage score and MPO activity were also detected, together with increased GSH content, pointing to positive effects (Ocete *et al.*, 1998).

Quercetin, 3,3',4',5,7-pentahydroxyflavone, is widespread in the human diet. Unlike its various positive *in vitro* effects, pre-treatment with quercetin, administered by oral route, generally results in modest to no effects in colitis models, probably because it is mostly absorbed before reaching the colon. In this respect, studies report no significant effect while others report protective effects, depending essentially on quercetin concentrations, period of treatment and vehicle used, even for the same species and similar experimental setups (Dodda *et al.*, 2014; Milackova *et al.*, 2015; Sotnikova *et al.*, 2013). Kwon and colleagues described no positive effect on colon length or levels of proinflammatory cytokines in CD1/ICR mice exposed to 5% DSS and pre-treated with quercetin rich diet (Kwon *et al.*, 2005). In another study, 2h before colitis induction, Swiss mice were orally administered quercetin dissolved in a Tween 80 solution or contained in controlled release microcapsules (Guazelli *et al.*, 2013). After acetic acid-induction of colitis, no significant amelioration was found in the group that received quercetin dissolved in solution. However, in the group receiving microcapsules, the authors reported amelioration in colon weight/length, reduction of neutrophil infiltration, decreased levels of proinflammatory IL-1β and -33, and anti-inflammatory IL-10; as well as increased levels of GSH and consequently the overall antioxidant capacity.

Hyperoside, quercetin 3-galactoside, pre-treatment (80, 120 mg/kg BW) 14 days before the induction of colitis with DSS in C57BL/6 mice, ameliorated colon length, decreased DAI, histological score, MDA content, protein levels of NF-κB p65, caspase 3 and Bax. A decrease of TNF, IL-6, and -4 gene expression levels was also reported. Moreover, hyperoside pre-treatment increased gene expression of IL-10, Bcl-2, Nrf-2, SOD, heme oxygenase-1 (HO-1), and, likewise, increased the protein levels of Bcl-2 (Yang *et al.*, 2017). Overall, hyperoside improved the antioxidant system of the gut, while attenuating apoptosis and inflammation.

Isoquercitrin, quercetin 3-glucoside, another quercetin glycoside, in Wistar rats exposed to DSS, ameliorated colon shortening and decreased proinflammatory COX-2 expression, when administered (1, 10 mg/kg BW) 14 days previously to colitis induction, and during the last 7 days that rats drank DSS solution (Cibicek *et al.*, 2016).

Quercitrin, quercetin-3-rhamnoside, is mostly hydrolysed to quercetin by α-rhamnosidases from the colonic microbiome. In a TNBS-induction model in Wistar rats, pre-treatment with quercitrin (1–5 mg/kg BW) 2h prior to the induction, caused the amelioration of colon weight, decreased damage score, as well as NOX1 expression, iNOS and COX-2 gene and protein expression, and reduced TNF and IL-1β gene expression (Romero *et al.*, 2017; Sanchez de Medina *et al.*, 2002).

Rutin, quercetin-3-rutinoside, has also been intensely studied as a pro-drug for quercetin delivery in the gut. Compared to quercetin pre-treatment, (0.1%) which resulted in significant changes in colon health parameters in CD1/ICR mice exposed to DSS; rutin pre-treatment (0.1%) during 2 weeks before colitis induction, induced amelioration of colon length, together with decreased levels of proinflammatory IL-1β and decreased gene expression of IL-1β and -6 (Kwon *et al.*, 2005). Additionally, in Wistar rats exposed to TNBS, rutin pre-treatment (5–100 mg/kg BW) 48, 24 and 1h before colitis induction, as well as 24h later, increased colonic GSH and decreased MPO activity (Cruz *et al.*, 1998). Other subsequent studies confirmed positive roles of rutin, e.g., decreased iNOS expression and increased expression of tight-junction (TJ) genes (Power *et al.*, 2016; Ye *et al.*, 2009). Importantly, rutin pre-treatment (0.025% in basal diet) for 2 weeks prior to and during colitis, ameliorated gut microbiota profile, with reported decrease in proteobacteria (comprising many pathogens) and increase in firmicutes, which represent the largest portion of healthy human gut microbiome (Power *et al.*, 2016).

Myricitrin, myricetin 3-*O*-rhamnoside, when administered as pre-treatment (1-10 mg/kg BW) to CDI/ICR mice, 1h before DSS administration, resulted in protective effects, as there was amelioration in colon length, and a reduction in DAI and in macroscopic damage score (Schwanke *et al.*, 2013). In this study, myricitrin prevented the activation of phosphatidylinositol 3-kinase (PI3K)/Akt signaling and NF-κB, compared to DSS control. Myricitrin also inhibited the iNOS and COX-2 gene expression, and reduced the levels of COX-2, IL-6, TNF, and CXCL1/KC (Schwanke *et al.*, 2013).

M10 is a synthetic myricetin derivative. This derivative (50–100 mg/kg BW) was given to C57BL/6 mice 5 days before colitis induction with DSS. It was shown that this compound decreased DAI and inflammation index, ameliorated colon length, and reduced TNF and IL-6 levels (F. Wang *et al.*, 2018).

Chloronaphthoquinone quercetin, 4'-(2-chloro-1,4-naphthoquinone-3-yl)-3,3',5,7-tetrahydroxyflavone, and monochloropivaloyl quercetin are synthetic quercetin derivatives. Pre-treatment with these compounds (2 × 50 mg/kg BW) in Wistar rats, 2h and 1h before the acetic acid rectal administration, ameliorated colon weight/length and disease score, however, it is still not known if these drugs act in similar manner to quercetin (Milackova *et al.*, 2015; Sotnikova *et al.*, 2013).

Flavanones

Naringenin, 4',5,7-trihydroxyflavanone, when administered over a 7-day period to Wistar rats, prevented some of the deleterious effects caused by administration of acetic acid (Al-Rejaie *et al.*, 2013). In this study, a decrease of colon inflammation, ulceration, hyperemia, necrosis, edema, and cellular infiltrate were observed. Moreover, naringenin pre-treatment resulted in increased mucus production and overall improvement of antioxidant status, evidenced by increased GSH, non-protein-SH, SOD activity and decreased MDA levels. Naringenin decreased the colonic levels of •NO, IL-1β, -6, TNF, and PGE_2. Additionally, in two distinct models of DSS-induced colitis, naringenin ameliorated colon length (Dou, Zhang, Sun, *et al.*, 2013; Guo *et al.*, 2015). In Wistar rats, upon naringenin treatment (50 mg/kg BW) 3 days former DSS-induced colitis and sustained until the finish of DSS treatment, NF-κB p65 was directly inactivated as evidenced by lower levels of p-p65, and NF-κB was also indirectly inactivated by increased levels of IκB-α, and decreased levels of inactive p-IκB-α (Dou, Zhang, Sun, *et al.*, 2013).

Hesperetin, 3',5,7-trihydroxy-4'-methoxyflavanone (100 mg/kg BW), 3 days pre-treatment in Wistar rats, resulted in amelioration of TNBS-induced colitis, confirmed by histopathological analyses. In this respect, a decrease in the number of positive cells for expression of TNF, CD45, caspase 3 and Bax was observed, suggesting anti-inflammatory and anti-apoptotic effect (Polat & Karaboga, 2018).

Farrerol, 6,8-dimethyl-4',5,7-trihydroxyflavanone, administration (45 mg/kg BW) 3 days prior to colitis induction by TNBS in C57BL/6 mice, resulted in amelioration of colon length and in a decrease of clinical and histological scores. At the molecular level, farrerol reduced the gene expression and levels of TNF, IL-1β and -6. Additionally, it increased the expression of the Mucin2 and TJ genes (X. Ran *et al.*, 2018).

Diplacone, 6-geranyl-3',4',5,7-tetrahydroxyflavanone, and mimulone, 6-geranylnaringenin, showed positive effects against DSS-induced colitis in Wistar rats, when administered 48 and 24h (each dose 25 mg/kg BW) before colitis induction. Both compounds decreased DAI and reduced COX-2 expression (Vochyanova *et al.*, 2015).

Hesperidin, hesperetin 7-rutoside, was found to have positive effects in a colitis model at low doses (5, 10 mg/kg) when administered prior to the colitis induction (1, 24 and 48h) by TNBS in Wistar rats. In contrast to higher doses (50 mg/kg), hesperidin, at 5 and 10 mg/kg, reduced colonic necrosis, hyperaemia, inflammation, and MPO activity. Moreover, it prevented MDA increase and GSH depletion caused by TNBS treatment (Crespo *et al.*, 1999).

Isoflavones

Genistein, 4',5,7-trihydroxy-isoflavone, and daidzein, 4',7-dihydroxyisoflavone, have hitherto not shown protective effects when administered before colitis induction. When administered at doses of 2–20 mg/kg BW, for 7 days before colitis induction by DSS in BALB/c mice, these isoflavones did not show any anti-inflammatory effect in the gut (Sakai *et al.*, 2011).

IN VIVO STUDIES OF IBD: HEALING EFFECTS OF FLAVONOIDS

In this section, an overview on the healing potential of different subclasses of flavonoids will be presented. In all cases, colitis was induced in mice or rats with DSS (1.5–5%), TNBS (10–100 mg/kg) or acetic acid (3–8%) and concomitantly or afterwards the flavonoids were administered (hours to days, various administration routes), at a dose ranging from 1 to 300 mg/kg BW. Unless otherwise stated, the parameters presented refer exclusively to the colon, including epithelial and immune cells.

Flavones

Several polyhydroxyflavones were studied as anti-colitic agents, and their effects are discussed below.

Chrysin, 5,7-dihydroxyflavone, (1–10 mg/kg BW) was orally administered to BALB/c mice, for 7 days, coordinated with the start of DSS exposure. It was observed an improvement of the disrupted architecture of the colon, a decrease in PGE_2 and •NO, and a remarkable reduction in colonic MPO activity. Chrysin prevented significant elevations in keratinocyte chemoattractant and MCP-1, IL-1β, -6, and -8 levels, without any effect on TNF (Shin *et al.*, 2009).

Luteolin (20, 50 mg/kg BW) significantly attenuated colon shortening, DAI, and the histological damages of DSS-induced UC, in a C57BL/6 mouse model. Moreover, luteolin administration decreased the expression of IL-6, iNOS, and TNF, and the colonic content of MDA. Luteolin treatment elevated colonic SOD and catalase activities and the levels of Nrf2 and its downstream targets, HO-1 and quinone oxidoreductase 1 (Li *et al.*, 2016).

Nobiletin, 3′,4′,5,6,7,8-hexamethoxyflavone [20, 40 mg/kg BW (Xiong *et al.*, 2015) and 50 mg/kg BW (Hagenlocher *et al.*, 2018)], cirsilineol, 4',5-dihydroxy-3',6,7-trimethoxyflavone (3–30 mg/kg BW) (Y. Sun *et al.*, 2010), and tangeretin, 5,6,7,8,4′-pentamethoxyflavone (10 and 20 mg/kg), have been studied as modulators of IBD in TNBS-induced experimental colitis model, and all the compounds ameliorated inflammation symptoms (Eun *et al.*, 2017). An increase in food intake and in body weight was observed, together with a decrease in the macroscopically visible damage, in the DAI, and in the colon weight/length ratio. In the case of nobiletin, these effects seem to be related to the downregulation of iNOS and COX-2 expression, to a decreased expression of NF-κB and myosin light chain kinase (MLCK), and to a decreased PI3K and Akt phosphorylation levels (Xiong *et al.*, 2015). The same compound was studied using another model, IL-$10^{-/-}$ colitic mice, that were fed with nobiletin for 11 weeks. This flavone was able to reduce colitis symptoms and promoted longer survival time and a reduction of histological scores of colitis. Mast cell number and degranulation was lower in the treated mice, and positively correlated with DAI (Hagenlocher *et al.*, 2018). The anti-inflammatory effect of cirsilineol seems to be related with a reduced activation and proliferation of the autoreactive T-cell. This may result from the selective inhibition of the IFN-γ signaling in colonic lamina propria $CD4^+$ T cells. Possibly intermediated by the downregulation of the activation of signal transducer and activator of transcription (STAT)1 and expression of T-bet which, in turn, could occur by the decrease in JAK2 activation, a vital kinase for the IFN-γ/STAT1 signaling. Interestingly, authors also reported an increase of the anti-inflammatory cytokines TGF-β and IL-10, which can modulate the IBD progression by defeating and counteracting the proinflammatory cytokines effects (Y. Sun *et al.*, 2010). The anti-inflammatory response of tangeretin, occurred by the inhibition of MAPK and NF-κB, through MPO activation. Furthermore, tangeretin inhibited the differentiation of Th1 and Th17 cells, as well as the expression of T-bet, RORγt, IFN-γ, IL-12, -17, and TNF. In turn, this flavone increased the differentiation of regulatory T cells and the production of anti-inflammatory mediators, as the expression of forkhead box protein P3 (Foxp3) and IL-10 (Y. Sun *et al.*, 2010).

Curiously, FVN625 and FVN1087 did not show an anti-colitic effect. These flavones were orally given to Wistar rats (5–25 mg/kg BW / day) before (2, 24 and 48 h) and after (24 h) TNBS colitis induction. None of the compounds barred the augmented colonic weight/length; abridged food intake; or altered the body weight when compared with colitic control rats. Despite the observed protection of GSH tissue content, none of the compounds inhibited the increased MPO and alkaline phosphatase (AP) activities and consequently none of them prevented the inflammatory response in rats (Seito *et al.*, 2015).

Baicalin, 5,6-dihydroxyflavone-7-*O*-glucuronide, is one of the most studied flavones. In general, and despite the differences found among the *in vivo* models, and the tested concentrations [100 mg/kg (Dai et al., 2012; Feng et al., 2014; Zou et al., 2015), and 1.25–5 mg/mL (Cui *et al.*, 2014)], the treatment of animals with this flavone originated consensual results, namely the amelioration of the inflammatory symptoms of induced colitis, through different pathways. The expression of toll-like receptor 4 (TLR4) was decreased, and consequently NF-κB p65 (Cui *et al.*, 2014; Feng *et al.*, 2014), myeloid differentiation primary response 88 (an upstream signal molecular of NF-κB signal pathway) (Cui *et al.*, 2014), and the macrophage migration inhibitory factor (MIF) were also decreased (Dai *et al.*, 2012). The level of oxidative stress was also reduced through the decrease of MPO activity (Zou *et al.*, 2015). In what concerns cytokines production, baicalin suppressed TNF, IL-6, -13 (Feng *et al.*, 2014), IL-12, -1β, IFN-γ (Zou *et al.*, 2015), macrophage inflammatory protein (MIP)-3a and MCP-1 (Dai *et al.*, 2012) expressions; while it elevated the expression of the anti-inflammatory cytokine IL-10 (Feng *et al.*, 2014; Zou *et al.*, 2015). It is also known that the pathologic response in IBD is regulated by the proinflammatory Th17 cells and the anti-inflammatory Treg cells, based on the production and function of the cytokines. Zou and colleagues (Zou *et al.*, 2015) stated that baicalin induced Th17/Treg imbalance, in the colon. It exerts this effect by the downregulation of the levels of retinoic acid receptor-related orphan receptor γ and IL-6 and -17; of the Th17 cells number; and by the increase of the number of Treg cells, IL-10, transforming growth factor- β, and forkhead box P3 levels (Zou *et al.*, 2015).

Wogonoside, 5,7-dihydroxy-8-methoxyflavone-7-glucuronide, (12.5–50 mg/kg BW), was intragastrically administrated for 10 days, simultaneously with DSS, to BALB/c mice (Y. Sun *et al.*, 2015). Wogonoside weakened the body weight loss and the shortening of the colon. Furthermore, it prevented the pathological damage of the colon and strongly prevented inflammatory cells infiltration. It also reduced the production of several inflammatory mediators as IFN-γ, MIP-1α, TNF, and IL-1β, -6, -18 in the colon, namely by the inhibition of the activities of iNOS, NF-κB, and MPO. The proposed underlying mechanisms for the observed protective effect was attributed to nucleotide-binding domain, leucine-rich-containing family, pyrin domain-containing-3 (NLRP-3) inflammasome activation in the colon (Y. Sun *et al.*, 2015).

The flavone oroxyloside (5,7-dihydroxy-6-methoxyflavone-7-*O*-β-D-glucuronide) (20–80 mg/kg BW), one of the main metabolites of oroxylin A, was used to treat colitis induced by DSS in C57BL/6 mice. In general, oroxyloside attenuated the colon length shortening, the pathological damage of the colon and the loss of body weight. The inhibition of NF-κB, by PPARγ activation, was also reported. Consequently, the levels of TNF, IL-1β, and -6 (proinflammatory), in serum and colon, were significantly reduced. Also, the activity of the oxidative stress mediators MPO and iNOS was reduced (X. Wang *et al.*, 2016).

DA-6034, a 7-carboxymethyloxy-3',4',5-trimethoxyflavone, a synthetic derivative, was orally administered in different IBD animal models: two chemically induced IBD rat models and one human leukocyte antigen (HLA)-B27 transgenic rat model. The latter does not need the use of exogenous agents, as it spontaneously develops colitis. An acetic acid solution was used to induce acute colitis in rats and DA-6034 was orally administered (0.3–3 mg/kg), two times/day, for 6 days. Chronic colitis was tempted by TNBS (intracolonic administration). One day after the injury DA-6034 was orally administered (1, 3 mg/kg BW): for the chronic phase, for 20 days; or for the acute phase, one time a day, for 6 days; or. DA-6034 (3 mg/kg BW) was orally given to HLAB27 transgenic rats two times a day, for 6 weeks. Differences were found among the used models and TNBS/ethanol was reported a better IBD experimental model than the one induced by acetic acid. In comparison with the colitis models induced by chemicals, the HLA-B27 transgenic rats just presented mild colitis. In general, DA-6034 was found to attenuate the colon damages (histological and macroscopic) in all used IBD models (Y. S. Kim *et al.*, 1999).

Dosmalfate, diosmin heptakis (hydrogensulfate) aluminium complex, was orally administered (400 and 800 mg/kg BW) for 7 days to DSS-treated BALB/c mice. Dosmalfate ameliorated severe colitis and reduced neutrophil infiltration, IL-1β levels, and increased PGE_2 synthesis in colon mucosa. However, the modulatory effect of dosmalfate in both PGE_2 and PGD_2 synthase expression remains unclear (Villegas, Alarcon de la Lastra, *et al.*, 2003).

Flavanols

The activity of few catechins were also studied against IBD models. Epicatechin, 3',4',5,7-tetrahydroxyflavanol, an isomer of catechin, (100–300 mg/kg BW) was administered orally in a DSS-induced acute UC, to C57BL/6 mice, for 7 days (Zhang *et al.*, 2016). Epicatechin clearly attenuated the acute intestinal injury and significantly relieved colon contracture and crypt damage, through several mechanisms. One of such mechanisms was the decrease of the release of proinflammatory cytokines as IL-6 and TNF. In what concerns oxidative stress, it was observed a decrease in the levels of •NO, MPO and MDA and an increase of the activity of the antioxidant enzymes SOD, GSH-Px and catalase. All of these alterations should be related with the inhibitory effect on the NF-κB activation (Zhang *et al.*, 2016).

EGCG was orally given (50 mg/kg BW) to Sprague-Dawley rats, after colitis induction by acetic acid, for 7 days. After the treatment with EGCG the disease progression was reduced and several symptoms ameliorated, as macroscopical lesion with edema, hematosis mucosa, superficial and small ulcers. EGCG elevated the SOD contents and reduced the MDA and •NO levels, in colonic tissues. The levels of TNF and IFN-γ were decreased and once again the decrease in NF-κB expression seems to play an important part in the anti-inflammatory activity of EGCG (Z. H. Ran *et al.*, 2008).

Kook and colleagues (Kook *et al.*, 2015) studied the intestinal activity of catechin-7-*O*-β-glucopyranoside (CGP) (1–10 mg/kg BW) through its daily administration, for 7 days, to Sprague–Dawley rats with TNBS-induced colitis. The highest tested concentration reduced MPO, NOS and COX-2 activities and MDA levels. The production of cytokines, IL-1β and TNF was also inhibited, possibly through the inhibition of the phosphorylation of p38MAPK and the NF-κB subunit IκB-α. The administration of CGP resulted in a decrease in MCP-1 and ICAM-1 mRNA levels and restored the expression of the mucins (MUC3 and MUC2) responsible for the regaining of the intestinal epithelial barriers functions (Kook *et al.*, 2015).

Flavonols

Quercetin, 3,3',4',5,7-pentahydroxyflavone, is ubiquitously found in its glycosylated forms (Comalada *et al.*, 2005). The ratio of these compounds in the intestine, as well as their anti-inflammatory effect, is still controversial.

Kim and colleagues (H. Kim *et al.*, 2005) induced the inflammatory process in Sprague-Dawley rats, using TNBS, followed by quercetin (rectal administration, 25–100 μM) or rutin (oral administration, 10 mg/kg BW), for 6 days. The authors reported that, in the large intestine, the sugar residue in rutin was rapidly deglycosylated to release quercetin, without significant biochemical loss in the upper intestine. Interestingly, both compounds significantly healed the damage of the colon and decreased the levels of MPO, an indicator of neutrophil infiltration. In contrast, Kwon and colleagues (Kwon *et al.*, 2005), who studied the effect of these two flavonols (6 mg/kg) 3 days after DSS-induced colitis and during 2 weeks, in ICR mice, reported that rutin ameliorated the inflammatory process by the suppression of IL-1β levels and colorectum shortening, without any effect of quercetin (Kwon *et al.*, 2005). Quercitrin, 3,3',4',5,7-pentahydroxyflavone-3-rhamnoside, (1 mg/kg BW) was described as ameliorating the evolution of the inflammatory process, as demonstrated by a substantial decrease in the DAI values, MPO (Camuesco *et al.*, 2004; Comalada *et al.*, 2005) and AP activities (Camuesco *et al.*, 2004), a decrease in the production of, IL-1β, TNF and LTB_4 (Camuesco *et al.*, 2004; Comalada *et al.*, 2005), a significant inhibition of iNOS expression (Camuesco *et al.*, 2004; Comalada *et al.*, 2005) and a downregulation of the NF-κB activity, but with no modification of the activity of JNK (Comalada *et al.*, 2005). The modulatory effect of quercitrin against these inflammatory mediators is related with the reduction of a macrophage infiltration in the inflamed tissue (Camuesco *et al.*, 2004). Interestingly, despite the anti-inflammatory activity of quercetin *in vitro*, quercetin did not show any anti-inflammatory activity using *in vivo* models. The paradoxical results obtained with quercetin and its glycoside quercitrin could be explained by the flavonoids' bioavailability. Generally, the literature describes aglycones as being absorbed in the small intestine, averting their beneficial effects in the inflamed colon. In contrast, the glycoside quercitrin reach the colon and exert its anti-inflammatory effect, because it is not absorbed in the gastrointestinal tract upper segments (Comalada *et al.*, 2005).

Following this rationale, Castangia and colleagues (Castangia *et al.*, 2015) encapsulated quercetin in polyethylene-glycol vesicles, coated by nutriose and chitosan. Those vesicles containing quercetin (9 mg/kg BW) were administered (oral gavage), one time a day, for 3 days, during days 3–5 (intense inflammation), after TNBS administration to Wistar rats (rectal). The group treated with non-entrapped quercetin or uncoated loaded vesicles presented severe colon damage, as in the group without treatment. The inflammatory profile changed when the vesicles containing quercetin. Quercetin accrues in the colon, exerting its local anti-inflammatory activity leading to an important improvement of the colitis indicators.

Morin was orally given daily at doses of 25 mg/kg, for 4 weeks, to Wistar rats previously subjected to a single colonic instillation of TNBS. Morin reduced macroscopic colonic damage and ameliorated the histological lesions. This flavonoid decreased the colonic MPO activity and reduced granulocyte infiltration, probably through the inhibition of LTB_4 synthesis. These effects were also related with an inhibition of the colonic production of IL-1β, which was persistent 3 weeks after the treatment, and may be responsible for the observed inhibition of colonic NOS activity (Galvez *et al.*, 2001).

Myricetin, 3,3',4',5,5',7-hexahydroxyflavone, was orally administered (50–200 mg/kg BW), for 10 days, to a murine model (BALB/c) of acute experimental colitis induced by DSS. It was observed that myricetin bettered the pathological DSS colitis indicators, possibly through the inhibition of •NO and MDA production, and the decrease of MPO activity, with the simultaneously increase of GSH-Px and SOD activities. Additionally, IL-6 and -1β levels were significantly decreased (Zhao *et al.*, 2013).

Isorhamnetin, 3'-methoxy-3,4',5,7-tetrahydroxyflavone, was tested (20 mg/kg BW) using two different IBD-induced models, one using DSS- and the other using TNBS, in C57BL/6 mice. In general, isorhamnetin abrogated inflammation through the inhibition of MPO activity, the reduction of iNOS, COX-2, ICAM-1, and IL-2 mRNA expression, and the levels of IL-6 and TNF. It was suggested that NF-κB played an important role in the anti-inflammatory effect of this flavonoid. Besides that, the authors reported that isorhamnetin can activate wild-type PXR. The observed upregulation of PXR constitutes another possible mechanism by which this flavonoid acts as anti-colitic agent (Dou *et al.*, 2014).

Icariin, an 8-prenyl derivative of kaempferol 3,7-*O*-diglucoside, is another flavonol glycoside that was studied in a C57BL/6 mice colitis model induced by DSS. Icariin (3, 10 mg/kg BW) was orally daily administered with DSS (Tao *et al.*, 2013). This flavonol showed an anti-colitic effect, by the modulation of different pathways, namely the inhibition of proinflammatory cytokines as IL-1β, -17F and -17A, IFN-γ, and TNF, and the inhibition of T lymphocytes proliferation and activation. STAT1 activation, the main transcription factor involved in the response of Th1 and of STAT3, which is a vital transcription factor in the response of Th17, were also inhibited by icariin (Tao *et al.*, 2013).

Flavanones

Azuma and colleagues (Azuma *et al.*, 2013) studied the effects of supplemental feeding with naringenin, 4',5,7-trihydroxyflavanone [0.3% (wt:wt)] in DSS-induced colitis in BALB/c mice, for 9 days. The study was performed at days 3, 6 and 9, counting from the day of disease induction, to better study the role of naringenin at the beginning and on the development of colitis. In general, naringenin totally or partially ameliorated the DSS-induced colitis, attenuating some typical symptoms as the colon shortening, the decrease in body weight, the increase in DAI score, possibly through the protection of the intestinal TJ barrier. Nevertheless, naringenin may suppress Th17 cells differentiation, as showed by the decrease of IL-17A gene expression and it is responsible for the suppression of further cytokines as IL-6, IFN-γ and MIP-2 (Azuma *et al.*, 2013).

Wogonin, 5,7-dihydroxy-8-methoxyflavanone, was given, by oral intake (20 mg/kg) for 2 weeks, after induction of colitis in BALB/c mice by DSS. Wogonin originated an increase in IgA and a reduction in IgE production by lymphocytes from the mesenteric lymph node. In this way, wogonin may improve the inflammatory response of the intestinal immune system. It was observed that wogonin increased Th1 cell cytokines as IFN-γ, IL-2 and TNF and decreased the Th2 cell cytokines IL-4, -5 and -10. As such, the authors concluded that wogonin can lessen the inflammation in DSS-induced colitis, modulating the abnormal Th2 response (Lim, 2004).

Hesperidin, 3',5,7-trihydroxy-4'-methoxyflavanone-7-rhamnoglucoside, (10–80 mg/kg BW) was orally administered to BALB/c mice once a day, for 7 days, beginning concomitantly with the exposure to DSS. Hesperidin ameliorated DSS-induced experimental colitis, through a decrease in MDA content, MPO activity, IL-6 levels, and DAI score. In turn, the anti-inflammatory cytokine IL-4 levels were not altered by the presence of this flavanone (Xu *et al.*, 2009).

Flavanonols

Ding and colleagues (Ding *et al.*, 2014) evaluated the anti-inflammatory effect of astilbin, taxifolin 3-rhamnoside, in an IBD model. For that purpose, different doses (25, 50 mg/kg BW) were administered, each day, through intraperitoneal injection, to C57BL/6 mice with acute colitis induced by DSS, for 7 days. The treatment with astilbin ameliorated the severity of colitis and originated an increase in the levels of IL-10 and TGF-β. Astilbin can modulate IBD by the regulation of dendritic cells (DCs) functions. It was demonstrated that treatment with astilbin, in mice with colitis, resulted in an augmented number of IL-10^+ DCs and TGF-β $^+$DCs and a decreased number of CD86$^+$DCs, IL-12 p40$^+$DCs and IL-1β $^+$DCs in the spleen (Ding *et al.*, 2014).

Isoflavones

Genistein, 4',5,7-trihydroxyisoflavone, is the best characterized isoflavone and one of the most abundant in the human diet. Genistein was studied in TNBS- (Seibel *et al.*, 2009) and DSS-induced colitis (Abron *et al.*, 2018) *in vivo* models. The treatment [10 mg/kg BW (Abron *et al.*, 2018) or 100 mg/kg BW (Seibel *et al.*, 2009)] started 24h after disease induction, once a day, for 14 days. Genistein diminished the extent and severity of the disease, resulting in a colon length and body weight increase, and in an inflammation score reduction. Some inflammatory mediators were studied and the obtained results showed that genistein reduced the COX-2 expression, the activity of MPO (Seibel *et al.*, 2009), and the production of IL-6, -1β TNF and MCP-1 (Abron *et al.*, 2018) whereas there was no significant inhibitory effect on the expression of proliferating cell nuclear antigen (Seibel *et al.*, 2009). Throughout the inflammatory process, macrophages are activated and produce several cytokines, varying among classical M1 (proinflammatory) or M2 (anti-inflammatory) phenotypes. The treatment with genistein modulated the ratio of M1/M2 macrophages, favoring the presence of the last group. Moreover, it was observed an increase of M2 dependent cytokines as IL-10 and arginase-1 (Abron *et al.*, 2018).

CONCLUSION

This chapter provides evidence that flavonoid compounds may be valuable both in the prevention and in the treatment of IBD (Figure 4). However, care should be taken in the interpretation of the published studies as the experimental conditions are variable in each model used. These variations are mostly related with times of exposure to both the flavonoid and the inflammatory stimuli used, doses and routes of administration. Despite these variables, *in vivo* studies performed for various flavonoids from different subclasses, depicted in this chapter, reveal that flavonoids' anti-inflammatory effects are wide and may include the modulation of several inflammatory mediators, both proinflammatory and anti-inflammatory, from TJ functionality to nuclear regulation.

Figure 2. Summary of the prophylactic and healing effects of flavonoids in in vivo studies of IBD. AcEGCG - peracetylated epigallocatechin gallate; CGP - catechin-7-O-β-glucopyranoside; CNQ – chloronaphthoquinone quercetin; DA-6034 - 7-carboxymethyloxy-3',4',5-trimethoxyflavone; FVN625 - 3'-Hydroxy-4',5,7-trimethoxyflavone; FVN1087 - 6-Hydroxy-5,7-dimethoxyflavone; M10 - myricetin derivative.

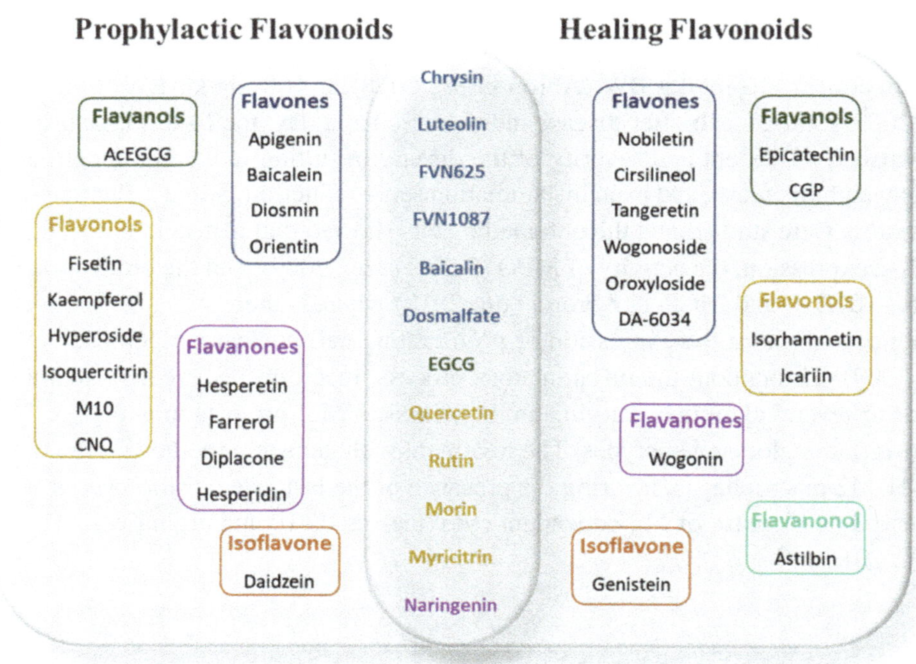

ACKNOWLEDGMENT

This work was supported by UIDB/50006/2020, UIDB/04378/2020, and UID/DTP/04138/2020 with funding from Fundação para a Ciência e Tecnologia / Ministério da Ciência, Tecnologia e Ensino Superior (FCT/MCTES) through national funds and also by the "Programa Operacional Competitividade e Internacionalização" (COMPETE) (POCI-01-0145-FEDER-029248). Daniela Ribeiro and Marisa Freitas acknowledge the financial support from the European Union [FEDER funds through the Operational Competitiveness Program (COMPETE)] (POCI-01-0145-FEDER-029253 and POCI-01-0145-FEDER-029248, respectively). FCT/MCT supported J.M.P. Ferreira de Oliveira (grant number SFRH/BPD/74868/2010) as defined by Decree-Law No. 57/2016, of 29 August, amended by Law No. 57/2017, of 19 July.

REFERENCES

Abron, J. D., Singh, N. P., Price, R. L., Nagarkatti, M., Nagarkatti, P. S., & Singh, U. P. (2018). Genistein induces macrophage polarization and systemic cytokine to ameliorate experimental colitis. *PLoS One*, *13*(7), e0199631. doi:10.1371/journal.pone.0199631 PMID:30024891

Al-Rejaie, S. S., Abuohashish, H. M., Al-Enazi, M. M., Al-Assaf, A. H., Parmar, M. Y., & Ahmed, M. M. (2013). Protective effect of naringenin on acetic acid-induced ulcerative colitis in rats. *World Journal of Gastroenterology*, *19*(34), 5633–5644. doi:10.3748/wjg.v19.i34.5633 PMID:24039355

Azuma, T., Shigeshiro, M., Kodama, M., Tanabe, S., & Suzuki, T. (2013). Supplemental naringenin prevents intestinal barrier defects and inflammation in colitic mice. *The Journal of Nutrition*, *143*(6), 827–834. doi:10.3945/jn.113.174508 PMID:23596159

Camuesco, D., Comalada, M., Rodriguez-Cabezas, M. E., Nieto, A., Lorente, M. D., Concha, A., Zarzuelo, A., & Gálvez, J. (2004). The intestinal anti-inflammatory effect of quercitrin is associated with an inhibition in iNOS expression. *British Journal of Pharmacology*, *143*(7), 908–918. doi:10.1038j.bjp.0705941 PMID:15533892

Castangia, I., Nacher, A., Caddeo, C., Merino, V., Diez-Sales, O., Catalan-Latorre, A., Fernàndez-Busquets, X., Fadda, A. M., & Manconi, M. (2015). Therapeutic efficacy of quercetin enzyme-responsive nanovesicles for the treatment of experimental colitis in rats. *Acta Biomaterialia*, *13*, 216–227. doi:10.1016/j.actbio.2014.11.017 PMID:25463498

Chiou, Y. S., Ma, N. J., Sang, S., Ho, C. T., Wang, Y. J., & Pan, M. H. (2012). Peracetylated (-)-epigallocatechin-3-gallate (AcEGCG) potently suppresses dextran sulfate sodium-induced colitis and colon tumorigenesis in mice. *Journal of Agricultural and Food Chemistry*, *60*(13), 3441–3451. doi:10.1021/jf300441p PMID:22409325

Cibicek, N., Roubalova, L., Vrba, J., Zatloukalova, M., Ehrmann, J., Zapletalova, J., Večeřa, R., Křen, V., & Ulrichová, J. (2016). Protective effect of isoquercitrin against acute dextran sulfate sodium-induced rat colitis depends on the severity of tissue damage. *Pharmacological Reports*, *68*(6), 1197–1204. doi:10.1016/j.pharep.2016.07.007 PMID:27657482

Comalada, M., Camuesco, D., Sierra, S., Ballester, I., Xaus, J., Galvez, J., & Zarzuelo, A. (2005). In vivo quercitrin anti-inflammatory effect involves release of quercetin, which inhibits inflammation through down-regulation of the NF-kappaB pathway. *European Journal of Nutrition*, *35*(2), 584–592. PMID:15668926

Crespo, M. E., Galvez, J., Cruz, T., Ocete, M. A., & Zarzuelo, A. (1999). Anti-inflammatory activity of diosmin and hesperidin in rat colitis induced by TNBS. *Planta Medica*, *65*(7), 651–653. doi:10.1055-2006-960838 PMID:10575379

Cruz, T., Galvez, J., Ocete, M. A., Crespo, M. E., de Medina, F. S., & Zarzuelo, A. (1998). Oral administration of rutoside can ameliorate inflammatory bowel disease in rats. *Life Sciences*, *62*(7), 687–695. doi:10.1016/S0024-3205(97)01164-8 PMID:9472728

Cui, L., Feng, L., Zhang, Z. H., & Jia, X. B. (2014). The anti-inflammation effect of baicalin on experimental colitis through inhibiting TLR4/NF-kappaB pathway activation. *International Immunopharmacology*, *23*(1), 294–303. doi:10.1016/j.intimp.2014.09.005 PMID:25239813

Dai, S. X., Zou, Y., Feng, Y. L., Liu, H. B., & Zheng, X. B. (2012). Baicalin down-regulates the expression of macrophage migration inhibitory factor (MIF) effectively for rats with ulcerative colitis. *Phytotherapy Research*, *26*(4), 498–504. doi:10.1002/ptr.3581 PMID:21887805

Ding, Y., Liang, Y., Deng, B., Qiao, A., Wu, K., Xiao, W., & Gong, W. (2014). Induction of TGF-beta and IL-10 production in dendritic cells using astilbin to inhibit dextran sulfate sodium-induced colitis. *Biochemical and Biophysical Research Communications*, *446*(2), 529–534. doi:10.1016/j.bbrc.2014.02.136 PMID:24613838

Dodda, D., Chhajed, R., & Mishra, J. (2014). Protective effect of quercetin against acetic acid induced inflammatory bowel disease (IBD) like symptoms in rats: Possible morphological and biochemical alterations. *Pharmacological Reports*, *66*(1), 169–173. doi:10.1016/j.pharep.2013.08.013 PMID:24905324

Dou, W., Mukherjee, S., Li, H., Venkatesh, M., Wang, H., Kortagere, S., Peleg, A., Chilimuri, S. S., Wang, Z.-T., Feng, Y., Fearon, E. R., & Mani, S. (2012). Alleviation of gut inflammation by Cdx2/Pxr pathway in a mouse model of chemical colitis. *PLoS One*, *7*(7), e36075. doi:10.1371/journal.pone.0036075 PMID:22815676

Dou, W., Zhang, J., Li, H., Kortagere, S., Sun, K., Ding, L., Ren, G., Wang, Z., & Mani, S. (2014). Plant flavonol isorhamnetin attenuates chemically induced inflammatory bowel disease via a PXR-dependent pathway. *The Journal of Nutritional Biochemistry*, *25*(9), 923–933. doi:10.1016/j.jnutbio.2014.04.006 PMID:24913217

Dou, W., Zhang, J., Sun, A., Zhang, E., Ding, L., Mukherjee, S., Wei, X., Chou, G., Wang, Z.-T., & Mani, S. (2013). Protective effect of naringenin against experimental colitis via suppression of Toll-like receptor 4/NF-kappaB signalling. *British Journal of Nutrition*, *110*(4), 599–608. doi:10.1017/S0007114512005594 PMID:23506745

Dou, W., Zhang, J. J., Zhang, E. Y., Sun, A. N., Ding, L. L., Chou, G. X., Wang, Z., & Mani, S. (2013). Chrysin Ameliorates chemically induced colitis in the mouse through modulation of a PXR/NF-kappa B signaling pathway. *The Journal of Pharmacology and Experimental Therapeutics*, *345*(3), 473–482. doi:10.1124/jpet.112.201863 PMID:23536316

Eun, S. H., Woo, J. T., & Kim, D. H. (2017). Tangeretin Inhibits IL-12 Expression and NF-kappaB Activation in Dendritic Cells and Attenuates Colitis in Mice. *Planta Medica*, *83*(6), 527–533. PMID:27806407

Feng, J., Guo, C., Zhu, Y., Pang, L., Yang, Z., Zou, Y., & Zheng, X. (2014). Baicalin down regulates the expression of TLR4 and NFkB-p65 in colon tissue in mice with colitis induced by dextran sulfate sodium. *International Journal of Clinical and Experimental Medicine*, *7*(11), 4063–4072. PMID:25550915

Flamant, M., & Roblin, X. (2018). Inflammatory bowel disease: Towards a personalized medicine. *Therapeutic Advances in Gastroenterology*, *11*, 1–15. doi:10.1177/1756283X17745029 PMID:29383027

Galvez, J., Coelho, G., Crespo, M. E., Cruz, T., Rodriguez-Cabezas, M. E., Concha, A., Gonzalez, M., & Zarzuelo, A. (2001). Intestinal anti-inflammatory activity of morin on chronic experimental colitis in the rat. *Alimentary Pharmacology & Therapeutics*, *15*(12), 2027–2039. doi:10.1046/j.1365-2036.2001.01133.x PMID:11736735

Geagea, A. G., Rizzo, M., Eid, A., Hussein, I. H., Zgheib, Z., Zeenny, M. N., & ... . (2017). Tea catechins induce crosstalk between signaling pathways and stabilize mast cells in ulcerative colitis. *Journal of Biological Regulators and Homeostatic Agents*, *31*(4), 865–877. PMID:29254289

Guan, F., Liu, A. B., Li, G., Yang, Z., Sun, Y., Yang, C. S., & Ju, J. (2012). Deleterious effects of high concentrations of (-)-epigallocatechin-3-gallate and atorvastatin in mice with colon inflammation. *Nutrition and Cancer*, *64*(6), 847–855. doi:10.1080/01635581.2012.695424 PMID:22716294

Guazelli, C. F., Fattori, V., Colombo, B. B., Georgetti, S. R., Vicentini, F. T., Casagrande, R., Baracat, M. M., & Verri, W. A. Jr. (2013). Quercetin-loaded microcapsules ameliorate experimental colitis in mice by anti-inflammatory and antioxidant mechanisms. *Journal of Natural Products*, *76*(2), 200–208. doi:10.1021/np300670w PMID:23347547

Guo, A., He, D. M., Xu, H. B., Geng, C. A., & Zhao, J. (2015). Promotion of regulatory T cell induction by immunomodulatory herbal medicine licorice and its two constituents. *Scientific Reports*, *5*(1), 14046. doi:10.1038rep14046 PMID:26370586

Hagenlocher, Y., Gommeringer, S., Held, A., Feilhauer, K., Köninger, J., Bischoff, S. C., & Lorentz, A. (2018). Nobiletin acts anti-inflammatory on murine IL-$10^{-/-}$ colitis and human intestinal fibroblasts. *European Journal of Nutrition*, 1391–1401. PMID:29525889

Karrasch, T., Kim, J. S., Jang, B. I., & Jobin, C. (2007). The flavonoid luteolin worsens chemical-induced colitis in NF-kappaB(EGFP) transgenic mice through blockade of NF-kappaB-dependent protective molecules. *PLoS One*, *2*(7), e596. doi:10.1371/journal.pone.0000596 PMID:17611628

Kim, H., Kong, H., Choi, B., Yang, Y., Kim, Y., Lim, M. J., Neckers, L., & Jung, Y. (2005). Metabolic and pharmacological properties of rutin, a dietary quercetin glycoside, for treatment of inflammatory bowel disease. *Pharmaceutical Research*, *22*(9), 1499–1509. doi:10.100711095-005-6250-z PMID:16132362

Kim, Y. S., Son, M., Ko, J. I., Cho, H., Yoo, M., Kim, W. B., Song, I. S., & Kim, C. Y. (1999). Effect of DA-6034, a derivative of flavonoid, on experimental animal models of inflammatory bowel disease. *Archives of Pharmacal Research*, *22*(4), 354–360. doi:10.1007/BF02979057 PMID:10489873

Kook, S.-H., Choi, K. C., Cho, S.-W., Cho, H.-K., Lee, K. D., & Lee, J.-C. (2015). Catechin-7-*O*-β-D-glucopyranoside isolated from the seed of Phaseolus calcaratus Roxburgh ameliorates experimental colitis in rats. *International Immunopharmacology*, *29*(2), 521–527. doi:10.1016/j.intimp.2015.10.003 PMID:26453508

Kwon, K. H., Murakami, A., Tanaka, T., & Ohigashi, H. (2005). Dietary rutin, but not its aglycone quercetin, ameliorates dextran sulfate sodium-induced experimental colitis in mice: Attenuation of pro-inflammatory gene expression. *Biochemical Pharmacology*, *69*(3), 395–406. doi:10.1016/j.bcp.2004.10.015 PMID:15652231

Li, Y., Shen, L., & Luo, H. (2016). Luteolin ameliorates dextran sulfate sodium-induced colitis in mice possibly through activation of the Nrf2 signaling pathway. *International Immunopharmacology*, *40*, 24–31. doi:10.1016/j.intimp.2016.08.020 PMID:27569028

Lim, B. O. (2004). Efficacy of wogonin in the production of immunoglobulins and cytokines by mesenteric lymph node lymphocytes in mouse colitis induced with dextran sulfate sodium. *Bioscience, Biotechnology, and Biochemistry*, *68*(12), 2505–2511. doi:10.1271/bbb.68.2505 PMID:15618621

Luo, X., Yu, Z., Deng, C., Zhang, J., Ren, G., Sun, A., Mani, S., Wang, Z., & Dou, W. (2017). Baicalein ameliorates TNBS-induced colitis by suppressing TLR4/MyD88 signaling cascade and NLRP3 inflammasome activation in mice. *Scientific Reports*, *7*(1), 16374. doi:10.103841598-017-12562-6 PMID:29180692

Manach, C., & Donovan, J. L. (2004). Pharmacokinetics and metabolism of dietary flavonoids in humans. *Free Radical Research*, *38*(8), 771–785. doi:10.1080/10715760410001727858 PMID:15493450

Mascaraque, C., Gonzalez, R., Suarez, M. D., Zarzuelo, A., Sanchez de Medina, F., & Martinez-Augustin, O. (2015). Intestinal anti-inflammatory activity of apigenin K in two rat colitis models induced by trinitrobenzenesulfonic acid and dextran sulphate sodium. *British Journal of Nutrition*, *113*(4), 618–626. doi:10.1017/S0007114514004292 PMID:25654996

Milackova, I., Prnova, M. S., Majekova, M., Sotnikova, R., Stasko, M., Kovacikova, L., Banerjee, S., Veverka, M., & Stefek, M. (2015). 2-Chloro-1,4-naphthoquinone derivative of quercetin as an inhibitor of aldose reductase and anti-inflammatory agent. *Journal of Enzyme Inhibition and Medicinal Chemistry*, *30*(1), 107–113. doi:10.3109/14756366.2014.892935 PMID:24666303

Mochizuki, M., & Hasegawa, N. (2005). Protective effect of (-)-epigallocatechin gallate on acute experimental colitis. *Journal of Health Science*, *51*(3), 362–364. doi:10.1248/jhs.51.362

Mochizuki, M., & Hasegawa, N. (2010). (-)-Epigallocatechin-3-gallate reduces experimental colon injury in rats by regulating macrophage and mast cell. *Phytotherapy Research*, *24*(S1), S120–S122. doi:10.1002/ptr.2862 PMID:19548282

Mullie, P., Clarys, P., Deriemaeker, P., & Hebbelinck, M. (2007). Estimation of daily human intake of food flavonoids. *Plant Foods for Human Nutrition (Dordrecht, Netherlands)*, *62*(3), 93–98. doi:10.100711130-007-0047-7 PMID:17597415

Nieman, D. C., Kay, C. D., Rathore, A. S., Grace, M. H., Strauch, R. C., Stephan, E. H., Sakaguchi, C., & Lila, M. (2018). Increased plasma levels of gut-derived phenolics linked to walking and running following two weeks of flavonoid supplementation. *Nutrients*, *10*(11), 1718. doi:10.3390/nu10111718 PMID:30423955

Nishitani, Y., Yamamoto, K., Yoshida, M., Azuma, T., Kanazawa, K., Hashimoto, T., & Mizuno, M. (2013). Intestinal anti-inflammatory activity of luteolin: Role of the aglycone in NF-kappa B inactivation in macrophages co-cultured with intestinal epithelial cells. *BioFactors (Oxford, England)*, *39*(5), 522–533. doi:10.1002/biof.1091 PMID:23460110

Ocete, M. A., Galvez, J., Crespo, M. E., Cruz, T., Gonzalez, M., Torres, M. I., & Zarzuelo, A. (1998). Effects of morin on an experimental model of acute colitis in rats. *Pharmacology*, *57*(5), 261–270. doi:10.1159/000028250 PMID:9742291

Olivera, P., Danese, S., Jay, N., Natoli, G., & Peyrin-Biroulet, L. (2019). Big data in IBD: A look into the future. *Nature Reviews. Gastroenterology & Hepatology*, *16*(5), 312–321. doi:10.103841575-019-0102-5 PMID:30659247

Park, M. Y., Ji, G. E., & Sung, M. K. (2012). Dietary kaempferol suppresses inflammation of dextran sulfate sodium-induced colitis in mice. *Digestive Diseases and Sciences*, *57*(2), 355–363. doi:10.100710620-011-1883-8 PMID:21901258

Polat, F. R., & Karaboga, I. (2018). Immunohistochemical examination of anti-inflammatory and anti-apoptotic effects of hesperetin on trinitrobenzene sulfonic acid induced colitis in rats. *Biotechnic & Histochemistry*, 1–8. PMID:30383440

Power, K. A., Lu, J. T., Monk, J. M., Lepp, D., Wu, W. Q., Zhang, C., Liu, R., Tsao, R., Robinson, L. E., Wood, G. A., & Wolyn, D. J. (2016). Purified rutin and rutin-rich asparagus attenuates disease severity and tissue damage following dextran sodium sulfate-induced colitis. *Molecular Nutrition & Food Research*, *60*(11), 2396–2412. doi:10.1002/mnfr.201500890 PMID:27349947

Radulovic, K., Normand, S., Rehman, A., Delanoye-Crespin, A., Chatagnon, J., Delacre, M., Waldschmitt, N., Poulin, L. F., Iovanna, J., Ryffel, B., Rosenstiel, P., & Chamaillard, M. (2018). A dietary flavone confers communicable protection against colitis through NLRP6 signaling independently of inflammasome activation. *Mucosal Immunology*, *11*(3), 811–819. doi:10.1038/mi.2017.87 PMID:29139477

Ran, X., Li, Y. H., Chen, G. X., Fu, S. P., He, D. W., Huang, B. X., Wei, L., Lin, Y., Guo, Y., & Hu, G. (2018). Farrerol ameliorates TNBS-induced colonic inflammation by inhibiting ERK1/2, JNK1/2, and NF-kappa B signaling pathway. *International Journal of Molecular Sciences*, *19*(7), 2037. doi:10.3390/ijms19072037 PMID:30011811

Ran, Z. H., Chen, C., & Xiao, S. D. (2008). Epigallocatechin-3-gallate ameliorates rats colitis induced by acetic acid. *Biomedicine and Pharmacotherapy*, *62*(3), 189–196. doi:10.1016/j.biopha.2008.02.002 PMID:18325726

Ribeiro, D., Freitas, M., Lima, J. L. F. C., & Fernandes, E. (2015). Proinflammatory pathways: The modulation by flavonoids. *Medicinal Research Reviews*, *35*(5), 877–936. doi:10.1002/med.21347 PMID:25926332

Ribeiro, D., Proenca, C., Rocha, S., Lima, J. L. F. C., Carvalho, F., Fernandes, E., & Freitas, M. (2018). Immunomodulatory effects of flavonoids in the prophylaxis and treatment of inflammatory bowel diseases: A comprehensive review. *Current Medicinal Chemistry*, *25*(28), 3374–3412. doi:10.2174/0929867325666180214121734 PMID:29446723

Rohr, M., Narasimhulu, C. A., Sharma, D., Doomra, M., Riad, A., Naser, S., & Parthasarathy, S. (2018). Inflammatory diseases of the gut. *Journal of Medicinal Food*, *21*(2), 113–126. doi:10.1089/jmf.2017.0138 PMID:29389238

Romero, M., Vera, B., Galisteo, M., Toral, M., Galvez, J., Perez-Vizcaino, F., & Duarte, J. (2017). Protective vascular effects of quercitrin in acute TNBS-colitis in rats: The role of nitric oxide. *Food & Function*, *8*(8), 2702–2711. doi:10.1039/C7FO00755H PMID:28703832

Sahu, B. D., Kumar, J. M., & Sistla, R. (2016). Fisetin, a dietary flavonoid, ameliorates experimental colitis in mice: Relevance of NF-kappaB signaling. *The Journal of Nutritional Biochemistry*, *28*, 171–182. doi:10.1016/j.jnutbio.2015.10.004 PMID:26878795

Sakai, T., Furoku, S., Nakamoto, M., Shuto, E., Hosaka, T., Nishioka, Y., & Sone, S. (2011). Soy isoflavone equol perpetuates dextran sulfate sodium-induced acute colitis in mice. *Bioscience, Biotechnology, and Biochemistry*, *75*(3), 593–595. doi:10.1271/bbb.100710 PMID:21389602

Sanchez de Medina, F., Vera, B., Galvez, J., & Zarzuelo, A. (2002). Effect of quercitrin on the early stages of hapten induced colonic inflammation in the rat. *Life Sciences*, *70*(26), 3097–3108. doi:10.1016/S0024-3205(02)01568-0 PMID:12008093

Schwanke, R. C., Marcon, R., Meotti, F. C., Bento, A. F., Dutra, R. C., Pizzollatti, M. G., & Calixto, J. B. (2013). Oral administration of the flavonoid myricitrin prevents dextran sulfate sodium-induced experimental colitis in mice through modulation of PI3K/Akt signaling pathway. *Molecular Nutrition & Food Research*, *57*(11), 1938–1949. doi:10.1002/mnfr.201300134 PMID:23861337

Seibel, J., Molzberger, A. F., Hertrampf, T., Laudenbach-Leschowski, U., & Diel, P. (2009). Oral treatment with genistein reduces the expression of molecular and biochemical markers of inflammation in a rat model of chronic TNBS-induced colitis. *European Journal of Nutrition*, *48*(4), 213–220. doi:10.100700394-009-0004-3 PMID:19234664

Seito, L. N., Sforcin, J. M., Bastos, J. K., & Di Stasi, L. C. (2015). Zeyheria montana Mart. (Bignoniaceae) as source of antioxidant and immunomodulatory compounds with beneficial effects on intestinal inflammation. *The Journal of Pharmacy and Pharmacology*, *67*(4), 597–604. doi:10.1111/jphp.12354 PMID:25556766

Shalkami, A. S., Hassan, M., & Bakr, A. G. (2018). Anti-inflammatory, antioxidant and anti-apoptotic activity of diosmin in acetic acid-induced ulcerative colitis. *Human and Experimental Toxicology*, *37*(1), 78–86. doi:10.1177/0960327117694075 PMID:29187079

Shin, E. K., Kwon, H. S., Kim, Y. H., Shin, H. K., & Kim, J. K. (2009). Chrysin, a natural flavone, improves murine inflammatory bowel diseases. *Biochemical and Biophysical Research Communications*, *381*(4), 502–507. doi:10.1016/j.bbrc.2009.02.071 PMID:19233127

Shivashankara, K. S., & Acharya, S. N. (2010). Bioavailability of dietary polyphenols and the cardiovascular diseases. *The Open Nutraceuticals Journal*, *3*(1), 227–241. doi:10.2174/1876396001003010227

Sotnikova, R., Nosalova, V., & Navarova, J. (2013). Efficacy of quercetin derivatives in prevention of ulcerative colitis in rats. *Interdisciplinary Toxicology*, *6*(1), 9–12. doi:10.2478/intox-2013-0002 PMID:24170973

Sun, A. N., Ren, G. Y., Deng, C., Zhang, J. L., Luo, X. P., Wu, X. J., Mani, S., Dou, W., & Wang, Z. (2016). C-glycosyl flavonoid orientin improves chemically induced inflammatory bowel disease in mice. *Journal of Functional Foods*, *21*, 418–430. doi:10.1016/j.jff.2015.12.029

Sun, Y., Wu, X. X., Yin, Y., Gong, F. Y., Shen, Y., Cai, T. T., Zhou, X.-B., Wu, X.-F., & Xu, Q. (2010). Novel immunomodulatory properties of cirsilineol through selective inhibition of IFN-gamma signaling in a murine model of inflammatory bowel disease. *Biochemical Pharmacology*, *79*(2), 229–238. doi:10.1016/j.bcp.2009.08.014 PMID:19698701

Sun, Y., Zhao, Y., Yao, J., Zhao, L., Wu, Z., Wang, Y., Pan, D., Miao, H., Guo, Q., & Lu, N. (2015). Wogonoside protects against dextran sulfate sodium-induced experimental colitis in mice by inhibiting NF-kappaB and NLRP3 inflammasome activation. *Biochemical Pharmacology*, *94*(2), 142–154. doi:10.1016/j.bcp.2015.02.002 PMID:25677765

Tao, F., Qian, C., Guo, W., Luo, Q., Xu, Q., & Sun, Y. (2013). Inhibition of Th1/Th17 responses via suppression of STAT1 and STAT3 activation contributes to the amelioration of murine experimental colitis by a natural flavonoid glucoside icariin. *Biochemical Pharmacology*, *85*(6), 798–807. doi:10.1016/j.bcp.2012.12.002 PMID:23261528

Villegas, I., Alarcon de la Lastra, C., Orjales, A., & La Casa, C. (2003). A new flavonoid derivative, dosmalfate, attenuates the development of dextran sulphate sodium-induced colitis in mice. *International Immunopharmacology*, *3*(13-14), 1731–1741. doi:10.1016/j.intimp.2003.07.002 PMID:14636824

Villegas, I., La Casa, C., Orjales, A., & Alarcon de la Lastra, C. (2003). Effects of dosmalfate, a new cytoprotective agent, on acute and chronic trinitrobenzene sulphonic acid-induced colitis in rats. *European Journal of Pharmacology*, *460*(2-3), 209–218. doi:10.1016/S0014-2999(02)02949-7 PMID:12559383

Vochyanova, Z., Bartosova, L., Bujdakova, V., Fictum, P., Husnik, R., Suchy, P., Šmejkal, K., & Hošek, J. (2015). Diplacone and mimulone ameliorate dextran sulfate sodium-induced colitis in rats. *Fitoterapia*, *101*, 201–207. doi:10.1016/j.fitote.2015.01.012 PMID:25623260

Wang, F., Song, Z. Y., Qu, X. J., Li, F., Zhang, L., Li, W. B., & Cui, S. X. (2018). M10, a novel derivative of myricetin, prevents ulcerative colitis and colorectal tumor through attenuating robust endoplasmic reticulum stress. *Carcinogenesis*, *39*(7), 889–899. doi:10.1093/carcin/bgy057 PMID:29757351

Wang, X., Sun, Y., Zhao, Y., Ding, Y., Zhang, X., Kong, L., Li, Z., Guo, Q., & Zhao, L. (2016). Oroxyloside prevents dextran sulfate sodium-induced experimental colitis in mice by inhibiting NF-kappaB pathway through PPARgamma activation. *Biochemical Pharmacology*, *106*, 70–81. doi:10.1016/j.bcp.2016.02.019 PMID:26947454

Weisshof, R., El Jurdi, K., Zmeter, N., & Rubin, D. T. (2018). Emerging therapies for inflammatory bowel disease. *Advances in Therapy*, *35*(11), 1746–1762. doi:10.100712325-018-0795-9 PMID:30374806

Xiong, Y., Chen, D., Yu, C., Lv, B., Peng, J., Wang, J., & Lin, Y. (2015). Citrus nobiletin ameliorates experimental colitis by reducing inflammation and restoring impaired intestinal barrier function. *Molecular Nutrition & Food Research*, *59*(5), 829–842. doi:10.1002/mnfr.201400614 PMID:25655748

Xu, L., Yang, Z. L., Li, P., & Zhou, Y. Q. (2009). Modulating effect of hesperidin on experimental murine colitis induced by dextran sulfate sodium. *Phytomedicine*, *16*(10), 989–995. doi:10.1016/j.phymed.2009.02.021 PMID:19386481

Yang, L., Shen, L., Li, Y., Li, Y., Yu, S., & Wang, S. (2017). Hyperoside attenuates dextran sulfate sodium-induced colitis in mice possibly via activation of the Nrf2 signalling pathway. *Journal of Inflammation*, *14*(1), 25. doi:10.118612950-017-0172-5 PMID:29162986

Ye, Z., Liu, Z. P., Henderson, A., Lee, K., Hostetter, J., Wannemuehler, M., & Hendrich, S. (2009). Increased CYP4B1 mRNA is associated with the inhibition of dextran sulfate sodium-induced colitis by caffeic acid in mice. *Experimental Biology and Medicine*, *234*(6), 605–616. doi:10.3181/0901-RM-1 PMID:19307459

Zhang, H., Deng, A., Zhang, Z., Yu, Z., Liu, Y., Peng, S., Wu, L. Q., Qin, H. L., & Wang, W. J. (2016). The protective effect of epicatechin on experimental ulcerative colitis in mice is mediated by increasing antioxidation and by the inhibition of NF-κB pathway. *Pharmacological Reports*, *68*(3), 514–520. doi:10.1016/j.pharep.2015.12.011 PMID:26878122

Zhao, J., Hong, T., Dong, M., Meng, Y., & Mu, J. (2013). Protective effect of myricetin in dextran sulphate sodium-induced murine ulcerative colitis. *Molecular Medicine Reports*, *7*(2), 565–570. doi:10.3892/mmr.2012.1225 PMID:23232835

Zhu, W., Jin, Z. S., Yu, J. B., Liang, J., Yang, Q. D., Li, F. J., Shi, X., Zhu, X., & Zhang, X. (2016). Baicalin ameliorates experimental inflammatory bowel disease through polarization of macrophages to an M2 phenotype. *International Immunopharmacology*, *35*, 119–126. doi:10.1016/j.intimp.2016.03.030 PMID:27039210

Zou, Y., Dai, S. X., Chi, H. G., Li, T., He, Z. W., Wang, J., Ye, C.-G., Huang, G.-L., Zhao, B., Li, W.-Y., Wan, Z., Feng, J.-S., & Zheng, X.-B. (2015). Baicalin attenuates TNBS-induced colitis in rats by modulating the Th17/Treg paradigm. *Archives of Pharmacal Research*, *38*(10), 1873–1887. doi:10.100712272-014-0486-2 PMID:25269538

Chapter 4
Diagnostic and Treatment Methods for Ulcerative Colitis and Colitis-Associated Cancer:
Natural Agents Therapy for Ulcerative Colitis – Elucidating the Mechanism of Action

Syed Nasar Rahaman
Central Leather Research Institute, India

Prathiba Sivaprakasam
B. S. Abdur Rahman Crescent Institute of Science and Technology, India

Ashok Kumar Pandurangan
https://orcid.org/0000-0003-2824-1757
B. S. Abdur Rahman Crescent Institute of Science and Technology, India

Suresh Kumar Anandasadagopan
https://orcid.org/0000-0001-5178-005X
Central Leather Research Institute, India

DOI: 10.4018/978-1-7998-3580-6.ch004

ABSTRACT

Ulcerative colitis (UC) is a serious health problem around the world. Inflammatory bowel disease (IBD) is comprised of both Crohn's disease (CD) and UC. IBD is a clinical condition referred as inflammation in the colon. So far there is no proper medication available to treat IBD. On the other hand, untreated UC can be developed as colitis associated cancer. Natural agents are diverse molecules possess many beneficial effects. Many researchers have proven that natural agents can be better option to treat UC. Natural agents such as chrysin, chelidonic acid, euphol, fish oil, diallyl trisulfide, embelin, isatin, and rutin were already reported to have anti-colitic activity. In this chapter, the authors documented the natural agents that were used as treatment for UC.

1. INTRODUCTION

1.1 Inflammatory Bowel Diseases (IBD) an Overview

Inflammatory bowel diseases (IBD) comprising of ulcerative colitis (UC) and Crohn's disease (CD) are severe chronic diseases affecting millions of people all over the globe with an increasing rate of incidence and have become more prevalent in the modern society (Molodecky *et al.,* 2012). Earlier in the ancient times there are reports by physicians that people suffered from chronic diarrhea dating back to Greek antiquity. During 4th Century BCE, Greek physician Hippocrates reported about patients suffered from diarrhea with symptoms of bloody, mucus-streaked stools (Tulchinsky, Hawley, & Nicholls, 2003). The Canon of Internal Medicine of ancient Chinese medicine described indications (abdominal pain, diarrhea, rectal bleeding) of a disease having resemblance like ulcerative colitis in Chinese population. In the first century CE, popular Roman physicians Aretaeus and Soranus reported about chronic diarrhea with bloody stools and an ulcerated bowel with a "distinct foul odour", with high incidence in female population than male (Kornbluth & Sachar, 2010). Similarly, Prince Charles (1745) of England suffered from ulcerative colitis and adopted a diet free of milk to avoid the complications of UC (G. *et al.,* 2014). Though reports of disease similar to UC were reported from a long time in literature, it was not termed as a distinct disease earlier to 1875.

In medical literature, the term ulcerative colitis was first reported in 1875 by two English physicians, Sir Samuel Wilks and Walter Moxon. Surprisingly for the first instance, they achieved to distinguish UC from other diarrheal diseases caused by pathogenic microbes from their case study conducted on a young woman who lost her life due to severe bloody diarrhea and her autopsy reports revealed ulceration and inflammation of the intestinal mucosa (Kirsner, 2001). Several reports of UC started to come from all over the regions of the world following the decades after 1909 and the UC was the major disease discussed at the Paris Congress of Medicine (1913).

1.2. Epidemiology of Inflammatory Bowel Disease

The prevalence of IBD has been in an alarming increase in developed nations since the mid of the 20th century, predominantly in the populations that adopted rapid changes in diet, hygiene and economy (Bager *et al.*, 2012). Interestingly, when a new group of population is identified with inflammatory bowel disease, ulcerative colitis always precedes Crohn's disease and has a higher rate of incidence. The prevalence of IBD is found to be least in the populations of continental Asia when compared to populations from western developed nations that have the highest incidence and prevalence of IBD. It is evident that the high prevalence of IBD in westernized environment is highly linked to the lifestyle attributes, which is associated with smoking, dietary content high in sugar and fat, frequent intake of medications having more side effects, mental stress, and high socioeconomic status (Danese & Fiocchi, 2006). Based on an article published in 2018 by Jobson Medical Information LLC, in United States the prevalence of CD was around 3.1 to 14.6 cases per 100,000 people annually and the incidence of UC was approximately 201 cases per 100,000 adults.

1.3 Prevalence of IBD in India

Since ancient times, IBD is thought to be a rare disease among Indian population. But due to varying lifestyle changes, now IBD is becoming very common in India. Among IBD, UC is seen more often in the subcontinent than CD. But in the recent years, Crohn's disease is being reported from all regions of India. The incidence of UC for the first time was reported from India in the year 1930, but a large number of case reports started to come following the decades after 1960's. A 1986 study conducted by Khosla *et al.*, from northern regions of India, reported that the community prevalence of UC was found to be around 42 per 100,000 people and a crude incidence rate of 6 per 100,000 persons. However, the first incidence of CD in India was recognized from the medical literature of 1972, which examined the surgical and pathological reports of the operated patients, i.e., approximately about three decades after the first documented UC reports. Further, a static prevalence has been observed from two previous population prevalence studies conducted 15 years apart, and there is a subjective viewpoint among gastroenterologists that the rate of incidence of CD has increased in the recent times in India (Desai & Gupte, 2005). Comparative analysis revealed that there is a prevalence of CD in about 50% of patients belonging to the southern parts of India when compared to only

26% from all the other regions. Moreover, this study unveiled that the likelihood of Crohn's disease is more persistent in southern regions of India compared to northern regions of India.

2. SYMPTOMS AND DIAGNOSIS OF ULCERATIVE COLITIS

2.1. Symptoms of Ulcerative Colitis

The common feature of UC is that it can affect people of any age groups, and various investigations conclude that the chances of acquiring UC is at peak from ages 15 to 30 and then again at ages 50 to70, further women and men are equally affected. The primary symptoms of active disease are abdominal discomfort with bloody diarrhea. In course of time anemia, fever and weight loss may also occur and symptoms may come slowly and shift from moderate to severe. Symptoms usually occur intermittently and tend to come and go with periods of remission and relapse. The period of remission can span for months or even years, in which patients may experience no sign of discomfort at all, although there may be relapse of these symptoms at any point of time. This unpredictable course of time may cause difficulty for clinicians to determine whether a specific treatment with certain medication has been effective or not. Other complications of UC may include megacolon, irritation of the eyes due to inflammation, kidney stones, liver disease, and osteoporosis which causes severe pain in the joints.

2.2 Diagnosis of Ulcerative Colitis

The evolution of modern techniques has become an important tool in the diagnosis of ulcerative colitis. Various techniques like endoscopic, radiological, histological and biochemical investigations were used in combination for the diagnosis of UC. At present scenario, the assessment of disease activity of UC and its degree of progression is determined by endoscopy along with histological techniques, which serves as a gold standard technique for the diagnosis of UC and has become a powerful method for probing and monitoring UC-associated colonic cancer. Endoscopic re-examination provides clinical significance about disease relapse, for refractory ulcerative colitis or steroid-dependent UC or when necessity arises for colectomy. Colonoscopy along with biopsy is commonly adopted technique to diagnose UC.

Other laboratory tests that are helpful to diagnose the disease condition include:

- Barium enema

- Performing complete blood count, Renal function tests, Liver function tests and quantifying electrolytes.
- Determination of Effective Sedimentation Rate (ESR)
- Measuring the level of C-Reactive protein
- X – ray examination
- Analysis of Stools
- Computed tomographic scan (CT)

2.3 Serological Markers in IBD

Studies reveal that quantitative measurement of serological markers like perinuclear Anti-Neutrophil Cytoplasmic Antibody (p-ANCA) and the anti-*Saccharomyces cerevisiae* antibody (ASCA) may act as effective diagnostic tools to investigate the genesis of inflammatory bowel diseases (IBD). Further, significant level of P-ANCA was detected in 50 to 80% of patients affected with UC and in 10 to 30% of patients affected with CD. Similarly, diagnostic levels of ASCA have been detected in 5 – 15% of UC patients and 40–70% in CD patients. Recently, a population-based study among IBD patients shows a positive p-ANCA and negative ASCA diagnostic results, which is helpful in prediction of about 75% of UC patients. Moreover, the predictive values obtained by measuring these serological markers to characterize the sub-class of IBD patients have been examined, and there is a different opinion concerning its association with a long lasting disease outcome.

3. ETIOLOGY AND PATHO-PHYSIOLOGY OF INFLAMMATORY BOWEL DISEASE

Ulcerative colitis is a severe chronic disorder that leads to inflammation and ulceration of the colon and rectum. The precise reason behind the cause of ulcerative colitis to date is still uncertain. Scientific evidences prove that the pathogenesis of IBD is a complicated one, as it involves various immunological, environmental, host genetic, and intestinal microbial factors (Figure 3A). In fact, in recent decades, extensive research has contributed to provide a better information about the disease condition and pathophysiology and provides a clear insight of the complex interactions among these factors which bring about in promoting the inflammation of the mucosa and thereby intensifying immune activation of the colonic mucosa can lead to the onset or development of IBD (Knights, Lassen, & Xavier, 2013).

The onset of ulcerative colitis usually initiates in the rectum, and spreads to the colon over time, in which the lining of the colon becomes inflamed and produces minute open sores, or ulcerations, that produce mucus and pus. This ulceration and inflammation can cause severe abdominal pain and recurrent emptying of the bowel in individuals suffering with UC. Moreover, inflammation in ulcerative colitis is normally restricted to the mucosal surface and can lead to the distraction of intestinal homeostasis and integrity.

3.1 Environmental Factors

Though genetic basis is one of the reasons behind the cause of IBD, it is unlikely to state that genetic drift in this short duration of time is the reason behind the cause of these two diseases, challenging the potential role of environmental factors with increased risk in stimulating the disease in genetically susceptible individuals. Further, these risk factors may affect individuals in numerous ways, but their action on the gut microbiota can result in the instability of host-microbe interactions, which may trigger the onset and pathogenesis of IBD. One of the main reasons contributing to the damage of the large intestine is hydrogen sulfide, a noxious gas considered as a cell poison, which is produced by bacteria present in the large intestine upon intake of dietary animal's meat and milk.

3.2 Peripartum Antibiotics

Worldwide the prescription of antibiotics has become common with unclear indications during pediatric ambulatory visits, almost 50% of the medications prescribed by physicians are broad spectrum antibiotics (Hersh, Shapiro, Pavia, & Shah, 2011). Often pregnant women and neonates are more frequently exposed to broad-spectrum antibiotics like cephalosporins in developed countries(Petersen, Gilbert, Evans, Ridolfi, & Nazareth, 2010). Further, several studies have shown a relationship between promiscuous use of antibiotics and inflammatory bowel diseases. Moreover during the initial stages of childhood, crucial events like development of the gastrointestinal microbiome and building of the immune system are likely to happen, which can be disturbed by the intake of antibiotics. A recent study aimed to determine the relationship between the temporal influence of the frequently administered antibiotic cefoperazone and IBD was performed in IL-10-deficient mice colitis model. The results hypothesize that severe gut dysbiosis was seen in offspring of cefoperazone exposed dams during the peripartum period and distortion of the host's self defense mechanism and increased susceptibility to spontaneous and DSS induced colitis. The transfer of gut dysbiosis from the mother treated with cefoperazone to the offspring is associated with the interruption in the building and progression of immune system and protective mechanisms that normally happens during the weaning time till maturity. Thus, exposure to antibiotics in the early stages of life, which is known to stimulate maternal dysbiosis during critical windows of development and assemblage of gut microbiome and immune programming induce a long-lasting effect and impose a greater risk of IBD in genetically susceptible offspring (Miyoshi *et al.*, 2017).

4. ROLE OF DIET AS A POTENTIAL RISK FACTOR IN CAUSING IBD

While nutrition and diet influence on health, their possible role in inflammatory bowel diseases have been investigated. Over the past decades, different aspects of nutrition and diet have been explored and their possible role in the etiology of IBD and how it can play a significant role in the management of these disorders. Further, in the last decade, the prevalence of IBD has been escalating not only in industrially developed western nations, but also in several countries, which were thought to have lower prevalence of this disease. The changes in dietary habit, similar to the western dietary style, which consist of high fat and proteins and lower amounts of fiber containing fruits and vegetables, are thought to be the major environmental factors contributing to the increasing occurrence of IBD and also plays an important role in the development and pathogenesis of IBD. Hou *et al* in 2011evaluated 19 studies involving about 2,600 IBD affected patients and reported that high dietary consumption of total fat, n-6 polyunsaturated fatty acids (PUFAs), omega-6 fatty acids, and intake of meat were linked with increased risk of UC and CD. However, intake of diet rich in fruits and high fiber were associated with decreased risk of Crohn's disease, while diet rich in high vegetable intake was associated with a decreased risk of ulcerative colitis. Further, studies reveal that there was no correlation between IBD risk and total carbohydrate intake.

5. ROLE OF IMMUNE SYSTEM IN IBD

Interestingly, immunity is a two-edged knife. Though, it affords the necessary weapon to safeguard the host from foreign pathogens, when uncontrolled it can attack the host immune system more aggressively, and leads to serious consequences which may be fatal. The important pathological feature of IBD is due to the infiltration of polymorphonuclear neutrophils and mononuclear cells into the gastrointestinal tissues. Further, monocyte and neutrophil migration inside the tissues is triggered by chemotactic agents of bacterial cell wall and cytokines produced locally (Suzuki *et al.*, 2001).

The epithelial cells lining the gastric mucosa separate the intestinal lumen that harbors the symbiotic commensal microbiota and food-borne pathogenic microbes from the body. There is a strict restriction by the mucosal immune system, that it does not trigger any hypersensitive reaction against the commensal microbes due to their oral tolerance. Further, the intestinal mucosa is safeguarded from the intestinal antigens by the presence of gut - associated lymphoid tissue (GALT), that mediates the protection by synthesizing secretory IgA and immunosuppressive cytokines like interleukin (IL)-10 and transforming growth factor (TGF) β.

It is noteworthy that the dendritic cells (DCs) of the intestine by protruding transepithelial dendrites and their sample intestinal contents capture intestinal foreign substances that come across the gut lumen. Further, macrophages, the main type of tissue-resident mononuclear phagocytic cells derived from monocytes, perform a major role in microbial identification by recognizing the toll-like receptors (TLR's) and their by elimination of the antigen and leads to the polarization of innate as well as adaptive immune mechanisms. Moreover, this intestinal macrophages secrete several types of anti-inflammatory cytokines like TGF-β, IL-10 and many proinflammatory cytokines like IFN-γ, TNF-α, IL-6, IL-23 and reactive oxygen species. Vedolizumab a monoclonal antibody used in the treatment of UC and CD inhibits integrin α4β7 a cell adhesion molecule present in the T-lymphocytes and used as an antagonist thereby preventing the production of proinflammatory cytokines (Figure 5A)

The role of T regulatory (Treg) cells performs a vital role in the progression and pathogenesis of IBD and other hypersensitivity reactions and autoimmune disorders. Interestingly, research have shown that patients affected with IBD harbor significantly decreased number of peripheral Treg cells and increased level of serum IL-2Rα. Further, substantial evidence supports the opinion that a change in the equilibrium among Foxp3+CD4+ T-regulatory cells and T- effector cells present in the intestinal microenvironment may influence the pathogenesis of inflammatory bowel disease (Mayne & Williams, 2013). Moreover, studies suggest that transferring Treg cells have the ability to control inflammatory lesions in IBD induced animal models.

5.1 Role of TNF α in Induction of Ulcerative Colitis

Proinflammatory mediators like TNF-α involves in an extremely crucial role in the progression of IBD. Further, expression of TNFα genes in adipocytes, platelets, activated monocytes, macrophages and T cells leads to the production of soluble TNFα, which binds to two TNFα receptors thereby mediating several biological effects like activating other macrophages, amplifying T cell immune response, stimulating the expression of endothelial adhesion molecules, recruiting neutrophils to the sites of inflammation, development of inflammatory edema; inactivating the coagulation process and stimulation of granuloma formation (Sandborn & Hanauer, 1999). Expression of adhesion molecules, several enzymes and cytokines are increased by a crucial transcription factor nuclear factor kappa beta (NF-κB), interestingly; these

NF-κB-dependent pathways were activated by TNFα which prolongs the inflammation by causing degradation and ulceration of the gastric mucosa by releasing matrix metalloproteinases (MMP). Further, increased production of TNFα and nuclear translocation of NF-κB have been observed in mononuclear cells of lamina propria obtained from both UC and CD patients. Moreover, a transcription factor called lipopolysaccharide-induced TNFα factor by binding to the TNFα gene promotes the transcription of TNFα gene in human macrophages, was found in the macrophages and intestinal tissue of both CD and UC affected patients, interestingly TNFα also upregulates the expression of other proinflammatory mediators like interleukin - 1β and interleukin - 6, thus intensifying the early sequences of the inflammatory cascade (Rossetti *et al.,* 2004).

5.2 ROS and Nitric Oxide Plays a Crucial Role in IBD

The formation of superoxide (O_2^-) radical in the gastrointestinal tract is mainly mediated by xanthine oxidase (XO), and this toxic O_2^- is ultimately converted to Hydrogen peroxide (H_2O_2) by the catalytic action of catalase and glutathione peroxidase. The H_2O_2 thus generated by the neutrophils is then used by myeloperoxidase (MPO) to generate hypochlorite ion (OCl^-). Interestingly, superoxide anion (O_2^-) is a very short living, highly unstable and highly reactive form of ROS, which makes it membrane impermeable and makes it to act locally near its place of origin leading to the oxidation of biomolecules which are in close proximity, while hydrogen peroxide can diffuse easily across the plasma membrane and oxidize the compounds situated inside it., Further, aquaporin 8 facilitates the diffusion of H_2O_2 inside the gastrointestinal tract (Te Velde *et al.*, 2008). More interestingly, the basal metabolic levels of ROS in the intestinal epithelial cells vary with decreased amounts of ROS in the small intestine and increased levels in the colon (Sanders *et al.,* 2004). These variations in the ROS production may influence the amount of oxidation of lipids, proteins and can cause DNA damage which can contribute to increased susceptibility of both these intestinal sites to gastrointestinal diseases (Figure 5.2 A).

Nitric oxide (NO) is a crucial multi-functional signaling molecule that contributes to the onset of inflammatory reactions. Under normal physiological conditions, nitric oxide functions like an anti-inflammatory substance and during abnormal conditions, it functions as a pro-inflammatory mediator that promotes inflammation due to its increased production. In the endothelial cells, NO is produced and released by the action of nitric oxide synthase that converts arginine into citrulline synthesizing NO during the course of reaction. NADPH and Oxygen are crucial cofactors during this conversion. Further, nitric oxide is thought to induce vasodilatation of cardiovascular system and also involves in immune reactions mediated by macrophages activated by cytokines, which release toxic nitric oxide in high concentrations. Moreover, nitric oxide is considered as a potent synaptic neurotransmitter and plays an active role in the regulation of cellular apoptosis and also contributes to the pathogenesis of inflammatory disorders of the gut, joint and lungs. Hence administration of NOS inhibitors account for the management of inflammatory disorders and acts as an important therapeutic advance. Moreover, it is proved that the use of synthetic arginine analogues and selective NO biosynthesis inhibitors can be used for the treatment of nitric oxide induced inflammation. Finally impaired production of nitric oxide causes undesired effects like inflammation vasoconstriction, and tissue damage.

6. NATURAL AGENTS IN TREATING INFLAMMATORY BOWEL DISEASES

6.1. Role of Herbal Compounds in Treatment of Inflammatory Bowel Diseases

In practice, the use of herbal plants or their medically potential bioactive components is in tremendous increase and the use of these natural products has become a most promising approach for the treatment of several inflammatory disorders like rheumatoid arthritis, multiple sclerosis and ulcerative colitis (Vitor *et al.,* 2009).

7. CHRYSIN AMELIORATE INFLAMMATORY BOWEL DISEASE

Many plant species contains natural polyphenolic compounds like flavonoids which plays a crucial role in the growth of plants and constitutes the average human diet. Chrysin chemically known as 5, 7-dihydroxyflavone is a naturally occurring flavonoid predominant in passion flowers, chamomile, honeycombs, and in certain mushrooms (Figure 1). The biological activity of chrysin is attributed to the absence of oxygenation in B and C-rings that makes it a potent anti-inflammatory and antitoxic agent. The existence of carbonyl group on 4th carbon atom and presence of double bond between 2nd and 3rd carbon atoms (30, 40 hydroxylation), makes chrysin to function as an important antioxidant compound.

Accumulation of neutrophils in the inflamed gut mucosa is a prominent characteristic in ulcerative colitis. The granules present in neutrophils contain a variety of proteolytic enzymes which includes myeloperoxidase, which upon stimulation along with other cytotoxic oxygen metabolites can contribute to damage of the intestinal tissue at sites of inflammation. The impact of chrysin in ameliorating IBD is attributed by its role in the downregulation of myeloperoxidase (MPO) activity, which results in the amelioration of colonic architecture from disruption and a considerable reduction in the synthesis of inflammatory mediators like prostaglandin E2 (PGE2), nitric oxide (NO) and other pro-inflammatory cytokines. Further, it is noteworthy that, in all inflammatory processes, nuclear factor NF-κB mediates a prominent role in the induction of inflammatory responses, which also serves as a crucial factor in the activation and progression of inflammatory bowel diseases.

Figure 1. Chrysin

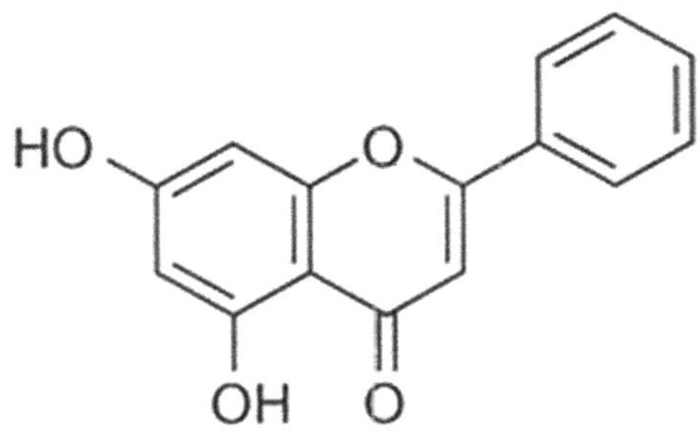

Moreover, studies prove that inhibition of p65 subunit of NF-κB protein complex in mice model induced with ulcerative colitis using antisense oligonucleotides reduced the disease activity, which implies the crucial role of NF-κB complex in promoting the inflammatory responses leading to the onset of UC (Spiik *et al.*, 2002). Interestingly, chrysin actively downregulates NF-κB mediated activation by suppressing the production of a variety of inflammatory cytokines and chemokines. Further, pretreatment of TNF-α-treated enterocytes (IEC-6 cells) with chrysin, significantly decreased the expression of p65 subunit of NF-κB in the nucleus of TNF-α-treated IEC-6 cells. Since, activation of NF-κB is considered to play a critical function in the regulation of transcription of pro-inflammatory genes (Ghosh & Hayden, 2008), and its suppression by the flavonoid chrysin may have an inhibitory effect on the initial steps of inflammation and modulate the upregulation of numerous pro-inflammatory genes as the binding sites of the transcription factors belonging to NF-κB superfamily are situated in the promoter as well as the enhancer regions of several genes, as well as the regions analogous to inflammatory molecules like chemokines, cytokines and various other growth factors associated to inflammatory response.

8. CHELIDONIC ACID A POTENT MOLECULE IN TREATING ULCERATIVE COLITIS

Chelidonic acid (CA), a novel pharmacologically effective phytochemical is an important constituent of *Chelidonium majus L.,* possess diverse beneficial effects on human health, which includes analgesic effects and antimicrobial properties (Figure 2).

Figure 2. Chelidonic acid

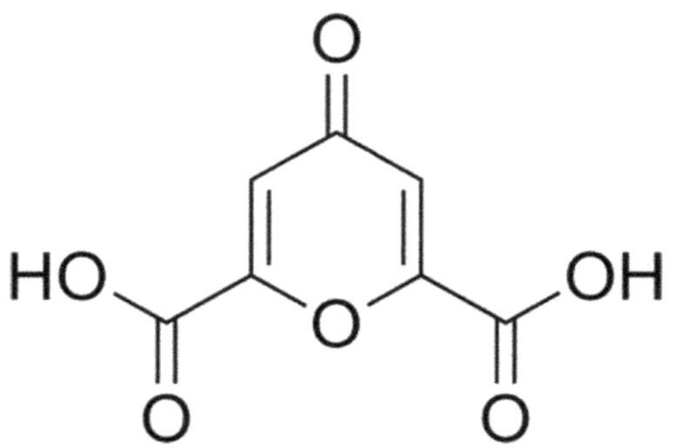

During inflammatory processes cycloxygenase-2 (COX-2) serves as a principal mediator of inflammatory reactions, and potentially involve in inducing the activation of macrophages. The main feature of COX-2 is that it acts an inducible enzyme and carries out important functions in some specific physiological processes, and found in low concentrations in healthy tissues. Several recent studies suggest that the levels of COX-2 are upregulated during inflammatory reactions and leads to the production of prostaglandins (PGs), by the reactions catalysed by COX-2, that contributes to inflammation leading to swelling and pain (Eisenach *et al.,* 2010). In addition, an elevated level of PGE2 and COX has been found in intestines of patients with IBD and are believed to be important mediators in ulcerative colitis.

A study conducted by Kim *et al* in 2012 suggests that chelidonic acid (CA) efficiently restore the severity of ulcerative colitis symptoms induced by DSS in mice model. They found that Chelidonic acid (CA) reduces IL-6 and TNF-α level in the serum of DSS induced mice, and thereby exerts an anti-inflammatory response. Further their studies revealed that CA suppressed both PGE2 production and COX-2 expression, which are potent inflammatory mediators in causing pain and swelling of the colon, and also they observed CA has a little inhibitory effect on the production of hypoxia inducing factor, which results in the hypoxic conditions of the colonic lesions. They also proved that anti-inflammatory effects of chelidonic acid were more effective as those of sulfasalazine (SFZ), a well known anti-inflammatory drug used in the treatment of IBD. They also observed, CA administration in DSS treated mice reduced clinical signs like shortening of the colon, weight loss and remarkable decrease in the DAI scores.

9. EUPHOL ACTS AGAINST INFLAMMATORY BOWEL DISEASE

The tetracyclic triterpene compound euphol is an important phytochemical constituent found in the sap of semi-arid plant *Euphorbia tirucalli,* a plant that belongs to the Euphorbiaceae family, and popularly known as aveloz in the Brazilian folk medicine (Figure 3). In the northeastern parts of Brazil, the milky latex obtained from *E. tirucalli* has been used in traditional folk medicine against syphilis, to treat cough, asthma, earache, cancer, sarcoma, skin tumors and epithelioma, to control intestinal parasites and also acts as a laxative agent. The latex obtained from bark of *E. tirucalli* is known to possess pharmacological activities that include anti-mutagenic, antiherpetic and molluscicidal activity (Betancur-Galvis *et al.,* 2002). It is also known to possess anti-carcinogenic and cocarcinogenic properties (Hecker, 1968).

Figure 3. Euphol

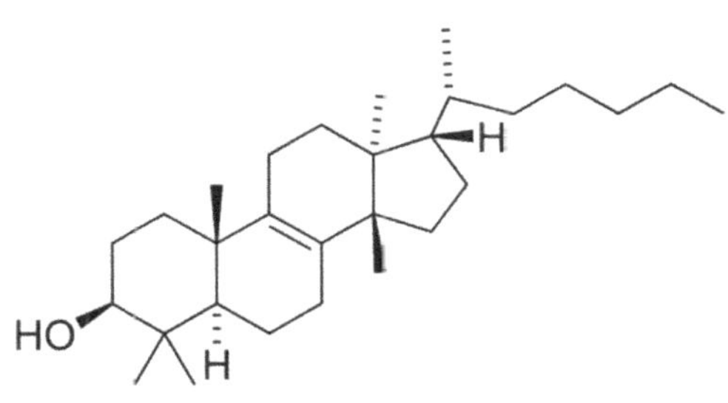

9.1 Preventive Effect of Euphol in Colonic NF-κB Activation and Inhibition of VEGF and NOS2 Expression

The effect of euphol in ameliorating the UC condition was studied in DSS induced murine colitis model that suggests pre-treatment of mouse orally with euphol leads to noticeable phosphorylation of p65 subunit of NF-κB complex in the tissues of the large intestine after seven days of euphol treatment, and it is noted that euphol administration at a dose of 30 mg/kg, orally by gavage considerably reduced the activation of p65 NF-κB mediated signaling pathway in the colonic tissue of mouse, thus strongly signifies that inhibitory action of euphol in NF-κB activation is likely to be the mode through which this molecule regulates intestinal inflammation. Further, it is found that in the intestinal mucosa, the up-regulated expression of nitric oxide synthase -2 (NOS2) intensifies the apoptotic process in the epithelial cells lining the gut mucosa (Yue *et al.,* 2001). Additionally, studies suggest that over expression of NOS2 also leads to prominent phenomenon called angiogenesis, which has been demonstrated recently as one of the key contributors in the progression of IBD (Danese *et al.,* 2006). Moreover, pretreatment of mice with euphol at a dose concentration of 30 mg/kg markedly blocked the excessive production of NOS2 and also the expression of VEGF (Vascular Endothelial Growth Factor) in colonic tissue of DSS induced colitis mice model. Notably, pretreatment of mice by administering euphol at a dose concentration of 10 and 30 mg/kg of body weight markedly reduced the colonic myeloperoxidase (MPO) levels in DSS-induced mice which normally show a surge in MPO levels. Further, it is speculated that the biological mechanisms associated with the anti-inflammatory property of euphol was likely to be related by its potential efficiency to inhibit the endothelial expression of cell adhesion molecules selectin and integrin due to the inhibition of NOS2, Ki67 and VEGF expression in the colonic tissue by regulating the action of nuclear transcription factor-κB (NF-κB).

10. *FICUS CARICA EXTRACT*, A POTENT SOURCE OF TREATING IBD

Fig trees (*Ficus Carica*) are considered to be sacred throughout the world and its dried fruit consumption is widespread, as drying of the fruit increases its shelf life and nutritive value. It has been reported that the dried fruits of *Ficus carica* is a good source of natural bioactive compounds that includes carbohydrates, flavonoid and phenolic compounds, and also contains high amount of fiber rich polysaccharides (as cellulose) and sugars (glucose, fructose, sucrose). The predominant monosaccharide's present in the dried fruit was fructose (56%) and glucose (43%), as determined by HPLC analysis. Further many studies conducted to evaluate the phenolic profile of dried fig fruits by adopting various phytochemical analysis tools, such as the HPLC-PDA system identified several phenolic components that include chlorogenic acid, gallic acid, syringic acid, rutin, (+)-catechin and (-)-epicatechin.

In vivo experiments have shown that *Ficus carica* extract (FCAE) remarkably ameliorated the gastric emptying process dose dependently when compared to the healthy control group (HC). Further, emptying of stomach is a complex process influenced by several factors that includes meal size, particle size, intake of water, composition of nutrients, calorific value of food, pharmaceutical administration, stress and state of health (Sadra *et al.,* 2017). In ulcerative colitis conditions, the results obtained demonstrated that the gastrointestinal motor activity, gastro intestinal transit time, was reduced in UC affected rats. Moreover it was observed that the loss of permeability and fluidity due to administration of dextran sodium sulfate (DSS) and loperamide (LOP) leads to the disruption of the equilibrium of the absorption/secretion process of water, nutrients and electrolytes, which in turn can lead to severe modifications in the physiological functions of the digestive tract like gastrointestinal transit time. These changes in the physiological function can be overcome by the administration of aqueous extracts of dried fruits of figs to the constipated and ulcerative-colitis mice models. Further, it is evaluated that FCAE shows notable laxative and protective activities through different mechanism of actions and ameliorated the architecture of gut mucosa and facilitated the progression of colonic contents (Sabiu & Ashafa, 2016)

11. FISH OIL AMELIORATES DSS-INDUCED INFLAMMATORY BOWEL DISEASE

Fish oil is the fat or oil extracted from oily fishes like salmon, mackerel, herring, tuna as well as anchovies. At certain occasions, fish oil is isolated from the livers of cod fish. Fish oil is considered as a nutritious food, due to its high ω-3 fatty acid content. Further, the oil obtained from fish is considered to be the most consumed dietary supplements globally.

Tumor necrosis factor α (TNF- α) is a proinflammatory cytokine that performs a pivotal role in the modulating the mucosal immune response during the pathogenesis of ulcerative colitis. TNF-α, being an important cytokine secreted in the gut mucosa during inflammation, another cytokine called IL-6 also plays an important role due to its various biological effects in the intestine and also in other tissues and organs (Sandborn & Hanauer, 1999). Yorulmaz *et al.*, in the year 2019 conducted a study in colitis induced rats and observed that the colonic tissue and serum levels of the proinflammatory cytokines IL-6 and TNF-α were reduced in separate and combinatorial use of mesalazine and fish oil compared to the control group in which IL-6 and TNF-α levels were increased. Further, combined administration of mesalazine and fish oil reduced the inflammation of intestinal mucosa of the rats induced with colitis and particularly their combinatorial use leads to remarkable recovery of colonic tissue by dramatically reducing the level of apoptotic bodies, decreasing vascular congestion and preventing the infiltration of inflammatory cells. Further, it is noted that supplementation of diet with fish oil in experimental colitis models has remarkably increased the incorporation of ω-3 fatty acids into the tissues of colonic mucosa and significantly reduced the inflammatory lesions of the colon in ulcerative colitis (Empey *et al.*, 1991). Studies also suggest that the administration of fish oil enemas also provide some degrees of retrogression in clinical indices in patients with moderate IBD (Tatar & Das, 2007). Recent studies also reported that the ameliorating effect of fish oil is mediated by its role in regulating the molecular mechanisms associated with redox reactions of important lipid metabolites (Sharma *et al.,* 2019).

12. DIALLYL TRISULFIDE (DATS) PREVENTS INFLAMMATORY BOWEL DISEASE

Garlic (*Allium sativum*) is a well known herb, used in herbal medicine from ancient times because of its protective effects on cardiovascular disease, microbial infection, immune suppression, and carcinogenesis (Rivlin, 2001). Studies revealed that these protective effects of garlic is due to the presence of several organosulfur compounds (OSCs) which includes diallyl sulphide, diallyl disulphide as well as diallyl trisulphide (Figure 4) DATS is one of the highly volatile compounds found in garlic oil, and reports suggest that it possess anti-carcinogenic, anti-inflammatory and antioxidant properties.

Figure 4. Organosulfur compounds (OSCs) a) Diallyl sulphide, b) Diallyl disulphide, c) Diallyl trisulphide

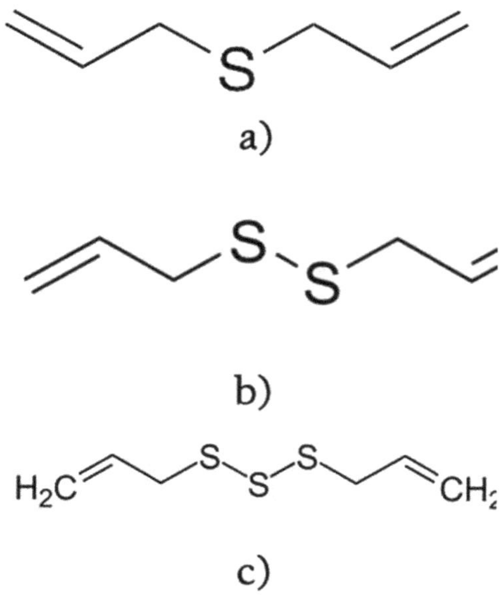

12.1 DATS Alleviated Colonic Expression of iNOS and COX-2 in DSS-Induced Colitis

Inhibitory nitric oxide synthase (iNOS) and cyclooxygenase-2 (COX-2) are often overexpressed in ulcerative colitis condition and known to play a crucial role in causing inflammation of the colon. It is evident from studies that the organosulfur compounds derived from garlic has been reported to have anti-inflammatory activity. Administration of DATS orally at a concentration of 10μmol decreased the colonic levels of both iNOS and COX-2 in DSS-induced colitis in mouse. This reduction iNOS and COX-2 levels is attributed to the obstruction of the NF-κB signaling pathway. One of the crucial events that take place in the NF-κB activation is its detachment from the inhibitory Iκ-Bα subunit, which occurs due to the phosphorylation of the Iκ-Bα subunit. Further, phosphorylation of Iκ-Bα rapidly ubiquitinate the protein at various sites and leads to subsequent degradation by proteasomes, there by releasing the free NF-κB protein, which will in turn translocate into the nucleus, where it can regulate the transcription of target genes. Studies conclude that DATS plays a major role by successfully inhibiting the phosphorylation of Iκ-Bα thereby preventing the formation of active NF-κB. In addition, a novel sulfur compound, thiacremonone (Figure 5) isolated from garlic actively blocked the expression of tumor necrosis factor-alpha (TNF-α) and TPA (Tetradecanoyl phorbol acetate) induced transcription of NF-κB and its DNA binding activity, both which are involved in inducing apoptosis in colonic cancer cells. Further, thiacremonone also reduced the expression of iNOS and COX-2 and other anti-apoptotic proteins like XIAP, cIAP1/2 and Bcl-2, that are considered as target proteins involved in NF-κB mediated downstream regulation (Jung *et al.*, 2007).

Figure 5. Thiacremonone

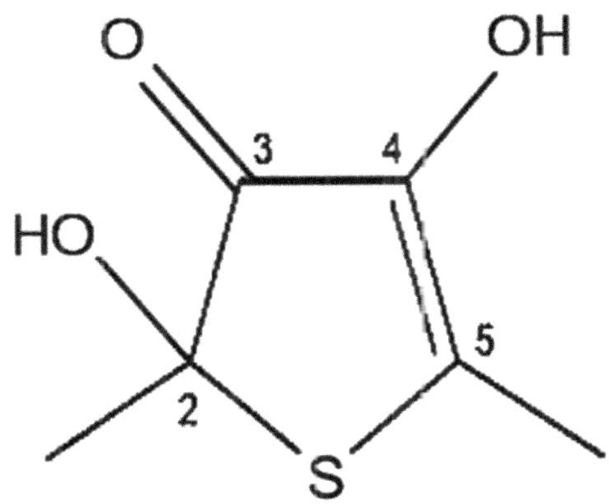

12.2 DATS Induced Inhibition of STAT3 and Transcription of its Target Protein

Studies suggest that as like NF-κB, inflammatory signals also stimulate the production of STAT3 (Signal transducer and activator of transcription 3) an apoptotic factor produced at the latent stage in the cytoplasm after DSS administration in mice model. STAT3, which also plays a vital role in the colonic inflammation, is generally activated through IL-6 - gp130 - JAK signaling pathway leading to the direct phosphorylation of the amino acid tyrosine 705 of the carboxy terminus end. Upon activation, STAT3 translocates into the nucleus, thereby regulating the genes that are involved in cellular apoptosis (Bcl-Xl), cell cycle progression (e.g., Cyclin D1, migration as well as survival, which depends on the cell type it acts on (Spano *et al.,* 2006). Further, Cyclin D1 is believed to be associated with ulcerative colitis-related neoplasia and inflammation (Pickert *et al.,* 2009) along with extracellular receptor kinase (ERK), which is known to play an important role in the activation of STAT3 by phosphorylating STAT3 protein at Tyrosine 705 (Aggarwal *et al.,* 2009). Moreover, administration of DATS at a concentration of 10μmol exerted a remarkable inhibitory effect on the DNA binding capacity of STAT3 induced by DSS and phosphorylation of STAT3 protein at Tyrosine 705 and thereby preventing the expression of cyclin D1, which is known to be the target protein of STAT3 and also prevents the stimulation of cell proliferation by cyclin D1. Molecular mechanisms involved behind the function of DATS and its suppressive effects on STAT3 and NF-κB is still unclear. Studies suggest that DATS contain an alkenyl functional group, which effectively reacts with the sulfhydryl (-SH) groups present in the cysteine molecule of cellular proteins (Chandra-Kuntal & Singh, 2010). Further, it is speculated that, cell cycle arrest upon DATS induction is likely due to the rapid disassembly of microtubules, which results due to the oxidative modification of certain cysteine residues found in the β-tubulin. Further, it is hypothesized that cysteinyl moieties present in STAT3 protein are considered as critical sites for the development of active therapeutic drugs (Buettner *et al.,* 2011) and the inhibitory property of DATS on STAT3 and NF-κB signaling mechanism is attributed to its role in directly modifying the cysteine residues found in both of the transcription factors.

13. EMBELIN TREATMENT AMELIORATE INFLAMMATORY BOWEL DISEASE

Embelin, chemically known as 2,5-dihydroxy-3-undecyl-1,4-benzoquinone is a naturally occurring phytocompound which possess an alkyl substituted hydroxyl benzoquinone compound is a component in the fruit of *Embelia ribes Burm* (Figure

6). Herbal extracts of this plant is extensively used in traditional herbal medicine for the ailment of various diseases. The fruit of this plant bears a bitter taste and is used as a febrifuge and also to treat various inflammatory and gastrointestinal disorders for more than thousands of years. Further, embelin is reported to have analgesic, antioxidant and anti-inflammatory activities and also aides in wound healing. Reports suggest that embelin impairs the inflammatory mechanism by effectively inhibiting NF-κB activity (Kwang, Sethi, & Aggarwal, 2007).

Figure 6. Embelin

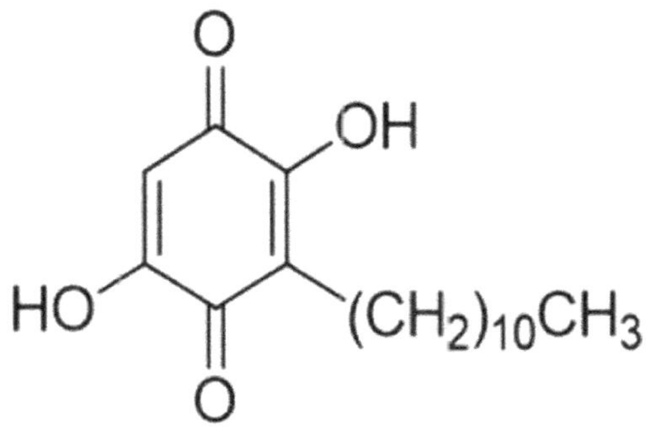

13.1 Embelin Treatment Impairs Lipid Peroxidation

Lipid peroxidase (LPO) is an active enzyme present in the tissues of the colon. Increased generation of these lipid peroxides leads to the production of abundant amounts of free radicals, which significantly deteriorates the cellular antioxidants like vitamin C and E and escalates the rate of progression of inflammation and ulceration. Further, studies expose that treatment with embelin loaded microspheres remarkably ameliorated the colonic oxidative stress in rat models induced with colitis using acetic acid. This remarkable amelioration is attributed to the reduction in the levels of malondialdehyde, an excellent indicator to determine lipid peroxidation. Moreover, administration of acetic acid intra rectally showed considerable elevation in the concentration of lipid peroxidase (166.3 μM of MDA/mg of colonic tissue), while treatment with embelin loaded microspheres prove a considerable reduction in the concentration of lipid peroxidase (101.33 μM of MDA/ mg of colonic tissue). Further, treatment of colitis induced rat models with plain embelin alone at a concentration of 50 mg/ kg of body weight significantly reduced the concentration of LPO to 126.3 μmol of MDA/mg of colonic tissue. Thus embelin coated microspheres can potentially reduce lipid peroxidase levels in colitis when compared to the control group (Nidhi *et al.,* 2017).

13.2 Embelin Lowers Glutathione and LDH Level in Colitis Induced rat Model

Reduced Glutathione (GSH) is an antioxidant mainly involved in the DNA synthesis and repair mechanisms, further it involves in facilitating the recycling of vitamin C and vitamin E and also prevents damage induced by free radicals and further enhances the antioxidant activity of vitamin C. Moreover, it is also involved in facilitating the transport of amino acids and performs a major role in the detoxification process carried out by liver (Chavan *et al.,* 2005). It is found that there is a steep reduction in the levels of GSH in acetic acid induced colitic rat models, while pretreatment with embelin inversed the depletion of reduced glutathione and restored the GSH levels to the normal conditions. In addition to it, during colitic conditions lactate dehydrogenase (LDH), a cytosolic enzyme found in almost all tissues that takes part in biochemical regulation mechanisms of the body fluids and tissues is increased in blood serum which makes a shift towards anaerobiosis in acetic acid induced colitic rats, that results in the surge of lactic acid production (Manna *et al.,* 2004). This condition is overcome by pre-treatment of the rats with embelin which altered the serum LDH level towards the normal in acetic acid induced colitis.

14. ANTI-INFLAMMATORY ACTION OF ISATIN AND INDIRUBIN AMELIORATES IBD.

Isatin, 1H-indole-2, 3-dione also known as tribulin, is a natural organic compound found in the plants of genus *Isatis* and also found in mammalian tissues and body fluids (Figure 7). It serves as a versatile building block and has the ability to construct a large number of heterocyclic compounds. The existence of several reaction centers in isatin and its derivatives make them competent to participate in a large number of reactions. Isatin and its derivatives have extensive applications in the medicinal and pharmacological fields like antifungal, antibacterial and antiviral activities. Isatin also known to possess enzyme inhibitory activity and serves as a potent cytotoxic agent against tumorogenic cells (Vine *et al.,* 2007). These pharmacological properties of isatin and its derivatives is attributed to the existence of bioactive indole moiety containing keto group at position 2 and lactum group in it.

Similarly, Indirubin, an indigo dye (Figure 8) is a phytochemical found in the shrub *Indigofera arrecta*. It is variously known as indigo red, indigo naturalis as well as Java indigo. It is also produced by the bacteria harboring urinary tract and present in the urine of humans and other mammals in trace amounts. *I. arrecta* has been used as a folk medicine in Africa and Asia for centuries. In particular, Congolese healers use it in combination with other herbs to treat epilepsy. Indirubin itself shows biological activity and has been studied as a treatment for diseases ranging from cancers to colitis.

Figure 7. Isatin

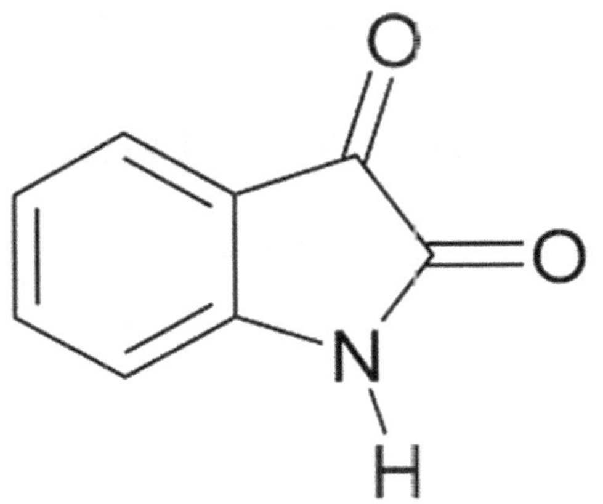

The pro-inflammatory cytokines like TNF-α, IFN-γ and IL-6 plays a critical role in promoting the progression of UC, whereas certain cytokines like IL-10 that possess anti-inflammatory activity can have a protective effect against UC. Similarly, nitric oxide produced from L-arginine by the action of iNOS and production of PGE2 from arachidonic acid by the reactions catalysed by COX-2, both of which acts as potent pro-inflammatory molecules (Hung *et al.*, 2017). Gao *et al.*, in 2018 demonstrated that isatin and indirubin can have a protective effect on the mice induced with ulcerative colitis using dextran sodium sulfate by stabilizing the anti-inflammatory and pro-inflammatory cytokines. Recent studies show that administration of isatin and indirubin alone or in combination reduced the concentrations of IFN-γ, TNF-α, COX-2, IL-6, PGE2, iNOS and nitric oxide (NO), while increased concentration of IL-10 was observed in DSS-induced colitis in rats. Further, it is evaluated that combinational treatment has more potentiality than single-agent therapy in inhibiting the inflammatory responses. Hence, it is suggested that isatin and indirubin as single administration or in combination can be capable to ameliorate ulcerative colitis because of their potent anti-inflammatory properties.

Consistently, studies also proved that isatin, indirubin alone or in combination can inhibit the apoptosis of epithelial cell lining the colon by effectively downregulating the expression of cleaved-caspase-3 and Bax and upregulating the expression of Bcl-2. Further mitogen activated protein kinase (MAPK's) including JNK 362, ERK and p38 plays a major role in orchestrating the generation of pro-inflammatory cytokines that leads to the progression of inflammatory bowel disease (Patterson *et al.*, 2014). Research suggests that isatin and indirubin remarkably blocked DSS-induced activation of the MAPK and NF-κB pathways. More so, the protective action of combinative therapy was higher than that of single-agent therapy and indicates that the blockade of MAPK and NF-κB signaling pathways may play a crucial in the protective effects of isatin and indirubin in ameliorating ulcerative colitis.

15. RUTIN ACTION INHIBITS DEVELOPMENT OF IBD

Flavonoids are a variety of numerous secondary metabolites commonly distributed throughout the plant kingdom; several studies have reported their anti-inflammatory and anti-oxidative properties in-vitro using cell lines and in murine models. These flavonoids are known for their effective role in the inhibition of variety of enzymes involved in certain inflammatory processes, while many cell types involved in the immune responses are down-regulated by the action of some specific flavonoids *in vitro*. Moreover, majority of flavonoids possess anti-oxidative and free radical scavenging properties. Rutin, chemically known as 3-O-rhamnosylglucosyl-quercetin is a naturally occurring flavonoid having a wide range of biological functions is widely present in variety of food substances like parsley, apricots, buckwheat and tomatoes (Figure 9).

Figure 8. Indirubin

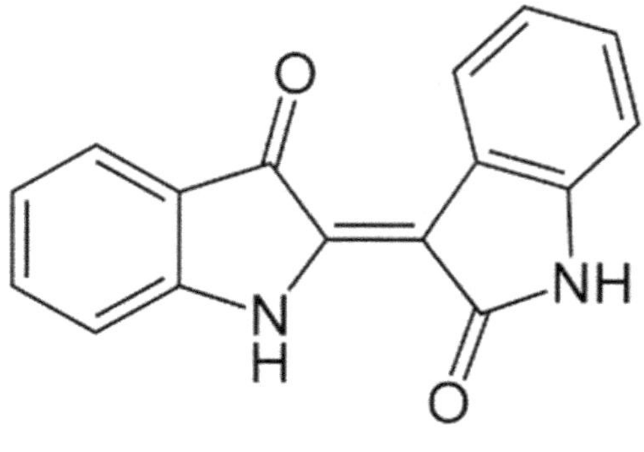

A study conducted by Kwon *et al* proved that dietary rutin, at very low dose concentration has been found to inhibit the biosynthesis of some crucial proinflammatory genes like IL-1b, IL-6 and GM-CSF and iNOS, thereby ameliorating the effect of dextran sodium sulfate induced colitis in mice. Further, rutin also remarkably ameliorated ulcerative colitis by following a specific therapeutic protocol. Considerably, as rutin is a commonly found phytochemical in various vegetables and fruits, the likelihood of using rutin-supplemented diet for therapeutic approach in colon carcinogenesis and IBD may be reasonable and promising (Kwon, Murakami, Tanaka, & Ohigashi, 2005).

16. CONCLUSION

In summary, various natural compounds described above possess a significant effect in ameliorating inflammatory bowel disease in animal models. This data suggest that there is a future for new herbal based therapies in the treatment of inflammatory bowel disease.

REFERENCES

Aggarwal, B. B., Kunnumakkara, A. B., Harikumar, K. B., Gupta, S. R., Tharakan, S. T., Koca, C., & Sung, B. (2009). Signal transducer and activator of transcription-3, inflammation, and cancer: How intimate is the relationship? *Annals of the New York Academy of Sciences*, *1171*(1), 59–76. Advance online publication. doi:10.1111/j.1749-6632.2009.04911.x PMID:19723038

Bager, P., Simonsen, J., Nielsen, N. M., & Frisch, M. (2012). Cesarean section and offspring's risk of inflammatory bowel disease: A national cohort study. *Inflammatory Bowel Diseases*, *18*(5), 857–862. Advance online publication. doi:10.1002/ibd.21805 PMID:21739532

Betancur-Galvis, L. A., Morales, G. E., Forero, J. E., & Roldan, J. (2002). Cytotocxic and antiviral activties of Colombian medicinal plant exatracts of the Euphorbia genus. *Memorias do Instituto Oswaldo Cruz*. Advance online publication. doi:10.1590/S0074-02762002000400017

Figure 9. Rutin

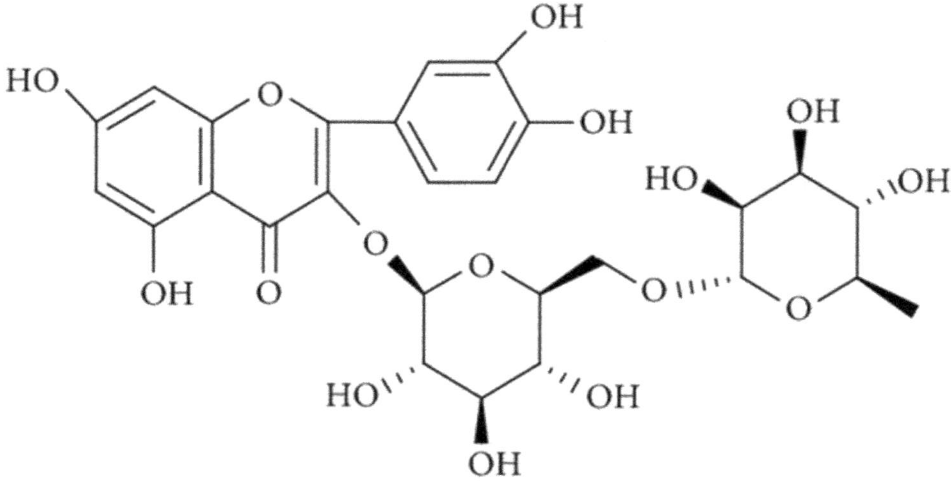

Buettner, R., Corzano, R., Rashid, R., Lin, J., Senthil, M., Hedvat, M., Schroeder, A., Mao, A., Herrmann, A., Yim, J., Li, H., Yuan, Y.-C., Yakushijin, K., Yakushijin, F., Vaidehi, N., Moore, R., Gugiu, G., Lee, T. D., Yip, R., ... Williams, J. C. (2011). Alkylation of cysteine 468 in stat3 defines a novel site for therapeutic development. *ACS Chemical Biology*, *6*(5), 432–443. Advance online publication. doi:10.1021/cb100253e PMID:21226522

Chandra-Kuntal, K., & Singh, S. V. (2010). Diallyl trisulfide inhibits activation of signal transducer and activator of transcription 3 in prostate cancer cells in culture and In vivo. *Cancer Prevention Research (Philadelphia, Pa.)*, *3*(11), 1473–1483. Advance online publication. doi:10.1158/1940-6207.CAPR-10-0123 PMID:20959517

Chavan, S., Sava, L., Saxena, V., Pillai, S., Sontakke, A., & Ingole, D. (2005). Reduced glutathione: Importance of specimen collection. *Indian Journal of Clinical Biochemistry*, *20*(1), 150–152. Advance online publication. doi:10.1007/BF02893062 PMID:23105514

Danese, S., & Fiocchi, C. (2006). Etiopathogenesis of inflammatory bowel diseases. *World Journal of Gastroenterology*, *12*(30), 4807. Advance online publication. doi:10.3748/wjg.v12.i30.4807 PMID:16937461

Danese, S., Sans, M., de la Motte, C., Graziani, C., West, G., Phillips, M. H., Pola, R., Rutella, S., Willis, J., Gasbarrini, A., & Fiocchi, C. (2006). Angiogenesis as a Novel Component of Inflammatory Bowel Disease Pathogenesis. *Gastroenterology*, *130*(7), 2060–2073. Advance online publication. doi:10.1053/j.gastro.2006.03.054 PMID:16762629

Desai, H. G., & Gupte, P. A. (2005). Increasing incidence of Crohn's disease in India: Is it related to improved sanitation? *Indian Journal of Gastroenterology*. PMID:15778522

Eisenach, J. C., Curry, R., Rauck, R., Pan, P., & Yaksh, T. L. (2010). Role of spinal cyclooxygenase in human postoperative and chronic pain. *Anesthesiology*, *112*(5), 1225–1233. Advance online publication. doi:10.1097/ALN.0b013e3181d94dc0 PMID:20395820

Empey, L. R., Jewell, L. D., Garg, M. L., Thomson, A. B. R., Clandinin, M. T., & Fedorak, R. N. (1991). Fish oil-enriched diet is mucosal protective against acetic acid-induced colitis in rats. *Canadian Journal of Physiology and Pharmacology*, *69*(4), 480–487. Advance online publication. doi:10.1139/y91-072 PMID:1647851

G., P., G., S., I., G., L., A., E., M., G., C., … R., T. (2014). Growing-up with an ileal-pouch: Adult-patient controlled and coetaneous population-based long-term evaluation of patients operated on in the developmental age in two Italian referral Centres. *Colorectal Disease*.

Gao, W., Zhang, L., Wang, X., Yu, L., Wang, C., & Gong, Y. (2018). The combination of indirubin and isatin attenuates dextran sodium sulfate induced ulcerative colitis in mice. *Biochemistry and Cell Biology*, *96*(5), 636–645. Advance online publication. doi:10.1139/bcb-2018-0041 PMID:29671340

Ghosh, S., & Hayden, M. S. (2008). New regulators of NF-κB in inflammation. *Nature Reviews. Immunology*, *8*(11), 837–848. Advance online publication. doi:10.1038/nri2423 PMID:18927578

Hecker, E. (1968). Cocarcinogenic Principles from the Seed Oil of Croton tiglium and from Other Euphorbiaceae. *Cancer Research*. PMID:5723975

Hersh, A. L., Shapiro, D. J., Pavia, A. T., & Shah, S. S. (2011). Antibiotic prescribing in ambulatory pediatrics in the United States. *Pediatrics*, *128*(6), 1053–1061. Advance online publication. doi:10.1542/peds.2011-1337 PMID:22065263

Hou, J. K., Abraham, B., & El-Serag, H. (2011). Dietary intake and risk of developing inflammatory bowel disease: A systematic review of the literature. *The American Journal of Gastroenterology*, *106*(4), 563–573. Advance online publication. doi:10.1038/ajg.2011.44 PMID:21468064

Hung, Y. L., Fang, S. H., Wang, S. C., Cheng, W. C., Liu, P. L., Su, C. C., Chen, C.-S., Huang, M.-Y., Hua, K.-F., Shen, K.-H., Wang, Y.-T., Suzuki, K., & Li, C. Y. (2017). Corylin protects LPS-induced sepsis and attenuates LPS-induced inflammatory response. *Scientific Reports*, *7*(1), 46299. Advance online publication. doi:10.1038rep46299 PMID:28397806

Jung, O. B., Dong, Y. Y., Koan, S. W., Tae, M. K., Ung, S. L., Jeong, H. S., ... Jin, T. H. (2007). Inhibition of cell growth and induction of apoptosis via inactivation of NF-κB by a sulfurcompound isolated from garlic in human colon cancer cells. *Journal of Pharmacological Sciences*, *104*(4), 374–383. Advance online publication. doi:10.1254/jphs.FP0070789

Kim, D. S., Kim, S. J., Kim, M. C., Jeon, Y. D., Um, J. Y., & Hong, S. H. (2012). The therapeutic effect of chelidonic acid on ulcerative colitis. *Biological & Pharmaceutical Bulletin*, *35*(5), 666–671. Advance online publication. doi:10.1248/bpb.35.666 PMID:22687399

Kirsner, J. B. (2001). Historical origins of current IBD concepts. *World Journal of Gastroenterology*, *7*(2), 175. Advance online publication. doi:10.3748/wjg.v7.i2.175 PMID:11819757

Knights, D., Lassen, K. G., & Xavier, R. J. (2013). Advances in inflammatory bowel disease pathogenesis: Linking host genetics and the microbiome. *Gut*, *62*(10), 1505–1510. Advance online publication. doi:10.1136/gutjnl-2012-303954 PMID:24037875

Kornbluth, A., & Sachar, D. B. (2010). Ulcerative colitis practice guidelines in adults: American college of gastroenterology, practice parameters committee. *The American Journal of Gastroenterology*, *105*(3), 501–523. Advance online publication. doi:10.1038/ajg.2009.727 PMID:20068560

Kwang, S. A., Sethi, G., & Aggarwal, B. B. (2007). Embelin, an inhibitor of X chromosome-linked inhibitor-of-apoptosis protein, blocks nuclear factor-κB (NF-κB) signaling pathway leading to suppression of NF-κB-regulated antiapoptotic and metastatic gene products. *Molecular Pharmacology*, *71*(1), 209–219. Advance online publication. doi:10.1124/mol.106.028787

Kwon, K. H., Murakami, A., Tanaka, T., & Ohigashi, H. (2005). Dietary rutin, but not its aglycone quercetin, ameliorates dextran sulfate sodium-induced experimental colitis in mice: Attenuation of pro-inflammatory gene expression. *Biochemical Pharmacology*, *69*(3), 395–406. Advance online publication. doi:10.1016/j.bcp.2004.10.015 PMID:15652231

Manna, S., Bhattacharrya, D., Basak, D. K., & Mandal, T. K. (2004). Single oral dose toxicity study of α-cypermethrin in rats. *Indian Journal of Pharmacology*.

Mayne, C. G., & Williams, C. B. (2013). Induced and natural regulatory T cells in the development of inflammatory bowel disease. *Inflammatory Bowel Diseases*, *19*(8), 1772–1788. Advance online publication. doi:10.1097/MIB.0b013e318281f5a3 PMID:23656897

Miyoshi, J., Bobe, A. M., Miyoshi, S., Huang, Y., Hubert, N., Delmont, T. O., Eren, A. M., Leone, V., & Chang, E. B. (2017). Peripartum Antibiotics Promote Gut Dysbiosis, Loss of Immune Tolerance, and Inflammatory Bowel Disease in Genetically Prone Offspring. *Cell Reports*, *20*(2), 491–504. Advance online publication. doi:10.1016/j.celrep.2017.06.060 PMID:28700948

Molodecky, N. A., Soon, I. S., Rabi, D. M., Ghali, W. A., Ferris, M., Chernoff, G., Benchimol, E. I., Panaccione, R., Ghosh, S., Barkema, H. W., & Kaplan, G. G. (2012). Increasing incidence and prevalence of the inflammatory bowel diseases with time, based on systematic review. *Gastroenterology*, *142*(1), 46–54.e42. Advance online publication. doi:10.1053/j.gastro.2011.10.001 PMID:22001864

Nidhi, D., Dadwal, A., Hallan, S. S., Sharma, S., & Mishra, N. (2017, August 18). A., Hallan, S. S., Sharma, S., & Mishra, N. (2017). Development of enteric-coated microspheres of embelin for their beneficial pharmacological potential in ulcerative colitis. *Artificial Cells, Nanomedicine, and Biotechnology*, *45*(6), 1092–1100. Advance online publication. doi:10.1080/21691401.2016.1202258 PMID:27388946

Patterson, H., Nibbs, R., Mcinnes, I., & Siebert, S. (2014). Protein kinase inhibitors in the treatment of inflammatory and autoimmune diseases. *Clinical and Experimental Immunology*, *176*(1), 1–10. Advance online publication. doi:10.1111/cei.12248 PMID:24313320

Petersen, I., Gilbert, R., Evans, S., Ridolfi, A., & Nazareth, I. (2010). Oral antibiotic prescribing during pregnancy in primary care: UK population-based study. *The Journal of Antimicrobial Chemotherapy*, *65*(10), 2238–2246. Advance online publication. doi:10.1093/jac/dkq307 PMID:20716554

Pickert, G., Neufert, C., Leppkes, M., Zheng, Y., Wittkopf, N., Warntjen, M., Lehr, H.-A., Hirth, S., Weigmann, B., Wirtz, S., Ouyang, W., Neurath, M. F., & Becker, C. (2009). STAT3 links IL-22 signaling in intestinal epithelial cells to mucosal wound healing. *The Journal of Experimental Medicine*, *206*(7), 1465–1472. Advance online publication. doi:10.1084/jem.20082683 PMID:19564350

Rivlin, R. S. (2001). Historical Perspective on the Use of Garlic. *The Journal of Nutrition*, *131*(3), 951S–954S. Advance online publication. doi:10.1093/jn/131.3.951S PMID:11238795

Rossetti, S., Actis, G. C., Fadda, M., Rizzetto, M., & Palmo, A. (2004). The use of the anti-tumour necrosis factor monoclonal antibody-infliximab-to treat ulcerative colitis: Implications and trends beyond the available data. *Digestive and Liver Disease*, *36*(6), 426–431. Advance online publication. doi:10.1016/S1590-8658(04)00088-X PMID:15248385

Sabiu, S., & Ashafa, O. T. A. (2016). Toxicological implications and laxative potential of ethanol root extract of Morella serrata in loperamide-induced constipated Wistar rats. *Pharmaceutical Biology*, *54*(12), 2901–2908. Advance online publication. doi:10.1080/13880209.2016.1193885 PMID:27267728

Sadra, A., Kweon, H. S., Huh, S. O., & Cho, J. (2017). Gastroprotective and gastric motility benefits of AD-lico/Healthy Gut™ Glycyrrhiza inflata extract. *Animal Cells and Systems*, *21*(4), 255–262. Advance online publication. doi:10.1080/19768354.2017.1357660 PMID:30460076

Sandborn, W. J., & Hanauer, S. B. (1999). Antitumor necrosis factor therapy for Inflammatory Bowel Disease: A review of agents, pharmacology, clinical results, and safety. *Inflammatory Bowel Diseases*, *5*(2), 119–133. Advance online publication. doi:10.1097/00054725-199905000-00008 PMID:10338381

Sharma, M., Kaur, R., Kaushik, K., & Kaushal, N. (2019). Redox modulatory protective effects of ω-3 fatty acids rich fish oil against experimental colitis. *Toxicology Mechanisms and Methods*, *29*(4), 244–254. Advance online publication. doi:10.1080/15376516.2018.1553220 PMID:30489199

Spano, J. P., Milano, G., Rixe, C., & Fagard, R. (2006). JAK/STAT signalling pathway in colorectal cancer: A new biological target with therapeutic implications. *European Journal of Cancer*, *42*(16), 2668–2670. Advance online publication. doi:10.1016/j.ejca.2006.07.006 PMID:16963263

Spiik, A. K., Ridderstad, A., Axelsson, L. G., Midtvedt, T., Björk, L., & Pettersson, S. (2002). Abrogated lymphocyte infiltration and lowered CD14 in dextran sulfate induced colitis in mice treated with p65 antisense oligonucleotides. *International Journal of Colorectal Disease*, *17*(4), 223–232. Advance online publication. doi:10.100700384-001-0366-3 PMID:12073070

Suzuki, K., Sugimura, K., Hasegawa, K., Yoshida, K., Suzuki, A., Ishizuka, K., ... Asakura, H. (2001). Activated platelets in ulcerative colitis enhance the production of reactive oxygen species by polymorphonuclear leukocytes. *Scandinavian Journal of Gastroenterology*. Advance online publication. doi:10.1080/003655201317097164 PMID:11761021

Tatar, E. L., & Das, K. M. (2007). Improvement in ulcerative colitis symptoms after use of fish oil enemas. *Gastroenterology & Hepatology*. PMID:21960787

Tulchinsky, H., Hawley, P. R., & Nicholls, R. J. (2003). Long-Term Failure after Restorative Proctocolectomy for Ulcerative Colitis. *Annals of Surgery*, *238*(2), 229–234. Advance online publication. doi:10.1097/01.sla.0000082121.84763.4c PMID:12894016

Vine, K. L., Locke, J. M., Ranson, M., Benkendorff, K., Pyne, S. G., & Bremner, J. B. (2007). In vitro cytotoxicity evaluation of some substituted isatin derivatives. *Bioorganic & Medicinal Chemistry*, *15*(2), 931–938. Advance online publication. doi:10.1016/j.bmc.2006.10.035 PMID:17088067

Vitor, C. E., Figueiredo, C. P., Hara, D. B., Bento, A. F., Mazzuco, T. L., & Calixto, J. B. (2009). Therapeutic action and underlying mechanisms of a combination of two pentacyclic triterpenes, aand B-amyrin, in a mouse model of colitis. *British Journal of Pharmacology*, *157*(6), 1034–1044. Advance online publication. doi:10.1111/j.1476-5381.2009.00271.x PMID:19508397

Yorulmaz, E., Yorulmaz, H., Gökmen, E. S., Altınay, S., Küçük, S. H., Zengi, O., Çelik, D. S., & Şit, D. (2019). Therapeutic effectiveness of rectally administered fish oil and mesalazine in trinitrobenzenesulfonic acid-induced colitis. *Biomedicine and Pharmacotherapy*, *118*, 109247. Advance online publication. doi:10.1016/j.biopha.2019.109247 PMID:31351432

Yue, G., Lai, P. S., Yin, K., Sun, F. F., Nagele, R. G., Liu, X., … Wong, P. Y. K. (2001). Colon epithelial cell death in 2,4,6-trinitrobenzenesulfonic acid-induced colitis is associated with increased inducible nitric-oxide synthase expression and peroxynitrite production. *Journal of Pharmacology and Experimental Therapeutics*.

Chapter 5
Nanoparticle-Mediated Therapeutic Approach for Ulcerative Colitis Treatment

Subhamoy Banerjee
B. S. Abdur Rahman Crescent Institute of Science and Technology, India

ABSTRACT

Ulcerative colitis is a chronic inflammation of the inner part of the colonic mucosa. It is a type of inflammatory bowel disease which is idiopathic in nature. It is multifactorial, debilitating disorder which may cause life threatening complications. Given to the architecture of colon, conventional medicines have limitation in treating the disease. Thus, the need for alternative methods of drug delivery is important. Nanoparticle is one of the preferred drug delivery system owing to its unique properties. Nanoparticles resist undesired and premature degradation of the drugs, increases bioavailability, and target specificity. Different nanoparticle-based drug delivery systems like metallic, liposome, silica, or polymeric nanoparticles have been designed to administer therapeutic agents through oral route to treat ulcerative colitis. Natural compounds and active components isolated from the plant extracts and other bioactive agents are also delivered by nanoparticle. In the current chapter, nanoparticle-mediated drug and phytochemicals delivery to treat ulcerative colitis are discussed.

DOI: 10.4018/978-1-7998-3580-6.ch005

1. INTRODUCTION

Ulcerative colitis (UC) is a type of inflammatory bowel disease (IBD). Another type of IBD is named as Crohn's disease. The two diseases can be easily separated by their clinical signatures such as endoscopic and histological analysis (Ordas *et al.*, 2012). UC is a chronic inflammation in colon caused by mucosal immune system towards the resident gut microbes. In brief, sustained inflammation in the innermost lining of colon and rectum for a very long time causes ulcer and leads to bloody diarrhea, pain and cramping and sometimes life threatening complications. According to Montreal classification, UC can be classified into following types (Ordas *et al.*, 2012; Silverberg *et al.*, 2005)-

1. E1 or Proctitis- inflammation confined in the area of rectum. May cause rectal bleeding and generally considered to be mildest.
2. E2 or distal left sided- inflammation in the area of sigmoid and descending colon. Symptoms are bloody diarrhea, left side cramping etc.
3. E3 or pancolitis- inflammation in entire colon. Symptoms are abdominal cramps and pain, severe diarrhea with blood etc.
4. S0 or remission- no symptoms
5. S1 or mild- four times or less stools per day with no blood sign and normal inflammatory markers.
6. S2 or moderate- minimum signs of disease symptoms.
7. 7. S3 or severe- several times of stools with profuse bleeding. Higher pulse rate and elevated body temperature and low hemoglobin count.

E= extent, S=severe

UC is found to happen worldwide. But latest reports indicate that the cases of UC are showing a downward trend in developed countries where once it was a major ailment. On the contrary, the number of UC patients is increasing in developing countries of Asia, Latin America and Eastern Europe. The population wide study shows a wide variation in global epidemiological data ranging from 0.5 to $31.5/10^5$ population (da Silva *et al.*, 2014). Asian population shows lower prevalence (5.3-$63.3/10^5$ population) compared to North America (37.5-$238/10^5$ population) (da Silva *et al.*, 2014). Among Asian population, it largely varies from country to country. In mainland China, UC burden ranges from 0.05-$1.09/10^5$ population whereas, Hong Kong shows comparatively higher prevalence of $1.25/10^5$ population. In India, the prevalence is comparatively higher and stands at $6.02/10^5$ population (Ng *et al.*, 2013).

1.1 Risk Factors Involving Ulcerative Colitis

UC is a multifactorial disorder with unknown etiology. The risk factors include age, race or ethnicity, genetic predisposition, environmental factors and habits. Despite several factors involved, the exact reasons are still not clear. The risk factors shall be discussed shortly-

a) Age- UC can be caused to any age group but young adults are found to be more susceptible. Generally the disease onset follows a bimodal distribution with two distict peaks based on the age group, the largest peak in the age group 18-30 years and a small but distinct peak at 50-70 years (Ordas *et al.*, 2012). The disease type found to differ with age group like older patients (>40 years) used to suffer from distal left sided colitis rather than pancolytis when compared to younger age group (Quezada & Cross, 2012). In general, older patients tend to suffer from less severe form of UC.
b) Ethnicity- The correlation between UC and ethnicity was studied hospital basis in different parts of the world. General observation suggest widely varies from study to another. One study in Thailand hospital suggested middle-east population has higher occurrence of UC than Caucasians (Permpoon *et al.*, 2016), other reports indicate higher occurrence in Caucasians (Afzali, 2019). Thus, UC can happen to any race or ethnicity but Ashkenazi Jews have comparatively higher predisposition of IBD (Roth *et al.*, 1989) due to some mutations specific to their genome.
c) Genetic mutation- UC is a polygenic disorder comprised of copy number variations comprised of insertion, deletion and duplication (Jostins *et al.*, 2012). SNP array analysis conducted on large cohort revealed two genes namely *ATP binding cassette, subfamily 4* (ABCC4) and *claudin 10* (CLDN10) undergoes deletion at its upstream region, 119 kb duplication at chromosome 7p22.1 encompassing genes namely *ring finer protein 216* (RNF216), *zinc finger protein 815* (ZNF815), *oncomodulin* (OCM) and *vacuolar fusion protein, human homologue* (CCZ1) which indicate genome wide rare copy number variation (Saadati *et al.*, 2016). Genome wide association study (GWAS) also found E cadherin, hepatocyte nuclear factor 4 (HNF4), laminin β1 subunit (LAMB1), guanine nucleotide binding protein α 12 (GNA12) as potential risk factor for UC (Feuerstein & Cheifetz, 2014).
d) Nutrition- Nutrition plays a very important role in pathology of UC. Undernourishment directly correlated with pathology of UC. Cohort study with 158 patients admitted in hospital shows unjustified underfeeding increase the disease flare (Gallinger *et al.*, 2017). Many patients remain malnourished to check the disease which in turn exacerbates the situation. A diet supplemented

with appropriate energy source, minerals, folic acid, Vitamin D and B12 shows control in the progression of the disease (Owczarek *et al.*, 2016).

e) Environmental factors- Environmental factors initiate UC for the genetically predisposed patients by starting immune response which finally resulted in chronic inflammation in the gastrointestinal tract (da Silva *et al.*, 2014). Smoking and appendectomy has well defined connection to UC in the predisposed patients (da Silva *et al.*, 2014). Intestinal microbiome is known to influence the functioning of immune system. The colonization of pathogenic microorganism in inner and outer lumen influences the host immune response like change in the secretion of mucin-2 (Muc-2) which results in decrease in the thickness of mucus layer. Also the colonization of harmful bacteria results in the imbalance in gut microbiome and induces dysbiosis and UC (Pei *et al.*, 2019).

1.2 Biology of Ulcerative Colitis

Intestinal epithelial barrier acts as the first line of defense against commensal microflora. The epithelium covered by mucinous layer separates microorganisms reside in the lumen from host immune cells. Also, mucinous layer secrete antimicrobial peptides (Ordas *et al.*, 2012). Thus, the balance between immune cells and microbiome is maintained. At present it is believed that UC is the result of an uncontrolled immune response caused by interleukin-13 (IL-13) secreted by T_h2 cells (de Souza & Fiocchi, 2016). The other theory suggest the involvement of epithelial cells which via thymic stromal lymphopoietin (TSLP) induces the immune cells like monocytes, dendritic cells and macrophages towards T_h2 cells (Fohlinger *et al.*, 2016). The activated T_h2 cells produces higher amount of mucus, epithelial cell hyperplasia and fibrosis. According to authors (Fohlinger *et al.*, 2016), two main conditions characterize the inflammation in UC. First, the 'acute' condition which is mediated by CD_{11b}+ macrophages and activator molecules like Thymus and activation regulated chemokines (TARC) and cytokine like hepatocyte growth factors (HGF) etc. Second, 'remodeling' condition characterized by Natural killer (NK) cells, CD_{14}+ monocytes and small molecules such as cytokine Transforming Growth Factor β (TGF β) and chemokine periostin. Genome wide association study (GWAS) indicated that polymorphism in Fc Gamma receptor 2A (FCGR2A) changes the binding affinity of the receptor towards its antibody (Jostins *et al.*, 2012). In another study, in the colonic mucosa of UC patients, researchers found the evidence of profound induction of inflammatory or anti-commensal IgG and activation of FcγRII receptors (Castro-Dopico *et al.*, 2019). Interleukin 1β (IL-1β) was found to be a key mediator of inflammation and effects on Th17 cell and γδ T cells. In a nutshell, various factors like cells, cytokines and chemokines, commensal microflora, genetic factors etc. are involved in modulating the inflammation in the epithelial lining of intestinal mucosa. Antigen presenting cells like dendritic cells and macrophages, different types of T helper cells, natural killer cells (NK cells) mediate the inflammation. Various cytokines like TNFα, TGFβ, IL-1, 3, 6, 10, 13 etc. induce and modulate the inflammation (Tatiya-Aphiradee *et al.*, 2018). The change in the types and number of microbes called dysbiosys and characterizes UC. Increase in *Escherichia spp., Campylobacter spp., Shigella spp., Helicobacter spp.* etc. and absence of *Lactobacillus spp., Pediococcus spp.* etc. are found in UC samples (Sasaki & Klapproth, 2012). The illustration of mechanism of UC is shown in Figure 1.

Figure 1. Mechanism of Ulcerative colitis. Cytokine upragulation and commensal microbes cause damage and alteration of epithelial cells which lead to uncontrolled inflammation. Different types of immune cells play pivotal role in pathogenesis of UC

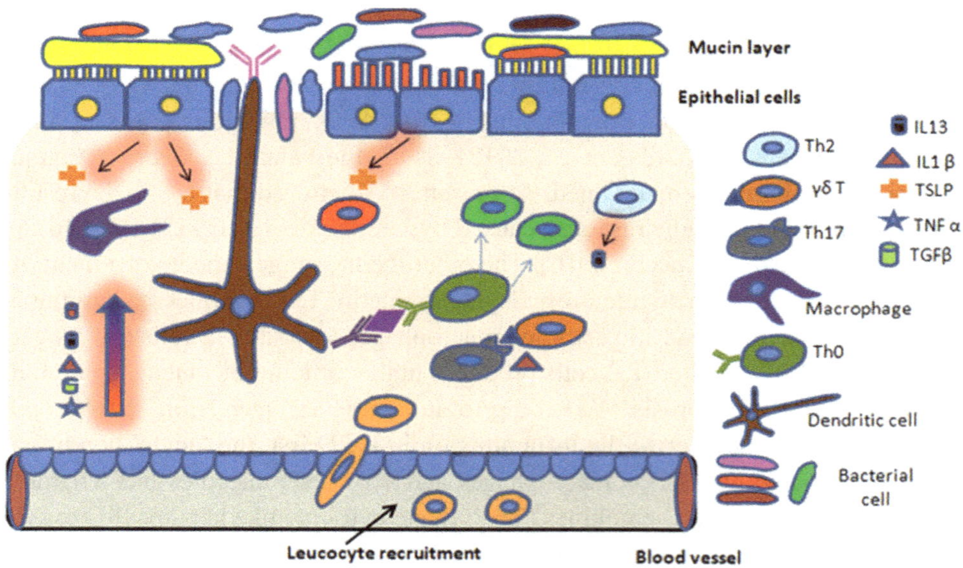

1.3 Therapeutic Approach Against Ulcerative Colitis

Being a chronic inflammation, generally therapeutic management of UC depends on several factors like stage of UC, localization, patient data like age, food habit etc. There are two aims of UC treatment- to target the root cause or etio-pathogenesis and treating the symptoms. The major goal is to initiate and sustain the remission process. Conventionally 5-Aminosalicylic acid (5-ASA) group of drugs like Balsalazide, Mesalamine, Olsalazine etc., corticosteroids, immunosuppressants like 6-Mercaptopurine, Azathioprine, Cyclosporine or tacrolimus are used to treat UC. When aforementioned conventional drugs fail to act against UC or UC becomes refractory against conventional therapies, the biological therapy found to act effectively. The biological agents like anti-TNF-α molecules, Janus kinase inhibitor or Integrin subtype blockers are found to be useful.

a) Anti-TNFα agents- Most commonly used biological agents are Infliximab Adalimumab and Golimumab. Infliximab is a mouse-human chimeric antibody and Adalimumab is humanized anti-TNFα IgG1 antibody. These antibodies bind to free TNFα in order to prevent it from binding to membrane bound TNFα receptors (TNFR 1 and 2) and inhibit the TNFα mediated inflammation (Seo & Chae, 2014). Infliximab is used for initiation and maintenance therapy. Adalimumab is a humanized monoclonal antibody used to treat mild to severe UC. Infliximab is administered intravenous route whereas Adalimumab is administered subcutaneously. Golimumab is also humanized monoclonal antibody approved to treat moderate to severe monoclonal antibody.
b) Anti-Integrin therapy- Integrin plays role in leukocyte adhesion to the vascular endothelial wall and migration to the site of inflammation. Thus, blocking integrin controls inflammation. Vedolizumab is a humanized monoclonal antibody approved for treatment of moderate to severe UC with Mayo score 6-12 (Arora & Shen, 2015). It specifically targets α4β7 integrin which is gut specific. Thus it plays as anti-adhesion therapeutic agent (Arijs *et al.*, 2018).
c) Janus kinase inhibitors- Most promising oral small molecule inhibitor is Janus Kinase (JAK) inhibitor tofacitinib. Tofacitinib is found to prefereably inhibit JAK 1 and JAK 3. Another JAK1 inhibitor in market is upadacitinib (X. Zhang *et al.*, 2019).

Other small molecule therapy for UC includes Ozanimod, an oral antagonist of sphingosine 1 subtype 1 and 5. Blocking its target, Ozanimod induces peripheral lymphocyte sequestration, thus inhibiting them from entering into GI tract (X. Zhang *et al.*, 2019).

The conventional therapeutic strategies suffer many obstacles like lack of target specificity, low residence time at the site of infection especially at the distant colon due to diarrhea etc. The lack of target specificity leads to many side effects like infections by opportunistic pathogens, autoimmunity, malignancies and cardiac complications (Stallmach *et al.*, 2010). Thiopurine group of drugs which are commonly used for UC treatments are reported to cross react with angiotensin converting enzyme inhibitors (used for cardiovascular diseases) and may cause hypersensitivity, nausea, malignancy and fertility complications. Biologics like TNF-α inhibitors are reported to cause multiple complications like heart failure, hypersensitivity, demyelination of nerve cells, fertility and pregnancy complications, opportunistic infections etc. Integrin antagonists are reported to cause progressive multifocal leucoencephalopathy, fertility complications etc. (Cohn *et al.*, 2017).

Nanoparticle (NP) mediated drug delivery has several advantages over conventional therapeutic system like high surface to volume ratio which enables NP to carry higher amount of drugs or more than one types of drug, longer circulation time in body, target specificity and controlled drug release capacity. Owing to these properties, NPs are gaining higher attention from the scientific community as a therapeutic strategy against ulcerative colitis. In this chapter, the scope of NPs as a therapeutic vehicle is discussed based on comprehensive literature review.

2. NANOPARTICLE MEDIATED THERAPY

NPs mediated therapy can be broadly classified into passive and active targeting methods. As the site of function of the therapeutic agents is gastrointestinal (GI) tract, thus NPs need to deliver the drug in epithelial or endothelial region of GI tract. The passive targeting is referred as NPs infiltrate the site of inflammation through its enhanced permeation and retention property. Different pro-inflammatory molecules like histamine, bradykinin, serotonin etc. increases the permeability of endothelial barrier, thus helps the nanoparticles to accumulate at the site of inflammation and release of bioactive agents. The size and surface charge of the NP play important role in penetration of lymphatic vessels. Active targeting involves targeting cell adhesion molecules on the cell surface, which plays role in the regulation of inflammation. The bioactive agents which are delivered through NPs are ranging from conventional drugs like budesonide (glucocorticoid) (Zhou & Qian, 2018) to natural compound extracts like ginger active compound 6-shogaol (M. Zhang *et al.*, 2018). The NPs can be delivered by intravenous or oral route. For GI tract infection, oral route for drug delivery is considered as attractive option as it is safer, patient compliant and cost effectieve. Ginger active compound 6-shogaol loaded in Poly L Lactic co Glycolic acid (PLGA)/ Poly L Lactic acid (PLA)-Polyethylene glycol (PEG) - folic acid (FA) was tested on dextran sulphate sodium (DSS) treated mouse model for ulcerative colitis. The levels pro-inflammatory cytokines like TNFα, IL-1β, IL-6 etc. found to be checked. The UC symptoms were alleviated and wound healing of colitis tissues accentuated (M. Zhang *et al.*, 2018).

2.1 Ginger Derived NPs

In another study, edible ginger derived nanoparticle (GDNPs 2) was synthesized and tested on co-culture of macrophage cell line RAW264.7 and colon-26 cell line and colitis induces mouse model (FVB/NJ mouse). Ginger derived NPs found to have 3 different sizes ranging from 200-300 nm based on bands obtained by sucrose gradient ultracentrifugation. Different types of biochemical analysis were conducted to estimate lipid and protein contents. c-DNA library formation followed by deep sequencing revealed 125 different mi-RNA is present in the GDNP. Oral administration of GDNPs 2 to mice showed the lower susceptibility of the mice to get UC upon DSS treatment. The pro-inflammatory cytokines like TNF-α, IL-6 and 1β etc. were found to down regulate upon treatment of GDNPs 2. The epithelial cell of colon and macrophages were found to internalize orally administered GDNPs 2 (M. Zhang *et al.*, 2016).

2.2 Curcumin Nanoformulation

Curcumin is considered as a broad spectrum bioactive agent and used in nanoparticle mediated delivery for different types of diseases. Porous PLGA based NPs have been synthesized with Pluronic F127 and curcumin was loaded into it. The hydrodynamic diameter of the NPs was found around 270 nm and PF127 was found to increase the cellular uptake. The UC mouse model treated with this NP showed higher inhibition of pro-inflammatory cytokines like TNFα, IL-6 and 12 etc. (Chen *et al.*, 2019). D-α-tocopherol PEG 1000 succinate (TPGS)-stabilized curcumin nanoparticle was synthesized by homogenization method. TPGS stabilized Curcumin NPs were orally administered to 2, 4, 6 trinitrobenzene sulfonic acid treated wistar rats. The anti-inflammatory effect of TPGS stabilized Curcumin NPs were observed on the wistar rat model (Rachmawati *et al.*, 2017). Targeting macrophages is an attractive strategy against UC. Silk fibroin (SF) based NP has been synthesized and curcumin was loaded into it followed by surface functionalization with chondroitin sulfate (CS) for controlled release. CS increases the chance of macrophages internalization of the NPs. Authors found that hence synthesized NPs show good responsiveness towards chemical stimuli like low pH, reduction by glutathione and reactive oxygen species (ROS) exerted by using hydrogen peroxide (H_2O_2). Orally administered SF-CS NPs loaded with fluorescent dye showed direct access to colonic mucosa. To save the NPs from harsh environment of GI tract, authors encapsulated it into chitosan/alginate hydrogel, results in crossing mucosal barrier. The NPs were tested against DSS treated mice and found to exert higher anti-inflammatory role. Although the GI tract species diversity found to be different in case of healthy mouse, DSS treated control and NPs treated UC model (Gou *et al.*, 2019). PLGA based porous and non porous NPs have been synthesized and curcumin was loaded into the NPs and tested *in vivo*. Porous NPs were synthesized in double emulsion technique where PVA used as emulsifier and Ammonium bicarbonate (ABC) as progen and curcumin was loaded into it. The synthesized Cur-PLGA NPs were tested on Kunming mice treated with DSS. The curcumin was found to exert anti-inflammatory effect on the inflamed colon and histopathological parameters shown to have improved (Chen *et al.*, 2017). Researchers tried to exert synergistic effect by adding drugs like celecoxib with curcumin. Celecoxib is a cycloxygenase-2 (COX-2) inhibitor and belongs to non steroidal anti inflammatory drugs (NSAID) group. The combinatorial effect of both curcumin and celecoxib were tested on Sprague-Dawley rats. The Eudragit™ S100 nanoparticle was synthesized and curcumin, celecoxib and curcumin-celecoxib in combination was loaded in nanoparticle. The tested rats showed decreased level of lipid peroxidation and myeloperoxidase where as superoxide dismutase level found to have increased (Gugulothu *et al.*, 2014).

2.3 Food Based NPs

Food derived nanoparticles for treating UC is gaining increased interest. As a part of it, broccoli derived NPs (BDN) were synthesized from fresh broccoli juice by sequential centrifugation and high pressure method. BDN were fed to mice for 10 days prior to DSS treatment for induction of colitis. BDN treated mouse was shown significantly less pro-inflammatory cytokine activation compared to untreated mouse (Deng *et al.*, 2017). Chinese herb *B. javanica* derived bioactive compound Brucein D (BD) is delivered by self nanoemulsifying drug delivery system (SNEDDS). The SNEDDS have been synthesized by Solutol HS 15, Medium chain triglyceride (MCT), polypropylene glycol and BD. Hence synthesized SNEDDS loaded with BD was tested on Sprague Dawley rats as UC model. BD SNEDDS was found to significantly ameliorate the UC which was proven by testing histochemical and biochemical markers line length of colon, ROS, TNFα, MPO etc. level in the infected tissue (Dou *et al.*, 2018). A specially designed polymer name Methoxy–poly (ethylene glycol) (mPEG) with hydrophobic hexyl substituted poly (lactic acid) (hexPLA) core was used to synthesize self-assembling nanocarriers in order to carry anti inflammatory hydrophobic drug Cyclosporine A (CsA) to site of inflammation of TNBS induced UC mouse model. Free CsA is found to be effective in remission of UC but acute nephro-toxicity as its side limits its efficacy. Encapsulating in self-assembling nanoparticle increases it efficiency. The nanocarriers quickly release the drugs when comes in contact with mucosal layer. The drug loaded nanocarrier was administered to healthy and diseased mouse through rectum. The reduction of inflammation was observed without any undesired toxicity (Courthion *et al.*, 2018). CsA also delivered to colon via Eudragit® FS30D/PLGA NP. Due to the presence of Eudragit and PLGA, the NP harnessed pH tunable and sustained release property respectively. The NP is synthesized by oil in water emulsion. CsA is loaded into the NPs and delivered to UC mouse model. Eudragit saved the burst release of CsA at low pH but at pH 7.4, the drug is released. The histological parameters and other molecular parameters were found to have improved in case of Eudragit NP based CsA delivery (Naeem, Bae, *et al.*, 2018). Embelin is an active component isolated from fruits of *Embelia riba* herb. It has a wide range of therapeutic effect. Lipid nanosphere has been synthesized by soya bean oil or virgin coconut oil stabilized by lecithin obtained from egg or soya bean. The mixture is homogenized at higher temperature followed by ultrasonication. Embelin is loaded into the lipid nanosphere and tested on acetic acid treated rat models suffering from UC. The biomarkers levels of UC (MPO, lactate dehydrogenase etc.) found to have decreased and the amount of reduced glutathione increased and histopathological signature improved (Badamaranahalli *et al.*, 2015). Resveratrol (Res) is obtained from grapes has been identified as a key polyphenol having anti-inflammatory, neuroprotective and anti tumor properties. Thus, Res has been tested against different diseases. Two different polymers poly (2-hydroxyethyl methacrylate) (pHEMA) and poly (*N*, *N*-dimethylaminoethyl methacrylate) (pDMAEMA) was used to synthesize NPs to encapsulate and deliver Res. Res loaded NPs were encapsulated in chitosan based hydrogel and release study was conducted in a simulated colonic environment (Iglesias *et al.*, 2019).

2.4 Nanocarrier Based Drug Delivery

Small molecule drugs are also loaded in NPs and delivered for UC therapy. Tacrolimus, an immunosuppressive agent, was loaded and delivered through cationic lipid assisted NPs (CLANs) and administered to DSS treated mouse. CLANs were composed of synthetic polymer PEG-block-PLA and cationic lipid 1, 2- dioleoyl-3-trimethylammonium-propanechloride (DOTAP). The other lipid component instead of DOTAP is N, N– bis (2-hydroxyethyl)- N- methyl- N- (2-cholesteryloxycarbonyl aminoethyl) ammonium bromide (BHEM-Chol). Hence synthesized CLANs accumulate in colon and internalized b epithelial cells and slowly release drug to the site. This nanosystem was found to attenuate UC (J. L. Wang *et al.*, 2018). Cyclosporine A (CsA) is a first line drug for UC. Lipid NPs synthesized by Precirol® ATO 5 loaded with CsA. The lipid NP was stabilized with 3 different chemicals viz. (i) Tween 80, (ii) L-α-phosphatidylcholine from egg yolk (Lec) and sodium taurocholate (TC) (3:1), and (iii) Pluronic® F127 (PL) and TC (1:1). Hence synthesized lipid NP loaded with CsA tested on mouse model of UC. But interestingly, authors found not much decrease of inflammation in terms of common markers like TNFα, myeloperoxidase etc. (Guada *et al.*, 2016).

2.5 Inorganic NPs Based UC Therapy

The effect of aqueous silver (Ag) NPs suspension was synthesized and tested against UC mouse model. Authors have synthesized two different types of AgNPs suspension AgNPs 1 and 2 with average hydrodynamic diameter 294 nm and 124 nm respectively. Mouse with UC was generated by standard protocol i.e. treatment with DSS and TNBS. The AgNPs treated mice shown anti-inflammatory activity. The colonic microbiota analysis showed AgNPs 2 has helped to decrease *Clostridium perfringens* and increase *Lactobacillus sp.* Thus, the Ag NP aqueous suspension showed promising result against UC (Siczek *et al.*, 2017). Previous report showed that nanocrystalline silver applied to UC rat model reduced the colonic inflammation by reducing the expression of MMP-9, TNFα, IL-1β (Bhol & Schechter, 2007).

Zinc oxide nanoparticle (ZnONP) has also been synthesized and tested on DSS treated mice to check its anti UC efficacy. Synthesized ZnONP showed high negative surface charge (-59.4±3.4 mV). The DSS treated UC affected mice were orally administered ZnONPs and tested for toxicity, anti inflammatory activity. It was found to be non toxic in nature and distinct anti-inflammatory effect was observed. The combination therapy of ZnONPs and 5-ASA which is a standard UC medication showed increased efficacy. Cytoprotective effect of transcription factor Nrf-2 is induced by ZnONPs. The transcriptional target of Nrf-2, antioxidant enzyme NQO-1 can attenuate oxidative stress. The combination effect of 5-ASA and ZnONP on the gut microflora was studied and it was found that *Enterobacterium spp., Enterococcus spp.* and *S. aureus* were decreased while *Lactobacillus spp.* and *Bifidobacteria spp.* population have increased (Li *et al.*, 2017).

5-ASA is a first line therapy for UC, it has been loaded into silicon oxide (SiO_2) to deliver at the site of inflammation. SiO_2 NPs had been synthesized by microemulsion technique and 5-ASA was loaded with help of acetonitrile in the SiO_2 NP. The 5-ASA-SiO_2 NPs were tested in vitro on Caco-2 cell line and in vivo on BALB/c mice. For experimentation purpose, authors have subdivided the mice in to 6 groups- healthy untreated, UC model untreated, UC model 5-ASA treated with normal dose and high dose, only SiO_2 NP treated and 5-ASA-SiO_2 NP treated group. The last group showed remission at low dose of 5-ASA which is comparable as high dose of free 5-ASA (Tang *et al.*, 2017).

Effect of gold (Au) NPs also tested on DSS treated mouse model. Authors have purchased the AuNPs with hydrodynamic diameter 7-20 nm. It was applied by intra-peretoneal injection for 2 weeks starting from 14th day to BALB/c mice at 2.5 mg/kg body weight/day basis. The histopathological signature was improved compared to untreated UC model. Also, IL-17β expression was found to be down regulated and the amount of Malondialdehyde (MDA) in tissue was also found to have significantly decreased compared to untreated mice having UC (Abdelmegid *et al.*, 2019). In another study, citrate and PVP stabilized AuNPs intragastrically applied to DSS treated mice. AuNPs was found to attenuate colonic inflammation based on the molecular markers e.g. myeloperoxidase, TNF-α, IL-6 and peripheral leucocyte and lymphocyte count. But, 16S rRNA sequencing indicated that AuNPs may induce gut dysbiosys (Zhu *et al.*, 2018).

2.6 Biomolecules Based Therapeutic Approaches

Cell based biological molecules like low molecular weight heparin (LMWH) has shown therapeutic efficacy against UC because of its anti inflammatory property, but the lack of suitable delivery vehicle has limit its therapeutic application. Polyethyl acrylate-co-methyl methacrylate-co-trimethyl ammonioethyl methacrylate chloride (PEMT) is used to synthesize the cationic nanoparticles for LMWH loading. *In vivo* higher dosage of LWMH loaded PEMT treatment showed distinct anti-inflammatory activity with significant reduction of pro-inflammatory cytokines considered as a marker for UC (Yazeji *et al.*, 2017). Naturally occurring tripeptide Lysine-proline-valine (KPV) is found to exert anti inflammatory effect on colonic tissue. The NP system was synthesized by double emulsion method (water in oil in water) followed by solvent evaporation. PLGA and chitosan was used to make the nanoparticle in two step method where poly vinyl alcohol (PVA) was used as stabilizing agent. KPV was loaded into the NP and hyaluronic acid (HA) was conjugated by formation of amide bond. Hence synthesized NP was fed to UC mouse model. It was found to promote mucosal healing besides its anti-inflammatory activity (Xiao *et al.*, 2017). They further loaded siRNA of CD98 molecule (siCD98) along with curcumin and functionalized hyaluronic acid (HA) on the surface of the PLGA-chitosan NPs and orally delivered it to the DSS treated mouse model. CD98 plays role in integrin related signaling and over expression of CD98 induce the disintegration of the epithelial layer. Down regulation of CD98 expression reduces the effect of UC in DSS treated mouse. So, siCD98 is used in combination of curcumin. Histopathological study, MPO activity and gene expression testing by RT PCR etc. indicated the remission of UC in mouse model (Xiao *et al.*, 2016). PLGA based NPs synthesized to deliver KPV tripeptide to target peptide transporter 1 (PepT1) along with CsA. The NP was synthesized by emulsion solvent evaporation method. CsA was loaded into PLGA NP and KPV was covalently liked with PLGA. Montmorillonite K10 (MMT) was used as surface modifying agent along low molecular weight chitosan or Pluronic F68. The synthesized NPs were tested on male BALB/c mice treated with DSS to induce colitis. The MPO level checked by biochemical analysis, proinflammatory cytokines expression was checked by RT PCR. The anti-inflammatory effect was favorable. The NPs were capable of target specific drug delivery in inflamed colon (Wu *et al.*, 2019). TNFα is one of the key mediators of inflammation and is found to be over expressed in UC. To tackle the inflammation, TNFα expression was targeted by siRNA designed against TNFα. The siTNFα was loaded into PLGA NP. The synthesized PLGA NP was grafted with galactosylated chitosan to make it target specific towards macrophage cells RAW 264.7. Further, when the NPs administered orally, the grafted NPs showed better remission over non grafted NPs. Colitis related parameters like weight loss, MPO activity etc. showed improvement and proved to be therapeutic approach against UC (Huang *et al.*, 2018). Dual delivery of siTNFα and anti inflammatory cytokine IL22 had been tested on UC model. Galactose functionalized with siTNFα loaded into PLGA NP. It was synthesized in double emulsion technique (water in oil in water). The nanoparticle is interwoven with PVA and chitosan and grafted with lactobionic acid. Hence synthesized NP loaded with siTNFα is loaded in hydrogel with IL22. The co-delivery of siTNFα and IL22 was tested on UC mouse model and Colon-26 cell line. The results of combination therapy showed higher macrophage engulfment due to presence of galactose, lower weight loss, reduced MPO activity etc. (Xiao *et al.*, 2018). Chitosan modified curcumin loaded PLGA NPs have been synthesized and modified with chondroitin sulphate to make it target specific for macrophages to treat UC. The uptake of NPs by macrophages was tested on RAW264.7 cell line. In order make the NPs suitable for oral administration, the NPs were coated in Chitosan/Alginate hydrogel. Upon feeding the hence synthesized NPs to UC mouse model; it was found to have a better therapeutic index for remission of UC (X. Zhang *et al.*, 2019).

2.7 Dendrimers

Most active form of vitamin E, α tocopheryl succinate (α-TOS), blocks the DNA binding activity of NFκB which is a pro-inflammatory inducible transcription factor. α-TOS has been loaded into generation 5 (G5) poly amido amine (NH_2) based dendrimer. Highly branched structure of dendrimer typically offers great advantage over other NPs in drug delivery. G5-NH_2 conjugated with α-TOS by amide bond. The free amide groups of G5-NH_2 were acetylated. The α-TOS loaded G5-NH_2 was administered along with DSS. The histopathological and other analysis suggested that α-TOS-G5-NH_2 dendrimer nanoparticle treated mice were least affected by UC upon DSS treatment (Y. Wang *et al.*, 2017). In another dendrimer based approach, poly amido amine (PAMAM) dendrimers were functionalized with folic acid to target macrophages where folate receptors are over expressed. In a two step synthesis, PAMAM was reacted with PEG2000 and PEG-PAMAM was formed. The folate was conjugated separately with PEG3500 and both were reacted to form folate conjugated PEG PAMAM dendrimer. Free amines were capped by anhydrous acetic acid. Folate capped dendrimers found have selectively targeted colonic macrophages in vivo and RAW264.7 cells in vitro. Thus, folate capped dendrimers act as a target specific drug delivery vehicle for UC (Poh *et al.*, 2017).

2.8 Tunable NPs

One of the key features of nanomedicine is its tunability. Based on specific physico-chemical influence, the nanocarrier is able to release the drug. To treat UC, pH triggered budesonide loaded surface charge reversing lipid NPs. The lipid NPs have been synthesized by Compritol and Phospholipon 90 G. Polyethylene imine (PEI) is used to add positive charge the on lipid NP. Then Eudragit S100 is added to make the lipid NP pH tunable. Imaging experiment suggest the selective accumulation of lipid NPs in the inflamed colon and due to pH change, charge reversal happened in the inflamed area and drug is released (Naeem, Oshi, *et al.*, 2018). In the inflamed colon, MPO is found in higher amount. Using MPO as a triggering agent, site specific drug delivery strategy has been devised. Human serum albumin (HAS) NPs has been synthesized and 5-ASA was loaded into it. The size and zeta potential of the NPs was suitable for the crossing the mucus layer and deposited on the mucosa. The interaction between HAS and MPO lead to the disintegration of NPs and release of 5-ASA at the site of inflammation, results in lowering inflammation of colon (Iwao *et al.*, 2018).

Application of different types of nanoparticle as therapeutic agent for UC has been shown in Figure 2.

Figure 2. Different types of nanoparticle mediated therapies for UC model (DSS treated rat/mouse)

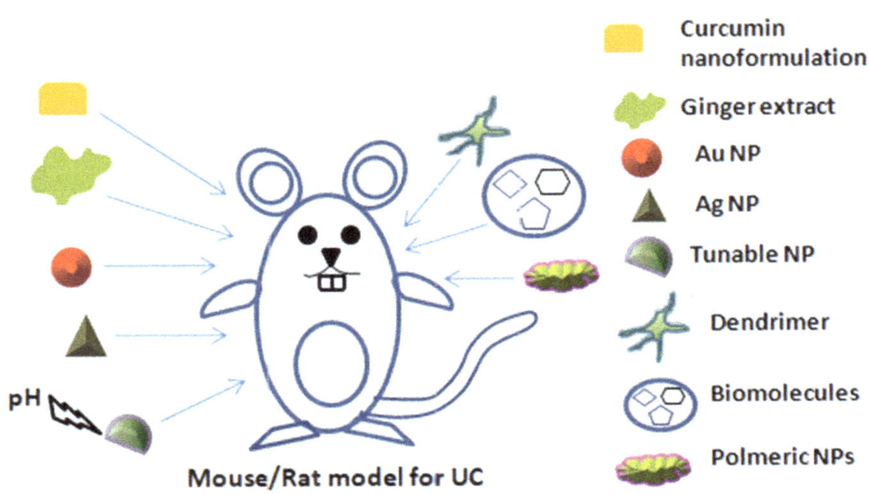

3. CONCLUSION

In conclusion, there is a significant shift in the therapeutic approaches towards UC can be observed. Instead of using free drugs, more emphasis is being given towards encapsulation of the drugs by NPs and hydrogels to save it in the oral route to colon (Jain *et al.*, 2017; Xiao *et al.*, 2017), especially, upper part of GI tract where a very pH environment is present. Thus, the bioavailabilities of the drugs are increased. Further, besides conventional drugs, there is an attention shift of the scientific community towards natural compounds like ginger derived active components, curcumin, reseveratrol etc. Nanoparticle enhances their bioactivities in different ways like increasing circulation half life, enhanced permeation and retention effect and solubility. Thus, using varieties of NPs like lipid NPs, polymeric NPs etc., the encapsulation and site specific delivery was possible (M. Zhang *et al.*, 2016). Also, drug delivery on demand and site specificity also increases the efficacy of the drug. Different surface modification made it possible to specifically target macrophages in the colon to attenuate inflammation (Naeem, Bae, *et al.*, 2018; Poh *et al.*, 2017; X. Zhang *et al.*, 2019). Further, 'on demand delivery' is a gold standard for any drug delivery system. In colon, pH tunable NPs are used for drug delivery (Naeem, Oshi, *et al.*, 2018; Zhou & Qian, 2018). Thus, NPs mediated drugs and natural compound delivery has opened a new avenue for ulcerative colitis therapy.

REFERENCES

Abdelmegid, A. M., Abdo, F. K., Ahmed, F. E., & Kattaia, A. A. A. (2019). Therapeutic effect of gold nanoparticles on DSS-induced ulcerative colitis in mice with reference to interleukin-17 expression. *Scientific Reports*, *9*(1), 10176. doi:10.103841598-019-46671-1 PMID:31308463

Afzali, A. (2019). The Impact of Racial and Ethnic Differences in Inflammatory Bowel Disease Phenotype in the United States. *e-WGN Expert Point of View Articles Collection.* https://www.worldgastroenterology.org/publications/e-wgn/e-wgn-expert-point-of-view-articles-collection/the-impact-of-racial-and-ethnic-differences-in-ibd-phenotype-in-the-us

Arijs, I., De Hertogh, G., Lemmens, B., Van Lommel, L., de Bruyn, M., Vanhove, W., Cleynen, I., Machiels, K., Ferrante, M., Schuit, F., Van Assche, G., Rutgeerts, P., & Vermeire, S. (2018). Effect of vedolizumab (anti-α4β7-integrin) therapy on histological healing and mucosal gene expression in patients with UC. *Gut*, *67*(1), 43–52. doi:10.1136/gutjnl-2016-312293 PMID:27802155

Arora, Z., & Shen, B. (2015). Biological therapy for ulcerative colitis. *Gastroenterology Report*, *3*(2), 103–109. doi:10.1093/gastro/gou070 PMID:25344680

Badamaranahalli, S. S., Kopparam, M., Bhagawati, S. T., & Durg, S. (2015). Embelin lipid nanospheres for enhanced treatment of ulcerative colitis - Preparation, characterization and in vivo evaluation. *European Journal of Pharmaceutical Sciences*, *76*, 73–82. doi:10.1016/j.ejps.2015.05.003 PMID:25957524

Bhol, K. C., & Schechter, P. J. (2007). Effects of nanocrystalline silver (NPI 32101) in a rat model of ulcerative colitis. *Digestive Diseases and Sciences*, *52*(10), 2732–2742. doi:10.100710620-006-9738-4 PMID:17436088

Castro-Dopico, T., Dennison, T. W., Ferdinand, J. R., Mathews, R. J., Fleming, A., Clift, D., Stewart, B. J., Jing, C., Strongili, K., Labzin, L. I., Monk, E. J. M., Saeb-Parsy, K., Bryant, C. E., Clare, S., Parkes, M., & Clatworthy, M. R. (2019). Anti-commensal IgG Drives Intestinal Inflammation and Type 17 Immunity in Ulcerative Colitis. *Immunity*, *50*(4), 1099–1114 e1010. doi:10.1016/j.immuni.2019.02.006 PMID:30876876

Chen, Q., Gou, S., Ma, P., Song, H., Zhou, X., Huang, Y., Kwon Han, M., Wan, Y., Kang, Y., & Xiao, B. (2019). Oral administration of colitis tissue-accumulating porous nanoparticles for ulcerative colitis therapy. *International Journal of Pharmaceutics*, *557*, 135–144. doi:10.1016/j.ijpharm.2018.12.046 PMID:30594685

Chen, Q., Si, X., Ma, L., Ma, P., Hou, M., Bai, S., Wu, X., Wan, Y., Xiao, B., & Merlin, D. (2017). Oral delivery of curcumin via porous polymeric nanoparticles for effective ulcerative colitis therapy. *Journal of Materials Chemistry. B, Materials for Biology and Medicine*, *5*(29), 5881–5891. doi:10.1039/C7TB00328E PMID:29081976

Cohn, H. M., Dave, M., & Loftus, E. V. Jr. (2017). Understanding the Cautions and Contraindications of Immunomodulator and Biologic Therapies for Use in Inflammatory Bowel Disease. *Inflammatory Bowel Diseases*, *23*(8), 1301–1315. doi:10.1097/MIB.0000000000001199 PMID:28708806

Courthion, H., Mugnier, T., Rousseaux, C., Moller, M., Gurny, R., & Gabriel, D. (2018). Self-assembling polymeric nanocarriers to target inflammatory lesions in ulcerative colitis. *Journal of Controlled Release*, *275*, 32–39. doi:10.1016/j.jconrel.2017.07.044 PMID:28774843

da Silva, B. C., Lyra, A. C., Rocha, R., & Santana, G. O. (2014). Epidemiology, demographic characteristics and prognostic predictors of ulcerative colitis. *World Journal of Gastroenterology*, *20*(28), 9458–9467. doi:10.3748/wjg.v20.i28.9458 PMID:25071340 de Souza, H. S., & Fiocchi, C. (2016). Immunopathogenesis of IBD: Current state of the art. *Nature Reviews. Gastroenterology & Hepatology*, *13*(1), 13–27. doi:10.1038/nrgastro.2015.186 PMID:26627550

Deng, Z., Rong, Y., Teng, Y., Mu, J., Zhuang, X., Tseng, M., Samykutty, A., Zhang, L., Yan, J., Miller, D., Suttles, J., & Zhang, H. G. (2017). Broccoli-Derived Nanoparticle Inhibits Mouse Colitis by Activating Dendritic Cell AMP-Activated Protein Kinase. *Molecular Therapy*, *25*(7), 1641–1654. doi:10.1016/j.ymthe.2017.01.025 PMID:28274798

Dou, Y. X., Zhou, J. T., Wang, T. T., Huang, Y. F., Chen, V. P., Xie, Y. L., Lin, Z.-X., Gao, J.-S., Su, Z.-R., & Zeng, H. F. (2018). Self-nanoemulsifying drug delivery system of bruceine D: A new approach for anti-ulcerative colitis. *International Journal of Nanomedicine*, *13*, 5887–5907. doi:10.2147/IJN.S174146 PMID:30319255

Feuerstein, J. D., & Cheifetz, A. S. (2014). Ulcerative colitis: Epidemiology, diagnosis, and management. *Mayo Clinic Proceedings*, *89*(11), 1553–1563. doi:10.1016/j.mayocp.2014.07.002 PMID:25199861

Fohlinger, M., Palamides, P., Mansmann, U., Beigel, F., Siebeck, M., & Gropp, R. (2016). Immunological profiling of patients with ulcerative colitis leads to identification of two inflammatory conditions and CD1a as a disease marker. *Journal of Translational Medicine*, *14*(1), 310. doi:10.118612967-016-1048-9 PMID:27809916

Gallinger, Z. R., Rumman, A., Pivovarov, K., Fortinsky, K. J., Steinhart, A. H., & Weizman, A. V. (2017). Frequency and Variables Associated with Fasting Orders in Inpatients with Ulcerative Colitis: The Audit of Diet Orders-Ulcerative Colitis (ADORE-UC) Study. *Inflammatory Bowel Diseases*, *23*(10), 1790–1795. doi:10.1097/MIB.0000000000001244 PMID:28906293

Gou, S., Huang, Y., Wan, Y., Ma, Y., Zhou, X., Tong, X., Huang, J., Kang, Y., Pan, G., Dai, F., & Xiao, B. (2019). Multi-bioresponsive silk fibroin-based nanoparticles with on-demand cytoplasmic drug release capacity for CD44-targeted alleviation of ulcerative colitis. *Biomaterials*, *212*, 39–54. doi:10.1016/j.biomaterials.2019.05.012 PMID:31103945

Guada, M., Beloqui, A., Alhouayek, M., Muccioli, G. G., Dios-Vieitez Mdel, C., Preat, V., & Blanco-Prieto, M. J. (2016). Cyclosporine A-loaded lipid nanoparticles in inflammatory bowel disease. *International Journal of Pharmaceutics*, *503*(1-2), 196–198. doi:10.1016/j.ijpharm.2016.03.012 PMID:26972380

Gugulothu, D., Kulkarni, A., Patravale, V., & Dandekar, P. (2014). pH-sensitive nanoparticles of curcumin-celecoxib combination: Evaluating drug synergy in ulcerative colitis model. *Journal of Pharmaceutical Sciences*, *103*(2), 687–696. doi:10.1002/jps.23828 PMID:24375287

Huang, Y., Guo, J., & Gui, S. (2018). Orally targeted galactosylated chitosan poly(lactic-co-glycolic acid) nanoparticles loaded with TNF-a siRNA provide a novel strategy for the experimental treatment of ulcerative colitis. *European Journal of Pharmaceutical Sciences*, *125*, 232–243. doi:10.1016/j.ejps.2018.10.009 PMID:30315858

Iglesias, N., Galbis, E., Diaz-Blanco, M. J., Lucas, R., Benito, E., & de-Paz, M. V. (2019). Nanostructured Chitosan-Based Biomaterials for Sustained and Colon-Specific Resveratrol Release. *International Journal of Molecular Sciences*, *20*(2), 398. Advance online publication. doi:10.3390/ijms20020398 PMID:30669264

Iwao, Y., Tomiguchi, I., Domura, A., Mantaira, Y., Minami, A., Suzuki, T., Ikawa, T., Kimura, S., & Itai, S. (2018). Inflamed site-specific drug delivery system based on the interaction of human serum albumin nanoparticles with myeloperoxidase in a murine model of experimental colitis. *European Journal of Pharmaceutics and Biopharmaceutics*, *125*, 141–147. doi:10.1016/j.ejpb.2018.01.016 PMID:29407223

Jain, S., Garg, T., Kushwah, V., Thanki, K., Agrawal, A. K., & Dora, C. P. (2017). alpha-Tocopherol as functional excipient for resveratrol and coenzyme Q10-loaded SNEDDS for improved bioavailability and prophylaxis of breast cancer. *Journal of Drug Targeting*, *25*(6), 554–565. doi:10.1080/1061186X.2017.1298603 PMID:28274130

Jostins, L., Ripke, S., Weersma, R. K., Duerr, R. H., McGovern, D. P., Hui, K. Y., Lee, J. C., Philip Schumm, L., Sharma, Y., Anderson, C. A., Essers, J., Mitrovic, M., Ning, K., Cleynen, I., Theatre, E., Spain, S. L., Raychaudhuri, S., Goyette, P., Wei, Z., ... Cho, J. H. (2012). Host-microbe interactions have shaped the genetic architecture of inflammatory bowel disease. *Nature*, *491*(7422), 119–124. doi:10.1038/nature11582 PMID:23128233

Li, J., Chen, H., Wang, B., Cai, C., Yang, X., Chai, Z., & Feng, W. (2017). ZnO nanoparticles act as supportive therapy in DSS-induced ulcerative colitis in mice by maintaining gut homeostasis and activating Nrf2 signaling. *Scientific Reports*, *7*(1), 43126. doi:10.1038rep43126 PMID:28233796

Naeem, M., Bae, J., Oshi, M. A., Kim, M. S., Moon, H. R., Lee, B. L., ... Yoo, J. W. (2018). Colon-targeted delivery of cyclosporine A using dual-functional Eudragit((R)) FS30D/PLGA nanoparticles ameliorates murine experimental colitis. *International Journal of Nanomedicine*, *13*, 1225–1240. doi:10.2147/IJN.S157566 PMID:29535519

Naeem, M., Oshi, M. A., Kim, J., Lee, J., Cao, J., Nurhasni, H., Im, E., Jung, Y., & Yoo, J. W. (2018). pH-triggered surface charge-reversal nanoparticles alleviate experimental murine colitis via selective accumulation in inflamed colon regions. *Nanomedicine (London)*, *14*(3), 823–834. doi:10.1016/j.nano.2018.01.003 PMID:29353017

Ng, S. C., Tang, W., Ching, J. Y., Wong, M., Chow, C. M., Hui, A. J., Wong, T. C., Leung, V. K., Tsang, S. W., Yu, H. H., Li, M. F., Ng, K. K., Kamm, M. A., Studd, C., Bell, S., Leong, R., de Silva, H. J., Kasturiratne, A., Mufeena, M. N. F., ... Chan, F. K. L. (2013). Incidence and phenotype of inflammatory bowel disease based on results from the Asia-pacific Crohn's and colitis epidemiology study. *Gastroenterology*, *145*(1), 158–165 e152. doi:10.1053/j.gastro.2013.04.007 PMID:23583432

Ordas, I., Eckmann, L., Talamini, M., Baumgart, D. C., & Sandborn, W. J. (2012). Ulcerative colitis. *Lancet*, *380*(9853), 1606–1619. doi:10.1016/S0140-6736(12)60150-0 PMID:22914296

Owczarek, D., Rodacki, T., Domagala-Rodacka, R., Cibor, D., & Mach, T. (2016). Diet and nutritional factors in inflammatory bowel diseases. *World Journal of Gastroenterology*, *22*(3), 895–905. doi:10.3748/wjg.v22.i3.895 PMID:26811635

Pei, L. Y., Ke, Y. S., Zhao, H. H., Wang, L., Jia, C., Liu, W. Z., Fu, Q., Shi, M., Cui, J., & Li, S. C. (2019). Role of colonic microbiota in the pathogenesis of ulcerative colitis. *BMC Gastroenterology*, *19*(1), 10. doi:10.118612876-019-0930-3 PMID:30642266

Permpoon, V., Pongpirul, K., & Anuras, S. (2016). Ethnic variations in ulcerative colitis: Experience of an international hospital in Thailand. *World Journal of Gastrointestinal Pharmacology and Therapeutics*, *7*(3), 428–433. doi:10.4292/wjgpt.v7.i3.428 PMID:27602244

Poh, S., Putt, K. S., & Low, P. S. (2017). Folate-Targeted Dendrimers Selectively Accumulate at Sites of Inflammation in Mouse Models of Ulcerative Colitis and Atherosclerosis. *Biomacromolecules*, *18*(10), 3082–3088. doi:10.1021/acs.biomac.7b00728 PMID:28863264

Quezada, S. M., & Cross, R. K. (2012). Association of age at diagnosis and ulcerative colitis phenotype. *Digestive Diseases and Sciences*, *57*(9), 2402–2407. doi:10.100710620-012-2081-z PMID:22370916

Rachmawati, H., Pradana, A. T., Safitri, D., & Adnyana, I. K. (2017). Multiple Functions of D-alpha-Tocopherol Polyethylene Glycol 1000 Succinate (TPGS) as Curcumin Nanoparticle Stabilizer: In Vivo Kinetic Profile and Anti-Ulcerative Colitis Analysis in Animal Model. *Pharmaceutics*, *9*(3), 24. Advance online publication. doi:10.3390/pharmaceutics9030024 PMID:28754010

Roth, M. P., Petersen, G. M., McElree, C., Feldman, E., & Rotter, J. I. (1989). Geographic origins of Jewish patients with inflammatory bowel disease. *Gastroenterology*, *97*(4), 900–904. doi:10.1016/0016-5085(89)91495-9 PMID:2777043

Saadati, H. R., Wittig, M., Helbig, I., Hasler, R., Anderson, C. A., Mathew, C. G., Kupcinskas, L., Parkes, M., Karlsen, T. H., Rosenstiel, P., Schreiber, S., & Franke, A. (2016). Genome-wide rare copy number variation screening in ulcerative colitis identifies potential susceptibility loci. *BMC Medical Genetics*, *17*(1), 26. doi:10.118612881-016-0289-z PMID:27037036

Sasaki, M., & Klapproth, J. M. (2012). The role of bacteria in the pathogenesis of ulcerative colitis. *Journal of Signal Transduction*, *704953*, 1–6. Advance online publication. doi:10.1155/2012/704953 PMID:22619714

Seo, G. S., & Chae, S. C. (2014). Biological therapy for ulcerative colitis: An update. *World Journal of Gastroenterology*, *20*(37), 13234–13238. doi:10.3748/wjg.v20.i37.13234 PMID:25309060

Siczek, K., Zatorski, H., Chmielowiec-Korzeniowska, A., Pulit-Prociak, J., Smiech, M., Kordek, R., Tymczyna, L., Banach, M., & Fichna, J. (2017). Synthesis and evaluation of anti-inflammatory properties of silver nanoparticle suspensions in experimental colitis in mice. *Chemical Biology & Drug Design*, *89*(4), 538–547. doi:10.1111/cbdd.12876 PMID:27696734

Silverberg, M. S., Satsangi, J., Ahmad, T., Arnott, I. D., Bernstein, C. N., Brant, S. R., . . . Warren, B. F. (2005). Toward an integrated clinical, molecular and serological classification of inflammatory bowel disease: report of a Working Party of the 2005 Montreal World Congress of Gastroenterology. *Can J Gastroenterol, 19 Suppl A*, 5A-36A. 10.1155/2005/269076

Stallmach, A., Hagel, S., & Bruns, T. (2010). Adverse effects of biologics used for treating IBD. *Best Practice & Research. Clinical Gastroenterology*, *24*(2), 167–182. doi:10.1016/j.bpg.2010.01.002 PMID:20227030

Tang, H., Xiang, D., Wang, F., Mao, J., Tan, X., & Wang, Y. (2017). 5-ASA-loaded SiO2 nanoparticles-a novel drug delivery system targeting therapy on ulcerative colitis in mice. *Molecular Medicine Reports*, *15*(3), 1117–1122. doi:10.3892/mmr.2017.6153 PMID:28138699

Tatiya-Aphiradee, N., Chatuphonprasert, W., & Jarukamjorn, K. (2018). Immune response and inflammatory pathway of ulcerative colitis. *Journal of Basic and Clinical Physiology and Pharmacology*, *30*(1), 1–10. doi:10.1515/jbcpp-2018-0036 PMID:30063466

Wang, J. L., Gan, Y. J., Iqbal, S., Jiang, W., Yuan, Y. Y., & Wang, J. (2018). Delivery of tacrolimus with cationic lipid-assisted nanoparticles for ulcerative colitis therapy. *Biomaterials Science*, *6*(7), 1916–1922. doi:10.1039/C8BM00463C PMID:29850666

Wang, Y., Shen, W., Shi, X., Fu, F., Fan, Y., Shen, W., Cao, Y., Zhang, Q., & Qi, R. (2017). Alpha-Tocopheryl Succinate-Conjugated G5 PAMAM Dendrimer Enables Effective Inhibition of Ulcerative Colitis. *Advanced Healthcare Materials*, *6*(14), 1700276. Advance online publication. doi:10.1002/adhm.201700276 PMID:28474434

Wu, Y., Sun, M., Wang, D., Li, G., Huang, J., Tan, S., Bao, L., Li, Q., Li, G., & Si, L. (2019). A PepT1 mediated medicinal nano-system for targeted delivery of cyclosporine A to alleviate acute severe ulcerative colitis. *Biomaterials Science*, *7*(10), 4299–4309. doi:10.1039/C9BM00925F PMID:31408067

Xiao, B., Chen, Q., Zhang, Z., Wang, L., Kang, Y., Denning, T., & Merlin, D. (2018). TNFalpha gene silencing mediated by orally targeted nanoparticles combined with interleukin-22 for synergistic combination therapy of ulcerative colitis. *Journal of Controlled Release*, *287*, 235–246. doi:10.1016/j.jconrel.2018.08.021 PMID:30107214

Xiao, B., Xu, Z., Viennois, E., Zhang, Y., Zhang, Z., Zhang, M., Han, M. K., Kang, Y., & Merlin, D. (2017). Orally Targeted Delivery of Tripeptide KPV via Hyaluronic Acid-Functionalized Nanoparticles Efficiently Alleviates Ulcerative Colitis. *Molecular Therapy*, *25*(7), 1628–1640. doi:10.1016/j.ymthe.2016.11.020 PMID:28143741

Xiao, B., Zhang, Z., Viennois, E., Kang, Y., Zhang, M., Han, M. K., Chen, J., & Merlin, D. (2016). Combination Therapy for Ulcerative Colitis: Orally Targeted Nanoparticles Prevent Mucosal Damage and Relieve Inflammation. *Theranostics*, *6*(12), 2250–2266. doi:10.7150/thno.15710 PMID:27924161

Yazeji, T., Moulari, B., Beduneau, A., Stein, V., Dietrich, D., Pellequer, Y., & Lamprecht, A. (2017). Nanoparticle-based delivery enhances anti-inflammatory effect of low molecular weight heparin in experimental ulcerative colitis. *Drug Delivery*, *24*(1), 811–817. doi:10.1080/10717544.2017.1324530 PMID:28509629

Zhang, M., Viennois, E., Prasad, M., Zhang, Y., Wang, L., Zhang, Z., Han, M. K., Xiao, B., Xu, C., Srinivasan, S., & Merlin, D. (2016). Edible ginger-derived nanoparticles: A novel therapeutic approach for the prevention and treatment of inflammatory bowel disease and colitis-associated cancer. *Biomaterials*, *101*, 321–340. doi:10.1016/j.biomaterials.2016.06.018 PMID:27318094

Zhang, M., Xu, C., Liu, D., Han, M. K., Wang, L., & Merlin, D. (2018). Oral Delivery of Nanoparticles Loaded With Ginger Active Compound, 6-Shogaol, Attenuates Ulcerative Colitis and Promotes Wound Healing in a Murine Model of Ulcerative Colitis. *Journal of Crohn's and Colitis*, *12*(2), 217–229. doi:10.1093/ecco-jcc/jjx115 PMID:28961808

Zhang, X., Ma, Y., Ma, L., Zu, M., Song, H., & Xiao, B. (2019). Oral administration of chondroitin sulfate-functionalized nanoparticles for colonic macrophage-targeted drug delivery. *Carbohydrate Polymers*, *223*, 115126. doi:10.1016/j.carbpol.2019.115126 PMID:31426992

Zhou, H., & Qian, H. (2018). Preparation and characterization of pH-sensitive nanoparticles of budesonide for the treatment of ulcerative colitis. *Drug Design, Development and Therapy*, *12*, 2601–2609. doi:10.2147/DDDT.S170676 PMID:30174414

Zhu, S., Jiang, X., Boudreau, M. D., Feng, G., Miao, Y., Dong, S., Wu, H., Zeng, M., & Yin, J. J. (2018). Orally administered gold nanoparticles protect against colitis by attenuating Toll-like receptor 4- and reactive oxygen/nitrogen species-mediated inflammatory responses but could induce gut dysbiosis in mice. *Journal of Nanobiotechnology*, *16*(1), 86. doi:10.118612951-018-0415-5 PMID:30384844

Chapter 6
Yoga Therapy on Digestive Function in Inflammatory Bowel Disease

Soccalingam Artchoudane
https://orcid.org/0000-0002-7826-0430
Center for Yogic Sciences, Aarupadai Veedu Medical College and Hospital, Vinayaka Mission's Research Foundation, India

ABSTRACT

Inflammatory bowel disease (IBD) is a psychosomatic disorder characterized by chronic inflammation of the gastrointestinal tract. Metabolism of an individual affected with IBD is equated to imbalance of jatharagni (digestive fire) which results in atijeernam (hyper digestive disorder), ajeernam (hypo digestive disorder), or kutajeernam (erroneous digestive disorder). Yoga stabilizes jatharagni that helps energy transformation of 1) food substances into nutritious substance, 2) nutritious substance into tissues. It improves anabolic and catabolic processes which help absorption of energy. Yogic cleansing techniques promote elimination of ama (toxic products) and kleda (waste products). Yoga therapy along with herbal medicine and lifestyle modification helps develop balanced state of doshas in individuals with IBD. Yoga practice has a healing effect on mind and body, reduces stress, increases emotional and physical self-awareness, and improves the ability to manage physical symptoms.

DOI: 10.4018/978-1-7998-3580-6.ch006

INTRODUCTION

Inflammatory Bowel Disease (IBD) is a psychosomatic disease characterized by chronic mental agitation or stress. It includes Crohn's disease (CD) which affects the entire digestive tract and Ulcerative colitis (UC) which affects the colon (large intestine). Both are the most common prolonged inflammation of the gastrointestinal tract (GIT) and an abnormal response to the body's immune system. India has the highest incidence and prevalence rates of IBD among Asian countries with CD more prominent in South India and UC in North India (Kedia and Ahuja, 2017). Although the disease prevalence in India is lower than in the West, the overall estimated IBD population in India came out to be 1.4 million. The rising incidence of IBD and prevalence of UC in India alone is 6.02/100,000 as per Asia-Pacific Crohn's and Colitis Epidemiologic Study (Kedia and Ahuja, 2017). Several studies consistently indicate that UC and CD are associated with a higher prevalence in India. The IBD survey reported that affected male and female ratio in India is 1:4 and 1:3 for UC and CD respectively.

UC has a slow and gradual effect and is not clinically severe until the consequences manifest, such as fulminant hepatitis, cancer, surgery and related complications. The other factors may be medically compliant high risk UC, development of polyps, low grade dysplasia (LGD), high grade dysplasia (HGD), dysplasia associated lesion or mass and CRC in the sequence followed by sporadic CRC. Unpredicted development of UC related colorectal cancer requires strict screening protocol. The chronic inflammations of the abdomen involve intestine, peritoneum, lymph nodes, or solid abdominal organs and an association of up to 50% of tuberculosis in patients with human immunodeficiency virus positivity (Sharma and Ahuja, 2009; Sharma and Mohan, 2004). Intestinal tuberculosis (ITB) may be localized to the bowel, terminal ileum and ileocecal junction that are the most common sites of involvement followed by the colon and jejunum (Tandon et al., 1986). The symptoms are common in patients with CD or ITB that include abdominal pain, chronic diarrhoea, recurrent bowel obstruction, rectal bleeding, fever, anorexia, weight loss, perianal fistula and in latter stage extraintestinal manifestations such as polyarthritis, uveitis and erythema nodosum. ITB and CD are chronic granulomatous disorders with phenotypic similarities and have close resemblance in the clinical, radiological, endoscopic, surgical, and histological features that make the differentiation between these two conditions challenging. Irritable bowel syndrome (IBS) is a condition with similar symptoms to IBD that does not cause inflammation, permanent damage to GI tract, increased risk of CRC, but affects the function and behavior of the intestines. Celiac disease is another condition with similar symptoms to IBD that are characterized by inflammation of the intestines and it is reversible with gluten free diet.

PATHOGENESIS OF IBD

The imbalance of higher bodies, energy, mental, wisdom and bliss bodies alter biofeedback mechanism and the association of psychosocial factors, sociocultural factors, smoking, dietary habits and repeated use of drugs affects genetic predisposition which may lead to abnormal communication of gut-brain axis. Undseth et al. (2014) found that altered gut-brain activity resulted in significantly lower postprandial levels of total short chain fatty acids (SCFAs like Faecali bacterium prausnitzii and Roseburia intestinalis), acetic acid, propionic acid and butyric acid (Venegas et al., 2019). Bacteroidetes (gram-negative) mainly produce acetate and propionate while Firmicutes (gram-positive) mostly produce butyrate; both are abundant phyla in the human intestine. The main substrates for bacterial fermentation and SCFA production are resistant starch, inulin, pectin, cellulose, wheat bran, oat bran and guar gum from the non-digestible dietary fibres (NDDF). Anaerobic fermentation occurs in the NDDF produced which split into carbohydrate polymers with three or more monomeric units, that are neither digested nor absorbed in the human gut.

The exaggerated pituitary-adrenal response to corticotrophin releasing hormone (CRH), elevated levels of plasma proinflammatory cytokines and gut mucosal immune attacking luminal antigens (probiotics, harmless viruses, fiber-rich protein) cause augmented visceral pain. Although other influences (including genetic, psychosocial, sociocultural and immunological factors) have subsequently been implicated to play a major role in the pathogenesis of IBD, several recent studies have suggested that the inflammation occurs bidirectionally. IBD patients with anxiety and depression were more likely to have elevated IL-6, tumor necrosis factor TNF-α, and the acute-phase protein, C-reactive protein (Santoft et al., 2020; Miłkowska et al., 2017). Thus psychiatric illnesses and stress cause increased intensity of disease in patients with IBD.

YOGIC OBSERVATION OF IBD

Yoga therapy is a holistic approach for treatment of stress and IBD. In the Bhagavad Gita (2.48) one of the definitions of yoga is given as, *yogasthah kuru karmani sangam tyaktva dhananjaya siddhyasiddhyoh samobhutva samatvam yoga uchyate,* (Vaniquotes, 2018) which means, to concentrate the mind upon the higher entity by controlling the ever disturbing senses. This is the approach on following which hypothalamic pituitary adrenal (HPA) and renin-angiotensin-aldosterone (RAA) axes are regulated. The balance of biofeedback mechanism has multiple benefits that improve strength, concentration and focus whereas lack of equilibrium brings the opposite. When an individual suffers or loses balance in life, besides bringing frustration it also damages quality of behavior and disturbs homeostasis which affects the digestive system.

According to Ayurveda, *sama dosha sama agnischa sama dhatu mala kriyaaha prasanna atma indriya manaha swastha iti abhidheeyate,* (Bhavanani, 2013) this means that the root cause of all disorders lies in poor digestion. Balance of the three *doshas* (*Vata, Pitta* and *Kapha*) governs all the physiological, psychological and spiritual aspects of one's life. Every food substance has certain predominant physical properties (*doshas*) and predominant subtle qualities (*guna*). *Vata* has dry and light properties and it is antagonistic to *Kapha* that is oily and heavy. Similarly the property of *Pitta* is heat and it is antagonistic to *Kapha* and *Vata* which are cold. Hence when two or three *doshas* are severely vitiated; they intertwine, interact and produce a toxic substance (*ama*) from dominant physical properties. The accumulation of toxins and impurities are mainly due to consumption of food containing a large amount of *pitta dosha*. *Vata dosha* is also vitiated due to lifestyle risk factors which cause imbalance in metabolism.

Metabolism can be equated to *agni* (digestive fire) which includes digestion, absorption, and assimilation. It is certain that imbalanced state of *agni* results in *atijeernam* (hyper digestive disorder), *ajeernam* (hypo digestive disorder), or *kutajeernam* (erroneous digestive disorder) that cause inflammatory bowel disease (IBD) which includes Crohn's disease (CD), ulcerative colitis (UC), irritable bowel syndrome (IBS). The *agni* activity takes place in accordance with physical property and subtle quality of food substance. The action of *agni* leads to energy transformation of i) food substances into nutritious substance, ii) nutritious substance into tissues. This process of *agni* activity is anabolic in which tissue substance is digested and disintegrated while its absorption for the liberation of heat and energy is a catabolic process. During disintegration of tissues, certain minute waste products are formed known as *kleda*. *Kleda* gets accumulated in the body which results in the formation of toxic substance known as *ama*.

The process of metabolism has an important role in formation of *sapta dhatu* (seven tissues). *Samadhatu* means balanced state of these tissues, *rasa* (plasma), *rakta* (blood), *mamsa* (muscle), *medha* (fat), *asthi* (bone), *majja* (bone marrow) and *shukra* (semen) in male / *artava* (ovum) in female, and finally *ojas* (vital force of the body) that is responsible for hormone secretion like serotonin (for wakefulness), melatonin (for sleep), or dopamine (for alertness). Imbalanced states of *dhatu* affect mental health, digestion, sleep cycle and thus cause risk factors for IBD. The imbalance in *doshas* results in *pitta atisara* (excess of pitta) and *rakta atisara* (excessive bleeding), its major symptoms that are relevant to IBD are diarrhoea, rectal bleeding, tenesmus, passing of mucus, crampy abdominal pain, loose stools, bloody stools, rectal bleeding, rectal urgency (sensation of incomplete evacuation despite an empty rectal vault) and proctitis. Other associated symptoms are anemia due to blood loss, fatigue, fever, nausea, weight loss, loss of appetite, abdominal sounds, mouth ulcers, loss of body fluids and nutrients, skin lesions and growth failure in children. It usually involves the rectum and extends proximally to involve all or part of the colon similar to UC and IBD. There are no biomarkers that have adequate diagnostic sensitivity and specificity for IBD.

Diet plays an active role in prevention and treatment of IBD. Modern science commonly recommends diets such as specific carbohydrate diets which consist of low-fermentable oligosaccharide, disaccharide, monosaccharide, polyol and anti-inflammatory agents for IBD patients (Knight-Sepulveda et al., 2015).

Lifestyle Risk Factors for IBD

Yogic principles state that the nature of diet influences human mind. The quantity and quality of food consumed by the body impacts the mind.

1. *Sattvik ahar* (sentient food): Food which increases subtle or high and pure quality of the mind and is conducive to physical and mental well-being. *Aharashuddhao Sattvashudhih* means sentient diet produces sentient body that emanates radiant auras (highly evolved being). Examples of sentient food are rice, wheat and barley, all kinds of pulses, fresh milk, fresh fruits, most green vegetables, etc.
2. *Rajasik ahar* (mutative food): Food which gives gross energy to the body and may not be good for the mind is mutative, for example, chilli, chocolate, tea, coffee etc.
3. *Tamasik ahar* (static food): Food which is harmful for the mind and imparts heaviness or sluggishness to the body is static food, for example, onion, garlic, mushroom, stale and rotten food, alcohol, eggs, meat of large animals such as buffaloes, etc.

The excessive intake of rajasik or tamasik ahar along with sedentary or sluggish lifestyle may influence both the risks of developing IBD and intestinal mucosal inflammation. Kaplan and Korelitz (1988); Buckley et al. (2015); Edwards et al. (2001); Sanford et al. (2014) have reported that IBD patients using narcotics were more likely to suffer from comorbid mental health illnesses compared to other IBD patients. Mantzouranis et al. (2018); Jowett et al. (2004); and Magee et al. (2005) have concluded that sedentary lifestyle along with high intake of sulfite which is a common additive in alcoholic drinks associated with increased risk of relapses and disease activity in patients with IBD. Lichtenstein et al. (2012); Kaplan and Korelitz (1988) have found IBD patients using narcotics to be a significant factor for IBD complications. Cohen et al. (2013) have studied that narcotics was used for analgesia among adult and young IBD patients which causes psychological dysfunction and impairs quality of life. Kerlin et al. (2018) found that narcotics was used as an alternative therapy or supplement to standard treatments in IBD patients. The addiction to alcohol is basically caused by a mental illusory state; the individual then consciously develops deleterious health effects, chronic inflammatory disorders like IBD. It not only affects the physical health but also affects mental health.

Risk Factors of IBD

Jatharagni (digestive fire or enzymes and hormones in second part of duodenum) is essential for complete and proper digestion of food. Due to low or high digestive fire, *ama* is created from *ajeerna* (diminished agni), *atijeerna* (increased agni), or *kutajeerna* (erroneous agni) that results in improperly digested food particles or toxic particles which accumulate wherever there is weakness in the body. Thus it affects elimination, gets retained in the intestine for a longer time and creates psychological imbalance. Due to this retention, fermentation or even putrefaction takes place. This is the root cause of all diseases and complication of diseases mainly in the intestines, lymphatic system, arteries and veins, capillaries, and genitourinary tract. Other nonphysical channels called *nadis* through which energy flows also get affected.

SOME APPROACHES OF MODERN SCIENCE ON IBD

Peripheral inflammation and psychiatric symptoms including anxiety and depression have become an important focus within biological psychiatry. Increased circulating TNF-α with immune activation is linked to the intensity of gastrointestinal symptoms of CD. Both depression and anxiety are more prevalent when IBD is active compared to when in remission. However psychological and gastrointestinal symptoms continue in a substantial proportion of patients despite mucosal healing. Characterized gastrointestinal symptoms are abdominal pain, malabsorption, diarrhea, rectal bleeding with resultant anemia, poor growth, nutritional deficiencies, and a host of other manifestations. Associations between negative mood and perceived stress with IBD relapse, hospitalization and risk of abdominal surgery suggest that stress reduction may improve the quality of life in individuals with IBD (Bannaga & Selinger, 2015; Sun et al., 2019).

The pathophysiology of IBD comprises multifactorial or multipart interplay between genetic predisposition, the gut microbiota, gut mucosal integrity, the immune system, and environmental triggers such as nutrition, psychosocial and sociocultural stressors. Conventional modern treatments consist of anti-inflammatory pharmacologic therapies, 5-aminosalicylic acid derivatives, corticosteroids and immunomodulators (6-mercaptopurine, methotrexate) (Bannaga & Selinger, 2015). Harris et al. (2016) and Hartman et al. (2016) found that oral administration of purified antibodies (anti-TNF drug AVX-470, molecular weight * 160-900 kDa) are inadequately absorbed in the systemic circulation and found clinically ineffective. Vermeire et al. (2011); Vermeire et al. (2017); and Sandborn et al. (2018) have analysed the failure of nti-adhesion drug, intolerance to anti-TNF or immunosuppressant drugs that are statistically insignificant. Sandborn et al. (2008) and Feagan et al. (2016) have studied immune modulation of IBD patients and found that the proliferation of type 1 and type 17 helper cells stimulated proinflammatory cytokines, interleukin 12 and 23 in moderate-to-severe CD as in psoriasis (Leonardi et al., 2008). Weisshof et al. (2018) have found that more number of therapies will emerge in time if supported by results of present clinical trials; this will enable physicians as well as patients to choose the best therapies, unhindered by limitations.

ROLE OF ALTERNATIVE THERAPIES ON IBD

Ayurvedic medicines derived from plants and other natural sources based on traditional system of medicine are potently effective for treatment of UC, CD, IBD. Major constituents of plant materials are extracted by the process of fermentation (*kasayam, arishtam, asava*) for IBD. The immunomodulatory properties of fruits of *terminalia chebula, terminalia belerica* and *emblica officinalis* present in fermented preparations are effective anti-inflammatory agents.

Anti-inflammatory agents present in *Terminalia chebula* are i) tannins: chebulinic acid (Lee et al., 2010), chebulagic acid, corilagin, neochebulinic acid (Reddy et al., 2009; Reddy et al., 2010), ellagic acid, gallic acid, punicalagin, terflavin-a, terchebin, ii) flavonoids: rutins, quercetin, luteolin (Suryaprakash et al., 2012), iii) phytochemicals: saponins, β-D-glucogallin, 1, 3, 6-trigalloyl glucose, anthraquinones, 1, 2, 3, 4, 6-penta-O-galloyl, and iv) other fatty acids, amino acids and carbohydrates (Rastogi & Mehrotra, Vol. 1:1990; Rastogi & Mehrotra, Vol. 3:1993; Rastogi & Mehrotra, Vol. 5:1995; Saleem et al., 2002; Gokhale, Kokate and Purohit, 2003; Juang and Sheu, 2005).

List of anti-inflammatory effects of *terminalia chebula* i) antifungal (Nagar et al., 2011; Dutta, Rahman & Das, 1998; Bajpai et al., 2010; Shinde et al., 2011), ii) antibacterial: Gram-positive and Gram-negative bacteria (Malekzadeh et al., 2001; Ghosh et al., 2008; Kannan, Ramadevi & Waheeta, 2009; Nagar et al., 2011), iii) antiviral: against cytomegalovirus, herpes simplex viruses, human immunodeficiency viruses, swine influenza A virus (Yukawa et al., 1996; Kim et al., 2001; Ma et al., 2010).

It is indicated that *treminalia chebula* has anti-inflammatory, anti-oxidant (Suchalatha, Srinivasulu & Devi, 2005; Chang & Lin, 2010), anti-mutagenic (Grover and Bala, 1992; Kaur et al., 2002), anti-nociceptive (Kaur and Jaggi, 2010), anti-anaphylactic properties and is effective in wound healing (Singh and Sharma, 2009; Choudhary, 2011). These properties act strongly against hepatitis B surface antigen, inhibits IL-1β, IL-6, TNF-α, IFN-β, and also additional neutrophils and macrophages at site of inflammation (Conforti et al., 2009). This inhibition and immunomodulation through TH1 and TH2 cytokines can be correlated with therapy for IBD (Mohan et al., 2011).

Terminalia bellerica acts as a rejuvenator, blood purifier and brain tonic. It contains i) gallotannins: gallic acid, ethylgallate, galloyl glucose, gallotannic acid, ellagic acid; ii) lignins: anolignan-B, termilignin, thannilignin; iii) oils (30-40%): linoleic, oleic, palmitic and stearic acid; iv) other: chebulaginic acid, anthraquinones, phenyllemblin, bellaricanin, carbohydrates; and v) effect: anti-inflammatory, anti-emetic, anti-pyretic, anti-diabetic, anti-diarrhoeal, anti-oxidant, astringent and analgesic (Tariq et al., 1977; Suthienkul et al., 1993; Shaila, Udupa AL, & Udupa SL, 1995; Anand et al., 1997; Ahmad, Mehmood & Mohammad, 1998; Aqil et al., 2005).

Emblica officinalis is highly beneficial for its properties such as gastroprotective (Al-Rehaily et al., 2002), hepatoprotective (Jeena, Joy & Kuttan, 1999; Jose & Kuttan, 2000), cytoprotective (Sairam et al., 2002), radioprotective (Singh et al., 2005). It helps protect against cataract (Suryanarayana et al., 2004), hyperthyroidism (Panda and Kar, 2003), hyperlipidemia (Mishra, Pathak & Khan, 1981; Thakur et al., 1988; Mathur et al., 1996; Kim et al., 2005), atherosclerosis (Bhattacharya et al., 2002; Rajak et al., 2004), and ulcer (Ghosh, Sharma & Talukder, 1992; Xia et al., 1997; Bandyopadhyay, Pakrashi & Pakrashi, 2000; Haque et al., 2001; Harikumar et al., 2004; Perianayagam et al., 2004; Suryanarayana et al., 2004; Sancheti et al., 2005; Duan & Zhang, 2005).

Ravishankar and Shukla (2007) have briefed the important role of Indian System of Medicine including Ayurveda, Siddha and Unani in providing health care. Belapurkar, Goyal and Tiwari-Barua (2014) have studied the immunomodulatory potential of *Terminalia bellerica*, *Terminalia chebula* and *Emblica officinalis*.

APPROACH OF YOGA THERAPY

Yoga therapy involves counseling, lifestyle modification, cleansing practices, breath movement coordination, breathing practices, incantation of certain sounds, pramitahara (balanced and nutritious diet), meditation or the continuous effortless linkage of the attention to a higher force, object or person. It brings about awareness of the root cause of disease and helps in healing. Yoga as an adjunct therapy for adolescents with IBD showed significant results in the management of chronic IBD and improved health outcomes (Arruda et al., 2018). Sharma et al. (2016) found that yoga improves state and trait anxiety levels and significantly reduces physical symptoms in patients with IBD. Yoga therapy consists of the following tools for IBD:

1. Adults With IBD

Lifestyle Modification: In younger individuals, the chaotic, stressed and hectic lifestyles have a direct effect on the digestive system. IBD is commonly caused by consumption of alcohol, drugs and smoking as well as lack of physical activity and unhealthy eating habits.

Yoga therapy recommends lifestyle modification through i) dietary changes: Lacto-vegetarian or vegetarian diet such as fruits, vegetables, green leaves, legumes, and also fresh sea food; ii) healthy-habits: regular physical exercise or yoga practices, avoiding alcohol and smoking (Chiba et al., 2010; Chiba et al., 2016). The physical *toxins* can be easily reduced by simply changing diet and lifestyle. Yogic lifestyle may reduce many several causes of IBD if the medical community effectively implements the choices for healthy lifestyle (Bodai et al., 2018). The medical community should strictly adhere to the Hippocratic Oath (*First do no harm*) for health. Yoga therapy establishes overall well-being by enhancing psychological health and longevity by means of observing codes of social-disipline (*yama*) and self-discipline (*niyama*).

CODE OF SOCIAL-DISCIPLINE

a. *Ahimsa* - guiding maxim is *do no harm*, adopt beneficent attitude, offer sincere service to those who deserve. It refers to an action done for the benefit of others:
    i. Honesty: one should have strict adherence to *yama* and *niyama*. Honesty and truthfulness are the psychological properties that deal with fear and anxiety. Acts such as deliberately misleading or deceiving others by selective omissions, overstatements, misrepresentations, partial truths, or any other means cause ever increasing mental imbalances.
    ii. Integrity: it demonstrates personal integrity which affects interpersonal and intrapersonal relationship, it is also a psychosocial factor that influences anxiety; principled, honorable and upright. It denotes that one should stand by one's principle and not exchange it for expediency, hypocrisy or unscrupulousness.

iii. Trustworthiness: the effort to fulfill the words and spirit of one's commitments brings psychological balance.

iv. Concern for others: caring, compassionate, benevolent and kind; help those in need, and seek to accomplish business objectives in a rational manner that causes no harm and for the greater good.

v. Reputation and morale: protect and take part in building a healthy society with good reputation and morale; help others to correct or prevent inappropriate conduct.

b. *Satya*: truthfulness
Pay importance to all human virtues and speak truth habitually. It teaches to think before speaking, thought-word-action must be in the same vein, communicate in an open and honest fashion, rational decisions and quick rectification.

c. *Asteya*: non-stealing
It enhances harmonious relationship of body, mind and emotion. It offers the gift of abundance and trust in an abundant universe.

d. *Brahmacharya*: non-sensuous
Yoga offers methods for managing sensory cravings and helps cultivation of self-awareness and transformation of habits.

e. *Aparigraha*: non-avarice
It teaches the virtue of non-possessiveness, non-grasping or non-greediness which is a significant aspect of psychology.

CODE OF SELF-DISCIPLINE

a. *Shauca*: cleanliness
It teaches of purity in mind, speech and body.

b. *Santosha*: contentment
It enables one to have satisfaction, both as an attitude and a state of deep inner peace. It helps to gain relief from cravings, desires and thus bestows the sense of freedom which is essential to pursue spiritual development.

c. *Tapah*: perseverance
It encourages steady discipline, complete and constant focus, and intense commitment necessary to overcome the impediments that keep us from being in true state of yoga.

d. *Svadhyaya*: introspection
It develops virtuous behavior in the practitioner by strict adherence to the principles that the human body is cleansed by water; the mind is cleansed by truth, and wisdom body is cleansed by self-study and meditation.

e. *Ishvara pranidhana*: contemplation
It inculcates commitment and empowerment of personality to succeed in every step of the individual's life.

Cleansing practices (shatkarma): The process of assimilation, digestion and elimination of food is affected because of unhealthy lifestyle in patients with IBD. Internal cleansing techniques are available only in yoga which cleanse and soothe the GI tract in patients with IBD. Cleansing practices can be performed under the supervision of yoga professionals. *Shatkarma* heals and also protects from further inflammation. It improves not only digestive function but also increases the efficiency of respiratory system & gut-brain activity. It is used to clear out *toxins* which might otherwise become stuck or stagnant. All the techniques work on removing physical *toxins* that come from consumption of food, drink, or drugs. These techniques also help psychosomatic disorders by cleansing the gathered mental and emotional *toxins* from thoughts and ideas in the mind. Yogic techniques are useful measures for mental digestion that increases awareness along with understanding and identification of emotions that are creating disturbances inside as a *mental toxin*. Some *shatkarma* techniques for IBD:

a. *Dhauti* (internal cleansing practice) is the method of rejuvenating and cleaning the digestive tract or gastrointestinal tract. Internal organs need cleansing for effective functioning just as a bath is necessary for cleanliness and freshness of the outer body. It eliminates accumulated rotten sludge, undigested food residue (*ama*) from the top of the alimentary canal to the colon through various techniques. *Gajakarani kriya* is one of the variations of *dhauti* which expels undigested content of the stomach from the deep trunk region.
b. *Nauli kriya* is a technique for maintaining and developing suppleness and relaxed state of muscles in the abdominal region and is also useful for decreasing mental stress. It works on the muscles, ligaments and tendons and also applies gentle pressure on the affected area. This helps increase blood flow, accelerates healing process and promotes a healthy digestive system.
c. *Basti kriya* is a technique for cleansing colon and lower intestine. It can be used therapeutically for working with a number of chronic problems including and similar to IBD. As regular bowel movements may stop, and the body can no longer eliminate efficiently the accumulated physical waste and toxins in turn give rise to emotional or mental *toxins*, by administration of *basti* one can easily expel these *toxins*. It enhances elimination of *ama* which helps heal IBD and prevents headache, constipation, piles, and worm infestation.

Strengthening: In chronic IBD, it is not only the digestive system but also respiratory and cardiovascular systems that are affected.

Recommended practices for IBD under the supervision of yoga therapist or yoga professionals:

a. Twisting postures – helps eliminate constipation.
   Eg. *Vakrasana, Ardhamatsyendrasana*
b. Backbending postures – relieves abdominal cramps and diarrhea.
   Eg. *Bhujangasana, Balasana*
c. Prone postures – improves circulation of blood to the abdominal organs.
   Eg. *Merusana, Shashahasana*
d. Supine postures – strengthens the abdominal organs.
   Eg. *Matsyamudra, Viparitakarani mudra*
e. Pranayama – relieves dryness and has soothing effect on wound in the stomach walls.
   Eg. *Sheetali pranayama, Chandra nadi pranayama*
f. Relaxation – enhances healing for body and mind.
   Eg. *Marmanasthana kriya, Shavasana*

Yoga helps heal the inflammation of alimentary canal and improves cardiovascular autonomic functions, eosinophilic cationic protein serum levels, interleukin- 2 soluble receptors, and ameliorates stress in patients with IBD (Sharma et al., 2015). Yoga can also improve significantly the vital capacity as a result of increased vagal modulation, decreased sympathetic activity and improved baroreflex sensitivity and quality of life in patients with IBD (Bhavanani et al., 2011; Artchoudane et al., 2018).

2. Elderly People With IBD

Loss of discipline in *aahar, vihar, aachar, vichar, or vyavahar* causes and aggravates IBD whereas yoga helps implement these disciplines in a proper way which allows healing of digestive disorders (Bhavanani, 2013).

a) *Aahar*: It includes intake of adequate drinking water; healthy, nourishing and balanced diet, fresh food, green salads, sprouts, unrefined cereals and fresh fruits. It is important to be aware of satvik diet, prepared and served with love and affection.
b) *Vihar*: The proper relaxation for body and mind is essential for good health. *Vasudev kutumbukkam* is the sense of transformation from individuality to universality.

c) *Aachar*: Daily practices of asana, pranayama and kriyas are essential healthy activities that improve the digestive system and enhance cardio-respiratory health.
d) *Vichar*: It emphasizes moral restraints and ethical observances which maintain balanced state of mind, right thoughts and right attitude.
e) *Vyavahar*: The development of proper psychological attitudes which improve interpersonal and intrapersonal relationship.

3. Special Children With IBD

IBD is one of the most common disorders with increased risk in children with autism and special needs (Losh et al., 2017). Sympathetic nervous system driven response in stress among special children is higher than normal which leads to atypical sensory process that includes increased heart rate and respiration, and diverts blood from the digestive system to the skeletal muscles in children with ASD (Marco et al., 2011).

Yoga practices improve relaxation response and increase parasympathetic activity which in turn reduces heart rate, blood pressure and respiratory rate which promotes digestion in children with ASD (Ditto et al., 2006; Jain et al., 2007; Artchoudane et al., 2019; Soccalingam et al., 2020).

CONCLUSION

Yoga Therapy regulates the function of *gunas, doshas* and *dhatus* bringing them into balance when affected. Yoga therapy along with herbal medicine and lifestyle modification helps protect and harmonize *doshas* in individuals with IBD. Yogic practices have a healing effect on mind and body, reduces stress, and improves emotional and physical self-awareness. Several studies have found that yoga improves quality of life and anxiety in individuals with IBD.

REFERENCES

Ahmad, I., Mehmood, Z., & Mohammad, F. (1998). Screening of some Indian medicinal plants for their antimicrobial properties. *Journal of Ethnopharmacology*, *62*(2), 183–193. doi:10.1016/S0378-8741(98)00055-5 PMID:9741890

Al-Rehaily, A. J., Al-Howiriny, T. S., Al-Sohaibanib, M. O., & Rafatullah, S. (2002). Gastroprotective effects of 'Amla' Emblica officinalis on in vivo test models in rats. *Phytomedicine*, *9*(6), 515–522. doi:10.1078/09447110260573146 PMID:12403160

Anand, K. K., Singh, B., Saxena, A. K., Chandan, B. K., Gupta, V. N., & Bhardwaj, V. (1997). 3,4,5,-Trihydroxy benzoic acid (gallic acid), the hepatoprotective principle in the fruits of Terminalia belerica-bioassay guided activity. *Pharmacological Research*, *36*(4), 315–321. doi:10.1006/phrs.1997.0236 PMID:9425622

Aqil, F., Khan, M. S., Owais, M., & Ahmad, I. (2005). Effect of certain bioactive plant extracts on clinical isolates of beta-lactamase producing methicillin resistant Staphylococcus aureus. *Journal of Basic Microbiology*, *45*(2), 106–114. doi:10.1002/jobm.200410355 PMID:15812867

Arruda, J. M., Bogetza, A. L., Vellankia, S., Wrenb, A., & Yehb, A. M. (2018). Yoga as adjunct therapy for adolescents with inflammatory bowel disease: A pilot clinical trial. *Complementary Therapies in Medicine*, *41*, 99–104. doi:10.1016/j.ctim.2018.09.007 PMID:30477870

Artchoudane, S., Bhavanani, A. B., Ramanathan, M., & Mariangela, A. (2019). Yoga as a therapeutic tool in autism: A detailed review. *Yoga Mimamsa*, *51*(1), 3–16. doi:10.4103/ym.ym_3_19

Artchoudane, S., Ranganadin, P., Bhavanani, A. B., Ramanathan, M., & Madanmohan, T. (2018). Effect of adjuvant yoga therapy on pulmonary function and quality of life among patients with Chronic Obstructive Pulmonary Disease: A randomized control trial. *SBV J Basic. Cli and Appl Health Science*, *2*, 117–122.

Bajpai, V. K., Rahman, A., Shukla, S., Shukla, S., Arafat, S. M., Hossain, M. A., & … . (2010). In vitro kinetics and antifungal activity of various extracts of Terminalia chebula seeds against plant pathogenic fungi. *Archiv für Phytopathologie und Pflanzenschutz*, *43*(8), 801–809. doi:10.1080/03235400802246887

Bandyopadhyay, S. K., Pakrashi, S. C., & Pakrashi, A. (2000). The role of antioxidant activity of Phyllanthus emblica fruits on prevention from indomethacin induced gastric ulcer. *Journal of Ethnopharmacology*, *70*(2), 171–176. doi:10.1016/S0378-8741(99)00146-4 PMID:10771207

Bannaga, A. S., & Selinger, C. P. (2015). Inflammatory bowel disease and anxiety: Links, risks, and challenges faced. *Clinical and Experimental Gastroenterology*, *8*, 111–117. doi:10.2147/CEG.S57982 PMID:25848313

Belapurkar, P., Goyal, P., & Tiwari-Barua, P. (2014). Immunomodulatory effects of triphala and its individual constituents: A review. *Indian Journal of Pharmaceutical Sciences*, *76*(6), 467–475. PMID:25593379

Bhattacharya, S. K., Bhattacharya, A., Sairam, K., & Ghosa, S. (2002). Effect of bioactive tannoid principles of Emblica officinalis on ischemia-reperfusion-induced oxidative stress in rat heart. *Phytomedicine*, *9*(2), 171–174. doi:10.1078/0944-7113-00090 PMID:11995952

Bhavanani, A. B. (2013). A closing word. In A. B. Bhavanani (Ed.), *Yoga Chikitsa: Application of yoga as a therapy* (1st ed.). Dhivyananda Creations.

Bhavanani, A. B., Sanjay, Z., & Madanmohan, T. (2011). Immediate Effect of Sukha Pranayama on Cardiovascular Variables in Patients of Hypertension. *International Journal of Yoga Therapy*, *21*(1), 73–76. doi:10.17761/ijyt.21.1.y007g51341634172 PMID:22398346

Bodai, B. I., Nakata, T. E., Wong, W. T., Clark, D. R., Lawenda, S., Tsou, C., & … . (2018). Lifestyle Medicine: A Brief Review of Its Dramatic Impact on Health and Survival. *The Permanente Journal*, *22*, 17–025. doi:10.7812/TPP/17-025 PMID:29035175

Buckley, J. P., Cook, S. F., Allen, J. K., & Kappelman, M. D. (2015). Prevalence of chronic narcotic use among children with inflammatory bowel disease. *Clinical Gastroenterology and Hepatology*, *13*(2), 310–315. doi:10.1016/j.cgh.2014.07.057 PMID:25117776

Chang, C. S., & Lin, C. S. (2010). Development of antioxidant activity and pattern recognition of Terminalia chebula Retzius extracts and its fermented products. *Hung Kuang J*, *61*, 115–129.

Chiba, M., Abe, T., Tsuda, H., Sugawara, T., Tsuda, S., Tozawa, H., & … . (2010). Lifestyle-related disease in Crohn's disease: Relapse prevention by a semi-vegetarian diet. *World Journal of Gastroenterology*, *16*(20), 2484–2495. doi:10.3748/wjg.v16.i20.2484 PMID:20503448

Chiba, M., Nakane, K., Takayama, Y., Sugawara, K., Ohno, H., Ishii, H., & … . (2016). Development and Application of a Plant-Based Diet Scoring System for Japanese Patients with Inflammatory Bowel Disease. *The Permanente Journal*, *20*(4), 16–019. doi:10.7812/TPP/16-019 PMID:27768566

Choudhary, G. P. (2011). Wound healing activity of ethanolic extract of Terminalia chebula Retz. *International Journal of Pharma and Bio Sciences*, *2*, 48–52.

Cohen, A. B., Lee, D., Long, M. D., Kappelman, M. D., Martin, C. F., Sandler, R. S., & Lewis, J. D. (2013). Dietary patterns and self-reported associations of diet with symptoms of inflammatory bowel disease. *Digestive Diseases and Sciences*, *58*(5), 1322–1328. doi:10.100710620-012-2373-3 PMID:22923336

Conforti, F., Sosa, S., Marrelli, M., Menichini, F., Statti, G. A., Uzunov, D., Tubaro, A., & Menichini, F. (2009). The protective ability of Mediterranean dietary plants against the oxidative damage: The role of radical oxygen species in inflammation and the polyphenol, flavonoid and sterol contents. *Food Chemistry*, *112*(3), 587–594. doi:10.1016/j.foodchem.2008.06.013

Ditto, B., Eclache, M., & Goldman, N. (2006). Short-term autonomic and cardiovascular effects of mindfulness body scan meditation. *Annals of Behavioral Medicine*, *32*(3), 227–234. doi:10.120715324796abm3203_9 PMID:17107296

Duan, W., Yu, Y., & Zhang, L. (2005). Antiatherogenic effects of Phyllanthus emblica associated with corilagin and it analogue. *Yakugaku Zasshi*, *125*(7), 587–591. doi:10.1248/yakushi.125.587 PMID:15997216

Dutta, B. K., Rahman, I., & Das, T. K. (1998). Antifungal activity of Indian plant extracts. *Mycoses*, *41*(11-12), 535–536. doi:10.1111/j.1439-0507.1998.tb00718.x PMID:9919899

Edwards, J. T., Radford-Smith, G. L., & Florin, T. H. (2001). Chronic narcotic use in inflammatory bowel disease patients: Prevalence and clinical characteristics. *Journal of Gastroenterology and Hepatology*, *16*(11), 1235–1238. doi:10.1046/j.1440-1746.2001.02468.x PMID:11903741

Feagan, B. G., Sandborn, W. J., Gasink, C., Jacobstein, D., Lang, Y., Friedman, J. R., Blank, M. A., Johanns, J., Gao, L.-L., Miao, Y., Adedokun, O. J., Sands, B. E., Hanauer, S. B., Vermeire, S., Targan, S., Ghosh, S., de Villiers, W. J., Colombel, J.-F., Tulassay, Z., ... Rutgeerts, P. (2016). Ustekinumab as Induction and Maintenance Therapy for Crohn's Disease. *The New England Journal of Medicine*, *375*(20), 1946–1960. doi:10.1056/NEJMoa1602773 PMID:27959607

Ghosh, A., Das, B. K., Roy, A., Mandal, B., & Chandra, G. (2008). Antibacterial activity of some medicinal plant extracts. *Journal of Natural Medicines*, *62*(2), 259–262. doi:10.100711418-007-0216-x PMID:18404337

Ghosh, A., Sharma, A., & Talukder, G. (1992). Relative protection given by extract of Phyllanthus emblica fruit and an equivalent amount of vitamin C against a known clastogen-caesium chloride. *Food and Chemical Toxicology*, *30*(10), 865–869. doi:10.1016/0278-6915(92)90052-M PMID:1427509

Gokhale, S. B., Kokate, C. K., & Purohit, A. P. (2003). Tannins. In Pharmacognosy (pp. 258–9). Pune, India: Nirali Prakashan.

Grover, I. S., & Bala, S. (1992). Antimutagenic activity of Terminalia chebula (myrobalan) in Salmonella typhimurium. *Indian Journal of Experimental Biology*, *30*, 339–341. PMID:1459604

Haque, R., Bin-Hafeez, B., Ahmad, I., Parvez, S., Panday, S., & Raisuddin, S. (2001). Protective effects of Emblica officinalis Gaertn. in cyclophosphamide-treated mice. *Human and Experimental Toxicology*, *20*(12), 643–650. doi:10.1191/096032701718890568 PMID:11936579

Harikumar, K. B., Sabu, M. C., Lima, P. S., & Kuttan, R. (2004). Modulation of haematopoetic system and antioxidant enzymes by Emblica officinalis Gaertn. and its protective role against gamma radiation induced damages in mice. *Journal of Radiation Research*, *45*(4), 549–554. doi:10.1269/jrr.45.549 PMID:15635265

Harris, M. S., Hartman, D., Lemos, B. R., Erlich, E. C., Spence, S., Kennedy, S., Ptak, T., Pruitt, R., Vermeire, S., & Fox, B. S. (2016). AVX-470, an Orally Delivered Anti-Tumour Necrosis Factor Antibody for Treatment of Active Ulcerative Colitis: Results of a First-in-Human Trial. *Journal of Crohn's and Colitis*, *10*(6), 631–640. doi:10.1093/ecco-jcc/jjw036 PMID:26822613

Hartman, D. S., Tracey, D. E., Lemos, B. R., Erlich, E. C., Burton, R. E., Keane, D. M., Patel, R., Kim, S., Bhol, K. C., Harris, M. S., & Fox, B. S. (2016). Effects of AVX-470, an Oral, Locally Acting Anti-Tumour Necrosis Factor Antibody, on Tissue Biomarkers in Patients with Active Ulcerative Colitis. *Journal of Crohn's and Colitis*, *10*(6), 641–649. doi:10.1093/ecco-jcc/jjw026 PMID:26802087

Jain, S., Shapiro, S. L., Swanick, S., Roesch, S. C., Mills, P. J., Bell, I., & Schwartz, G. E. R. (2007). A randomized controlled trial of mindfulness meditation versus relaxation training: Effects on distress, positive states of mind, rumination, and distraction. *Annals of Behavioral Medicine*, *33*(1), 11–21. doi:10.120715324796abm3301_2 PMID:17291166

Jeena, K. J., Joy, K. L., & Kuttan, R. (1999). Effect of Emblica officinalis, Phyllanthus amarus and Picrorrhiza kurroa on N-nitrosodiethylamine induced hepatocarcinogenesis. *Cancer Letters*, *136*(1), 11–16. doi:10.1016/S0304-3835(98)00294-8 PMID:10211933

Jose, J. K., & Kuttan, R. (2000). Hepatoprotective activity of Emblica officinalis and chyavanprash. *Journal of Ethnopharmacology*, *72*(1-2), 135–140. doi:10.1016/S0378-8741(00)00219-1 PMID:10967464

Jowett, S. L., Seal, C. J., Pearce, M. S., Phillips, E., Gregory, W., Barton, J. R., & … . (2004). Influence of dietary factors on the clinical course of ulcerative colitis: A prospective cohort study. *Gut*, *53*(10), 1479–1484. doi:10.1136/gut.2003.024828 PMID:15361498

Juang, L. J., & Sheu, S. J. (2005). Chemical identification of the sources of commercial Fructus chebulae. *Phytochemical Analysis*, *16*(4), 246–251. doi:10.1002/pca.823 PMID:16042149

Kannan, P., Ramadevi, S. R., & Waheeta, H. (2009). Antibacterial activity of Terminalia chebula fruit extract. *African Journal of Microbiological Research*, *3*, 180–184.

Kaplan, M. A., & Korelitz, B. I. (1988). Narcotic dependence in inflammatory bowel disease. *Journal of Clinical Gastroenterology*, *10*(3), 275–278. doi:10.1097/00004836-198806000-00010 PMID:2980762

Kaur, S., Arora, S., Kaur, K., & Kumar, S. (2002). The in vitro antimutagenic activity of Triphala an Indian herbal drug. *Food and Chemical Toxicology*, *40*(4), 527–534. doi:10.1016/S0278-6915(01)00101-6 PMID:11893411

Kaur, S., & Jaggi, R. K. (2010). Antinociceptive activity of chronic administration of different extracts of Terminalia bellerica Roxb. and Terminalia chebula Retz. fruits. *Indian Journal of Experimental Biology*, *48*(9), 925–930. PMID:21506501

Kedia, S., & Ahuja, V. (2017). Epidemiology of Inflammatory Bowel Disease in India: The Great Shift East. *Inflammatory Intestinal Diseases*, *2*(2), 102–115. doi:10.1159/000465522 PMID:30018961

Kerlin, M., Long, M., Kappelman, M., Martin, C., & Sandler, R. S. (2018). Profiles of patients who use marijuana for inflammatory bowel disease. *Digestive Diseases and Sciences*, *63*(6), 1600–1604. doi:10.100710620-018-5040-5 PMID:29594968

Kim, H. J., Yokozawa, T., Kim, H. Y., Tohda, C., Rao, T. P., & Juneja, L. R. (2005). Influence of amla (Emblica officinalis Gaertn.) on hypercholesterolemia and lipid peroxidation in cholesterol-fed rats. *Journal of Nutritional Science and Vitaminology*, *51*(6), 413–418. doi:10.3177/jnsv.51.413 PMID:16521700

Kim, T. G., Kang, S. Y., Jung, K. K., Kang, J. H., Lee, E., Han, H. M., & Kim, S. H. (2001). Antiviral activities of extracts isolated from Terminalis chebula Retz., Sanguisorba officinalis L., Rubus coreanus Miq. and Rheum palmatum L. against hepatitis B virus. *Phytotherapy Research*, *15*(8), 718–720. doi:10.1002/ptr.832 PMID:11746867

Knight-Sepulveda, K., Kais, S., Santaolalla, R., & Abreu, M. T. (2015). Diet and Inflammatory Bowel Disease. *Gastroenterology & Hepatology, 11*(8), 511–520. PMID:27118948

Lee, H. S., Koo, Y. C., Suh, H. J., Kim, K. Y., & Lee, K. W. (2010). Preventive effects of chebulic acid isolated from Terminalia chebula on advanced glycation end product-induced endothelial cell dysfunction. *Journal of Ethnopharmacology, 131*(3), 567–574. doi:10.1016/j.jep.2010.07.039 PMID:20659546

Leonardi, C. L., Kimball, A. B., Papp, K. A., Yeilding, N., Guzzo, C., Wang, Y., Li, S., Dooley, L. T., & Gordon, K. B. (2008). Efficacy and safety of ustekinumab, a human interleukin-12/23 monoclonal antibody, in patients with psoriasis: 76-week results from a randomised, double-blind, placebo-controlled trial (PHOENIX 1). *Lancet, 371*(9625), 1665–1674. doi:10.1016/S0140-6736(08)60725-4 PMID:18486739

Lichtenstein, G. R., Feagan, B. G., Cohen, R. D., Salzberg, B. A., Diamond, R. H., Price, S., Langholff, W., Londhe, A., & Sandborn, W. J. (2012). Serious infection and mortality in patients with Crohn's disease: More than 5 years of follow-up in the TREAT™ registry. *The American Journal of Gastroenterology, 107*(9), 1409–1422. doi:10.1038/ajg.2012.218 PMID:22890223

Losh, M., Martin, G. E., Lee, M., Klusek, J., Sideris, J., Barron, S., & Wassink, T. (2017). Developmental Markers of Genetic Liability to Autism in Parents: A Longitudinal, Multigenerational Study. *Journal of Autism and Developmental Disorders, 47*(3), 834–845. doi:10.100710803-016-2996-x PMID:28070788

Ma, H., Diao, Y., Zhao, D., Li, K., & Kang, T. (2010). A new alternative to treat swine influenza A virus infection: Extracts from Terminalia chebula Retz. *African Journal of Microbiological Research, 4*, 497–499.

Magee, E. A., Edmond, L. M., Tasker, S. M., Kong, S. C., Curno, R., & Cummings, J. H. (2005). Associations between diet and disease activity in ulcerative colitis patients using a novel method of data analysis. *Nutrition Journal, 4*(1), 7. doi:10.1186/1475-2891-4-7 PMID:15705205

Malekzadeh, F., Ehsanifar, H., Shahamat, M., Levin, M., & Colwell, R. R. (2001). Antibacterial activity of black myrobalan (Terminalia chebula Retz) against Helicobacter pylori. *International Journal of Antimicrobial Agents, 18*(1), 85–88. doi:10.1016/S0924-8579(01)00352-1 PMID:11463533

Mantzouranis, G., Fafliora, E., Saridi, M., Tatsioni, A., Glanztounis, G., Albani, E., & … . (2018). Alcohol and narcotics use in inflammatory bowel disease. *Annals of Gastroenterology, 31*(6), 649–658. doi:10.20524/aog.2018.0302 PMID:30386114

Marco, E. J., Hinkley, L. B. N., Hill, S. S., & Nagarajan, S. S. (2011). Sensory processing in autism: A review of neurophysiologic findings. *Pediatric Research, 69*(5 Pt 2), 48R–54R. doi:10.1203/PDR.0b013e3182130c54 PMID:21289533

Mathur, R., Sharma, A., Dixit, V. P., & Varma, M. (1996). Hypolipidaemic effect of fruit juice of Emblica officinalis in cholesterol-fed rabbits. *Journal of Ethnopharmacology, 50*(2), 61–68. doi:10.1016/0378-8741(95)01308-3 PMID:8866725

Miłkowska, P., Popko, K., Demkow, U., & Wolańczyk, T. (2017). Pro-inflammatory Cytokines in Psychiatric Disorders in Children and Adolescents: A Review. *Advances in Experimental Medicine and Biology, 1021*, 73–80. doi:10.1007/5584_2017_32 PMID:28405892

Mishra, M., Pathak, U. N., & Khan, A. B. (1981). Emblica officinalis Gaertn and serum cholesterol level in experimental rabbits. *British Journal of Experimental Pathology, 62*, 526–528. PMID:7295546

Mohan, K., Paramasivam, R., Chandran, P., Veerasami, V., Gnanasekaran, A., Shanmugam, A., & ... . (2011). Inhibition of Hepatitis B virus DNA polymerase and modulation of TH1 and TH2 cytokine secretion by three Indian medicinal plants and its correlation with antiviral properties. *Journal of Pharmacy Research, 4*, 1044–1046.

Nagar, S., Belapurkar, P., Barua, P. T., & Goyal, P. (2011). Antimicrobial and phytochemical analysis of Triphala and comparison with its individual constituents. *National Journal of Life Sciences, 8*, 101–103.

Panda, S., & Kar, A. (2003). Fruit extract of Emblica officinalis ameliorates hyperthyroidism and hepatic lipid peroxidation in mice. *Die Pharmazie, 58*, 753–755. PMID:14609291

Perianayagam, J. B., Sharma, S. K., Joseph, A., & Christina, A. J. (2004). Evaluation of anti-pyretic and analgesic activity of Emblica officinalis Gaertn. *Journal of Ethnopharmacology, 95*(1), 83–85. doi:10.1016/j.jep.2004.06.020 PMID:15374611

Rajak, S., Banerjee, S. K., Sood, S., Dinda, K. A., Gupta, Y. K., & Maulik, S. K. (2004). Emblica officinalis causes myocardial adaptation and protects against oxidative stress in ischemic-reperfusion injury in rats. *Phytotherapy Research, 18*(1), 54–60. doi:10.1002/ptr.1367 PMID:14750202

Rastogi, R. P., & Mehrotra, B. N. (1991). Indian Medicinal Plants. In Compendium of Indian Medicinal plants - vol 1, (pp.1960-69). Central Drug Research Institute (CDRI), Lucknow and Publication and Information Directorate, Council of Scientific and Industrial Research (CSIR), New Delhi.

Rastogi, R. P., & Mehrotra, B. N. (1993). Indian Medicinal Plants. In Compendium of Indian Medicinal Plants - vol III, (pp.1985-89). Central Drug Research Institute (CDRI), Lucknow and Publication and Information Directorate, Council of Scientific and Industrial Research (CSIR), New Delhi.

Rastogi, R. P., & Mehrotra, B. N. (1995). Indian Medicinal Plants. In Compendium of Indian Medicinal Plants - vol IV, (pp.1985-89). Central Drug Research Institute (CDRI), Lucknow and Publication and Information Directorate, Council of Scientific and Industrial Research (CSIR), New Delhi.

Ravishankar, B., & Shukla, V. J. (2007). Indian systems of medicine: A brief profile. *AJTCAM*, *4*(3), 319–337. doi:10.4314/ajtcam.v4i3.31226 PMID:20161896

Reddy, D. B., Reddy, T. C., Jyotsna, G., Sharan, S., Priya, N., Lakshmipathi, V., & Reddanna, P. (2009). Chebulagic acid, a COX-LOX dual inhibitor isolated from the fruits of Terminalia chebula Retz., induces apoptosis in COLO-205 cell line. *Journal of Ethnopharmacology*, *124*(3), 506–512. doi:10.1016/j.jep.2009.05.022 PMID:19481594

Reddy, T. C., Aparoy, P., Babu, N. K., Kumar, K. A., Kalangi, S. K., & Reddanna, P. (2010). Kinetics and docking studies of a COX-2 inhibitor isolated from Terminalia bellerica fruits. *Protein and Peptide Letters*, *17*(10), 1251–1257. doi:10.2174/092986610792231537 PMID:20441561

Sairam, M., Neetu, D., Yogesh, B., Anju, B., Dipti, P., Pauline, T., Sharma, S. K., Sarada, S. K. S., Ilavazhagan, G., Kumar, D., & Selvamurthy, W. (2002). Cyto-protective and immunomodulating properties of Amla (Emblica officinalis) on lymphocytes: An in vitro study. *Journal of Ethnopharmacology*, *81*(1), 5–10. doi:10.1016/S0378-8741(01)00421-4 PMID:12020921

Saleem, A., Husheem, M., Harkonen, P., & Pihlaja, K. (2002). Inhibition of cancer cell growth by crude extract and the phenolics of Terminalia chebula Retz fruit. *Journal of Ethnopharmacology*, *81*(3), 327–336. doi:10.1016/S0378-8741(02)00099-5 PMID:12127233

Sancheti, G., Jindal, A., Kumari, R., & Goyal, P. K. (2005). Chemopreventive action of Emblica officinalis on skin carcinogenesis in mice. *Asian Pacific Journal of Cancer Prevention*, *6*, 197–201. PMID:16101333

Sandborn, W. J., Feagan, B. G., Fedorak, R. N., Scherl, E., Fleisher, M. R., Katz, S., Johanns, J., Blank, M., & Rutgeerts, P. (2008). A randomized trial of Ustekinumab, a human interleukin-12/23 monoclonal antibody, in patients with moderate-to-severe Crohn's disease. *Gastroenterology*, *135*(4), 1130–1141. doi:10.1053/j.gastro.2008.07.014 PMID:18706417

Sandborn, W. J., Lee, S. D., Tarabar, D., Louis, E., Klopocka, M., Klaus, J., Reinisch, W., Hébuterne, X., Park, D.-I., Schreiber, S., Nayak, S., Ahmad, A., Banerjee, A., Brown, L. S., Cataldi, F., Gorelick, K. J., Cheng, J. B., Hassan-Zahraee, M., Clare, R., & D'Haens, G. R. (2018). Phase II evaluation of anti-MAdCAM antibody PF-00547659 in the treatment of Crohn's disease: Report of the OPERA study. *Gut*, *67*(10), 1824–1835. doi:10.1136/gutjnl-2016-313457 PMID:28982740

Sanford, D., Thornley, P., Teriaky, A., Chande, N., & Gregor, J. (2014). Opioid use is associated with decreased quality of life in patients with Crohn's disease. *Saudi Journal of Gastroenterology*, *20*(3), 182–187. doi:10.4103/1319-3767.133020 PMID:24976282

Santoft, F., Hedman-Lagerlof, E., Salomonsson, S., Lindsater, E., Ljotsson, B., & Kecklund, G. (2020). Inflammatory cytokines in patients with common mental disorders treated with cognitive behavior therapy. *Brain, Behavior, & Immunity – Health*. (in press)

Shaila, H. P., Udupa, A. L., & Udupa, S. L. (1995). Preventive actions of Terminalia belerica in experimentally induced atherosclerosis. *International Journal of Cardiology*, *49*(2), 101–106. doi:10.1016/0167-5273(95)02285-5 PMID:7628881

Sharma, M. P., & Ahuja, V. (2009). Abdominal (gastrointestinal tract) tuberculosis in adult. In H. S. Schaaf, A. Zumla, & J. M. Grange (Eds.), *Tuberculosis: A comprehensive clinical reference (pp* (pp. 424–431). Saunders/Elsevier. doi:10.1016/B978-1-4160-3988-4.00039-1

Sharma, P., Poojary, G., Dwivedi, S. N., & Deepak, K. K. (2015). Effect of Yoga-Based Intervention in Patients with Inflammatory Bowel Disease. *International Journal of Yoga Therapy*, *25*(1), 101–112. doi:10.17761/1531-2054-25.1.101 PMID:26667293

Sharma, S. K., & Mohan, A. (2004). Extrapulmonary tuberculosis. *The Indian Journal of Medical Research*, *120*, 316–353. PMID:15520485

Shinde, L., More, S. M., Junne, S. B., & Wadje, S. S. (2011). The antifungal activity of five Terminalia species checked by paper disk method. *Int J Pharma Res Dev*, *3*, 36–40.

Singh, I., Sharma, A., Nunia, V., & Goyal, P. K. (2005). Radioprotection of Swiss albino mice by Emblica officinalis. *Phytotherapy Research*, *19*(5), 444–446. doi:10.1002/ptr.1600 PMID:16106381

Singh, M. P., & Sharma, C. S. (2009). Wound healing activity of Terminalia chebula in experimentally induced diabetic rats. *International Journal of Pharm Tech Research*, *1*, 1267–1270.

Soccalingam, A., Ramanathan, M., & Bhavanani, A. B. (2020). Yoga therapy on Cognitive function in Neurodevelopmental disorders. In T. Wadhera & D. Kakkara (Eds.), *Interdisciplinary Approaches to Altering Neurodevelopmental Disorders* (pp. 143–161). IGI-Global. doi:10.4018/978-1-7998-3069-6.ch009

Suchalatha, S., Srinivasulu, C., & Devi, S. C. (2005). Antioxidant activity of ethanolic extract of Terminalia chebula fruit against isoproterenol-induced oxidative stress in rats. *Indian Journal of Biochemistry & Biophysics*, *42*, 246–249. PMID:23923550

Sun, Y., Li, L., Xie, R., Wang, B., Jiang, K., & Cao, H. (2019). Stress Triggers Flare of Inflammatory Bowel Disease in Children and Adults. *Frontiers in Pediatrics*, *7*, 432. doi:10.3389/fped.2019.00432 PMID:31709203

Suryanarayana, P., Kumar, P. A., Saraswat, M., Petrash, J. M., & Reddy, G. B. (2004). Inhibition of aldose reductase by tannoid principles of Emblica officinalis: Implications for the prevention of sugar cataract. *Molecular Vision*, *10*, 148–154. PMID:15031705

SuryaPrakash, D.V., Satya, N.S., Avanigadda, S., & Vanglapati, M. (2012). Pharmacological review on Terminalia chebula. *International Journal of Research in Pharmaceutical and Biomedical Sciences*, *3*, 679–683.

Suthienkul, O., Miyazaki, O., Chulasiri, M., Kositanont, U., & Oishi, K. (1993). Retroviral reverse transcriptase inhibitory activity in Thai herbs and spices: Screening with Moloney murine leukemia viral enzyme. *The Southeast Asian Journal of Tropical Medicine and Public Health*, *24*, 751–755. PMID:7524165

Tandon, R. K., Sarin, S. K., Bose, S. L., Berry, M., & Tandon, B. N. (1986). A clinic-radiological reappraisal of intestinal tuberculosis–Changing profile? *Gastroenterologia Japonica*, *21*(1), 17–22. doi:10.1007/BF02775935 PMID:3699397

Tariq, M., Hussain, S. J., Asif, M., & Jahan, M. (1977). Protective effect of fruit extracts of Emblica officinalis (Gaertn.) and Terminalia belerica (Roxb.) in experimental myocardial necrosis in rats. *Indian Journal of Experimental Biology*, *15*, 485–486. PMID:598885

Thakur, C. P., Thakur, B., Singh, S., Sinha, P. K., & Sinha, S. K. (1988). The Ayurvedic medicines Haritaki, Amala and Bahira reduce cholesterol induced atherosclerosis in rabbits. *International Journal of Cardiology*, *21*(2), 167–175. doi:10.1016/0167-5273(88)90219-7 PMID:3225068

Undseth, R., Berstad, A., Kløw, N. E., Arnljot, K., Moi, K. S., & Valeur, J. (2014). Abnormal accumulation of intestinal fluid following ingestion of an unabsorbable carbohydrate in patients with irritable bowel syndrome: An MRI study. *Neurogastroenterology and Motility*, *26*(12), 1686–1693. doi:10.1111/nmo.12449 PMID:25271767

Vaniquotes. (2018). Chapter 02.48. *Bhagavad Gita*. Retrieved 10 March 2020, from https://vaniquotes.org/wiki/BG_02.48_yoga-sthah_kuru_karmani..._cited

Venegas, D. P., Fuente, M. K. D., Landskron, G., González, M. J., Quera, R., Dijkstra, G., & … . (2019). Short Chain Fatty Acids (SCFAs)-Mediated Gut Epithelial and Immune Regulation and its relevance for Inflammatory Bowel Diseases. *Frontiers in Immunology*, *10*, 277. doi:10.3389/fimmu.2019.00277 PMID:30915065

Vermeire, S., Ghosh, S., Panes, J., Dahlerup, J. F., Luegering, A., Sirotiakova, J., Strauch, U., Burgess, G., Spanton, J., Martin, S. W., & Niezychowski, W. (2011). The mucosal addressin cell adhesion molecule antibody PF-00547,659 in ulcerative colitis: A randomised study. *Gut*, *60*(8), 1068–1075. doi:10.1136/gut.2010.226548 PMID:21317177

Vermeire, S., Sandborn, W. J., Danese, S., Hébuterne, X., Salzberg, B. A., Klopocka, M., Tarabar, D., Vanasek, T., Greguš, M., Hellstern, P. A., Kim, J. S., Sparrow, M. P., Gorelick, K. J., Hinz, M., Ahmad, A., Pradhan, V., Hassan-Zahraee, M., Clare, R., Cataldi, F., & Reinisch, W. (2017). Anti-MAdCAM antibody (PF-00547659) for ulcerative colitis (TURANDOT): A phase 2, randomised, double-blind, placebo-controlled trial. *Lancet*, *390*(10090), 135–144. doi:10.1016/S0140-6736(17)30930-3 PMID:28527704

Weisshof, R., El-Jurdi, K., Zmeter, N., & Rubin, D. T. (2018). Emerging Therapies for Inflammatory Bowel Disease. *Advances in Therapy*, *35*(11), 1746–1762. doi:10.100712325-018-0795-9 PMID:30374806

Xia, Q., Xiao, P., Wan, L., & Kong, J. (1997). Ethnopharmacology of Phyllanthus emblica L. *Zhongguo Zhongyao Zazhi*, *22*, 515–574. PMID:11038937

Yukawa, T. A., Kurokawa, M., Sato, H., Yoshida, Y., Kageyama, S., Hasegawa, T., Namba, T., Imakita, M., Hozumi, T., & Shiraki, K. (1996). Prophylactic treatment of cytomegalovirus infection with traditional herbs. *Antiviral Research*, *32*(2), 63–70. doi:10.1016/0166-3542(95)00978-7 PMID:8891165

Chapter 7
Dysbiosis in Microbiome Leading to Colitis-Associated Cancer:
Gut Microbiome Correlation With CAC

Priyamvada Priyamvada
Banaras Hindu University, India

ABSTRACT

Colitis-associated cancers are a metastatic form of inflammatory bowel disease considered a vital health associated risk factor causing the death of approximately five lacs people every year throughout the world. There are trillions of bacteria that are associated with our gut as a part of our healthy microbiome. The microbiota plays a plethora of important role in determining the normal physiological processes of the cells and, subsequently, the body. The imbalance in microbiome diversity (dysbiosis) due to abnormal dietary habitats, hectic lifestyle, and other factors thus alters the normal physiological processes of the body, thereby causing several chronic diseases. Therefore, it is essential to maintain the homeostasis between the host and their gut microbiome. So, based on the facts mentioned above, this chapter is entirely devoted to providing an overview of colitis-associated cancer and their relation with the dysbiosis of a healthy microbiome. Moreover, the mechanism involved in the development of colorectal cancer and its preventive insights has also been addressed.

DOI: 10.4018/978-1-7998-3580-6.ch007

1. INTRODUCTION

The human body is colonized by a vast array of microbes, especially bacteria. This gut microbiome plays a crucial role in health and diseases. In the past decades, exposure to microbiota research is at a peak, mainly to study how the microbiomes are associated with cancer. Various studies have estimated that the gastrointestinal tract contains bacteria which are same in number to the cells present in the human body. The gut microbiome plays a vital role in maintaining the epithelium growth in intestine, the release of antimicrobial substances which regulate the immune system in concordance with the various physiological functions (Sartor, 2008). There are sum trillions of the microbiome existing in our gastrointestinal tract. Microbiome shows different kinds of symbiotic relationships with the hosts viz. commensalism and mutualism. Now, it has been predicted that the alteration in gut microbiome balance might also play an essential role in regulating the development of cancer, such as colitis-associated cancer and inflammatory bowel diseases (IBD). Therefore, it is mandatory to recognize the mechanism which is being established between the bacteria and the host. And study about the association of these microbiomes with the development of IBD, in association with colitis-associated cancer (CAC).

IBD, a collective term used for both Ulcerative Colitis (UC) and Crohn's disease (CD). This disease has been increasing in number in the last few decades and ultimately leading to CAC (Itzkowitz and Yio, 2004; Eaden *et al.*, 2001). CAC is a complex multifactorial disease involving an interaction between genetic landscape and environmental factors that plays out the interface between the immune system and the resident microbiota. On behalf of the abovementioned background, the present chapter demonstrates the establishment of microbes in the gut. Alteration in these microbiomes leads to the development of IBD and CAC. Further moving, in this chapter, there is brief information regarding the treatments, which helps in modulating the existing microbiome that has been altered during IBD and CAC development.

2. KNOWING MORE ABOUT GUT MICROBIOTA

Gut microbiota of small intestine shows a dynamic deviation from the microbes present in the colon concerning their affluence and distribution. Small intestine deals with the conversion of lower carbohydrates and also adapting to the overall nutrient available. Whereas, microbiota present in the colon is effectively driven by the breakdown of indigestible complex carbohydrates (Marchesi *et al.*, 2016). Understanding more about the gut microbiota, it is desirable to classify these bacteria according to the phylum where they are placed. Mainly five phyla represent the bacteria present in gut microbiota. It is around 160 spp. in the colon of an individual (Rajilić-Stojanović and de Vos, 2014) which include some gram-negative bacteria as well as some gram-positive bacteria. In the case of gram-negative bacteria, the phylum which has been given the first position is *Fusobacteria.* These consist of anaerobic, non-spore-forming bacteria *Bacteroidetes*, these are also distributed fully in GIT. The phylum which has got more than 200 genera is *Proteobacteria* that includes *Salmonella*, *E. coli*, *H. pylori* etc. (Fierer *et al.*, 2007). Talking about gram-positive bacteria, this includes *Actinobacteria* (aerobic) and *Firmicutes.*

Figure 1. Pie chart depicts the distribution of different phyla. Colonic microbiota includes Firmicutes and Bacteroidetes, which are predominant bacteria (57.2% and 32.0%, respectively). Other phyla that are present in the colon are Proteobacteria, Actinobacteria, Fusobacteria constituting 2.81%, 2.22%, and 2.20%, respectively. *Data provided by (Wang et al., 2012.)*

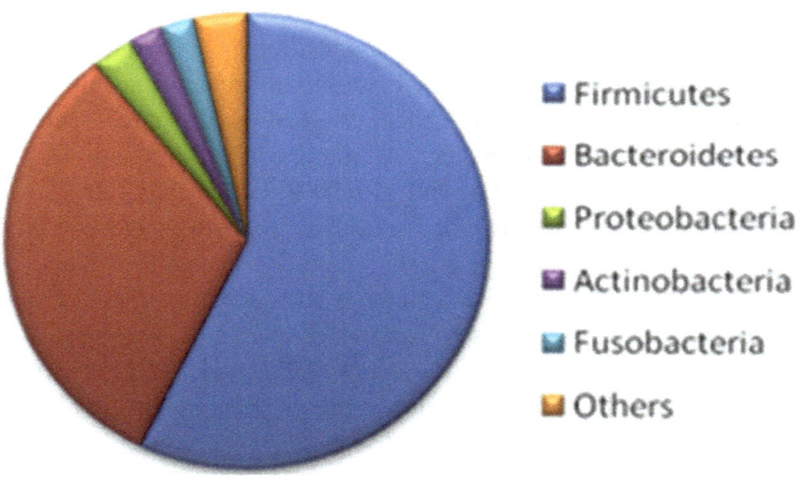

3. INFLAMMATORY BOWEL DISEASE

IBD is a chronic, idiopathic, inflammatory disease that affects the colon, leading to colitis-associated cancer. IBD is known to be a multifactorial disease which triggers the dysbiosis of luminal mucosal homeostasis. As there is an alteration between the regulatory mediator and inflammatory mediator, this contributes to the inappropriate inflammatory responses. Colitis associated cancer is mainly caused due to dysfunction of the microfloral integrity (Tomasello *et al.*, 2014). IBD deals with two major entities, i.e., CD and UC. Both have overlapping symptoms which include diarrhoea, rectal bleeding, and loss of weight.

CD is associated with the inflammation in any part of the intestine mostly in the ileum and colon section. It is characterized by the spreading of aggregates of lymphoid in the mucosal and submucosal membrane. At the beginning stage, infiltrates of neutrophils are observed in the epithelial layer and with due time in crypts. With due time it destroys crypts leading to colonic atrophy. There is also a formation of non-necrotizing granulomas resulting from chronic inflammation. These small changes later lead to series of complications which include abdominal pain, diarrhoea, rectal bleeding and also there is malabsorption which may occur due to inflammation in the ends of the ileum (Chandrasekar and Venu, 2015). The leading cause of CD inflammation is the Th17 response. The responses include the production of IL-17 and IFN-γ, TNF-α, IL-6, IL-1, which are immediate effectors of inflammation.

UC is also the same kind of inflammatory disease mainly in colonic mucosa and submucosa, which begins in the rectum. This inflammatory disease can even extend its effect to proximal parts with the course of the disease. In severe cases, there is dilatation of colon, necrosis, and perforation that occur along with massive haemorrhage. UC can even result in crypt abscession with neutrophils infiltrates in the crypts. Symptoms are same like rectal bleeding and excessive discharge of mucus, abdominal pain, malaise (Husssein et al., 2008). Cytokines which predominate in Ulcerative Colitis is mainly of the Th2 pattern of adaptive immune responses. Ultimately releases many different kinds of pro-inflammatory cytokines, such as IL-4, 5 and 13 (Basso et al., 2014).

4. HOW GENOME IS ALTERED IN CASE OF SOPADIC COLORECTAL CANCER AND COLITIS ASSOCIATED CANCER

CRC is the third most common type of cancer in the world. In the case of female, it is the leading cause of death. The risk factors mainly include male sex, genetic history, high BMI, and less activity. Sporadic colorectal cancer mainly develops from adenoma, which is premalignant through any kind of gene mutation such as APC, K-RAS, p53. Studies show that eight genes are most frequently mutated. Genes include APC, K-RAS, PIK3CA, SMAD4, NRAS, TCF7L2, NRAS, and p53. Another pathway in sporadic CRC consists of a mutation in PI3K and RAS-MAPK. This mutation has been found in 93% of the tumour (Sigel *et al.*, 1999).

Table 1. Local and Systematic effect of the gut microbiome on physiological functions, non- neoplastic pathology, cancer and its therapies

Local effect of gut microbiome	Systemic effect of gut microbiome
1. Physiological effects	
i) Absorption of nutrients ii) Vitamin synthesis iii) Bile metabolism iv) Carbs fermentation v) Morphogenesis vi) Strengthening of barrier	i) Functions such as neurological, behavioral and cognitive ii) Functions of cardiovascular and musculoskeletal iii) Hematopoiesis and functioning of myeloid cell iv) Circadian rhythm v) Inflammation
2. Non- neoplastic pathology	
i) IBD ii) Gastric ulcers	i) Cardiovascular diseases ii) Non-alcoholic steatohepatitis iii) Insulin resistance
3. Cancer	
i) Colorectal cancer ii) Gallbladder carcinoma iii) Stomach cancer	i) Pancreatic cancer ii) Prostate cancer iii) Ovarian cancer
4. Cancer therapy	
i) Cancer therapy gastrointestinal toxicity	i) Chemotherapy, immunotherapy ii) Cancer toxicity

Figure 2. Depiction of which all different environmental factors contributes to the development of IBD

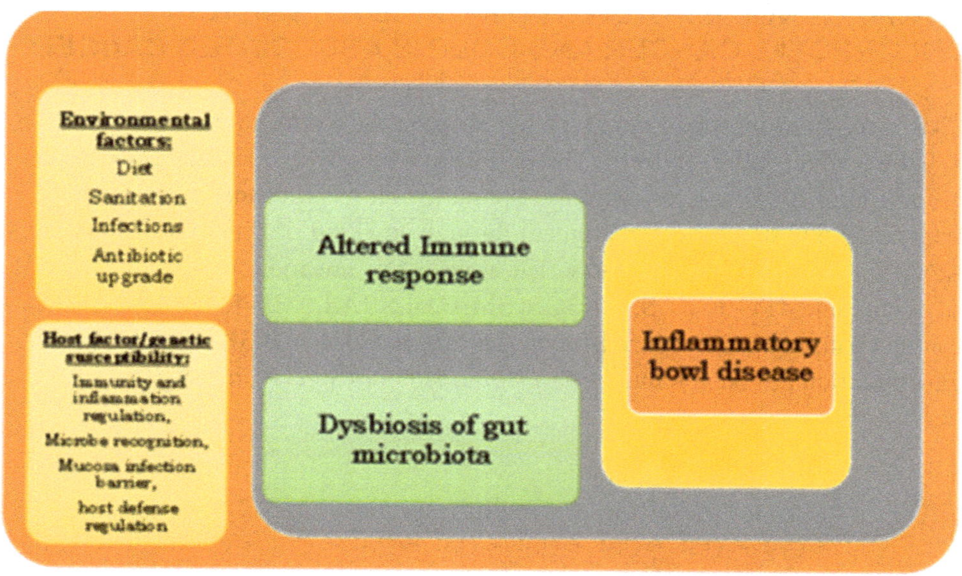

The patience with colitis-associated cancer have increased β- catenin transcriptional level and may also show a contribution to increased CL1 gene expression. When compared to sporadic CRC specific genes are mutated such as RAC1, DOCK2, DOCK3 and RADIL. These genes are mainly responsible for cell motility and remodelling of the cytoskeleton. The most frequent mutation was found primarily on EP300 and TRRAP. Sporadic CRC and colitis-associated cancer both have similar missense mutation, which was studied within the DNA binding domain of p53 only difference are in the molecular distribution of single substitution mutation.

Figure 3. Pathway and the genetic target leading to sporadic colon cancer. APC plays an essential role in early adenoma as if there is any mutation such as aneuploidy, methylation. Whereas, in late adenoma, DCC/DPC4 shows the changes. Finally leading to carcinoma condition.

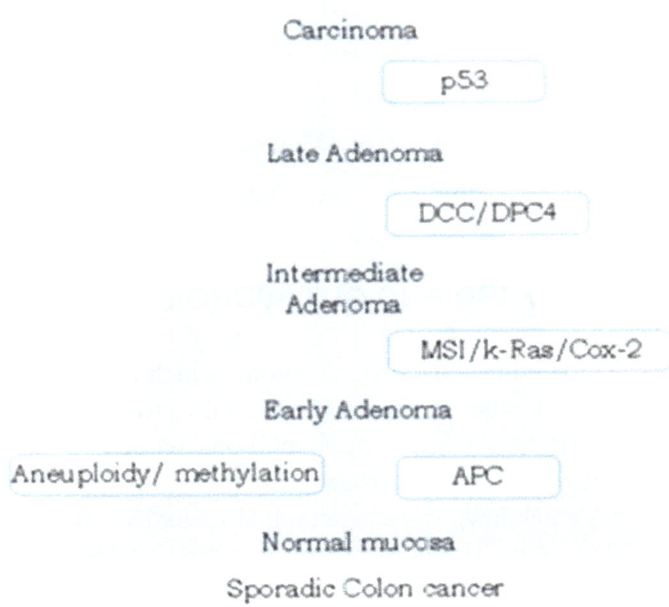

Figure 4. Pathway in which p53 is playing a crucial role in the development of early adenoma. Here DCC/DPC4 is leading to low-grade dysplasia, and APC leads to cancer

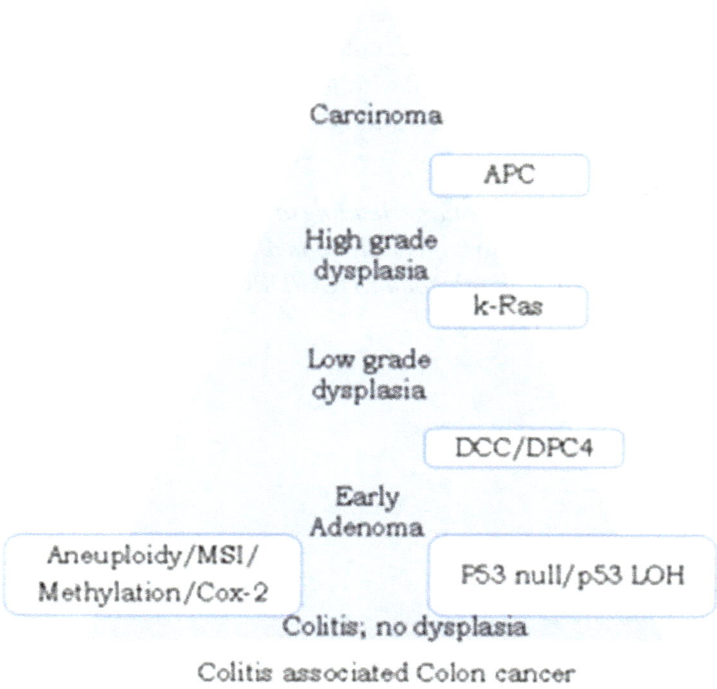

5. ASSOCIATION OF IBD AND GUT MICROBIOME

IBD is one of the chronic intestinal inflammations, which is mediated by immune responses. IBD is driven either by the environmental factors and genetic changes. IBD includes CD and UC, which affects millions of people worldwide. For IBD development, there is a definite change in the healthy gut microbiome, and also there is there a breakdown of host-microbial mutualism. These changes are linked to either CD or UC. The most crucial difference is lowering the number of Firmicutes which is balanced by an increase in the number of members of the phylum Bacteroidetes (Frank *et al.,* 2011). In patients with CD, studies have shown that there is a reduction in *F. prausnitzii* as compared to control. Together with phyla Firmicutes and Bacteriodetes there is also change in the member of phylum Proteobacteria. Proteobacteria increases in the case of IBD and has an active role in causing cancer (Mukopadhya *et al.,* 2011). This phylum has a role in the initiation of chronic inflammation in patients with IBD. It has been documented that ileal

CD has an increased number of *E.coli*. It has been shown that it is associated with alteration in the metabolism of bacterial carbohydrate. There is an interaction between the bacteria and host by secreting an enzyme by the host. There is depletion in the biosynthesis of SCFAs and amino acids. In an inflammatory condition such as T2D, there is a shift in microbial metabolic. Recent studies have shown that there is a crucial role of viruses in colitis-associated colorectal cancer with the expansion of *Caudovirales* bacteriophage.

6. HOW THIS BACTERIAL PHYLUM CHANGES DURING COLITIS ASSOCIATED CANCER

6.1. Firmicutes

This phylum plays a significant role in maintaining health and disease. Family such as *Staphylococcaceae* was found to be high in the patient suffering from CRC. While a class of gram-positive bacteria, *Clostridiales* was negatively regulated in the case of CRC (Baxter *et al.*, 2014). Temporal stability of species such as *Clostridium coccoides* and *C.leptum* show significant lowering in the case of CRC patients (Scanlan *et al.*, 2008). *Eubacteriaceae* belonging to order *Clostridiales* have been studied, which was found to be increased in the patients (Wu *et al.*, 2013). Probiotics species *Lactobacillus* (p=0.064) and *Ruminococcus* belonging to this phylum also seem to diminish. According to the study made by Wang et al. (*Faecalibacteriumprausnitzii* and (butyrate-producing genera) also gets lowered in CRC patients.

6.2. Bacteroidetes

Wu *et al.* observed it. That there was not only an increase in density in CRC patients but, also mentioned that there was a positive relationship between frequency and the disease. *Bacteroidesfragilis* of this phylum express a gene that encodes for the toxin that is related to IBD and CRC patients (Boleij *et al.*, 2015). In CRC patients, *the Prevotella* genus belonging to this phylum is overregulated (p=0.009) studied by Sobhani *et al.* (2011).Family *Porphyromonadaceae* composed by genera *Phorphyromonas* and *Dysgonomas*is less prevalent in healthy individuals.

6.3. Proteobacteria

This phylum turns to be overregulated in conditions of adenoma (Shen *et al.*, 2010). *Enterobacteriaceae* family belongs to this phylum which constitutes microorganism which is harmless and has been studied that these are intensified in patients who have cancer. But there is controversy with a member of this family such as *Kluyvera* sp., *Shigella* sp., *Cronobacter* sp., *Serratia* sp., *and Salmonella* sp., which have been lowered or lessened in cancer tissue (Marchesi *et al.*, 2011). Another family *Camphylobacteraceae* of this phylum is less prevalent in control. One of the commensal bacterial, which is commonplace in the gut of humans, is *E. coli*. Some strains of these bacteria have shown extreme relevance to inflammation and also in producing toxin cylomodulin. In advance stages of cancer cylomodulin, positive pathogenic strains were found to be prevalent.

6.4. Actinobacteria

Actinobacteria include gram-positive bacteria *Bifidobacterium,* which is ubiquitous and colonizes the oral cavity, gastrointestinal tract. Higher in healthy individuals as compared to colorectal cancer patients (Mira-Pascual *et al*., 2015). *Coriobacteridae* is demonstrated to be enhanced in colorectal cancer tissue.

6.5. Fusobacteria

Genera *Fusobacterium* belonging to this phylum is highly prevalent in the individual with Colorectal Cancer (p=0.001) (Zhu *et al.*, 2014). The high abundance of *Fusobacterium* was more likely to have adenoma. A study made by McCoy *et al.* (2013) supported that there is a link between the presence of *Fusobacterium* in colonic mucosa and adenoma. This link suggests that this plays an essential role in mucosal inflammation.

7. INTERACTION BETWEEN THE GUT MICROBIOME AND HOST MUCOSAL MEMBRANE

The interaction between the microbiota and host has got a physical barrier in the form of mucous membranes along with antimicrobial peptides and IgA (Yang and Jobin, 2017). Goblet cells are present in the mucosal membrane, where they secret various types of mucins such as MUC2, MUC3, MUC4, which help in protecting the mucosal layer. Mucus has a gel-like texture due to the presence of glycan's, which are bound carbohydrates. The deficiency of MUC2 in mice leads to the up-regulation of the defence factor RELM-β which enhances the production of colonic antimicrobial lectin REGIIIβ. This antimicrobial lectin targets lactobacillus species which produces short-chain fatty acids. In the case of MUC2 mutant mice, when lactobacilli are administered through oral gavage, it reduces RELM-β and REGIIIβ, which help in relieving spontaneous colitis (Morampudi *et al.*, 2016). Whereas

MUC4 stimulates Colitis Associated Cancer, it has been studied that, MUC4 mutant mice are not prone to ulcerative Colitis. UC might be due to the up-regulation of MUC2 and MUC3.

Table 2. Group of bacteria from different phylum, which plays a role in Colitis associated cancer. The presence of these bacterium has been studied in a different subject. Accordingly, the effect has been considered.

Phylum and species to which they belong	Abundance to cancer	Subject on with it has been studied
	Gram-Negative Bacteria	
1. Phylum: *Fusobacteria*		
Fusobacterium	High	Human, Animal
Fusobacteriumnucleatum	High	Human, Animal
2.Phylum: *Bacteroides*		
Prevotellaceae	Low	Animal
Prevotella	High	Human
Alistipes	High	Animal
Porphyromonadaceae	-	-
Porphyromonas	High	Human
Dysgonomonas	High	Human
Odoribacter	High	Animal
Parabacterioides	High	Animal
Gram-Positive Bacteria		
1. Phylum: *Actinobacteria*		
Bifidobacterium	Low	Human
Coriobacteridae	High	Human
Slackia	High	Human
Collinsella	High	Human
2. Phylum: *Firmicutes*		
Clostridiales	Low	Animal
Eubacteriaceae	High	Human
Eubacterium	Low	Animal
Staphylococcaceae	High	Human
Lactobacillus	Low	Human, Animal
Ruminococcus	Low	Animal

IgA is one of the important intestinal immunoglobulins which is defensive against enteric microbiota. IgA is produced by B cells which can be enhanced together by IL-33 and TGF-β. IL-33 mutant mice are more receptive to have colitis Associated cancer. It can be extricated by inhibiting IL-1α (Malik *et al.,* 2016)

Antimicrobial proteins, such as Lipocalin 2 (LCN2) limits the acquisition of iron. Lcn2 mutated mice show a dysbiosis in the bacterial population in the intestine. In this case, there is an immense increase in Bacteroidetes and a decrease in Tenericutes. This dysregulation in microbiota leads to Colitis Associated Cancer.

8. MECHANISMS OF THE GUT MICROBIOME IN COLON CANCER

Many studies show that the microbiome present in the colon plays a vital role in causing sporadic CRC. The increase in diversity in the faecal sample of the host as well as reduced stability shows a relation with colorectal cancer (Ou *et al.,* 2013). The oncogenic microbiome has been identified and categorized as the bacterial sp. based on metagenomic and transcriptomic. These bacteria colonize the cells of the gastrointestinal tract in the case of the tumour. Through various processes, these microbial strains promote the progression of cancer. The bacterial strain act through the biosynthesis of genotoxin, which interferes with the regulation of the cell cycle by interfering with the cell surface receptor. Production of the toxic metabolite is exceptionally effective in the case of cancer. Taking an example of toxin released by *E.coli* strain which is colibactin toxin causes a break in double-stranded DNA leading to the accumulation of chromosomal anomalies. There is a risk of developing cancer by the process of mutation, stimulation of cell proliferation, together with angiogenesis, inhibiting apoptosis. Bacterial translocation and activation of innate and adaptive component result in inflammatory disease (Ivanov *et al.*, 2009). Innate and adaptive response results in increased release of cytokines such as IL-12, IL-23, TNF-α, and INFγ by various cells like Macrophages (M φ), Dendritic cells (DC) Natural killer (NK) cells. Subsequently activates cells of the adaptive immune system such as lymphocytes (T-cells and B-cells). Inflammatory responses, such as activation of various transcription factors NF-KB and STAT3. Which ultimately leads to oxidative stress, DNA damage, the release of different reactive oxygen and nitrogen compound, resulting in the development of colorectal cancer (Tian et al., 2003).

There have been many theories proposed against how the colonic microbiome regulates CRC. Keystone-pathogen hypothesis and α–bug hypothesis: Both of these hypothesis states the same, i.e. members such as *B. fagilis* (enterotoxigenic) show low abundance and have virulent traits such as pro-oncogenic. This enterotoxigenic bacteria also enhance immune responses and remodels the microbiome in epithelial cells of the colon (Sears and Pardoll, 2011). Drive passenger model: Tjalsma *et al.*(2012) proposed that indigenous bacteria in colon damage DNA were contributing to the initiation of colorectal cancer. Damage induces niches alteration in the intestine, which favours the growth of bacteria which is opportunistic one like anaerobic gram-negative bacteria (Warren *et al.*, 2013). Strategies made by mucosal defensive have been managed to a greater extent, such as, expression of α-defensin increases in case of adenoma, which results in an increment of antibacterial activity. There are many members of pathobionts which have shown a link with CRC and adenoma. These are *Enterococcus faecalis, Bacteriales fragilis*, and *E. coli,* which are enriched and expresses gene for oncogenesis mainly includes translocation of M cell and angiogenesis (Prorok-Hamon *et al.*, 2014).

To study the mechanism of how *F. nucleatum* is involved in the stimulation of cell proliferation. It has got cell adhesion molecule, i.e. fadA which adhere and invade epithelial cell in human and elicit an inflammatory response (Han *et al.*, 2000). Salmonella release a product AvrA which activates the signalling of β- cantenin, which in turn enhances colonic tumour (Lu *et al.*, 2014). Work has been done focusing on the metabolic functioning of the gut microbiome. The metagenomic study has shown that there is a constant reduction of microbes which produces butyrate. Also, it plays an essential role in the metabolism of sulfate through its assimilatory reduction to cysteine and methionine, which are amino acid. While, dissimilatory reduction produces H2S, in turn, contribute to colon associated cancer (Carbonero *et al.*, 2012). Variation in the genotype of the host affects the landscape of carbohydrate affect the composition and function of microbes which resides in the intestine (Kashyap *et al.*, 2013). So, it might be possible that patient with CRC has modified bacteria, which are metabolically active, determined by the gene of the host, effect of diet and environment.

Due to the metabolism of nutrient to small molecules by various gut microbes leads to the development of neoplastic cells in the bowel. Studies have shown that intestinal bacteria also have a role in the metabolism of bile acid, where cholic acid is turned into deoxycholic acid while chenodeoxycholic acid into lithocholic acid. The deoxycholic acid contributes to ROS and genomic instability which may show a crucial effect on colon cancer (Rubin *et al.,* 2012). Incase if there high intake of protein in diet then their fermentation product will also increase in the colon. Waste such as sulfide nitrate, ammonium, and amides resulting from the digestion of protein, enhances the growth of *Desulfovibrio* sp. and *Desulfomonas* sp., (sulfate-reducing bacteria). The end product of protein metabolism is H2S which increases in the case of CRC patients (Kanazawa *et al.*, 1996).

A biomarker Ki67 is used for cancer risk. This increases or decreases due to intervention of diet having high fiber, high fat. This intervention leads to reciprocal changes, causing changes in the gene expression of the microbes.

9. APPROACHES TO MODULATE THE MICROBIOTA FOR CAC TREATMENT

Recent studies have shown that how microbiome profile is associated with the development and progression of cancer. The microbiome in intestine remains constant or stable for years but can change in response to exposure to pathogens, diet composition which has been altered, or any antibiotics treatment (Chevalier *et al.*, 2015; Kamdar *et al.*, 2016). Therefore, to modulate, there are many therapeutics that effectively treat IBD and CRC. The microbiome affects various characters ranging from mood to metabolism (Schmidt, 2015). The clinical approaches are still challenging, and more efforts should be made on the way to evaluate the effectiveness of the methods.

9.1. Prebiotics

These are component of food which helps in facilitating the growth of gut microbes. In turn, it maintains the homeostasis and also reduces the chances of developing colitis-associated colorectal cancer (Macfarlane and Cummings, 1999;Gustaw *et al.*, 2011). Through the process of fermentation prebiotics such as polydextrose, trans-galactooligosaccharide and inulin help in enriching the gut short-chain fatty acids (SCFAs) in the gut. Prebiotics has got many benefits such as microbiota composition can be altered and also increase in abundance of *Bifidobacterium sp*. regulates and inhibit proliferation of epithelial cell (Weitkunat *et al.*, 2015; Vinolo *et al.*, 2011). It has got great potential to treat many diseases such as CRC and IBD.

9.2. Faecal Microbiota Transplantation (FMT)

There is an exchange of gut microbiota in between individual who is healthy and another who is diseased. The clinical remission rate after treatment is 36% (Lopez and Grinspan, 2016). Infection with *C. difficile* and IBD in individuals can be treated by using faecal microbiota transplantation (Moayyedi *et al.*, 2015). FMT even help in reducing colorectal cancer, studied in mice. But, there are challenges to be taken under consideration, such as how they can be administered; another critical criterion is patient selection, together with patient sample (Rossen *et al.*, 2015). It's still unclear it is worth in case of tumour progression in humans as there is a difficulty at the level of knowing the variation in microbiota in a healthy person. FMT could be advantageous as it can balance the microbiota hence the chance of long term reset. An alternative to Faecal microbiota transplantation could be using a defined microbe with known benefits.

9.3. Probiotics

Naturally occurring non- pathogenic bacteria in our body are beneficial bacteria that maintain homeostasis in the gastrointestinal tract. Probiotics are live microbes which, when administered, can confer the benefit to host health. They are defensive against pathogens to protect any disorder in GI. It has been shown in (Fig. 5) that how probiotics play an essential role in the cause of IBD. It helps in enhancing immunity either it can be innate or adaptive. In Strains of *Lactobacillus (*lactic acid bacteria) and *Bifidobacterium* is predominant probiotic organisms.

a) Isolates of *Lactobacillus* such as *L. casei, L. plantarum, L. rhamnosus, L. acidophilus* are effective in cancer. They work through various mechanisms, like activation of the natural killer cell (NK Cell), maturation of dendritic cell (DC), the release of derivative of probiotics, i.e. ferrichrome (it is an iron scavenger). *Lactobacillus* sp. exerts a cancer-specific suppression of tumours through the apoptosis-inducing JNK signalling.

b) *B.fragilis* has been found of either type enterotoxigenic or non-enterotoxigenic. Enterotoxigenic type raises the TH17 cells (pro-inflammatory) which in turn accelerates carcinogenesis in prone condition. Whereas, in enterotoxin producing, strains have anti-cancer properties w.r.t. anti-CTLA4 immunotherapy (Vétizou*et al*., 2015). This immunotherapy is unsuccessful in reducing the growth of colon cancer in antibiotic-treated (germ-free) mice. *B. fragilis* can be used to treat this defect.

c) *Bifidobacteriales* are found naturally in the colon and also in many dairy products. In the case of reduced growth of transplantable melanomas and diminished CTL-mediated immune surveillance, it has found the abundance of Bifidobacterium. The introduction or transfer of *B. breve* or *B. longum* has reduced the growth of melanoma and also help in restoring the anti-melanoma CTL responses. They also stimulate maturation of dendritic cells in turn help in priming of tumour-specific CTLs. These strains help in responding better to immunotherapy.

Figure 5. Depicting the role of probiotics on IBD and CRC. Probiotics activate the cytokines such as IL-10 which has a role in the anti-inflammatory process. TLR4 has an inhibitory effect on inflammation which leads to inhibition of IBD and CRC.

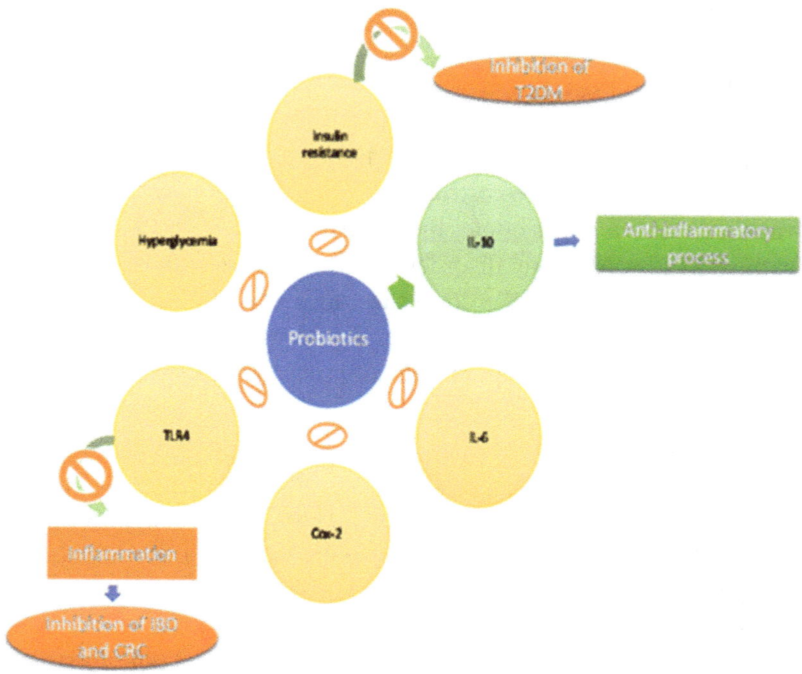

10. HOW MICROBIAL PRODUCT MODULATE CANCER

These are some bacteria which release various molecules, which modulate the survival of the cancer cell and even can affect the anti-cancer immunosurveillance. These are toxin which may have direct anti-cancer property ligands of PRRs, which affect the immune response and bacteria metabolites affecting host metabolism. Phenazine secreted by *Pseudomonas aeruginosa* and phthiocol from *M. tuberculosis* binds on hydrocarbon receptor (functions as TFs) and N-acetylglucosamine (bacterial peptidoglycan layer). It acts on hexokinase to activate inflammation (Wolf *et al.*, 2016).

10.1. Toxin Production

A variety of bacteria produces different types of toxin. Toxins help the bacterial species to compete with others to sustain it in a particular area (Becattini *et al.*, 2016). Streptomyces sp. produces toxin anthracycline, which directly shows the anticancerous effect. Doxorubicin is also used widely as anticancerous chemotherapy and can even induce anti-cancer immune responses (Kroemer *et al.*, 2013). Toxin such as Colicin are peptide with a structure of β- helix containing cationic charges, and this allows them to lyse non protected bacteria membrane. LTX-315 is one who kills the cancerous cell by lysis of mitochondria (Ellerby *et al.,* 1999). There can even be fused with motifs that target protein on surface-expressed explicitly by tumour epithelial and vascular endothelium membrane, e.g. GRP78, IL-11R (Arap *et al.,* 2004)

10.2. PRRs Ligands

PRRs recognize pathogen-associated molecular patterns. Lipopolysaccharide (LPS) being one of the components of the outer membrane of G-ve bacteria, is one of the well-known PAMP which interacts with TLR4. Through breaches in the intestine, the bacteria enters the systemic circulation) and LPS in bacterial membrane how can stimulate the inflammatory response. This condition may emerge after its use in radiation therapy for cancer treatment and also, helps in the inhibition of tumour growth by activating T-cells. PAMPs can even be used as vaccine adjuvants which elicit an immune response mainly against the viruses which can cause cancer. E.g. Monophosphoryl lipid A (MPL), is a derivative of *Salmonella enterica* subspecies entericaserovar.

10.3. Metabolite Production

Half of the metabolites in plasma are of bacterial origin which has got a role in metabolism. Various products like secondary bile acids, vitamins, polyamines and SCFAs are synthesized by microbes present in our gut. These metabolites affect the development of cancer and the effectiveness of antineoplastic therapies. Through our dietary- fiber, polysaccharides, and many metabolites such as acetate, propionate, and butyrate are produced in the colon. Clostridium clusters IV and XIVa of phylum Firmicutes along with species of genera *Eubacterium, Faecalibacterium* and *Roseburia,* are evolved in generating SCFAs. Propionate and butyrate favour the differentiation of regulatory T- cells. It starts accumulating, which mediates the anti-inflammatory effect. Butyrate and propionate have a crucial role in the inhibition of histone deacetylase (HDACs. It acts as an agonist of GPCRs which possess an oncosuppressive effect.

Apoptosis, in the case of colorectal cancer and lymphoma cells, is induced by butyrate (Jan *et al.*, 2002). In addition to it, butyrate has a negative role in the proliferation and regeneration of the potential stem cells. Studies have shown that in patients of colorectal cancer, butyrate-producing bacteria are less in number as compared to a healthy person. So, there is a need to increase the butyrate in our colon. To accomplish that, we need to take butyrogenic diet, i.e. fermentable carbohydrates (Gutiérrez-Díaz*et al.*, 2016). Secondary bile acids such as lithocholic acid and deoxycholic acid have produced from primary bile acid. These acid has got potential in DNA damaging and hence, showing carcinogenic effect. It can affect metabolism by showing an increased affinity for bile acid receptors. Gut microbiota has also altered by secondary bile assets either directly or indirectly through activation of the immune system.

In the case of colitis-associated cancer, there is low expression of enzymes that are related to the transport of polyamine. Bifidobacterium animalis subspecies lactis LKM512 is a strain which increases intestinal luminal polyamine concentration. Vitamins are not sufficiently produced by our cell; that's why there is a need to provide it by diet, or our gut microbiome can synthesize it. Interestingly, the human gut microbiome has the potential to synthesize at a minimum of eight vitamin B such as biotin, cobalamine, niacin, and pyridoxine are some of them. It has been known that pyridoxine stimulates anti-cancer immunosurveillance concerning cisplatin-based chemotherapy against lung cancer. Ulcerative Colitis, associated cancer, and sporadic colorectal cancer are marked by an increase in the expression of enzymes that catabolizes all-trans-retinoic acid (atRA). It is related to intestinal inflammation induced by the gastrointestinal microbiome. All trans-retinoic acid (atRA) reduces the burden of tumour formation, colitis-associated colorectal cancer (Bhattacharya *et al.*, 2016). Vitamin A derivatives have also found useful in the treatment of colorectal cancer.

11. THERAPIES WHICH CAUSES SHIFT IN GUT MICROBIOME

In the case of germ-free mice, studies have shown that chemo and immunotherapeutics have less effect in reducing the growth of the tumour. Removal of the microbiome has a negative impact as it eliminates cytotoxic T lymphocyte, which protects against cancer. Also, there is a reduction in innate and adaptive immune responses. The host genome, way of lifestyle affect indirectly in the case of cancer and respond to therapies through a change in the composition of the microbiota. In recent studies, progress has been in the area of treatments out of which immunotherapies are more promising.

11.1. Chemotherapy and its Effect on Microbiota

Mustards showed a cytotoxic effect during World War II. From that time, only this cytotoxic drug has been used as a chemotherapeutic agent. Classification of the cytotoxic drug is made based on the mechanism of action. They act as antitumors by interacting with the integrity of the target DNA strand and cell, which are dividing or involved in cell division. These drugs show the effect on semi-autonomous organelle i.e. mitochondria and also on the cell membrane.

11.1.1. Metabolism of the Drug

The gut microbiome has got an effect on the drug, its anti-cancer activity and toxic at different levels (Spanogiannopoulos et al., 2018). The absorption rate of drugs depends on its exposure to the host gut and enzyme secreted by the bacteria (Li and Jia, 2013). Gene expression of the microbiome present in the gut is modulated or changed by Xenobiotics which are chemical molecules that are not produced naturally and are foreign. The microbiome biotransform drugs through chemical reaction such as hydrolysis, reduction of the compound. Removal of functional group and cleavage of nitrogen oxides along with denitration, acetylation, NH3 formation are other ways of modification of drugs (Haiser *et al.,* 2013). The microbes bind to the drugs physically, which are used in chemotherapy and lead to a decrease in its absorption (Carmody *et al.*, 2014). These gut microbiome also affects the metabolism indirectly by modulating the gene expression of the mucosal barrier (Bjorkholm *et al.*, 2009). When the liver is germ-free, a member of the Cyp 450 gene is increased along with Cyp 2a, Cyp 2b, Cyp 3a which are involved in the metabolism of steroids. While Cry 4a, which is associated with the metabolism of fatty acid (arachidonic acid). Also, there is constant overexpression of gene which encodes for receptor and transcription factors like constitutive androstane receptor, also called Nrli3. Alteration of these genes resulted in faster metabolism of Xenobiotics.

Drugs that are introduced intravenously are metabolized in the liver before they are excreted in the gut. In the gut, they are well exposed to the gut microbiome, which further helps in their metabolism and reabsorption. Irinotecan is one such drug that is introduced intravenously and used in treatment for colorectal cancer. Carboxylesterase converts irinotecan into its active form and further detoxified into its active form which is SN-38 G by UDP-glucuronosyltransferase in the liver. It can be reverted by bacterial enzyme β-glucuronidase (Fujita *et al.*, 2010). In tumourigenic rat these chemotherapic drug increases the composition of the bacterium – clostridium and Enterobacteriaceae in colon shows that there is an alteration in microbiota and it directly affects the inflammation or the bacteria possessing the β-glucuronidase enzyme (Lin *et al.*, 2012). The use of antibiotics decreases the number of these bacteria, which produce glucuronidase. Probiotics also have shown a clinical effect, i.e., a decrease in irinotecan induced diarrhoea. Irinotecan has got severe impact as they are intestinal toxic and hence, are dose limited. So, there is a need for the development of inhibitors of β-glucuronidase to reduce the toxic condition.

11.1.2. Response to Chemotherapies

Chemotherapeutic drugs have got direct interaction with the bacteria. These drugs can either inhibit bacterial growth or enhance. Studies have shown that E.coli (G-ve bacteria) and L.welshimeri (G+ve bacteria) is inhibited with the use of the drug (Lehouritis *et al.,* 2015). These interactions are studied by HPLC and mass spectrometer, which show the result of the biotransformation of drugs. Antineoplastic drugs like Oxaliplatin and Cisplatin are a platinum compound which kills tumour cells. These drugs act by inhibiting DNA replication and also targets cell membrane and organelle mitochondria (Galluzzi *et al.*, 2014). The drug leads to DNA double-strand breaks. Together with the killing of tumour cells; this also disrupts the integrity of the blood-brain barrier and ototoxicity, leading to hearing loss. Barrier breaching causes the microbes and pathogens easy access to the lymphatic node and even in blood circulation leading to septicemia (Hopper *et al.,* 2010).

Acidophilus, which is a probiotic bacterial species, help in restoring cisplatin-induced inflammation and anticancerous effect. *L. acidophilus* prime in the myeloid cells, for the production of ROS in response to platinum drugs. It is mainly dependent on the signalling pathway via myeloid differentiation primary response (MYD88) associated with PRRs. In germ-free mice, the genotoxic effect, as well as the cytotoxic effect of platinum compound and oxaliplatin, is decreased. (Lida *et al.*, 2013).

11.1.3. Toxicity Induced by Drug

Combination of living *L. acidophilus* and *B. bifidum*is lyophilized are used in the prevention of intestinal toxicity when treated with radiotherapy or cisplatin. *L. acidophilus* shows a positive response to the anticancerous effect of cisplatin. It may prevent the toxic side effects of drugs used. The gut microbiome can even regulate the β- cells of the pancreas, inflammation of the adipose tissue leading to induced obesity

11.2. Radiotherapy and its Effect on Microbiota

Radiotherapy is the use of ionized radiation therapy (RTX) for the treatment of cancer. Ionized radiation target nucleus and cause DNA damage due to the production of ROS by dissociation of water molecules. Ionization Radiation can also affect non-irradiated cells such as systemic radio- adaptive responses, including inflammatory and genomic instability. These are secondary to DNA damage and mediated by disruption of the protein involved in cell-cell interaction. Therefore, radiation is also associated with the infection of the pathogen.

11.2.1. Response to Ionization Radiation Therapy (RTX)

Microbiome in gut regulates the response to ionization radiation therapy. Effects of RTX are stimulative as well as suppressive response and even be ineffective in activating an anti-cancer immune response (Kroemer *et al.,* 2013). The gut microbiome has shown an effect in immune response which is induced by the death of an immunogenic cell in both cases, i.e. chemotherapic and immunotherapeutic. It is hypothesized that the gut microbiome has also got a role in the immunostimulatory effect of Ionisation Radiation Therapy (RTX).

11.2.2. Toxicity of RTX

Severe effects of RTX may induce enteropathy, which leads to incompletion of therapy. Probiotics have shown to be beneficial in the case of enteropathy. It contains *L. acidophilus, B. bifidum, L. casei* which has been found protective against gut toxicity. Studies have shown that circadian rhythm affects apoptosis and activation of p53. As this show association with both diurnal variation in gut microbial composition and short-chain fatty acid production, this results in oscillation in several circulating inflammatory cell.

11.3. Immunotherapy and its Effect on Microbiota

In most of the patients, cancer therapies are becoming resistant, and the chance of reoccurrence is increased. Immunotherapy has the potential to treat solid cancer, and as studies have shown how gut microbiome affect inflammation. These microbes can even modulate the immunotherapy responses, which seem to improve the efficacy of immunotherapy.

11.3.1. IntratumoralCpG–oligodeoxynucleotidetherapy (ODN)

CpG-oligodeoxynucleotides (OND), when combined with antibody, neutralizes IL-10 signalling, which helps in treating subcutaneous tumour (Backhed *et al.,* 2015). After treatment with OND, there is a significant difference seen in the gene expression, notably, which encodes for inflammatory products like TNF and IL-12. It is also found a reduction in response to OND in TLR-4 deficient condition. The change in the bacterial count of genera of Alistipes (Gram-negative bacteria) and Ruminococcus (gram-positive) genera show a positive relation with TNF production. On the other hand, *L. murinum, L. intestinalis* and *L. fermentum* are negatively related. Indicates that different gut microbiome has a different response when treated with the OND.

11.3.2. Inhibitors of Immune Checkpoints

CTLA4 is expressed on the activated effector T cell. On anti-CTLA-4 treatment species of *Bacteroidales* decreases but species of *Clostridiales* increases. Moreover, *Bacteroidesfragilis* doesn't change (Veitzou). This increased frequency of *Bacteroidetes* has shown a relation with resistance to Colitis. If *B. fragilis* and *B. cepacia* is administered, then there is restoring of therapeutic response to anti-CTLA4.

12. CONCLUSION

The gut microbiome plays an essential role in Colitis associated cancer. Crohn's disease and Ulcerative Colitis are two main entities of IBD which also show their relation with the dysbiosis of microbiome. By the use of fewer carbohydrates in our diet leading to less production of SCFAs and further reduces colon polyps. Gut microbiota responds to therapies such as chemo, radio and immune that are made in case of the tumour. The challenge is how to modify the gut microbiota in patients with CRC. Studies have shown that therapeutics have targeted microbiome and able to recolonize the microbiome, which is ready to fight against the antibiotic resistance.

REFERENCES

Arap, M. A., Lahdenranta, J., Mintz, P. J., Hajitou, A., Sarkis, Á. S., Arap, W., & Pasqualini, R. (2004). Cell surface expression of the stress response chaperone GRP78 enables tumor targeting by circulating ligands. *Cancer Cell, 6*(3), 275–284. doi:10.1016/j.ccr.2004.08.018 PMID:15380518

Bäckhed, F., Roswall, J., Peng, Y., Feng, Q., Jia, H., Kovatcheva-Datchary, P., ... Khan, M. T. (2015). Dynamics and stabilization of the human gut microbiome during the first year of life. *Cell Host & Microbe, 17*(5), 690–703. doi:10.1016/j.chom.2015.04.004 PMID:25974306

Basso, P. J., Fonseca, M. T. C., Bonfá, G., Alves, V. B. F., Sales-Campos, H., Nardini, V., & Cardoso, C. R. B. (2014). Association among genetic predisposition, gut microbiota, and host immune response in the etiopathogenesis of inflammatory bowel disease. *Brazilian Journal of Medical and Biological Research, 47*(9), 727–737. doi:10.1590/1414-431X20143932 PMID:25075576

Baxter, N. T., Zackular, J. P., Chen, G. Y., & Schloss, P. D. (2014). Structure of the gut microbiome following colonization with human feces determines colonic tumor burden. *Microbiome*, *2*(1), 20. doi:10.1186/2049-2618-2-20 PMID:24967088

Becattini, S., Taur, Y., & Pamer, E. G. (2016). Antibiotic-induced changes in the intestinal microbiota and disease. *Trends in Molecular Medicine*, *22*(6), 458–478. doi:10.1016/j.molmed.2016.04.003 PMID:27178527

Bhattacharya, N., Yuan, R., Prestwood, T. R., Penny, H. L., DiMaio, M. A., Reticker-Flynn, N. E., ... Tolentino, L. (2016). Normalizing microbiota-induced retinoic acid deficiency stimulates protective CD8+ T cell-mediated immunity in colorectal cancer. *Immunity*, *45*(3), 641–655. doi:10.1016/j.immuni.2016.08.008 PMID:27590114

Björkholm, B., Bok, C. M., Lundin, A., Rafter, J., Hibberd, M. L., & Pettersson, S. (2009). Intestinal microbiota regulate xenobiotic metabolism in the liver. *PLoS One*, *4*(9), e6958. doi:10.1371/journal.pone.0006958 PMID:19742318

Boleij, A., Hechenbleikner, E. M., Goodwin, A. C., Badani, R., Stein, E. M., Lazarev, M. G., ... Platz, E. A. (2015). The Bacteroides fragilis toxin gene is prevalent in the colon mucosa of colorectal cancer patients. *Clinical Infectious Diseases*, *60*(2), 208–215. doi:10.1093/cid/ciu787 PMID:25305284

Carbonero, F., Benefiel, A. C., Alizadeh-Ghamsari, A. H., & Gaskins, H. R. (2012). Microbial pathways in colonic sulfur metabolism and links with health and disease. *Frontiers in Physiology*, *3*, 448. doi:10.3389/fphys.2012.00448 PMID:23226130

Carmody, R. N., & Turnbaugh, P. J. (2014). Host-microbial interactions in the metabolism of therapeutic and diet-derived xenobiotics. *The Journal of Clinical Investigation*, *124*(10), 4173–4181. doi:10.1172/JCI72335 PMID:25105361

Chandrasekar, V. T., & Venu, N. (2015). So What Is Crohn's Disease and Ulcerative Colitis? Pathophysiology of Crohn's Disease and Ulcerative Colitis. In *Inflammatory Bowel Disease* (pp. 15–23). Springer.

Eaden, J. A., Abrams, K. R., & Mayberry, J. F. (2001). The risk of colorectal cancer in ulcerative Colitis: A meta-analysis. *Gut*, *48*(4), 526–535. doi:10.1136/gut.48.4.526 PMID:11247898

Ellerby, H. M., Arap, W., Ellerby, L. M., Kain, R., Andrusiak, R., Del Rio, G., ... Bredesen, D. E. (1999). Anti-cancer activity of targeted pro-apoptotic peptides. *Nature Medicine*, *5*(9), 1032–1038. doi:10.1038/12469 PMID:10470080

Fierer, N., Bradford, M. A., & Jackson, R. B. (2007). Toward an ecological classification of soil bacteria. *Ecology*, *88*(6), 1354–1364. doi:10.1890/05-1839 PMID:17601128

Frank, D. N., Robertson, C. E., Hamm, C. M., Kpadeh, Z., Zhang, T., Chen, H., ... Pace, N. R. (2011). Disease phenotype and genotype are associated with shifts in intestinal-associated microbiota in inflammatory bowel diseases. *Inflammatory Bowel Diseases*, *17*(1), 179–184. doi:10.1002/ibd.21339 PMID:20839241

Fujita, K. I., & Sparreboom, A. (2010). Pharmacogenetics of irinotecan disposition and toxicity: A review. *Current Clinical Pharmacology*, *5*(3), 209–217. doi:10.2174/157488410791498806 PMID:20406168

Galluzzi, L., Vitale, I., Michels, J., Brenner, C., Szabadkai, G., Harel-Bellan, A., Castedo, M., & Kroemer, G. J. C. D. (2014). Systems biology of cisplatin resistance: Past, present and future. *Cell Death & Disease*, *5*(5), e1257–e1257. doi:10.1038/cddis.2013.428 PMID:24874729

Gustaw, W., Kordowska-Wiater, M., & Kozioł, J. (2011). The influence of selected prebiotics on the growth of lactic acid bacteria for bio-yoghurt production. *Acta Scientiarum Polonorum. Technologia Alimentaria*, *10*(4), 455–466. PMID:22230927

Gutiérrez-Díaz, I., Fernández-Navarro, T., Sánchez, B., Margolles, A., & González, S. (2016). Mediterranean diet and faecal microbiota: A transversal study. *Food & Function*, *7*(5), 2347–2356. doi:10.1039/C6FO00105J PMID:27137178

Haiser, H. J., & Turnbaugh, P. J. (2013). Developing a metagenomic view of xenobiotic metabolism. *Pharmacological Research*, *69*(1), 21–31. doi:10.1016/j.phrs.2012.07.009 PMID:22902524

Han, Y. W., Shi, W., Huang, G. T. J., Haake, S. K., Park, N. H., Kuramitsu, H., & Genco, R. J. (2000). Interactions between periodontal bacteria and human oral epithelial cells: Fusobacterium nucleatum adheres to and invades epithelial cells. *Infection and Immunity*, *68*(6), 3140–3146. doi:10.1128/IAI.68.6.3140-3146.2000 PMID:10816455

Hooper, L. V., & Macpherson, A. J. (2010). Immune adaptations that maintain homeostasis with the intestinal microbiota. *Nature Reviews. Immunology*, *10*(3), 159–169. doi:10.1038/nri2710 PMID:20182457

Hussein, I. A. H., Tohme, R., Kassem Barada, M. H. M., Freund, J. N., Jurjus, R. A., Karam, W., & Jurjus, A. (2008). Inflammatory bowel disease in rats: Bacterial and chemical interaction. *World Journal of Gastroenterology: WJG*, *14*(25), 4028. doi:10.3748/wjg.14.4028 PMID:18609687

Itzkowitz, S. H., & Yio, X. (2004). Inflammation and cancer IV. Colorectal cancer in inflammatory bowel disease: The role of inflammation. *American Journal of Physiology. Gastrointestinal and Liver Physiology*, *287*(1), G7–G17. doi:10.1152/ajpgi.00079.2004 PMID:15194558

Ivanov, K., Kolev, N., Tonev, A., Nikolova, G., Krasnaliev, I., Softova, E., & Tonchev, A. (2009). Comparative analysis of prognostic significance of molecular markers of apoptosis with clinical stage and tumor differentiation in patients with colorectal cancer: A single institute experience. *Hepato-Gastroenterology*, *56*(89), 94–98. PMID:19453036

Jan, G. B. A. S., Belzacq, A. S., Haouzi, D., Rouault, A., Metivier, D., Kroemer, G., & Brenner, C. (2002). Propionibacteria induce apoptosis of colorectal carcinoma cells via short-chain fatty acids acting on mitochondria. *Cell Death and Differentiation*, *9*(2), 179–188. doi:10.1038j.cdd.4400935 PMID:11840168

Kamdar, K., Khakpour, S., Chen, J., Leone, V., Brulc, J., Mangatu, T., ... Young, G. (2016). Genetic and metabolic signals during acute enteric bacterial infection alter the microbiota and drive progression to chronic inflammatory disease. *Cell Host & Microbe*, *19*(1), 21–31. doi:10.1016/j.chom.2015.12.006 PMID:26764594

Kanazawa, K., Konishi, F., Mitsuoka, T., Terada, A., Itoh, K., Narushima, S., Kumemura, M., & Kimura, H. (1996). Factors influencing the development of sigmoid colon cancer: Bacteriologic and biochemical studies. *Cancer: Interdisciplinary International Journal of the American Cancer Society*, *77*(8), 1701–1706. doi:10.1002/(SICI)1097-0142(19960415)77:8<1701::AID-CNCR42>3.0.CO;2-0 PMID:8608565

Kashyap, P. C., Marcobal, A., Ursell, L. K., Smits, S. A., Sonnenburg, E. D., Costello, E. K., ... Knight, R. (2013). Genetically dictated change in host mucus carbohydrate landscape exerts a diet-dependent effect on the gut microbiota. *Proceedings of the National Academy of Sciences of the United States of America*, *110*(42), 17059–17064. doi:10.1073/pnas.1306070110 PMID:24062455

Kroemer, G., Galluzzi, L., Kepp, O., & Zitvogel, L. (2013). Immunogenic cell death in cancer therapy. *Annual Review of Immunology*, *31*(1), 51–72. doi:10.1146/annurev-immunol-032712-100008 PMID:23157435

Lehouritis, P., Cummins, J., Stanton, M., Murphy, C. T., McCarthy, F. O., Reid, G., Urbaniak, C., Byrne, W. L., & Tangney, M. (2015). Local bacteria affect the efficacy of chemotherapeutic drugs. *Scientific Reports*, *5*(1), 14554. doi:10.1038rep14554 PMID:26416623

Li, H., & Jia, W. (2013). Cometabolism of microbes and host: Implications for drug metabolism and drug-induced toxicity. *Clinical Pharmacology and Therapeutics*, *94*(5), 574–581. doi:10.1038/clpt.2013.157 PMID:23933971

Lida, N., Dzutsev, A., Stewart, C. A., Smith, L., Bouladoux, N., Weingarten, R. A., ... Dai, R. M. (2013). Commensal bacteria control cancer response to therapy by modulating the tumor microenvironment. *Science*, *342*(6161), 967–970. doi:10.1126cience.1240527 PMID:24264989

Lin, X. B., Dieleman, L. A., Ketabi, A., Bibova, I., Sawyer, M. B., Xue, H., Field, C. J., Baracos, V. E., & Gänzle, M. G. (2012). Irinotecan (CPT-11) chemotherapy alters intestinal microbiota in tumour bearing rats. *PLoS One*, *7*(7), e39764. doi:10.1371/journal.pone.0039764 PMID:22844397

Lopez, J., & Grinspan, A. (2016). Fecal microbiota transplantation for inflammatory bowel disease. *Gastroenterology & Hepatology*, *12*(6), 374. PMID:27493597

Lu, R., Wu, S., Zhang, Y. G., Xia, Y., Liu, X., Zheng, Y., ... Li, L. (2014). Enteric bacterial protein AvrA promotes colonic tumorigenesis and activates colonic beta-catenin signaling pathway. *Oncogenesis*, *3*(6), e105. doi:10.1038/oncsis.2014.20 PMID:24911876

Macfarlane, G. T., & Cummings, J. H. (1999). Probiotics and prebiotics: Can regulating the activities of intestinal bacteria benefit health? *BMJ (Clinical Research Ed.)*, *318*(7189), 999–1003. doi:10.1136/bmj.318.7189.999 PMID:10195977

Malik, A., Sharma, D., Zhu, Q., Karki, R., Guy, C. S., Vogel, P., & Kanneganti, T. D. (2016). IL-33 regulates the IgA-microbiota axis to restrain IL-1α–dependent Colitis and tumorigenesis. *The Journal of Clinical Investigation*, *126*(12), 4469–4481. doi:10.1172/JCI88625 PMID:27775548

Marchesi, J. R., Adams, D. H., Fava, F., Hermes, G. D., Hirschfield, G. M., Hold, G., ... Thomas, L. V. (2016). The gut microbiota and host health: A new clinical frontier. *Gut*, *65*(2), 330–339. doi:10.1136/gutjnl-2015-309990 PMID:26338727

Marchesi, J. R., Dutilh, B. E., Hall, N., Peters, W. H., Roelofs, R., Boleij, A., & Tjalsma, H. (2011). Towards the human colorectal cancer microbiome. *PLoS One*, *6*(5), e20447. doi:10.1371/journal.pone.0020447 PMID:21647227

McCoy, A. N., Araujo-Perez, F., Azcarate-Peril, A., Yeh, J. J., Sandler, R. S., & Keku, T. O. (2013). Fusobacterium is associated with colorectal adenomas. *PLoS One*, *8*(1), e53653. doi:10.1371/journal.pone.0053653 PMID:23335968

Mira-Pascual, L., Cabrera-Rubio, R., Ocon, S., Costales, P., Parra, A., Suarez, A., Moris, F., Rodrigo, L., Mira, A., & Collado, M. C. (2015). Microbial mucosal colonic shifts associated with the development of colorectal cancer reveal the presence of different bacterial and archaeal biomarkers. *Journal of Gastroenterology*, *50*(2), 167–179. doi:10.100700535-014-0963-x PMID:24811328

Moayyedi, P., Surette, M. G., Kim, P. T., Libertucci, J., Wolfe, M., Onischi, C., Armstrong, D., Marshall, J. K., Kassam, Z., Reinisch, W., & Lee, C. H. (2015). Fecal microbiota transplantation induces remission in patients with active ulcerative Colitis in a randomized controlled trial. *Gastroenterology*, *149*(1), 102–109. doi:10.1053/j.gastro.2015.04.001 PMID:25857665

Morampudi, V., Dalwadi, U., Bhinder, G., Sham, H. P., Gill, S. K., Chan, J., ... Gibson, D. L. (2016). The goblet cell-derived mediator RELM-β drives spontaneous Colitis in Muc2-deficient mice by promoting commensal microbial dysbiosis. *Mucosal Immunology*, *9*(5), 1218–1233. doi:10.1038/mi.2015.140 PMID:26813339

Mukhopadhya, I., Hansen, R., Nicholl, C. E., Alhaidan, Y. A., Thomson, J. M., Berry, S. H., Pattinson, C., Stead, D. A., Russell, R. K., El-Omar, E. M., & Hold, G. L. (2011). A comprehensive evaluation of colonic mucosal isolates of Sutterella wadsworthensis from inflammatory bowel disease. *PLoS One*, *6*(10), e27076. doi:10.1371/journal.pone.0027076 PMID:22073125

Ou, J., Carbonero, F., Zoetendal, E. G., DeLany, J. P., Wang, M., Newton, K., Gaskins, H. R., & O'Keefe, S. J. (2013). Diet, microbiota, and microbial metabolites in colon cancer risk in rural Africans and African Americans. *The American Journal of Clinical Nutrition*, *98*(1), 111–120. doi:10.3945/ajcn.112.056689 PMID:23719549

Prorok-Hamon, M., Friswell, M. K., Alswied, A., Roberts, C. L., Song, F., Flanagan, P. K., ... Hall, N. (2014). Colonic mucosa-associated diffusely adherent afaC+ Escherichia coli expressing lpfA and pks are increased in inflammatory bowel disease and colon cancer. *Gut*, *63*(5), 761–770. doi:10.1136/gutjnl-2013-304739 PMID:23846483

Rajilić-Stojanović, M., & de Vos, W. M. (2014). The first 1000 cultured species of the human gastrointestinal microbiota. *FEMS Microbiology Reviews*, *38*(5), 996–1047. doi:10.1111/1574-6976.12075 PMID:24861948

Rossen, N. G., MacDonald, J. K., de Vries, E. M., D'Haens, G. R., de Vos, W. M., Zoetendal, E. G., & Ponsioen, C. Y. (2015). Fecal microbiota transplantation as novel therapy in gastroenterology: A systematic review. *World journal of gastroenterology. WJG*, *21*(17), 5359. doi:10.3748/wjg.v21.i17.5359 PMID:25954111

Rubin, D. C., Shaker, A., & Levin, M. S. (2012). Chronic intestinal inflammation: Inflammatory bowel disease and colitis-associated colon cancer. *Frontiers in Immunology*, *3*, 107. doi:10.3389/fimmu.2012.00107 PMID:22586430

Sartor, R. B. (2008). Microbial influences in inflammatory bowel diseases. *Gastroenterology*, *134*(2), 577–594. doi:10.1053/j.gastro.2007.11.059 PMID:18242222

Scanlan, P. D., Shanahan, F., Clune, Y., Collins, J. K., O'Sullivan, G. C., O'Riordan, M., Holmes, E., Wang, Y., & Marchesi, J. R. (2008). Culture-independent analysis of the gut microbiota in colorectal cancer and polyposis. *Environmental Microbiology*, *10*(3), 789–798. doi:10.1111/j.1462-2920.2007.01503.x PMID:18237311

Sears, C. L., & Pardoll, D. M. (2011). Perspective: Alpha-bugs, their microbial partners, and the link to colon cancer. *The Journal of Infectious Diseases*, *203*(3), 306–311. doi:10.1093/jinfdis/jiq061 PMID:21208921

Shen, X. J., Rawls, J. F., Randall, T. A., Burcall, L., Mpande, C., Jenkins, N., Jovov, B., Abdo, Z., Sandler, R. S., & Keku, T. O. (2010). Molecular characterization of mucosal adherent bacteria and associations with colorectal adenomas. *Gut Microbes*, *1*(3), 138–147. doi:10.4161/gmic.1.3.12360 PMID:20740058

Sigel, J. E., Petras, R. E., Lashner, B. A., Fazio, V. W., & Goldblum, J. R. (1999). Intestinal adenocarcinoma in Crohn's disease: A report of 30 cases with a focus on coexisting dysplasia. *The American Journal of Surgical Pathology*, *23*(6), 651–655. doi:10.1097/00000478-199906000-00003 PMID:10366146

Sobhani, I., Tap, J., Roudot-Thoraval, F., Roperch, J. P., Letulle, S., Langella, P., Corthier, G., Van Nhieu, J. T., & Furet, J. P. (2011). Microbial dysbiosis in colorectal cancer (CRC) patients. *PLoS One*, *6*(1), e16393. doi:10.1371/journal.pone.0016393 PMID:21297998

Spanogiannopoulos, P., & Turnbaugh, P. J. (2018). Broad collateral damage of drugs against the gut microbiome. *Nature Reviews. Gastroenterology & Hepatology*, *15*(8), 457–458. doi:10.103841575-018-0028-3 PMID:29752457

Tian, J., Lin, X., Zhou, W., & Xu, J. (2003). Hydroxyethyl starch inhibits NF-κB activation and prevents the expression of inflammatory mediators in endotoxic rats. *Annals of Clinical and Laboratory Science*, *33*(4), 451–458. PMID:14584760

Tjalsma, H., Boleij, A., Marchesi, J. R., & Dutilh, B. E. (2012). A bacterial driver–passenger model for colorectal cancer: Beyond the usual suspects. *Nature Reviews. Microbiology*, *10*(8), 575–582. doi:10.1038/nrmicro2819 PMID:22728587

Tomasello, G., Tralongo, P., Damiani, P., Sinagra, E., Di Trapani, B., Zeenny, M. N., ... Leone, A. (2014). Dismicrobism in inflammatory bowel disease and colorectal cancer: Changes in response of colocytes. *World Journal of Gastroenterology: WJG*, *20*(48), 18121. doi:10.3748/wjg.v20.i48.18121 PMID:25561781

Vétizou, M., Pitt, J. M., Daillère, R., Lepage, P., Waldschmitt, N., Flament, C., ... Poirier-Colame, V. (2015). Anticancer immunotherapy by CTLA-4 blockade relies on the gut microbiota. *Science*, *350*(6264), 1079–1084. doi:10.1126cience.aad1329 PMID:26541610

Vinolo, M. A., Rodrigues, H. G., Nachbar, R. T., & Curi, R. (2011). Regulation of inflammation by short chain fatty acids. *Nutrients*, *3*(10), 858–876. doi:10.3390/nu3100858 PMID:22254083

Wang, T., Cai, G., Qiu, Y., Fei, N., Zhang, M., Pang, X., Jia, W., Cai, S., & Zhao, L. (2012). Structural segregation of gut microbiota between colorectal cancer patients and healthy volunteers. *The ISME Journal*, *6*(2), 320–329. doi:10.1038/ismej.2011.109 PMID:21850056

Warren, R. L., Freeman, D. J., Pleasance, S., Watson, P., Moore, R. A., Cochrane, K., & Holt, R. A. (2013). Co-occurrence of anaerobic bacteria in colorectal carcinomas. *Microbiome*, *1*(1), 16. doi:10.1186/2049-2618-1-16 PMID:24450771

Weitkunat, K., Schumann, S., Petzke, K. J., Blaut, M., Loh, G., & Klaus, S. (2015). Effects of dietary inulin on bacterial growth, short-chain fatty acid production and hepatic lipid metabolism in gnotobiotic mice. *The Journal of Nutritional Biochemistry*, *26*(9), 929–937. doi:10.1016/j.jnutbio.2015.03.010 PMID:26033744

Wolf, A. J., Reyes, C. N., Liang, W., Becker, C., Shimada, K., Wheeler, M. L., Cho, H. C., Popescu, N. I., Coggeshall, K. M., Arditi, M., & Underhill, D. M. (2016). Hexokinase is an innate immune receptor for the detection of bacterial peptidoglycan. *Cell*, *166*(3), 624–636. doi:10.1016/j.cell.2016.05.076 PMID:27374331

Wu, N., Yang, X., Zhang, R., Li, J., Xiao, X., Hu, Y., & Luan, C. (2013). Dysbiosis signature of fecal microbiota in colorectal cancer patients. *Microbial Ecology*, *66*(2), 462–470. doi:10.100700248-013-0245-9 PMID:23733170

Yang, Y., & Jobin, C. (2017). Novel insights into microbiome in Colitis and colorectal cancer. *Current Opinion in Gastroenterology*, *33*(6), 422–427. doi:10.1097/MOG.0000000000000399 PMID:28877044

Zhu, Q., Jin, Z., Wu, W., Gao, R., Guo, B., Gao, Z., & Qin, H. (2014). Analysis of the intestinal lumen microbiota in an animal model of colorectal cancer. *PLoS One*, *9*(3), e90849. doi:10.1371/journal.pone.0090849 PMID:24603888

Chapter 8
Mathematical Approach in Colitis-Related Colon Cancer Genomics:
Inflammatory Bowel Disease (IBD)

Pervaiz Iqbal
B. S. Abdur Rahman Crescent Institute of Science and Technology, India

Rubeena Khaliq
B. S. Abdur Rahman Crescent Institute of Science and Technology, India

Aadil Rashid Sheergojri
B. S. Abdur Rahman Crescent Institute of Science and Technology, India

ABSTRACT

Ulcerative colitis or Crohn's illness patients are in danger of colon cancer due to chronic inflammation, resulting from the reaction of the immune system to bacterial disease caused by genetic alterations in the colonic mucosa. Somatic cells gain genomic changes, such as TP53 that regulates MUC2 production and APC alterations linked with β-catenin and MUC1 contribution in the slight proliferation of cells. Mathematical modeling describes developmental modifications and uses the phrases to link parameter to curves of age-dependent incidence of epidemiological cancer. By using the long-lasting investigation of IBD patients to gather the genomic estimations for increasingly exact computations of IBD-explicit developmental parameters as initiation, birth, and death. Colon cancer genetic trajectory follows the structure of the composition of functions that leads to malignancies. Models of population level can be utilized to consolidate epidemiological information and in this manner describe malignant growth advancement in a population with IBD.

DOI: 10.4018/978-1-7998-3580-6.ch008

INTRODUCTION

In idiopathic inflammatory bowel disorder (IBD), UC and CD are two types of chronic disorders categorized in a way that turns out to be worse with time having disease symptoms and acquired by severe signs which don't cease or vanish completely. The distinctions between inflammatory bowel disease, ulcerative colitis, and Crohn's disease are confusing for many individuals. On the other hand, roughly 10% of patients cannot be measured accurately in either classification and are classified as having indeterminate colitis. The brief answer is that IBD is the shelter word for both UC and CD. But there is a lot more to the tale, of course (Gillen et al., 1994).

Both illnesses comprise of inflammation of the intestine or bowel cap - hence the name resulting in inflamed, enlarged bowel, and that develop ulcers. Inflammation and its effects on UC and CD are distinct. The inflammation causes abdominal discomfort, diarrhea, and intestinal bleeding to varying degrees. Both illnesses can lead to severe digestive issues, and are characterized by the body's immune system's unusual reaction and may share certain signs (Feakins, 2013). There are also significant variations, though. These differences include mainly the place of diseases in the body of the gastrointestinal (GI) and how each disease reacts to therapy. Understanding these characteristics is essential for a gastroenterologist to obtain a correct diagnosis. For genetically susceptible individuals subjected to environmental risk factors, IBD is thought to result from an excessive and inadequate immune response to gut luminal microbes. Although recent progress has shed a great deal of light on its molecular pathogenesis, IBD's exact cause(s) remains elusive (Hendrickson et al., 2002).

1.1. IBD (Inflammatory Bowel Disorder)

IBD (Inflammatory Bowel Disorder) is a severe state of unknown origin that is defined by intense inflammation and intestinal mucosal deterioration. Inflammatory Bowel Disease is a set of intestinal disorders that cause long-term digestive tract inflammation, which includes the throat, esophagus, stomach, small intestine, and large intestine and is accountable for breaking down food products, reducing nutrients, and recycling unusable materials and waste products (Axelrad et al., 2016; Baumgart & Carding, 2007).

IBDs are a prominent illustration of the connection between chronic inflammation and cancer, and an enhanced likelihood of creating colorectal cancer is one result of constant inflammation of the colon or ulcerative colitis (Abdulkhaleq et al., 2018). Animal models that replicate many elements of this human disease have given important hints as to the key functions of inflammatory mediators and associated molecular occurrences contributing to the growth of colon cancer ().

Long ahead, the increase of enhanced sanitation and metropolinization in the early 20th decade, IBD was rarely seen. It is still discovered today primarily in advanced countries like the US. Similar to additional self-immune and sensitive illnesses, it is thought that the absence of growth of germ resistance has led in part to illnesses like IBD (Kappelman et al., 2007).

In individuals with IBD, the immune system scans for overseas objects food, bacteria, or other products in the GI tract and reacts by bringing WBC's into the bowel border. The outcome of the assault by the immune system makes it persistent for infection. The term inflammation itself arises from the flames of the Greek phrase. It implies literally "being put on flame" (Alberts, 1994).

IECs are physical obstacles for bacteria and other antigens entering the bloodstream from the lumen of the intestine. An intact mucosal obstacle is based on junctions inside the cells that help to seal the gap between neighboring epithelial cells and tense junctions that are the main seal components. The paracellular space has increased permeability in inflammatory bowel disease, and to govern the close junctions is deficient (). These phenomena may be caused by a primary barrier function defect or may arise from inflammation.

1.2. Main Types of IBD

Included in this IBD umbrella term are many diseases. UC and CD are the two most prevalent circumstances. Both diseases comprise of inflammation of the bowel or intestine wall-hence the name-leading to inflammation, swelling, and ulcers in the bowel. In UC and CD, the swelling and its effects are distinct. The inflammation leads to abdominal discomfort, diarrhea, and intestinal bleeding in different degrees. Both illnesses can cause severe digestive issues (Gillen et al., 1994).

1.2.1. UC (Ulcerative Colitis)

UC is a type of IBD, the umbrella word for a disorder causing small intestine and colon inflammation. IBD includes a cluster of gastrointestinal tract-affected illnesses. Diagnosing UC is difficult as the signs are close to additional intestinal disorders as well as another form of IBD called Crohn's disease (CD), which varies because it induces greater inflammation in the intestinal wall (transmural) and may happen in other areas of the digestive system including the mouth, esophagus, small intestine, and stomach ().

UC happens when your large intestine lining (also known as the colon) rectum or both becomes inflamed. This inflammation turns out small sores on the lining of your colon called ulcers. Usually, it starts in the rectum and extends upwards and can contain your entire colon. The inflammation leads your intestine to progress quickly and frequently empty its contents. As cells die on your bowel's lining surface, ulcers form. The ulcers can induce mucus and pus to bleed and release ().

UC is a chronic disease that can lead from asymptomatic moderate swelling to severe colon infection, leading to regular bloody stools, tissue destruction and, potentially permanent fibrosis, colonic motility dysfunction, complete symptoms, and surgical need.

UC is classified according to the severity of the symptom and the nature of the disease. Severity is characterized as mild, moderate, extreme or fulminant depending on the symptoms, the number of stools per day, changes in the level of erythrocyte sedimentation, and toxicity signs (Feuerstein & Cheifetz, 2014).

On the basis of the location of inflammation in the intestines, UC may be defined as:

a) **Ulcerative proctitis:** If the rectum or lower portion of the colon is inflamed. It is usually the mildest type of ulcerative colitis
b) **Proctosigmoiditis:** This involves the inflammation in the rectum and the sigmoid colon, which is the lower end of the colon.
c) **Pancolitis:** when the whole colon is affected. Continuous inflammation starts at the rectum and spreads beyond the splenic bending.
d) **Left-sided or distal colitis:** Continuous inflammation starts at the rectum in this type of ulcerative colitis and spreads to the colon with endpoint as the splenic flexure that is a spot where the bowel bends near the spleen.

I. Symptoms of Ulcerative Colitis

Diarrhea is typically the first sign of ulcerative colitis. Feces slowly become looser, and cramped abdominal pain and an extreme urge to move stools may occur. Diarrhea may start slowly or suddenly. Symptoms depend on inflammation severity and distribution.

The most common symptoms that patients may also experience are as follows:

- Body moisture loss (diarrhea) and nutrition loss (weight loss).
- Anemia was due to bleeding, causing tiredness as less count in red blood cells.
- Eye puffiness and redness
- Articular ache (arthritis).
- Skin sores and rash.
- Illness in lung and liver.

Over months or years at a time, symptoms may be mild or absent. These usually return without intervention, however, and vary depending on the section of the affected colon.

II. Causes of Ulcerative Colitis

Accurately, the cause of UC is unclear. Investigators consider that the immune system of the body responds towards bacteria and viruses, leading to cause intestinal wall inflammation. On the other hand, many researchers declared that UC may be the immune reaction, not the cause (). Ulcerative Colitis can be caused by the following factors:

a) **Familial history or genetic factors:** Approximately one-fifth of the population has a close relation with UC, because of inheritance or hereditary factors. Research studies have shown that in people with ulcerative colitis, several unusual genes may exist. However, researchers were unable to demonstrate a strong association between ulcerative colitis and unusual genes.
b) **Infectious agents or toxins from the atmosphere:** Some studies suggest that some environmental issues, such as smoking, diet, air pollution, poor hygiene, may increase a person's risk of ulcerative colitis, although the overall possibility of developing the disease is small.
c) **Immune System:** Many immune system changes have been reported as leading to inflammatory disease of the intestine. The body can respond to a viral or bacterial infection in a manner that causes ulcerative colitis-related inflammation.
d) **Psychological factors:** A few studies indicate that stress or emotional distress may raise the outbreak of UC in people. Such factors may cause symptoms in some people.

III. Diagnosis of Ulcerative Colitis

UC is treated with numerous tests. The first steps are generally a physical examination and medical history ().

A health care provider has the following diagnosis of ulcerative colitis:

- Family history and medical history.
- Physical examination.
- Laboratory examinations.
- Large-intestinal endoscopies.

1.2.2. CD (Crohn's Disease)

Dr. Burrill B. Crohn and his team in 1932, first identified CD is an IBD, a common name for conditions that cause inflammation or swelling of the intestines. CD is a condition of uncertain etiology characterized by gastrointestinal (GI) transmural inflammation. CD might include a few or all segments of the whole GIT from the oral cavity to the perianal zone; however, the perianal zone and terminal ileal show it typically. The inflammation it induces may reach deep into the wall of the affected areas of the digestive tract, resulting in swelling and formation of wounds that can cause symptoms such as diarrhea and pain (Feakins, 2013).

The condition of CD impacts both genders alike and appears to be running in some home members. Approximately 20% of individuals having CD have an ancestral history by a type of IBD, often shown in siblings, and a father/mother or a kid. CD may happen at all ages of people; however, it has been detected most commonly in people aged 20 to 30. Persons of are at the high-risk zone of getting a CD with Jewish heritage while as European countries are at lower risk of developing the same disorder (Baumgart & Sandborn, 2012; Kappelman et al., 2007)

Based on the affected part of the intestines, the CD may be defined as ():

- **Ileocolitis:** This is the most common type of CD. This affects the ileum and colon of the small intestine. Ileocolitis is diagnosed in about 50% of people.
- **Ileitis:** The ileum is affected by this form of CD, caused by bacterium Lawsonia intracellularis.
- **Gastroduodenal CD:** By this process, the stomach, the duodenum and the initial segment of the small bowel are affected and damaged.
- **Jejunoileitis:** A form of the disease that triggers infection in the jejunum area, which is the middle part of the small intestine.
- **Crohn's (Granulomatous) Colitis:** Large intestine (colon) is affected in this type of CD.

I. Symptoms of Crohn's Disease

The symptoms present are quite complex, but they can correlate to some degree with the pathology and position of the disease. CD can cause a wide range of symptoms that may differ in form as well as severity (Kaplan & Ng, 2017).

The most serious symptoms of CD include cramping, nausea, and pain in the belly and weight loss. Other signs include

- Bleeding from the rectum.
- Fever.

- Nausea, vomiting.
- Proper nutrient shortage, inadequacy in vitamins.
- Common dullness.
- Social disorders like stress, anxiety, and complications in coping, children might also have some problems with their lifestyle and physical appearance.

CD in Children can experience late and stunted growth. Not only symptoms are the sole guide for decisions on management (Gasparetto & Guariso, 2014), but subjective findings from biochemical markers, endoscopy, or radiological reports should be interrelated with objective findings of disease activity ().

II. Causes of Crohn's Disease

No unified theory describes the pathogenesis and inflammatory processes of CD (). Experts believe that CD can be caused by the following factors ().

a) **Autoimmune reaction:** An autoimmune reaction may be one cause of CD i.e. when your healthy cells are badly attacked by the immune system in your body. The immune system of humans consists of various proteins and cells that prevent people against infection. The major common theory states that the immune system of the body responds abnormally, foods, mistaking bacteria, and other foreign substances in people with CD. Erythema nodosum, Arthritis, iritis, and other extraintestinal symptoms seen in victims with CD and UC are probably responsible for antigen-antibody reactions in the skin, joints, and ears.
b) **Genes:** Sometimes CD may be genetic. If family members are affected by CD, there is a high chance of developing CDs or a high-risk zone of developing the same disease. Approximately 10–15% of CD patients have a family history of the disorder. Identical twins have a concordance of at least 53% for CD; even there is a similar possibility for fraternal twins as having a family history.
c) **Other factors:** Several reports indicate other factors can increase the risk of CD.
    - Smoking acts as a bad prognostic factor as it doubles the possibility of promoting the CD.
    - CD can be caused by Non-steroidal anti-inflammatory drugs (NSAIDs) like ibuprofen or aspirin, birth control pills, and antibiotics which in turn speed up the risk of CD.
    - Additionally, a high intake of fat full diet also increases the chance of having a CD. However, consuming some foods shows no exacerbation towards CD.

III. Diagnosis of Crohn's Disease

Since the symptoms of CD are not barefaced at its infancy showing high complications while diagnosis. So, doctors usually make use of different screening tools as well as different treatment methodologies to detect and treat CD respectively, which are the same as those used in UC (Geboes, 2001).

2. EPIDEMIOLOGY OF INFLAMMATORY BOWEL DISEASE

2.1. United States Statistics

According to United States Statistics, till 1960 UC was leading and was much higher than that of CD, but current demography reflects that CD victims are tending to UC incidence rate. In addition in 2015, the U.S. reported 1.3% of adults (3 million) IBD (either CD or UC) diagnosed, which was a substantial raise from 1999 (0.9% or 2 million adults). Annually, IBD accounts for an additional seven lakh doctor visits and one lakh hospitalizations. Around 1-2 million residents of the United States have UC and CD, with a frequency of 70-150 occurrences every one lakh population. In Olmstead County, Minnesota, the frequency of UC in people of European origin was about 7.3 reports every one lakh population every annum, with a rate of one hundred sixteen reports every one lakh population every year; the frequency of CD was 5.8 reports every one lakh population every annum, with a rate of one hundred thirty-three clients every one lakh population every year (Kappelman et al., 2007).

Depending on data from the National Inpatient Survey, there was no substantial improvement in medication rate from 2003 to 2013 when CD was the main diagnosis. However, over this time the medication rate raised dramatically from 44.2 to 59.7 every one lakh people when it was identified as an ordinary diagnosis. The estimated medication cost for CD was $11,345 and UC was $13,412. Total hospitalization costs for CD rose by 3% per year from 2003 to 2008 and UC by 4% but remained unchanged for both diseases from 2008 to 2014 ().

In the pediatric population, the estimated incidence of CD, UC and gross IBD was 43, 28, and 71 for every one lakh respectively, and the estimated incidence was two lakh twelve hundred thirty-eight and four hundred forty-four for CD, UC, and full IBD, respectively for adults. Residents of America are suffering from CD and have about four lakh thirty-six thousands (one hundred fifty-one per one lakh) and five lakh twelve thousands have UC (one hundred seventy-eight per one lakh) after setting these incidence levels by the definite gender, age and a geographic sketch of U.S. population in 2005. About forty-five thousands three hundred (fifty-seven per one lakh) suffered patients are children under the age of twenty (twenty-seven thousands three hundred CD and eighteen thousands UC) (Kappelman et al., 2007).

2.2. International Statistics

It is believed that the highest IBD rates are in highly advanced nations and that the lowest is in growing environments; colder weather areas and metropolitan areas have higher IBD rates than warmer weather areas and far-flung areas. Globally, the prevalence of IBD is about 0.5-24.5 events of UC for every one lakh person-years and 0.1-16 events of CD for every one lakh person-years. Generally, IBD is found in three hundred ninety-six cases one lakh people per year (Kaplan & Ng, 2017).

An IBD study found that CD occurrence throughout North America was three hundred nineteen among one lakh people, whereas in Europe; it was three hundred twenty-two among one lakh people. The occurrence rates for UC throughout North America were two hundred forty-nine among one lakh people and in Europe five hundred five among one lakh people. CD average prevalence was 20.2 every one lakh person-years throughout North America, 12.7 for one lakh person-years throughout Europe, and 5.0 per one lakh person-years in Asia and the Middle East, while UC prevalence's remained 19.2 among one lakh person-years throughout North America, 24.3 per one lakh person-years of Europe, and 6.3 per one lakh person-years of the Middle East and Asia. Analyzes of the time pattern revealed statistically relevant changes in IBD prevalence with time.

The few studies measuring race/ethnicity recorded the highest IBD incidence among white and Jewish people. Nevertheless, it has been shown that the incidence of IBD among Hispanic and Asian people is growing; research has also shown that persons emigrating via weak prevalence areas (e.g., Asia) towards stronger prevalence areas (e.g., England) will be at higher risk of having IBDs, especially of first-generation children ().

Basically, IBD incidence in every area of the world is rising or stable. Since IBD mortality is small and the disorder is frequently detected in young people, these results reflect that IBD's global occurrence will increase continuously. The increasing prevalence of IBD throughout the 20th century can be explained by ecological changes arising from growing urbanization; yet, this rise might be due to raised understanding of IBD by specialists and the people, along with improvements in diagnostic methods of IBD (Alatab et al., 2020).

3. SOCIO-DEMOGRAPHIC FACTORS OF IBD

CD and UC incidence in both adolescent and elderly communities were significantly associated with age, area, and Medicaid status (da Silva et al., 2015).

a) **Effect of age:** The age distribution for recently diagnosed cases of IBD is bell-like; the highest occurrence happens in people at its infancy of the second phase of life, with the huge number of new diseases in people between the ages of 15 and 40 years. Second, lower occurrence increase arises and is increasing in patients aged 55-65 years. In IBD around 10% of victims come less than 18 years of age group. The prevalence of CD decreases after 30 years of age, while the prevalence tends to increase in older people. For CD, the rise in incidence decreased after the age of 30; whereas, the incidence for UC continues to enhance in older people.

b) **Effect of sex:** As for every chronic low-mortality disease, CD and UC incidence increased with growing age. For UC and CD, the male-to-female ratio is about 1:1, but reporting a significantly greater frequency with females. For young adults, UC and CD both are mostly reported (i.e., late puberty to the third phase of life).

c) **Geographic area influence:** Regional variations are important for both children and adults with UC and CD. For both conditions, the incidence in the South was lower than in all other areas. There was major geographic variability for both children as well as adults with UC and CD. The incidence was weaker in the South for both factors relative to all other areas.

d) **Racial effect:** It is estimated that the prevalence and incidence of IBD among African descent Americans are the same as the occurrence of European origin Americans, with the maximum percentage among middle European origin Jewish groups. There is a greater incidence in the Middle East and Asia along a North-South continuum, while trends suggest that the difference is narrowing.

e) **Impact of an insurance policy:** Kids with health insurance are more likely to be treated with CD or UC as compared to those who don't have any Medicaid insurance. This was also well valid in adults; though, the scale of the outcome was lower.

The comparative impacts of gender, age, insurance policy and geographic area on the occurrence of IBD didn't alter considerably with less use of stringent operational case definitions (Duricova et al., 2014).

4. SIGNALING PATHWAYS OF COLITIS ASSOCIATED COLON (CAC) CANCER

4.1. Oxidative Stress: CAC Damage Caused by DNA

Several genetic pathways, like nuclear factor-κB/tumor necrosis factor or interleukin 6/signal transducer and transcription 3 signaling activator, are being reported as significant factors to CAC development and might be essential clinical strategies for CAC treatment and prevention. Displacement of different oncogenes is needed for tumor initiation to allow subsequent tumor growth, including mutations resulting in apoptosis resistance and the acquisition of malignant potential. Likewise, when CAC progresses slowly, a series of different alterations develop. It may be named the carcinoma–inflammation–dysplasia pathway, describing the origin of substandard carcinoma in the history of abdominal infection, with eventual escalation to carcinoma in situ and eventually advanced nonmelanoma skin cancers. Alterations within spontaneous CRC are attributable to multiple types of genomic and biochemical volatility like CG island methylator phenotype, chromosomal volatility, global hypomethylation, and imbalance genetic abnormalities which results in nucleotide insecurity. Even though such genetic and biochemical modifications also arise in CAC, confirmation suggests a key function in infection (Fearon & Vogelstein, 1990).

Oxidative stress occurs by inequality in the production and removal of Reactive oxygen species (ROS) and reactive nitrogen species (RNS) (Gorrini et al., 2013). Enhanced oxidative stress is one of the main characteristics of continual infection when innate immune system cells release different types of reactive oxygen and nitrogen species (RONS) into the tissue microenvironment involving hyperoxide, peroxide, single oxygen, hydroxide ions, and nitrogen monoxide. Research shows that higher RONS associate with human IBD disease development, along with decreased antioxidant levels. Sohnet et al identified a number of proteins such as (phospho-checkpoint kinase 2, Histon gamma H2A.X) and senescence (Heterochromatin protein 1 gamma) markers in growing order of DDR for IBD patients with infectious tissue samples. In UC specimens, DDR and senescence increased as a possible source of RONS associated with macrophage infiltration promoting the use of apoptosis as a malignant shielding apparatus (Avdagić et al., 2013; Baskol et al., 2008; Jackson & Loeb, 2001).

4.2. NF-κB Pathway

As for as, NF-κB is concerned, this pathway is a main inflammatory receptor and could be regulated by a wide range of signals, consisting of constituents of bacteria, mainly pro-inflammatory cytokines like TNF-α and IL-1, lipopolysaccharides (LPS), agents and viruses that lead to damage of DNA (Karin & Greten, 2005). Many proinflammatory cytokines (like IL-1, IL-6, and TNF-α) expressed via a track with specified genes lead to inflammatory tissue destruction, and are correlated with growth and development of the tumor. TNF-α, e.g., was shown as a powerful mutagen that leads to the activation of the tumor through the activation of reactive oxygen species (ROS) development and the promotion of DNA destruction (). Expanded development and induction of proinflammatory cytokines such as TNF-α, IL-1, and IL-6 have been reported in IBD cases, particularly in mucosal macrophages and epithelial cells (Atreya et al., 2008). This can also encourage cancer growth and agitation by explicitly or implicitly developing both the VEGF, IL-8 and, COX-2, to induce new blood vessel development called angiogenesis (). In summary, the NF-κB pathway acts as a multi-atomic connection of tumorigenesis and inflammation because of its potential promoting the production of antiapoptotic genes, having the capability of promoting infection, proteases and blood vessels formation factors that encourage tumor activation and secure the future proliferation of malignant cells and invasion.

In animal experiments, a connection of NF-κB pathway and the colitis-associated CRC pathogenesis was reported. The design of the CA-CRC of an animal model was developed by AOM dose accompanied by regular oral intake of DSS, causing persistent infection to resemble IBD (Greten et al., 2004). Removal of IKKβ drastically reduced the occurrence of tumors infected with colitis, while significant increases in histological inflammation levels and proinflammatory cytokines were reported. AOM and DSS administration resulted in the IKK production and the secretion of BCL-XL, which is an anti-apoptotic protein that is missing in the IKKβ knockout mouse. The removal of enterocytes from IKKβ too enhanced programmed cell death by controlling the production of proapoptotic proteins Bak and Bax. Such findings suggest that in epithelial cells the NF-kB signaling pathway stimulates tumor growth by blocking apoptosis, instead of resolving proinflammatory gene transcription. The NF-κB pathway collectively promotes the growth of cancer in animal studies however, the signaling pathway to inhibit programmed cell death or pro-inflammatory cytokines are triggered that rely on the type of cell (Atreya et al., 2008; Greten et al., 2004; Karin & Greten, 2005). Mouse models in colitis-associated CRC were recognized by joint treatment of DSS and AOM, increased appearance of TNF-α was verified. TNF-Rp55 knockout or TNF-α antagonist etanercept treatment decreases the infiltration of mucosal inflammatory cells, tumor occurrence, and tumor volume (). TNF-α is, above all, a primary risk zone for the production of colitis-associated CRC within the NF-kB pathway

4.3. CTGF (Connective Tissue Growth Factor): Intervene Signaling Pathway

In UC, the CTGF-intervene signaling pathway alters infectious factors and abdominal flora (). CTGF is a form of CCN family-owned 38-kDa cysteinerich mysterious polypeptide (consisting of fisp12/CTGF, Nov, cry61/Cef10), that too may be directly persuaded by TGF-β (Chen et al., 2001). In collagenous colitis, research recently identified the upregulation of CTGF that too was observed to be an increment in ethanol-induced colitis/TNBS, which is considered the main frequently used model of CD (Günther et al., 2010). In order to persuade the experimental model of UC, a sulfated polysaccharide synthesized with sucrose, DSS was commonly used with anti-carcinogenic or anti-immunodeficiency effects (Bhattacharyya et al., 2009). In the intestinal mucosa of patients with UC, CTGF was found up-regulated in connection to severity and level. In addition, patients having UC displayed increased expression of ERK/p-ERK and TNF-α, MPO, IL-1β, IL-6, increased B. fragilis and E. coli, and decreased lactobacillus and bifidobacterium (di Mola et al., 2004).

4.4. Interleukin-13's Pathway

Interleukin (IL)-13 belongs to Th aid (Th) 2 cytokine members along with IL-4 and IL-5. In a huddle of cytokine families of genes like IL-3, IL-4, IL-5, and GM-CSF in human chromosome 5q31, IL-13 is located (). The GATA3 transcription factor Th2 modulates IL-13 transcription, that holds together to two cell shallow promoters however essentially transmits just via one (). Generally, type 1 IL-13R receptor is formed by the IL-13 receptor (IL-13R) α1 when dimerized with IL-4Rα, which raises its attraction to IL-13 and transmits signals inside the cells by phosphorylating the STAT 6 by nonreceptor tyrosine kinases called Janus kinase. The receptor type 1 IL-4Rα/IL-13Rα1 holds together by IL-4Rα not only to IL-13 but also to IL-4. In addition to STAT6, the activation of other Type 1 IL-13R signaling molecules like PI3-K, STAT3, and MAPK was observed in various in vitro cell models (Atherton et al., 2003; Hecker et al., 2010; Iwashita et al., 2003). Besides, IL-13R type 2, occurs primarily as a building block of proteins called monomer and holds together IL-13 having greater rapport compared to IL-13R type 1 dimeric (Andrews et al., 2002). Type 2 IL-13R acts usually as an IL-13 receptor that can recognize and join particular cytokines/growth factors called decoy receptors, attaching it and making the cytokine inaccessible for IL-13 type 1 receptor activation not triggering its transportation inside the cell. IL-13Rα2-communicating cells are referred to be IL-13 scavengers because of their ability to remove them from the growth medium and therefore restrict IL-13 activity (Kasaian et al., 2011).

At different levels, IL-13 expression and pathway are regulated. Both GATA3 and the Hedgehog (Hh) signaling pathway positively regulate transcription and growth, while it is negatively managed by IFN-α (). Furthermore, the receptor IL-13Rα2 may be referred to as an adverse manager of the IL-13 signaling pathway, because its transportation is persuaded with IFN-γ or Interleukin-13 itself, thus moving the promotor within the cell to cell shallow. So, in IBD pathogenesis overabundance of infectious cytokines acts crucially, in which the key players are IL-23, IL-12, and IL-10. The p40 subunit is shared by IL-12 and IL-23 cytokines while their respective receptors share the IL-12Rβ1 link, indicating that the above-mentioned cytokines might distribute general pathways. Nevertheless, when triggering the signaling route of the receptor IL-12/IL-12, the Th1 response is guided and IFN-γ production, the IL-23/IL-23 pathway rides the Th17 feedback resulting in the development of cytokines namely IL-22, IL-17A, and IL-17F. The receptor IL-12 and IL-23 could worsen the swelling of the intestines. For example, in the colitis mouse model of DSS, the inoculation of IL-12 cDNA raises infection and caused colitis to escalate and exacerbate. Additionally to IL-12 and IL-23 the receptor IL-10 is a further important pathway involving abdominal stability and IBD development. In humans, the high threat of acquiring UC and CD is associated with the occurrence of different forms in the IL10/IL-10R signaling pathway and different elements in IL-10R leading to the severity of colitis. IL-10 also plays a pivotal role in intestinal equilibrium and the depletion of the IL-10 signaling pathway was involved in the initial commencement of IBD (Daines & Hershey, 2002; Giuffrida et al., 2019).

4.5. IL-6/STAT3 Pathway

A key pathogenic function in IBD is the proinflammatory cytokine IL-6. IL-6 levels in IBD patient's serum and intestinal mucosa are clearly escalated and strongly related to the extent of the infection (Atreya & Neurath, 2005). The traditional IL-6 signaling pathway is activated through attaching with its (IL-6R) membrane-receptor to form a complex receptor IL-6R/IL-6, that triggers the enrollment and formation of two identical polypeptides called homodimer of two submolecular of gp130 to trigger the signal inside the cell, involving ERK/Ras, JAK / STAT, and PI3 K /Akt pathway. Several studies have shown that IL-6 pro-inflammatory activity is mediated by trans-signaling (Chalaris et al., 2012; Jones et al., 2010). Excessive circulating rates of IL-6/sIL-6R and sIL-6R combinations have been identified in patients having IBD, where STAT3 activation induced by the combination of complexes of IL-6/ sIL-6R and subunits of gp130 increases the anti-apoptotic element production such as BCL-2 and BCL-XL inducing programmed cell death tolerance in co-receptor of T cells and leading towards the continuation of persistent infection of the bowel. The signaling pathway IL-6/STAT3 will improve the viability and multiplication of those intestinal epithelial cells (IEC) or tissue that are imposed to become malignant which we called precancer or premalignant. Current research has revealed that the signaling pathway IL-6/STAT3 axis is a key driver of tumors in cancer infected with colitis (Grivennikov et al., 2009).

In CAC animal models, which merged the cure of DSS and AOM, IL-6 was conveyed mostly through macrophages infiltration, accessory cells, and T cells during oncogenesis (Becker et al., 2004). Colitis induced in DSS, IBD, and multiple cancers, STAT3 was strongly activated. For cell proliferation, STAT3 signaling target genes sometimes plays an essential role, such as cyclin D and PCNA, which were down-regulated in IL- $6^{-/-}$ mice (Becker et al., 2006; Bollrath et al., 2009; Fu, 2006). Moreover, the CA-CRC oncogenesis has shown a correlation among TGF-β, IL-6/STAT3 signaling pathways. Many lines of evidence support TGF-β's defensive function in producing the CRC. Mutations have been found in receptor TGF-βRII in CRC victims. Over appearance of receptor TGF-βR in the dysplastic epithelium was identified in DSS/ AOM -treated mice ().

4.6. NF-κB and STAT3 Crosstalk Pathway

Also, a link between two transportations attributes NF-kB and STAT3 are known to be the key regulatory factors connecting swelling to the tumor. NF-κB plays a pivotal function in governing the nonspecific defense and antigen-specific immune and infectious activities by amplifying the production of many infectious chemokines and cytokines and thereby managing the rapid increase and development of malignant cells. Furthermore, decreased NF-κB development is a trademark of several kinds of cancers. NF-κB has been often reported aberrantly triggering in CAC growth. STAT proteins, on the other hand, are responsible for regulating the growth, survival, and differentiation of cells. The STAT family has 7 CAC development members, namely STAT1, STAT2, STAT3, STAT4, STAT5A, STAT5B, and STAT6 (DiDonato et al., 2012).

STAT3 is termed as the influential one which is triggered by family members of IL-6 and engaged cell regulation, progression, and apoptosis among all STAT families. The related JAK1 and JAK2 tyrosine kinases proteins are triggered and consequently, STAT3 tyrosine-705 phosphorylation is stimulated, the functional type of STAT3, which is transported from the membrane to the core where it can trigger the production of antiapoptotic genes such as Bcl-xL, Bcl-2, and Mcl-1 including essential growth factors such as c-fos, c-jun, and c-myc and cell cycle regulation genes. STAT3 and NF-κB are impactful collaborative duo which enhances the pathogenesis of CRC. The association and crosstalk between STAT3 and NF-κB perform a significant duty in fostering the production and growth of epithelial oncogenesis by regulating the interaction of microenvironmental inflammatory or immune cells and malignant cells (Du et al., 2012).

4.7. COX-2/PGE2 Pathway

COX-2 has a major function in tumorigenesis and colonic infection. Increased COX-2 production was found in about 85% of CRCs and associated with lower endurance. COX-2 in IBD was found through an aggressive infection and abnormal growth in cells called neoplasm infected with colitis. COX-2 can stimulate tumor growth by its talent to enhance the anti-apoptotic protein production such as BCL-2 and contributing to apoptosis tolerance. Additionally, a high standard of MMPs and migration of cancerous cells are associated with COX-2 over-expression (Gupta & DuBois, 2001). As a result, in IBD and CRC, COX-2; PGE2 stimulates the results of COX-2. PGE 2 works by a unique EP cell shallow receptor consisting of four EP1, EP2, EP3, and EP4 subtypes. In CRC, current research has shown that PGE 2 could interrelate on dendritic cells with receptors EP2/EP4 to persuade IL-23 appearance and worsen experimental colitis. This is proposed EP4 may stimulate the tumor-proceeding effects of PGE2 (). In addition, AOM-treated mice have also shown a crucial function of EP1 in colon carcinogenesis, where genetic or medicinal removal of EP1 substantially inhibited the production of tumors.

Additionally, PGE2 can also facilitate tumor development by triggering the production of a proangiogenic chemokine CXCL1, having the capability of stimulating vascular endothelial cell displacement and the creation of the tube to facilitate cancer increase and aggression. In addition, PGE2 cancer-promoting actions are implicated in the transmutation of nuclear hormone receptor PPARs. In the PGE2/COX-2 signaling pathways, PPARs are considered as one of the downstream destinations. However, in colonic cancer cells, the COX-2 expression might be persuaded by the creation of PPARs. PGE2 derived from COX-2 encourages the production of pre infectious cytokines that devote to cancer associated with colitis. PGE2 is suggested to mediate the crosstalk among colonic tumorigenesis and systemic inflammation through an auto-amplifying process among PPARs and the receptor COX-2/PGE2 ().

5. MATHEMATICAL MODELING IN CAC: A NOVEL APPROACH

Real-life issues arise from different disciplines like life science, social science, education, finance, and Information Technology, etc. Mathematical modeling is the application of mathematics to:

- describe our opinions of how the world works

- investigate key questions about the observed universe
- explain the phenomenon of the real world
- check your thoughts
- make real-world predictions

Mathematical biological modeling has a long history as it makes it possible to study and simulate complex biological dynamic systems at a low price. A mathematical model based on scientific or medical evidence may be utilized to build and examine theories, raise questions about "what if" and direct future research and confirmation in silico Experiments. These models can help to define and even provide information into the processes that trigger modifications in complex systems. Although a mathematically formulated model could never surpass definite examinations, it may play nicely with the examination that really secures time and energy by recognizing examinational circumstances which are improbable to yield desirable results and by implementing optimization criteria to find the most similar studies. Mathematical modeling can lead to a superior grip on the metabolic remodeling of cancer and to the discovery of the latest probable methods of therapeutic intervention. In the biological context, mathematical modeling can be done either by top-down or bottom-up methods. According to Shahzad and Loor, the top-down method requires a five-stage flow chart of work.

a) Sample selection and laboratory tests to acquire the initial data set.
b) High-performance "omic" assays to enlarge the data set to be examined.
c) Examination of the obtained data.
d) Usage of functional enrichment and modeling of bioinformatics applications.
e) Data analysis and extraction/inference of newly discovered data is the final critical step.

There is a lateral communication of information in this top-down approach from "omes" (transcriptome, proteome, metabolome ...) to the flow of metabolites through metabolic network pathways. at the next end, there includes a four-step bioinformatics-driven process in the bottom-up methodology that uses comprehensive knowledge from kinetic, biochemical, and metabolic datasets, from publication studies, and latest findings from biochemical biomarkers as the input collection from which a drafted design reconstruction takes place in the first step. The third phase transforms the treated array into mathematically formulated models after intensive manual treatment work in the second phase. Eventually, the model should be tested and improved in the fourth step resulting in a last design of computation. Such quantitative metabolism models can be designed on various scales with specific degrees of precision, forming extremely brief designs of specified metabolic signaling pathways depending on the deep knowledge gained of the reactive information of each and every persons reaction participating in the course, not so comprehensive mid-range designs focused on the analysis of flux balance, to worldwide genetic-scaling. The model of mammalian polyamine metabolism is a counterexample of a mathematical metabolic model pathway depending on extensive energetic data. This model represented the key characteristics of these two cyclic pathway and was later identified by the other groups in experimentation with the primary regulating and regulated proteins of the pathway (Al Bakir et al., 2018).

The stochastic existence of genetic changes needs sufficient time almost in years for oncogenesis to proceed phenotype of healthy cells to cancerous cells in the body of humans. Carcinogenesis pursues the Darwinian development principles, whereby germ cells gain genetic changes, such as TP53 which regulates MUC2 production and APC mutations linked with β-catenin and MUC1 contribution in the slight proliferation of cells. We can develop mathematical statements that explain these genetic mutations and then use the phrases to link this developmental parameter to curves of age-dependent incidence of epidemiological cancer. By using the long-lasting investigation of IBD cases to gather the genetic estimations for increasingly exact computations of IBD-explicit developmental inputs as the birth, beginning, and death ().

The theory is centered on calculating both the degree and rate of genetic changes as a measure of whether the cells have developed "close to cancer. In IBD, mathematically formulated models of oncogenesis are in its early stages. Various kinds of modeling methods can be fruitful to implement measurements of the developmental cycles into IBD models of tumor growth for estimation and forecasting of victim-unique paths. Continuum growth models can be utilized to forecast basic changes in the group of cells that can assess the consequences of spatial sampling bias on the identification of unusual sub descendant, but the refinement of such formulations involves neglecting certain bio information. Models at the population level could also be implemented to integrate epidemiological information (e.g. pre-malignant prevalence, cancer occurrence) and thus explain the development of cancer in an IBD population. The choice of the right model (or type of model) is not obvious and shows dependency on the value, the model is looking for. By using multi-stage computational model equations with approximate parameter values, we may then identify these frames by optimizing the probabilities (numerically and analytically) that a person would most probably have a pre-malignant or cancerous injury of a scan-distinguishable scale at diagnosis/endoscopic screening, and after that using the results for each test to calculate the development of evolution. Recent research in CAC shows the geometry of colonic crypt and by mathematical modeling simplification of geometry by reverting to 1-D geometry in which the epithelium apical membrane is a smooth surface x=0. Also, the level of replication of tumor cells by the mixed β-catenin and NF-κB has been shown ().

The genetic history of colon cancer matches the composition structure of functions that contribute to malignancies as the gene is a region of DNA that encodes chromosomes in a sequence that follows a genetic pathway with an increase in the number of chromosomes under mapping. Genetic pathways like TP53, NF-KB, and β-catenin, MUC1; MUC2has been mathematically expressed using ordinary differential equations. Moreover, the RAS pathway can be described mathematically in CAC. One research article showed a mathematical model that ties CRC growth to exosomal miRs concentration. Among CRC exosomal miRs, MiR-21, miR-23a, miR-92a, and miR-1246 are the most over-expressed miRs of CRC patients focused on the gene network in the blood that consists the signal pathways through which these miRs connect to proceed CRC invasion. System simulations yield quantitative relationships of a tumor dynamics with increasing the full radius and the rising lump of the miRs mentioned above ().

6. CONCLUSION

IBD Patients have an elevated chance of experiencing colorectal cancer, and this change is correlated with the frequency, period, and accumulated burden of infection of the disease. A noteworthy figure of colon cancer arising from UC and CD is related to chronic infection. This inflection is caused by the reaction of the immune system to a bacterial disease that arises in the gastrointestinal wall as hereditary mutations appear. For natural sciences including cancer biology, mathematical models are used. It may help to explain the system, study the effects of various components, and make predictions of behavior. Our study describes a number of mathematical models that can be used in the CAC, such as probability models, population-based models, time series models, and statistical models.

Table 1. Abbreviations

Abbreviated form	Explanation
IBD	Inflammatory Bowel Disorder
UC	Ulcerative Colitis
CD	Crohn's Disease
MUC	Mucin
GI	Gastro Intestinal
WBC	White Blood Cells
IEC	Intestinal Epithelial Cells

continues on following page

Table 1. Continued

Abbreviated form	Explanation
U.S	United States
CAC	Colitis Associated Cancer
DNA	Deoxyribonucleic Acid
CRC	Colorectal Cancer
NSAIDs	Non - Steroidal Anti - Inflammatory Drugs
ROS	Reactive Oxygen Species
RNS	Reactive Nitrogen Species
RONS	Reactive Oxygen and Nitrogen Species
DDR	DNA Damage Response
NF-κB	Nuclear Factor Kappa B cells
TNF-α	Tumor Necrosis Factor - *Alpha*
IL	Interleukin
LPS	Lipopolysaccharides
VEGF	Vascular Endothelial Growth Factor
COX-2	Cyclooxygenase-2,
CA-CRC	Colitis Associated- Colorectal Cancer
IKKβ	Inhibitor of κB kinase β
AOM	Azoxymethane
DSS	Dextran Sulfate Sodium
TNF-Rp55	Tumor Necrosis Factor - Receptor Protein 55
CTGF	Connected Tissue Growth Factor
MPO	Myeloperoxidase
GM-CSF	Granulocyte - Macrophage Colony - Stimulating Factor
STAT	Signal Transducer and Activator Of Transcription
MAPK	Mitogen - Activated Protein Kinase
Hh	Hedgehog
IFN-α	Interferon Alpha
cDNA	Complementary DNA
ERK	Extracellular Signal - Regulated Kinase
JAK	Janus Kinase
BCL-XL	B-Cell Lymphoma-Extra Large
PCNA	Proliferating Cell Nuclear Antigen
TGF-β	Tumor Growth Factor- β
PGE2	Prostaglandin E2
MMPs	Matrix metallopeptidases

continues on following page

Table 1. Continued

Abbreviated form	Explanation
CXCL	Chemokines (C-X-C motif) Ligand 1
PPARs	Peroxisome Proliferator - Activated Receptors
TP53	Tumor Protein53
ExomiRs	Exosomal *Micro RNAs*

REFERENCES

Abdulkhaleq, L. A., Assi, M. A., Abdullah, R., Zamri-Saad, M., Taufiq-Yap, Y. H., & Hezmee, M. N. M. (2018). The crucial roles of inflammatory mediators in inflammation: A review. *Veterinary World*, *11*(5), 627–635. doi:10.14202/vetworld.2018.627-635 PMID:29915501

Al Bakir, I., Curtius, K., & Graham, T. A. (2018). From colitis to cancer: An evolutionary trajectory that merges maths and biology. *Frontiers in Immunology*, *9*, 2368. doi:10.3389/fimmu.2018.02368 PMID:30386335

Alatab, S., Sepanlou, S. G., Ikuta, K., Vahedi, H., Bisignano, C., Safiri, S., & Naghavi, M. (2020). The global, regional, and national burden of inflammatory bowel disease in 195 countries and territories, 1990–2017: A systematic analysis for the Global Burden of Disease Study 2017. *The Lancet. Gastroenterology & Hepatology*, *5*(1), 17–30. doi:10.1016/S2468-1253(19)30333-4 PMID:31648971

Alberts, B. (1994). Cell junctions, cell adhesion and the extracellular matrix. *Molecular Biology of the Cell*, 949–1009.

Andrews, A. L., Holloway, J. W., Puddicombe, S. M., Holgate, S. T., & Davies, D. E. (2002). Kinetic analysis of the interleukin-13 receptor complex. *The Journal of Biological Chemistry*, *277*(48), 46073–46078. doi:10.1074/jbc.M209560200 PMID:12354755

Atherton, H. C., Jones, G., & Danahay, H. (2003). IL-13-induced changes in the goblet cell density of human bronchial epithelial cell cultures: MAP kinase and phosphatidylinositol 3-kinase regulation. *American Journal of Physiology. Lung Cellular and Molecular Physiology*, *285*(3), L730–L739. doi:10.1152/ajplung.00089.2003 PMID:12794003

Atreya, I., Atreya, R., & Neurath, M. F. (2008). NF-κB in inflammatory bowel disease. *Journal of Internal Medicine*, *263*(6), 591–596. doi:10.1111/j.1365-2796.2008.01953.x PMID:18479258

Atreya, R., & Neurath, M. F. (2005). Involvement of IL-6 in the pathogenesis of inflammatory bowel disease and colon cancer. *Clinical Reviews in Allergy & Immunology*, *28*(3), 187–195. doi:10.1385/CRIAI:28:3:187 PMID:16129903

Avdagić, N., Zaćiragić, A., Babić, N., Hukić, M., Šeremet, M., Lepara, O., & Nakaš-Ićindić, E. (2013). Nitric oxide as a potential biomarker in inflammatory bowel disease. *Bosnian Journal of Basic Medical Sciences*, *13*(1), 5. doi:10.17305/bjbms.2013.2402 PMID:23448603

Axelrad, J. E., Lichtiger, S., & Yajnik, V. (2016). Inflammatory bowel disease and cancer: The role of inflammation, immunosuppression, and cancer treatment. *World Journal of Gastroenterology*, *22*(20), 4794. doi:10.3748/wjg.v22.i20.4794 PMID:27239106

Baskol, M., Baskol, G., Koçer, D., Ozbakir, O., & Yucesoy, M. (2008). Advanced oxidation protein products: A novel marker of oxidative stress in ulcerative colitis. *Journal of Clinical Gastroenterology*, *42*(6), 687–691. doi:10.1097/MCG.0b013e318074f91f PMID:18574392

Baumgart, D. C., & Carding, S. R. (2007). Inflammatory bowel disease: Cause and immunobiology. *Lancet*, *369*(9573), 1627–1640. doi:10.1016/S0140-6736(07)60750-8 PMID:17499605

Baumgart, D. C., & Sandborn, W. J. (2012). Crohn's disease. *Lancet*, *380*(9853), 1590–1605. doi:10.1016/S0140-6736(12)60026-9 PMID:22914295

Becker, C., Fantini, M. C., & Neurath, M. F. (2006). TGF-beta as a T cell regulator in colitis and colon cancer. *Cytokine & Growth Factor Reviews*, *17*(1-2), 97–106. doi:10.1016/j.cytogfr.2005.09.004 PMID:16298544

Becker, C., Fantini, M. C., Schramm, C., Lehr, H. A., Wirtz, S., Nikolaev, A., & Neurath, M. F. (2004). TGF-β suppresses tumor progression in colon cancer by inhibition of IL-6 trans-signaling. *Immunity*, *21*(4), 491–501. doi:10.1016/j.immuni.2004.07.020 PMID:15485627

Bhattacharyya, S., Dudeja, P. K., & Tobacman, J. K. (2009). ROS, Hsp27, and IKKβ mediate dextran sodium sulfate (DSS) activation of IκBa, NFκB, and IL-8. *Inflammatory Bowel Diseases*, *15*(5), 673–683. doi:10.1002/ibd.20821 PMID:19085995

Bollrath, J., Phesse, T. J., von Burstin, V. A., Putoczki, T., Bennecke, M., Bateman, T., & Greten, F. R. (2009). gp130-mediated Stat3 activation in enterocytes regulates cell survival and cell-cycle progression during colitis-associated tumorigenesis. *Cancer Cell*, *15*(2), 91–102. doi:10.1016/j.ccr.2009.01.002 PMID:19185844

Chalaris, A., Schmidt-Arras, D., Yamamoto, K., & Rose-John, S. (2012). Interleukin-6 trans-signaling and colonic cancer associated with inflammatory bowel disease. *Digestive Diseases (Basel, Switzerland)*, *30*(5), 492–499. doi:10.1159/000341698 PMID:23108305

Chen, Y., Segarini, P., Raoufi, F., Bradham, D., & Leask, A. (2001). Connective tissue growth factor is secreted through the Golgi and is degraded in the endosome. *Experimental Cell Research*, *271*(1), 109–117. doi:10.1006/excr.2001.5364 PMID:11697887

da Silva, B. C., Lyra, A. C., Mendes, C. M. C., Ribeiro, C. P. O., Lisboa, S. R. O., de Souza, M. T. L., Portela, R. C., & Santana, G. O. (2015). The demographic and clinical characteristics of ulcerative colitis in a northeast Brazilian population. *BioMed Research International*, *2015*, 2015. doi:10.1155/2015/359130 PMID:26509150

Daines, M. O., & Hershey, G. K. K. (2002). A novel mechanism by which interferon-γ can regulate interleukin (IL)-13 responses: Evidence for intracellular stores of IL-13 receptor α-2 and their rapid mobilization by interferon-γ. *The Journal of Biological Chemistry*, *277*(12), 10387–10393. doi:10.1074/jbc.M108109200 PMID:11786536

di Mola, F. F., Di Sebastiano, P., Gardini, A., Innocenti, P., Zimmermann, A., Büchler, M. W., & Friess, H. (2004). Differential expression of connective tissue growth factor in inflammatory bowel disease. *Digestion*, *69*(4), 245–253. doi:10.1159/000079845 PMID:15256831

DiDonato, J. A., Mercurio, F., & Karin, M. (2012). NF-κB and the link between inflammation and cancer. *Immunological Reviews*, *246*(1), 379–400. doi:10.1111/j.1600-065X.2012.01099.x PMID:22435567

Du, W., Hong, J., Wang, Y. C., Zhang, Y. J., Wang, P., Su, W. Y., & Fang, J. Y. (2012). Inhibition of JAK2/STAT3 signalling induces colorectal cancer cell apoptosis via mitochondrial pathway. *Journal of Cellular and Molecular Medicine*, *16*(8), 1878–1888. doi:10.1111/j.1582-4934.2011.01483.x PMID:22050790

Duricova, D., Burisch, J., Jess, T., Gower-Rousseau, C., & Lakatos, P. L. (2014). Age-related differences in presentation and course of inflammatory bowel disease: An update on the population-based literature. *Journal of Crohn's and Colitis*, *8*(11), 1351–1361. doi:10.1016/j.crohns.2014.05.006 PMID:24951261

Feakins, R. M. (2013). Inflammatory bowel disease biopsies: Updated British Society of Gastroenterology reporting guidelines. *Journal of Clinical Pathology*, *66*(12), 1005–1026. doi:10.1136/jclinpath-2013-201885 PMID:23999270

Fearon, E. R., & Vogelstein, B. (1990). A genetic model for colorectal tumorigenesis. *Cell, 61*(5), 759-767.

Feuerstein, J. D., & Cheifetz, A. S. (2014, November). Ulcerative colitis: Epidemiology, diagnosis, and management. *Mayo Clinic Proceedings*, *89*(11), 1553–1563. doi:10.1016/j.mayocp.2014.07.002 PMID:25199861

Fu, X. Y. (2006). STAT3 in immune responses and inflammatory bowel diseases. *Cell Research*, *16*(2), 214–219. doi:10.1038j.cr.7310029 PMID:16474436

Gasparetto, M., & Guariso, G. (2014). Crohn's disease and growth deficiency in children and adolescents. *World Journal of Gastroenterology: WJG*, *20*(37), 13219. doi:10.3748/wjg.v20.i37.13219 PMID:25309059

Geboes, K. (2001). Crohn's disease, ulcerative colitis or indeterminate colitis—how important is it to differentiate? *Acta Gastro-Enterologica Belgica*, *64*(2), 197–200. PMID:11475135

Gillen, C. D., Walmsley, R. S., Prior, P., Andrews, H. A., & Allan, R. N. (1994). Ulcerative colitis and Crohn's disease: A comparison of the colorectal cancer risk in extensive colitis. *Gut*, *35*(11), 1590–1592. doi:10.1136/gut.35.11.1590 PMID:7828978

Giuffrida, P., Caprioli, F., Facciotti, F., & Di Sabatino, A. (2019). The role of interleukin-13 in chronic inflammatory intestinal disorders. *Autoimmunity Reviews*, *18*(5), 549–555. doi:10.1016/j.autrev.2019.03.012 PMID:30844559

Gorrini, C., Harris, I. S., & Mak, T. W. (2013). Modulation of oxidative stress as an anticancer strategy. *Nature Reviews. Drug Discovery*, *12*(12), 931–947. doi:10.1038/nrd4002 PMID:24287781

Greten, F. R., Eckmann, L., Greten, T. F., Park, J. M., Li, Z. W., Egan, L. J., & Karin, M. (2004). IKKβ links inflammation and tumorigenesis in a mouse model of colitis-associated cancer. *Cell*, *118*(3), 285–296. doi:10.1016/j.cell.2004.07.013 PMID:15294155

Grivennikov, S., Karin, E., Terzic, J., Mucida, D., Yu, G. Y., Vallabhapurapu, S., Scheller, J., Rose-John, S., Cheroutre, H., Eckmann, L., & Karin, M. (2009). IL-6 and Stat3 are required for survival of intestinal epithelial cells and development of colitis-associated cancer. *Cancer Cell*, *15*(2), 103–113. doi:10.1016/j.ccr.2009.01.001 PMID:19185845

Günther, U., Bateman, A. C., Beattie, R. M., Bauer, M., MacDonald, T. T., & Kaskas, B. A. (2010). Connective tissue growth factor expression is increased in collagenous colitis and coeliac disease. *Histopathology, 57*(3), 427–435. doi:10.1111/j.1365-2559.2010.03652.x PMID:20840672

Gupta, R. A., & DuBois, R. N. (2001). Colorectal cancer prevention and treatment by inhibition of cyclooxygenase-2. *Nature Reviews. Cancer, 1*(1), 11–21. doi:10.1038/35094017 PMID:11900248

Hecker, M., Zasłona, Z., Kwapiszewska, G., Niess, G., Zakrzewicz, A., Hergenreider, E., & Morty, R. E. (2010). *Dysregulation of the Interleukin 13 Receptor System: A Novel Pathomechanism in Pulmonary Arterial Hypertension*. Academic Press.

Hendrickson, B. A., Gokhale, R., & Cho, J. H. (2002). Clinical aspects and pathophysiology of inflammatory bowel disease. *Clinical Microbiology Reviews, 15*(1), 79–94. doi:10.1128/CMR.15.1.79-94.2002 PMID:11781268

Iwashita, J., Sato, Y., Sugaya, H., Takahashi, N., Sasaki, H., & Abe, T. (2003). mRNA of MUC2 is stimulated by IL-4, IL-13 or TNF-α through a mitogen-activated protein kinase pathway in human colon cancer cells. *Immunology and Cell Biology, 81*(4), 275–282. doi:10.1046/j.1440-1711.2003.t01-1-01163.x PMID:12848848

Jackson, A. L., & Loeb, L. A. (2001). The contribution of endogenous sources of DNA damage to the multiple mutations in cancer. *Mutation Research. Fundamental and Molecular Mechanisms of Mutagenesis, 477*(1-2), 7–21. doi:10.1016/S0027-5107(01)00091-4 PMID:11376682

Jones, G. W., McLoughlin, R. M., Hammond, V. J., Parker, C. R., Williams, J. D., Malhotra, R., & Jones, S. A. (2010). Loss of CD4+ T cell IL-6R expression during inflammation underlines a role for IL-6 trans signaling in the local maintenance of Th17 cells. *Journal of Immunology (Baltimore, Md.: 1950), 184*(4), 2130–2139. doi:10.4049/jimmunol.0901528 PMID:20083667

Kaplan, G. G., & Ng, S. C. (2017). Understanding and preventing the global increase of inflammatory bowel disease. *Gastroenterology, 152*(2), 313–321. doi:10.1053/j.gastro.2016.10.020 PMID:27793607

Kappelman, M. D., Rifas–Shiman, S. L., Kleinman, K., Ollendorf, D., Bousvaros, A., Grand, R. J., & Finkelstein, J. A. (2007). The prevalence and geographic distribution of Crohn's disease and ulcerative colitis in the United States. *Clinical Gastroenterology and Hepatology, 5*(12), 1424–1429. doi:10.1016/j.cgh.2007.07.012 PMID:17904915

Karin, M., & Greten, F. R. (2005). NF-κB: Linking inflammation and immunity to cancer development and progression. *Nature Reviews. Immunology*, *5*(10), 749–759. doi:10.1038/nri1703 PMID:16175180

Kasaian, M. T., Raible, D., Marquette, K., Cook, T. A., Zhou, S., Tan, X. Y., & Tchistiakova, L. (2011). IL-13 antibodies influence IL-13 clearance in humans by modulating scavenger activity of IL-13Rα2. *Journal of Immunology (Baltimore, Md.: 1950)*, *187*(1), 561–569. doi:10.4049/jimmunol.1100467 PMID:21622864

Kaser, A., Molnar, C., & Tilg, H. (1998). Differential regulation of interleukin 4 and interleukin 13 production by interferon α. *Cytokine*, *10*(2), 75–81. doi:10.1006/cyto.1997.0270 PMID:9512896

Klampfer, L. (2008). The role of signal transducers and activators of transcription in colon cancer. *Frontiers in Bioscience*, *13*(1), 2888–2899. doi:10.2741/2893 PMID:17981761

Konstantinidis, A. K., Puddicombe, S. M., Mochizuki, A., Sheth, P. D., Yang, I. A., Yoshisue, H., ... Holloway, J. W. (2008). Cellular localization of interleukin 13 receptor alpha2 in human primary bronchial epithelial cells and fibroblasts. *Journal of Investigational Allergology & Clinical Immunology*, *18*(3), 174–180. PMID:18564628

Lai, X., & Friedman, A. (2017). Exosomal microRNA concentrations in colorectal cancer: A mathematical model. *Journal of Theoretical Biology*, *415*, 70–83. doi:10.1016/j.jtbi.2016.12.006 PMID:27993628

Lee, S. H., Kwon, J., & Cho, M.-L. (2018). Immunological pathogenesis of inflammatory bowel disease. *Intestinal Research*, *16*(1), 26. doi:10.5217/ir.2018.16.1.26 PMID:29422795

Lo, W. C., Martin, E. W. Jr, Hitchcock, C. L., & Friedman, A. (2013). Mathematical model of colitis-associated colon cancer. *Journal of Theoretical Biology*, *317*, 20–29. doi:10.1016/j.jtbi.2012.09.025 PMID:23026764

Luo, C., & Zhang, H. (2017). The role of proinflammatory pathways in the pathogenesis of colitis-associated colorectal cancer. *Mediators of Inflammation*, *2017*, 2017. doi:10.1155/2017/5126048 PMID:28852270

Ma, J., Liu, J., Wang, Z., Gu, X., Fan, Y., Zhang, W., & Cai, D. (2014). NF-kappaB-dependent microRNA-425 upregulation promotes gastric cancer cell growth by targeting PTEN upon IL-1β induction. *Molecular Cancer*, *13*(1), 1–11. doi:10.1186/1476-4598-13-40

Mahdi, B. M. (2018). Introductory Chapter: Inflammatory Bowel Disease. In New Concepts in Inflammatory Bowel Disease. IntechOpen.

Mahlich, J., Matsuoka, K., Nakamura, Y., & Sruamsiri, R. (2017). The relationship between socio-demographic factors, health status, treatment type, and employment outcome in patients with inflammatory bowel disease in Japan. *BMC Public Health, 17*(1), 1–7. doi:10.118612889-017-4516-0 PMID:28676039

McKenzie, A. N., Li, X., Largaespada, D. A., Sato, A., Kaneda, A., Zurawski, S. M., & Copeland, N. G. (1993). Structural comparison and chromosomal localization of the human and mouse IL-13 genes. *Journal of Immunology (Baltimore, Md.: 1950), 150*(12), 5436–5444. PMID:8099936

Medina, M. Á. (2018). Mathematical modeling of cancer metabolism. *Critical Reviews in Oncology/Hematology, 124*, 37–40. doi:10.1016/j.critrevonc.2018.02.004 PMID:29548484

Metcalf, C. (2002). Crohn's disease: an overview. *Nursing Standard, 16*(31), 45.

Mirsepasi-Lauridsen, H. C., Du, Z., Struve, C., Charbon, G., Karczewski, J., Krogfelt, K. A., & Wells, J. M. (2016). Secretion of alpha-hemolysin by Escherichia coli disrupts tight junctions in ulcerative colitis patients. *Clinical and Translational Gastroenterology, 7*(3), e149. doi:10.1038/ctg.2016.3 PMID:26938480

Molodecky, N. A., & Kaplan, G. G. (2010). Environmental risk factors for inflammatory bowel disease. *Gastroenterology & Hepatology, 6*(5), 339. PMID:20567592

Molodecky, N. A., Soon, S., Rabi, D. M., Ghali, W. A., Ferris, M., Chernoff, G., & Kaplan, G. G. (2012). Increasing incidence and prevalence of the inflammatory bowel diseases with time, based on systematic review. *Gastroenterology, 142*(1), 46–54. doi:10.1053/j.gastro.2011.10.001 PMID:22001864

Mutoh, M., Watanabe, K., Kitamura, T., Shoji, Y., Takahashi, M., Kawamori, T., ... Wakabayashi, K. (2002). Involvement of prostaglandin E receptor subtype EP4 in colon carcinogenesis. *Cancer Research, 62*(1), 28–32. PMID:11782353

O'Connor, P. M., Lapointe, T. K., Beck, P. L., & Buret, A. G. (2010). Mechanisms by which inflammation may increase intestinal cancer risk in inflammatory bowel disease. *Inflammatory Bowel Diseases, 16*(8), 1411–1420. doi:10.1002/ibd.21217 PMID:20155848

Panizza, P. S. B., Viana, P. C. C., Horvat, N., dos Santos, V. R., de Araújo, D. A. P., Yamanari, T. R., & Cerri, G. G. (2017). Inflammatory bowel disease: current role of imaging in diagnosis and detection of complications: gastrointestinal imaging. *Radiographics*, *37*(2), 701–702. doi:10.1148/rg.2017160050 PMID:28287943

Panizza, P. S. B., Viana, P. C. C., Horvat, N., dos Santos, V. R., de Araújo, D. A. P., Yamanari, T. R., Leite, C. C., & Cerri, G. G. (2017). Inflammatory bowel disease: current role of imaging in diagnosis and detection of complications: gastrointestinal imaging. *Radiographics*, *37*(2), 701–702. doi:10.1148/rg.2017160050 PMID:28287943

Pithadia, A. B., & Jain, S. (2011). Treatment of inflammatory bowel disease (IBD). *Pharmacological Reports*, *63*(3), 629–642. doi:10.1016/S1734-1140(11)70575-8 PMID:21857074

Podolsky, D. K. (1991). Inflammatory bowel disease. *The New England Journal of Medicine*, *325*(13), 928–937. doi:10.1056/NEJM199109263251306 PMID:1881418

Popivanova, B. K., Kitamura, K., Wu, Y., Kondo, T., Kagaya, T., Kaneko, S., & Mukaida, N. (2008). Blocking TNF-α in mice reduces colorectal carcinogenesis associated with chronic colitis. *The Journal of Clinical Investigation*, *118*(2), 560–570. doi:10.1172/JCI32453 PMID:18219394

Rabe, B., Chalaris, A., May, U., Waetzig, G. H., Seegert, D., Williams, A. S., & Scheller, J. (2008). Transgenic blockade of interleukin 6 transsignaling abrogates inflammation. *Blood*, *111*(3), 1021–1028. doi:10.1182/blood-2007-07-102137 PMID:17989316

Ray, G. (2016). Inflammatory bowel disease in India-Past, present and future. *World Journal of Gastroenterology*, *22*(36), 8123. doi:10.3748/wjg.v22.i36.8123 PMID:27688654

Rogan, D. F., Cousins, D. J., Santangelo, S., Ioannou, P. A., Antoniou, M., Lee, T. H., & Staynov, D. Z. (2004). Analysis of intergenic transcription in the human IL-4/IL-13 gene cluster. *Proceedings of the National Academy of Sciences of the United States of America*, *101*(8), 2446–2451. doi:10.1073/pnas.0308327100 PMID:14983029

Romano, M., Sironi, M., Toniatti, C., Polentarutti, N., Fruscella, P., Ghezzi, P., & Mantovani, A. (1997). Role of IL-6 and its soluble receptor in induction of chemokines and leukocyte recruitment. *Immunity*, *6*(3), 315–325. doi:10.1016/S1074-7613(00)80334-9 PMID:9075932

Sartor, R. B. (2006). Mechanisms of disease: Pathogenesis of Crohn's disease and ulcerative colitis. *Nature Clinical Practice. Gastroenterology & Hepatology*, *3*(7), 390–407. doi:10.1038/ncpgasthep0528 PMID:16819502

Segal, A. W. (2016). Making sense of the cause of Crohn's–a new look at an old disease. *F1000 Research*, 5. PMID:28105308

Seher, A., Nickel, J., Mueller, T. D., Kneitz, S., Gebhardt, S., ter Vehn, T. M., & Sebald, W. (2011). Gene expression profiling of connective tissue growth factor (CTGF) stimulated primary human tenon fibroblasts reveals an inflammatory and wound healing response in vitro. *Molecular Vision*, *17*, 53. PMID:21245951

Sheibanie, A. F., Yen, J. H., Khayrullina, T., Emig, F., Zhang, M., Tuma, R., & Ganea, D. (2007). The proinflammatory effect of prostaglandin E2 in experimental inflammatory bowel disease is mediated through the IL-23 IL-17 axis. *Journal of Immunology (Baltimore, Md.: 1950)*, *178*(12), 8138–8147. doi:10.4049/jimmunol.178.12.8138 PMID:17548652

Sheng, H., Shao, J., Morrow, J. D., Beauchamp, R. D., & DuBois, R. N. (1998). Modulation of apoptosis and Bcl-2 expression by prostaglandin E2 in human colon cancer cells. *Cancer Research*, *58*(2), 362–366. PMID:9443418

Song, R., Li, Y., Hao, W., Wang, B., Yang, L., & Xu, F. (2018). Identification and analysis of key genes associated with ulcerative colitis based on DNA microarray data. *Medicine*, *97*(21), e10658. doi:10.1097/MD.0000000000010658 PMID:29794741

Song, Z. M., Liu, F., Chen, Y. M., Liu, Y. J., Wang, X. D., & Du, S. Y. (2019). CTGF-mediated ERK signaling pathway influences the inflammatory factors and intestinal flora in ulcerative colitis. *Biomedicine and Pharmacotherapy*, *111*, 1429–1437. doi:10.1016/j.biopha.2018.12.063 PMID:30841458

Sonnenberg, A., McCarty, D. J., & Jacobsen, S. J. (1991). Geographic variation of inflammatory bowel disease within the United States. *Gastroenterology*, *100*(1), 143–149. doi:10.1016/0016-5085(91)90594-B PMID:1983816

Souza, R. F., Lei, J., Yin, J., Appel, R., Zou, T. T., Zhou, X., & Meltzer, S. J. (1997). A transforming growth factor beta 1 receptor type II mutation in ulcerative colitis-associated neoplasms. *Gastroenterology*, *112*(1), 40–45. doi:10.1016/S0016-5085(97)70217-8 PMID:8978341

Syn, W. K., Witek, R. P., Curbishley, S. M., Jung, Y., Choi, S. S., Enrich, B., Omenetti, A., Agboola, K. M., Fearing, C. M., Tilg, H., Adams, D. H., & Diehl, A. M. (2009). Role for hedgehog pathway in regulating growth and function of invariant NKT cells. *European Journal of Immunology*, *39*(7), 1879–1892. doi:10.1002/eji.200838890 PMID:19544307

Takiishi, T., Fenero, C. I. M., & Câmara, N. O. S. (2017). Intestinal barrier and gut microbiota: Shaping our immune responses throughout life. *Tissue Barriers*, *5*(4), e1373208. doi:10.1080/21688370.2017.1373208 PMID:28956703

Tan, Y., & Zheng, C. (2018). Effects of alpinetin on intestinal barrier function, inflammation and oxidative stress in dextran sulfate sodium-induced ulcerative colitis mice. *The American Journal of the Medical Sciences*, *355*(4), 377–386. doi:10.1016/j.amjms.2018.01.002 PMID:29661352

Tandon, H. D., & Prakash, A. (1972). Pathology of intestinal tuberculosis and its distinction from Crohn's disease. *Gut*, *13*(4), 260–269. doi:10.1136/gut.13.4.260 PMID:5033841

Ungaro, R., Colombel, J. F., Lissoos, T., & Peyrin-Biroulet, L. (2019). A treat-to-target update in ulcerative colitis: A systematic review. *The American Journal of Gastroenterology*, *114*(6), 874–883. doi:10.14309/ajg.0000000000000183 PMID:30908297

Viennois, E., Chen, F., & Merlin, D. (2013). NF-κB pathway in colitis-associated cancers. *Translational Gastrointestinal Cancer*, *2*(1), 21. PMID:23626930

Vilela, E. G., da Gama Torres, H. O., Martins, F. P., de Abreu Ferrari, M. D. L., Andrade, M. M., & da Cunha, A. S. (2012). Evaluation of inflammatory activity in Crohn's disease and ulcerative colitis. *World journal of gastroenterology. WJG*, *18*(9), 872. doi:10.3748/wjg.v18.i9.872 PMID:22408345

Vogelstein, B., Fearon, E. R., Hamilton, S. R., Kern, S. E., Preisinger, A. C., Leppert, M., Smits, A. M. M., & Bos, J. L. (1988). Genetic alterations during colorectal-tumor development. *The New England Journal of Medicine*, *319*(9), 525–532. doi:10.1056/NEJM198809013190901 PMID:2841597

Waldner, M. J., & Neurath, M. F. (2012). Potential avenues for immunotherapy of colitis-associated neoplasia. *Immunotherapy*, *4*(4), 397–405. doi:10.2217/imt.12.15 PMID:22512634

Wang, D., Wang, H., Brown, J., Daikoku, T., Ning, W., Shi, Q., Richmond, A., Strieter, R., Dey, S. K., & DuBois, R. N. (2006). CXCL1 induced by prostaglandin E2 promotes angiogenesis in colorectal cancer. *The Journal of Experimental Medicine*, *203*(4), 941–951. doi:10.1084/jem.20052124 PMID:16567391

Watanabe, K., Kawamori, T., Nakatsugi, S., Ohta, T., Ohuchida, S., Yamamoto, H., ... Wakabayashi, K. (1999). Role of the prostaglandin E receptor subtype EP1 in colon carcinogenesis. *Cancer Research*, *59*(20), 5093–5096. PMID:10537280

Wright, K., Kolios, G., Westwick, J., & Ward, S. G. (1999). Cytokine-induced apoptosis in epithelial HT-29 cells is independent of nitric oxide formation: Evidence for an interleukin-13-driven phosphatidylinositol 3-kinase-dependent survival mechanism. *The Journal of Biological Chemistry*, *274*(24), 17193–17201. doi:10.1074/jbc.274.24.17193 PMID:10358077

Xavier, R. J., & Podolsky, D. K. (2007). Unravelling the pathogenesis of inflammatory bowel disease. *Nature*, *448*(7152), 427–434. doi:10.1038/nature06005 PMID:17653185

Yamashiro, T., Fukunaga, T., Kobashi, N., Kamioka, H., Nakanishi, T., Takigawa, M., & Takano-Yamamoto, T. (2001). Mechanical stimulation induces CTGF expression in rat osteocytes. *Journal of Dental Research*, *80*(2), 461–465. doi:10.1177/00220345010800021201 PMID:11332533

Yu, H., Kortylewski, M., & Pardoll, D. (2007). Crosstalk between cancer and immune cells: Role of STAT3 in the tumour microenvironment. *Nature Reviews. Immunology*, *7*(1), 41–51. doi:10.1038/nri1995 PMID:17186030

Zisman, T. L., & Rubin, D. T. (2008). Colorectal cancer and dysplasia in inflammatory bowel disease. *World journal of gastroenterology. WJG*, *14*(17), 2662. doi:10.3748/wjg.14.2662 PMID:18461651

Chapter 9
Role of Cancer Stem Cells in Colitis-Associated Colorectal Cancer

Vasudevan Sekar
University of Madras, India

ABSTRACT

Colorectal cancer the third-leading cause of cancer mortality Worldwide; it's a well characterised model at molecular level among various cancera. Chronic ulcerative colitis is one of the causes of colorectal cancer. Recent cancer research focuses on tumor-initiating cells which are the cause of tumor initiation, invasions, drug-resistant, recurrence, and metastasis. Emerging research findings support the presence of colon cancer stem cells in sporadic colorectal cancer and in colitis-associated colorectal cancer. Colitis-associated cancer cells exhibit increased colon cancer stem cell marker expression along with activated developmental signaling pathways. Also, emerging reports exhibit that inhibition stem cell markers in chronic ulcerative colitis cells impedes progression of cancer in genetically engineered animal models and primary samples. This chapter deals of colitis-cancer transition, microenvironment of colitis-associated colorectal cancer, and articulates that cancer stem cells are ideal targets for colorectal cancer.

1. INTRODUCTION

Colitis associated colorectal cancer is known as extensive and long-lasting chronic inflammation, the complication of inflammatory bowel diseases with cancer development in colon cancer rectum. Inflammatory bowel diseases are group of

DOI: 10.4018/978-1-7998-3580-6.ch009

chronic inflammation in the gastrointestinal tract, which is caused by an inflammatory response in the gastrointestinal microbiome.(Eaden, Abrams, & Mayberry, 2001; Shacter & Weitzman, 2002) There are two distinct well known inflammatory bowel diseases are Crohn's diseases and ulcerative colitis. Crohn's diseases will affect anywhere in the gastrointestinal tract from mouth to the anus, mostly dominant in the small intestine. Ulcerative colitis will affect in the colon. Colitis is also known as an inflammation of the colon. Ulcerative colitis is characterised by relapsing and remitting mucosal inflammation from the rectum to proximal colon, resulting in bloody diarrhea, colonic motility dysfunction, and colonic tissue damage.(Al Bakir, Curtius, & Graham, 2018; Romano *et al.,* 2016) Patient with ulcerative colitis are at increased risk of colorectal cancer. Colitis associated colorectal cancer is one of the most serious consequences of ulcerative colitis. In 1925 Crohn and Rosenberg reported the first case of adenocarcinoma in ulcerative colitis patient.(Dobbins, 1984) The major risk factors are the degree of inflammation, diagnosis of young age ulcerative, long duration of ulcerative colitis, family history of Colorectal cancer, accumulation of inflammatory changes associated with colonic epithelial injury, repair, and regeneration.(Beaugerie & Itzkowitz, 2015; Pinczowski, Ekbom, Baron, Yuen, & Adami, 1994; Velayos *et al.,* 2006) Colitis associated-colorectal cancer developed from non-dysplastic mucosa to indefinite dysplasia, low-grade dysplasia, high-grade dysplasia and finally to invasive adenocarcinoma.(Yashiro, 2014) Ulcerative colitis-associated colorectal cancer contributes to 1% of overall colorectal cancer. The incidence of colitis associated-colorectal cancer is ten times greater than sporadic colorectal cancer. Colitis associate-colorectal cancer diagnosed at an advanced stage.(Baars *et al.,* 2011; Gyde *et al.,* 1982) The cancer stem cells theory demonstrates, cancer stem cells are small subpopulation present in the tumour bulk, which possesses the self-renewal and differential capability. Cancer stem cells are causes for tumor initiation, progression, drug resistance and metastasis of cancer. Cancer stem cells are have similar characteristics as normal stem cells. (Bu & Cao, 2012; Dhawan, Ahmad, Srivastava, & Singh, 2011; Zhou *et al.,* 2018) The cancer stem cells were first identified in hematological malignancy and later in solid tumor.(Bonnet & Dick, 1997) The cancer stem cells identified and isolated by using cell surface marker such as CD133, CD24, CD44, CD166, lgr5 etc. also functional markers ALDH and stem cell transcription factors Oct,SOX, Nanog, etc. Colon cancer stem cells were identified using the cell surface markers CD133, CD44, CD166 Lgr5 and ALDH.(Gabriela Pop, 2019; Munro, Wickremesekera, Peng, Tan, & Itinteang, 2018) Based on the cancer stem cells theory, several establish reports exhibits that the cancer stem cells involved in the tissue regeneration and carcinogenesis of sporadic cancer. Where as in ulcerative colitis associated-colorectal cancer, role of cancer stem cells in the inflammation dysplasia carcinoma sequence has not fully understood. In this chapter, its stand to reason that role of cancer stem cells influence in the ulcerative colitis associate-colorectal cancer which may lay a platform for early diagnostic and identification of therapeutic targets.

2. INFLAMMATORY BOWEL DISEASE

Inflammatory bowel diseases represent group of non-specific chronic inflammation in the digestive tract, which is caused by an inappropriate inflammatory response in intestinal microbiome often results in continuous epithelial injury, leads to erosions, and ulceration. The dysfunctional defects of epithelium such as epithelial-cell development, barrier function, cell-matrix adhesion, endoplasmic reticulum stress, and epithelial restitution after injury also caused for inflammatory bowel disease. (Cosnes, Gower–Rousseau, Seksik, & Cortot, 2011; Loftus, 2004) The pathogenesis of inflammatory bowel disease remains unclear. The well-known inflammatory bowel disease, such as Crohn's disease and ulcerative colitis. Crohn's diseases will affect anywhere in the gastrointestinal tract. Ulcerative colitis will affect the colon and rectum. Ulcerative colitis having the highest prevalence in the world. Inflammatory bowel diseases are well known as Western disease, about 50–200 per 100,000 persons suffering Crohn's disease also 120–200 per 100,000 persons for Ulcerative colitis. The incidence of inflammatory bowel disease high in Western countries and now the rate of incidence and prevalence have shown to be increasing in Asia and African countries due to Western lifestyle adaptation.(Ng *et al.,* 2018)

3. ULCERATIVE COLITIS

Ulcerative colitis is a relapsing and remitting disease with chronic idiopathic inflammation of the colon. Ulcerative colitis resulting in frequent bloody diarrhea, colonic motility dysfunction, potentially permanent fibrosis and colonic damage. Ulcerative colitis caused reduced the crypt density, altered crypt architecture, and decreased the mucosal secretion. Also, continuous ulcerative colitis causes the loss of normal vascular pattern, granularity, erosion, bleeding and ulceration in colonic tissue, which increase the risk of colorectal cancer.(Torres, Billioud, Sachar, Peyrin-Biroulet, & Colombel, 2012; Ungaro, Mehandru, Allen, Peyrin-Biroulet, & Colombel, 2017) Several risk factors are abnormal immune response genetics, microbiome and environmental for ulcerative colitis but till now specific cause of that are not well characterised. Ulcerative colitis affects all age group of people, most commonly adults 30-40 year aged. There is no sex predominance in ulcerative colitis, incidence and prevalence have been increasing Worldwide.(Ananthakrishnan, 2015) The pathogenesis of ulcerative colitis is multifactorial, such as hereditary, epithelial barrier defects, dysfunctional immune response, also environmental factors. Ulcerative colitis increased risk of colorectal cancer. Ulcerative colitis contributed 1% of overall colorectal cancer.(Ungaro *et al.,* 2017; Yashiro, 2014) The molecular mechanism involved colitis to cancer transition sequence is not well understood. Patients with ulcerative colitis, are substantially increased risk of developing a form of colorectal cancer (CRC) known as colitis-associated colorectal cancer. Colitis associated colorectal cancer is molecularly distinct from the common sporadic colorectal cancer.

4. COLORECTAL CANCER

Colon cancer, more commonly known as colorectal cancer or large bowel cancer, which includes cancer growth in colon and rectum. Colon and rectum last are part of the digestive system also called the gastrointestinal system. Cancer develops in colon and rectum more frequent than the small intestine. The ascending and transverse colon collective knew as proximal colon, tumor in the proximal colon is more common in woman and older patients. Descending and sigmoid colon are referred to as distal colon tumor in the distal colon more common among men. Younger patients are known as the proximal colon; the tumor in the proximal colon is more common in woman and older patients. Descending and sigmoid colon is referred as distal colon tumor in distal colon more common among men and younger patients(Nawa *et al.,* 2008) Most of the colon cancer arises from the adenomatous polyps, adenomatous polyps are visible glandular projections lining in the surface of the colon and rectum. The presence of polyps doubles the risk of subsequent colon cancer. Cancer arises from the glandular cells is called adenocarcinoma. All the adenomas have the capacity to become cancerous. Most of the colon cancer are adenocarcinomas.(Dame *et al.,* 2010; Levine & Ahnen, 2006; Risio, 2010) The molecular mechanism of the multistage progression and development of colon cancer. Colonic tissue undergoes orderly progression from polyps to the development of carcinoma through continuous, and series gene mutations cause activation of the proto-oncogene and the loss of tumor suppressor genes(Fearon & Vogelstein, 1990). These mutational changes in colonocyte lead to the proliferation of colonic stem cells in glandular crypts is normally restricted in one-third of the crypts, whereas in polyps proliferative activity migrates upwards and form the microadenoma. Then its progress and develops into visible adenomas these proliferative cells fail to undergo normal maturation and bypass the cell death pathways this leads to focal growth dysplastic colonic mucosa in aberrant crypt foci.(Vogelstein *et al.,* 1988) The colon cancer progression and development involves various genetic and molecular changes in cell proliferation cell survival, resistance to apoptosis and metastasis. The mutational changes in the APC gene, loss of function and inactivation of GSK-3 causes the stabilization of the, and its nuclear localization constitute to activate the Wnt/β-catenin signaling pathway which subsequently activates the downstream gene which is involved in tumorigenesis like cyclin D1, myc, VEGF and matrix metalloproteases(Li, Mizukami, Zhang, Jo, & Chung, 2005; Segditsas & Tomlinson, 2006). Also, the k-ras mutations result in the activation of Ras and its downstream effectors MAPK and PI3k /Akt pathways. EGFR and TGF pathways also involved in upregulation of hyperproliferative ACF. (Giehl, 2005) The progression of the colon cancer characterized by histologically distinct like colonic crypt hyperplasia, dysplasia adenoma, adenocarcinoma and distinct metastasis. ACF putative preneoplastic lesions believed to be a histological biomarker of colon cancer.

Research updates in the colon cancer suggested four major tenets derives for the pathogenesis of colon cancer they are, genetic and epigenetic alterations, the multistep progression of the molecular and morphological level, molecular instability, and also the hereditary defects. The progressive accumulation of mutations in genes of APC, (adenomatous polyposis coli) K-RAS (kristein rat sacroma), P53 (tumor protein-53) and DCC (deleted in colon cancer) leads to transformation of normal colonic mucosa into adenoma and carcinoma and results to colon cancer (Kheirelseid, Miller, & Kerin, 2013) APC is mutated with up to 70% of all sporadic colon adenocarcinoma(Chung, 2000; Miyaki *et al.*, 1994). K-RAS is mutated in 31-41% of the colon carcinoma occurs in early colon cancer formation(Arber *et al.*, 2000; Bos *et al.*, 1987). In primary human cancer, P53 is mutated 50%. DCC is one of the most frequent gene mutations in advanced colorectal cancer loss of heterozygosity in DCC. (Somasundaram, 2000) The role of epigenetic alteration such as hypo and hypermethylation in DNA related to activation and inhibition, respectively in oncogene and tumor suppressor. In colon cancer are classified three categories of genetic mutations related to the hereditary influence Sporadic colon cancer (60%) comprises with no inherited gene mutation, familial colorectal cancer(30%) alteast one blood-related gene mutation in colonic adenoma, and hereditary colon cancer (10%) with result of germline inheritance of mutations(Ivanovich, Read, Ciske, Kodner, & Whelan, 1999).

5. COLITIS ASSOCIATED-COLORECTAL CANCER

Colitis associated colon cancer as a complication of ulcerative colitis with malignancy developing in colon and rectum with chronic inflammation.(Yashiro, 2014) The major causes of colitis-associated cancer are prolonged inflammatory bowel diseases, familial history, and increased severity of colitis, pseudo polyps, and dysplasia. In colitis-associated colorectal cancer, the chronic inflammation leads to genetic alterations through oxidative stress, increased secretion of inflammatory mediators, and alteration in the immune receptor. The ulcerative colitis-associated colorectal cancer involved progression from non-neoplastic inflammatory epithelium to dysplasia to cancer. Ulcerative colitis colorectal more frequent in younger age, they have multiple cancer lesion, mucinous carcinoma as compared to sporadic colorectal cancer.(Chambers, Warren, Jewell, & Mortensen, 2005; Isbell & Levin, 1988) Ulcerative colitis-associated colorectal cancer contributes 1-2% of colorectal cancer overall population. Compare to sporadic colorectal cancer colitis-associated colorectal cancer, poor prognosis and high mortality. In colitis-associated colorectal cancer, inflammation is an important initial factor. The relapsing and remitting chronic inflammation, colonic mucosal repair stimulate the oxidative stress in the inflammatory microenvironment.(Grivennikov, 2013; Shacter & Weitzman, 2002) These stress cumulatively impair the DNA induce mutation leads to tumor initiation. Colitis associated colorectal carcinogenesis is progressed by various molecular alteration such as aneuploidy, p53 mutation, chromosomal and microsatellite instability.(Kavanagh *et al.,* 2014) There are more than 300 cancer-related mutations were found in the colitis-associated colorectal cancer. NGS and TCGA database showed 6.2 genomic alterations per tumour. *TP53* (89%), *APC* (21%), *KRAS* (40%), *SMAD4* (17%), *MYC* (26%), *GNAS* (13%), and *IDH* (11%) genomic alteration were found in colitis-associated colorectal cancer. Among them, TP53, MYC, APC and IDH were more frequent.(Romano *et al.,* 2016; Velayos *et al.,* 2006) Also, the MYC and TGF-β components of the WNT signaling pathway were mutated in the colitis-associated cancer patients. IDH mutation was increased in colitis-associated colon cancer compared the sporadic colon cancer.(O'Connor, Lapointe, Beck, & Buret, 2010)

6. CANCER STEM CELLS

Cancer stem cells are small subpopulations of tumor cells; they are immortal tumor-initiating cells, possess self-renewal and pluripotent capacity. Cancer stem cells are the basis for tumor initiation, development, metastasis, recurrence and drug resistance(Clarke *et al.,* 2006; Han, Shi, Gong, Zhang, & Sun, 2013; Koch, Krause, & Baumann, 2010; Reya, Morrison, Clarke, & Weissman, 2001). Cancer stem cells based research has recently attracted much attention due to the potential development and discovery of cancer stem cell-related therapies. Cancer stem cell hypothesis was first formulated in 1800, by the Rudolf Virchow's cellular Pathalogie and a case report by Julius Cohnheim in 1875, Later on, Pierce and Speers proposed a hierarchical model for the development and propagation of cancer states the tumor are caricatures of normal tissue development. In 1997 Bonnet and Dick were provided with the first evidence for the existence of cancer stem cells in acute leukaemia using the $CD33^+$ /$CD38^-$ cells in NOD/SCID mice to initiate hematopoietic malignancy(Bonnet & Dick, 1997). Then Al-Hajj reported cancer stem cells in the solid tumor using $CD44^+$/ $CD24^-$ in breast cancer(Al-Hajj, Wicha, Benito-Hernandez, Morrison, & Clarke, 2003). To date cancer stem cells have been identified in various solid tumors including lung cancer(Eramo *et al.,* 2008), colon cancer(Ricci-Vitiani *et al.,* 2007), prostate cancer(Maitland & Collins, 2008), gastric carcinoma(Takaishi, Okumura, & Wang, 2008), head and neck squamous cell cancer(Prince *et al.,* 2007), brain cancer(Singh *et al.,* 2004), liver carcinoma(Yang *et al.,* 2008) and others etc. Cancer stem cells were identified based on cell surface markers CD44, CD133, CD24, CD166, LGR5 and intracellular molecules ALDH1. Over the past several years, cancer research was targeting the cancer stem cells for the development of the new drugs, based on the cell surface molecular markers and various signaling pathways. New cancer stem cell-targeted therapeutic strategies focused on cancer treatment. A variety of signaling mechanism involved in the regulation of cancer stem cell such as Wnt/β-catenin, BMP pathway, Notch pathway, sonic hedgehog signaling pathways.(Blanco Calvo *et al.,* 2009; Cochrane, Szczepny, Watkins, & Cain, 2015; Holland, Klaus, Garratt, & Birchmeier, 2013; Pannuti *et al.,* 2010)

7. ROLE OF CANCER STEM CELLS IN COLITIS TO COLORECTAL CANCER TRANSITION

The common colorectal cancer sporadic colon cancer is well-characterised cancer model at the molecular level, whereas colitis-associated colorectal cancer the mechanism involved is not well characterised. The sequence of colitis associated-colorectal cancer may involve inflammation-dysplasia-carcinoma, as compared to the sporadic colorectal cancer it is unclear. The transition of colitis to cancer involves mutational events, epigenetic modification and the inflamed microenvironment.(Al Bakir *et al.,* 2018) The sequence of colitis associate-colorectal cancer is distinct from sporadic colorectal cancer. P53 mutation and chromosomal instability areas early events of colitis-associated colorectal cancer, further the APC and K-RAS mutations less ubiquitous as compare to common sporadic cancer. The transition of adenoma to carcinoma the sporadic colorectal cancer the APC gene mutated at the early event, which is tumour suppressor gene negatively regulate Wnt signaling.(Baker *et al.,* 2019) APC is a component of the destruction complex in the Wnt/β-catenin signaling pathway, and which stabilize the cytoplasmic and leads the β-catenin translocation into the nucleus. Activated Wnt signaling subsequent transcript Wnt targeted genes including *axin2, LGR5, c-Myc,* and *cyclin D1*. (Clevers, 2006) The mutation in any one of the components of Wnt constitutive activation of this pathway, as observed in cases of sporadic colorectal cancer. The aberrant Wnt signaling activation in the sporadic colon cancer has been shown to mark the cancer stem cells compartment. (Vermeulen *et al.,* 2010) Established reports supported that sporadic colorectal cancer is initiated by a rare population of crypt cells called colon cancer stem cells which showed increased Wnt activation and the normal colonic stem cells marker. The cancer stem cells in the colitis associated-colorectal cancer are still unclear. Several molecular consequences, such as the generation of reactive oxygen species, microsatellite instability, telomere shortening, and chromosomal instability, have been attributed to inflammation-driven genomic stress that leads to colorectal cancer. (Thorsteinsdottir, Gudjonsson, Nielsen, Vainer, & Seidelin, 2011) The emerging studies exhibiting that high Wnt signaling activity could be drives colitis to cancer transition. Also, ALDH expression of colon cancer stem cells leads to the tumorigenesis in the colitis to cancer transition, these results suggest that colitis and sphere and/or xenograft formation will be useful to survey colitis patients at risk of developing cancer.(Carpentino *et al.,* 2009; Huang *et al.,* 2009) The ALDH + and high Wnt more specific marker to screening for colon cancer stem cell in patients with colitis, recent findings indicate that evaluation of both CD133 and p53 expression by immunohistochemistry may be a useful diagnostic tool or biomarker for early detection of ulcerative colitis-associated colorectal cancer and demonstrated that CD133 expression was positively associated with ulcerative colitis-associated colorectal dysplasia and ulcerative colitis-associated colon cancer tumor grade. (Shenoy *et al.,* 2012) The common thread is activating mutations in components of the Wnt/β-catenin signaling pathway, which occur commonly as early events in sporadic colorectal cancer. The possible associations between Wnt/β-catenin signaling and colitis to cancer transition based on the cancer stem cell model shows that Wnt/β-catenin immunostaining indicated that ulcerative colitis patients have a level of Wnt-pathway active cells that is intermediate between a normal colon and colorectal cancer. These ulcerative cells exhibiting activation of the Wnt pathway constituted a major subpopulation 52% of the colonic epithelial cells positive for ALDH, a putative marker of colon cancer stem cells. Further, this subpopulation of colon cancer stem cells were successive passages, expresses the highest Wnt activity which exhibited higher clonogenic and tumorigenic potential. The Wnt signaling activity in driving cancer stem cells properties in ulcerative colitis-associated colorectal cancer transition. Notably, 5/20 single cell injected results high-Wnt cancer stem cells resulted in tumor formation, suggesting a correlation with colitis to cancer transition. Attenuation of Wnt/β-catenin in high-Wnt cancer stem cells by shRNA-mediated downregulation or pharmacological inhibition significantly reduced tumor growth rates. Overall, these studies exhibit that early activation of Wnt/β-catenin signaling is critical for colitis to cancer transition, high levels of Wnt/β-catenin signaling can further demarcate ALDH+ tumor-initiating cells in the non-dysplastic epithelium of ulcerative colitis patients.(Carpentino *et al.*, 2009) LGR5 may play an important role in tumor development in the context of the inflammation–dysplasia–carcinoma sequence. With respect to LGR5 expression, that LGR5-positive may play a critical role in the development of ulcerative colitis-associated colorectal cancer in the setting of p53 loss of function. The loss of p53 function in LGR5 + stem cells enables colonic tumor formation only when combined with DNA damage and chronic inflammation in the colitis associate colorectal cancer model studies.(Davidson *et al.*, 2015)

8. CANCER STEM CELLS AND COLITIS-ASSOCIATED COLORECTAL CANCER

Cancer stem cells are small sub-population, are the basis for tumor initiation, development, metastasis, recurrence and drug resistance. The colon cancer stem cells were identified initially by the surface marker such as CD133 (Ricci-Vitiani *et al.*, 2007). The colon cancer stem cells were well established in the common sporadic cancer. Whereas it's untested in cases of inflammation-associated cancers such as colitis-associated cancer. The benign colonic mucosa progresses into colon cancer is known as the adenoma to carcinoma sequence whereas in colitis-associated cancers is believed the accumulation of genetic alterations to proceed via a pathway known as the inflammation-dysplasia-cancer progression. The evaluation molecular mechanism involved of colitis to cancer transition reveals that activation of the Wnt signaling pathway constituted a major subpopulation (52%+7.21) of the colonic epithelial cells positive for aldehyde dehydrogenase ALDH, a putative marker of cancer stem cells.(Carpentino *et al.*, 2009; Shenoy *et al.*, 2012) Also, the colon cancer stem cells marker CD44 was increased in colitis-associated colon cancer as compared to the sporadic colon cancer. The CD44 and the variant of the CD44 expression whereas CD133 in unregulated in the colitis. Wnt signaling were upregulated in the colitis-associated colon cancer patient, which is downstream of CD44(Hynes, Huang, & Huang, 2009). Emerging research shreds of evidence exhibit that surface markers such as CD44+, CD166+, CD133+ and functional ALDH+ cells from the colitis patient and AOM and DSS model derived cells and enriched cells from xenografts in mice, recapitulate human tumour and set as the functional characteristics of colon cancer stem cells.(Carpentino *et al.*, 2009; Huang *et al.*, 2009)

9. CANCER STEM CELLS SIGNALING PATHWAYS IN COLITIS-ASSOCIATED COLORECTAL CANCER

Cancer stem cells small subpopulation of tumor possess similar properties to the normal stem cells, and the evidence suggests that altered developmental signaling pathways such as Wnt Notch, Hedgehog etc. these signalings play an important role in maintaining cancer stem cells and thereby the tumor itself. Wnt signaling is a key player in the normal and pathological intestinal mucosa for maintenance epithelial homeostasis, the inhibition of this signaling in the intestine, colonic crypt loss and tissue degeneration, which is an evolutionarily conserved tissue regeneration program.(Clevers, 2006) The APC mutation which activated the Wnt signaling and induced the rapid proliferation of colon cancer stem cells. Whereas in Colitis associate colorectal cancer, the chronic inflammation-mediated tissue damage activates Wnt signaling.(Shenoy *et al.,* 2012) Wnt signaling is not generally considered an inflammatory pathway; the mounting evidence exhibits as a driver of injury repair in the colitis-associated colorectal cancer. Also, colitis to cancer transition the Wnt signaling highly expressed exhibits that increased cancer stem cell proliferation observed in the non-dysplastic epithelium of ulcerative colitis patients. (Romano *et al.,* 2016) Emerging evidence exhibits that Wnt signaling pathway used as a diagnostic marker and therapeutic target for the early event of colitis to cancer transition in colitis-associated colorectal cancer.

Notch signaling pathway is a highly conserved developmental pathway that regulates a vital role in proliferation, stem cell maintenance, differentiation, and homeostasis of the multicellular organism. Notch pathway plays a major role in the embryonic stem cell and Cancer stem cells self-renewal, also the maintenance of intestinal stem cells for a proper balance of differentiation between secretory and absorptive cell lineages. Notch signaling as a gatekeeper of the intestinal progenitor compartment (Fre *et al.,* 2005; Wang, Li, Banerjee, & Sarkar, 2009) Notch signaling is initiated by ligand binding to Notch receptor leads to the proteolytic cleavage of ADAM family protease and γ-secretase and releasing the NICD, which translocate and activate Notch target gene. Notch signaling is reported to 10-30 fold increase in colon cancer stem cells. Blocking the notch signaling induces apoptosis and loss of proliferating stem and progenitor cells and global secretory cell hyperplasia in the intestine.(Sikandar *et al.,* 2010) In chronic inflammatory bowel activated Notch, 1 mediate the cell proliferation, goblet cell depletion, and ectopic expression of PLA2G2A, thereby contributing to the regeneration of the damaged epithelia. Notch I and NICD increased expression was found in ulcerative colitis. Increased Notch signaling may be linked to the increased susceptibility of colon cancer development in precancerous conditions. Emerging reports support that notch signaling activated in the ulcerative colitis involved in intestinal tissue regeneration.(Okamoto *et al.,* 2009)

Hedgehog signaling plays a critical role in the growth differentiation and patterning of various tissue, including the gastrointestinal tract. Hedgehog signaling initiates by binding of ligands and leads to the release of the suppressed transmembrane protein Smoothened (Smo). The release of Smo subsequently activates the Gli transcription factors Hh signaling pathway has been implicated in the pathogenesis of various human cancers.(Cochrane *et al.,* 2015) The hedgehog signaling pathway is involved in the continuous renewal of the intestinal epithelial cells in adults, which leads to the speculation that dysfunctional of hedgehog signaling pathway would cause pathological hyperplasia of intestinal epithelial cells and contribute to the generation and progression of malignancies. But the role of the hedgehog signaling pathway in colorectal cancer remains controversial. The controversy due to the currently available data, most of the studies shows a correlation between the hedgehog and colorectal cancer (98 out of 101 studies), also few researches that claimed that hedgehog is not, or at least not directly, related to colorectal cancer. (Papadopoulos *et al.,* 2016) Inflammation triggers the tissue regeneration through numerous external clue cytokines growth factors, decides the homeostasis maintenance of epithelium during colitis. Also, the molecular level the clue are transduced by conserved signaling pathways. The inflammatory microenvironment of the ulcerative colitis hedgehog pathway stimulation exerts its effects. Genetic augmentation of the Hedgehog respons, and small-molecules potently ameliorate colitis and restrain initiation and progression of colitis-induced adenocarcinoma. In the DSS-induced colitis, Hedgehog pathway significantly reduced also the pharmacological activation of SAG21k which ameliorates the severity of colitis as well as progression to colitis-associated adenocarcinoma.(Lee *et al.,* 2016)

10. CONCLUSION

Colitis associated colorectal cancer incidence and mortality increasing worldwide, it's growing alarmingly in the Asian countries due to the western lifestyle adaptation. Therapeutic approaches improve the quality of the ulcerative colitis-associated colorectal cancer patients. Recent therapeutic research approaches to identify new drug target for the complete cure, cancer stem cells and the developmental signaling pathway in the colitis-associated colorectal cancer have not been fully elucidated understanding the intricate molecular will leads to exploring the ideal target for diagnosis and treatment.

REFERENCES

Al Bakir, I., Curtius, K., & Graham, T. A. (2018). From Colitis to Cancer: An Evolutionary Trajectory That Merges Maths and Biology. *Frontiers in Immunology*, *9*, 2368. doi:10.3389/fimmu.2018.02368 PMID:30386335

Al-Hajj, M., Wicha, M. S., Benito-Hernandez, A., Morrison, S. J., & Clarke, M. F. (2003). Prospective identification of tumorigenic breast cancer cells. *Proceedings of the National Academy of Sciences of the United States of America*, *100*(7), 3983–3988. doi:10.1073/pnas.0530291100 PMID:12629218

Ananthakrishnan, A. N. (2015). Epidemiology and risk factors for IBD. *Nature Reviews. Gastroenterology & Hepatology*, *12*(4), 205–217. doi:10.1038/nrgastro.2015.34 PMID:25732745

Arber, N., Shapira, I., Ratan, J., Stern, B., Hibshoosh, H., Moshkowitz, M., Gammon, M., Fabian, I., & Halpern, Z. (2000). Activation of c-K-ras mutations in human gastrointestinal tumors. *Gastroenterology*, *118*(6), 1045–1050. doi:10.1016/S0016-5085(00)70357-X PMID:10833479

Baars, J. E., Looman, C. W. N., Steyerberg, E. W., Beukers, R., Tan, A. C. I. T. L., Weusten, B. L. A. M., Kuipers, E. J., & van der Woude, C. J. (2011). The risk of inflammatory bowel disease-related colorectal carcinoma is limited: Results from a nationwide nested case-control study. *The American Journal of Gastroenterology*, *106*(2), 319–328. doi:10.1038/ajg.2010.428 PMID:21045815

Baker, A.-M., Cross, W., Curtius, K., Al Bakir, I., Choi, C.-H. R., Davis, H. L., Temko, D., Biswas, S., Martinez, P., Williams, M. J., Lindsay, J. O., Feakins, R., Vega, R., Hayes, S. J., Tomlinson, I. P. M., McDonald, S. A. C., Moorghen, M., Silver, A., East, J. E., ... Graham, T. A. (2019). Evolutionary history of human colitis-associated colorectal cancer. *Gut*, *68*(6), 985–995. doi:10.1136/gutjnl-2018-316191 PMID:29991641

Beaugerie, L., & Itzkowitz, S. H. (2015). Cancers Complicating Inflammatory Bowel Disease. *The New England Journal of Medicine*, *373*(2), 195. doi:10.1056/NEJMc1505689 PMID:26154801

Blanco Calvo, M., Bolós Fernández, V., Medina Villaamil, V., Aparicio Gallego, G., Díaz Prado, S., & Grande Pulido, E. (2009). Biology of BMP signaling and cancer. *Clinical & Translational Oncology*, *11*(3), 126–137. doi:10.1007/S12094-009-0328-8 PMID:19293049

Bonnet, D., & Dick, J. E. (1997). Human acute myeloid leukemia is organized as a hierarchy that originates from a primitive hematopoietic cell. *Nature Medicine*, *3*(7), 730–737. doi:10.1038/nm0797-730 PMID:9212098

Bos, J. L., Fearon, E. R., Hamilton, S. R., Verlaan-de Vries, M., van Boom, J. H., van der Eb, A. J., & Vogelstein, B. (1987). Prevalence of ras gene mutations in human colorectal cancers. *Nature*, *327*(6120), 293–297. doi:10.1038/327293a0 PMID:3587348

Bu, Y., & Cao, D. (2012). The origin of cancer stem cells. *Frontiers in Bioscience (Scholar Edition)*, *4*, 819–830. PMID:22202093

Carpentino, J. E., Hynes, M. J., Appelman, H. D., Zheng, T., Steindler, D. A., Scott, E. W., & Huang, E. H. (2009). Aldehyde dehydrogenase-expressing colon stem cells contribute to tumorigenesis in the transition from colitis to cancer. *Cancer Research*, *69*(20), 8208–8215. doi:10.1158/0008-5472.CAN-09-1132 PMID:19808966

Chambers, W. M., Warren, B. F., Jewell, D. P., & Mortensen, N. J. M. (2005). Cancer surveillance in ulcerative colitis. *British Journal of Surgery*, *92*(8), 928–936. doi:10.1002/bjs.5106 PMID:16034807

Chung, D. C. (2000). The genetic basis of colorectal cancer: Insights into critical pathways of tumorigenesis. *Gastroenterology*, *119*(3), 854–865. doi:10.1053/gast.2000.16507 PMID:10982779

Clarke, M. F., Dick, J. E., Dirks, P. B., Eaves, C. J., Jamieson, C. H. M., Jones, D. L., Visvader, J., Weissman, I. L., & Wahl, G. M. (2006). Cancer stem cells—perspectives on current status and future directions: AACR Workshop on cancer stem cells. *Cancer Research*, *66*(19), 9339–9344. doi:10.1158/0008-5472.CAN-06-3126 PMID:16990346

Clevers, H. (2006). Wnt/beta-catenin signaling in development and disease. *Cell*, *127*(3), 469–480. doi:10.1016/j.cell.2006.10.018 PMID:17081971

Cochrane, C. R., Szczepny, A., Watkins, D. N., & Cain, J. E. (2015). Hedgehog Signaling in the Maintenance of Cancer Stem Cells. *Cancers (Basel)*, *7*(3), 1554–1585. doi:10.3390/cancers7030851 PMID:26270676

Cosnes, J., Gower–Rousseau, C., Seksik, P., & Cortot, A. (2011). Epidemiology and Natural History of Inflammatory Bowel Diseases. *Gastroenterology*, *140*(6), 1785–1794.e4. doi:10.1053/j.gastro.2011.01.055 PMID:21530745

Dame, M. K., Bhagavathula, N., Mankey, C., DaSilva, M., Paruchuri, T., Aslam, M. N., & Varani, J. (2010). Human colon tissue in organ culture: Preservation of normal and neoplastic characteristics. *In Vitro Cellular & Developmental Biology. Animal*, *46*(2), 114–122. doi:10.100711626-009-9247-9 PMID:19915935

Davidson, L. A., Callaway, E. S., Kim, E., Weeks, B. R., Fan, Y.-Y., Allred, C. D., & Chapkin, R. S. (2015). Targeted Deletion of p53 in Lgr5-Expressing Intestinal Stem Cells Promotes Colon Tumorigenesis in a Preclinical Model of Colitis-Associated Cancer. *Cancer Research*, *75*(24), 5392–5397. doi:10.1158/0008-5472.CAN-15-1706 PMID:26631266

Dhawan, P., Ahmad, R., Srivastava, A. S., & Singh, A. B. (2011). Cancer stem cells and colorectal cancer: An overview. *Current Topics in Medicinal Chemistry*, *11*(13), 1592–1598. doi:10.2174/156802611796117694 PMID:21446911

Dobbins, W. O. III. (1984). Dysplasia and malignancy in inflammatory bowel disease. *Annual Review of Medicine*, *35*(1), 33–48. doi:10.1146/annurev.me.35.020184.000341 PMID:6372661

Eaden, J. A., Abrams, K. R., & Mayberry, J. F. (2001). The risk of colorectal cancer in ulcerative colitis: A meta-analysis. *Gut*, *48*(4), 526–535. doi:10.1136/gut.48.4.526 PMID:11247898

Eramo, A., Lotti, F., Sette, G., Pilozzi, E., Biffoni, M., Di Virgilio, A., Conticello, C., Ruco, L., Peschle, C., & De Maria, R. (2008). Identification and expansion of the tumorigenic lung cancer stem cell population. *Cell Death and Differentiation*, *15*(3), 504–514. doi:10.1038j.cdd.4402283 PMID:18049477

Fearon, E. R., & Vogelstein, B. (1990). A genetic model for colorectal tumorigenesis. *Cell*, *61*(5), 759–767. doi:10.1016/0092-8674(90)90186-I PMID:2188735

Fre, S., Huyghe, M., Mourikis, P., Robine, S., Louvard, D., & Artavanis-Tsakonas, S. (2005). Notch signals control the fate of immature progenitor cells in the intestine. *Nature*, *435*(7044), 964–968. doi:10.1038/nature03589 PMID:15959516

Gabriela Pop, M. (2019). Stem Cell Markers in Colon Cancer. In M. Gabriela Pop (Ed.), *Basic Principles and Practice in Surgery*. doi:10.5772/intechopen.84315

Giehl, K. (2005). Oncogenic Ras in tumour progression and metastasis. *Biological Chemistry*, *386*(3), 193–205. doi:10.1515/BC.2005.025 PMID:15843165

Grivennikov, S. I. (2013). Inflammation and colorectal cancer: Colitis-associated neoplasia. *Seminars in Immunopathology*, *35*(2), 229–244. doi:10.100700281-012-0352-6 PMID:23161445

Gyde, S., Prior, P., Dew, M. J., Saunders, V., Waterhouse, J. A., & Allan, R. N. (1982). Mortality in ulcerative colitis. *Gastroenterology*, *83*(1 Pt 1), 36–43. doi:10.1016/S0016-5085(82)80281-3 PMID:7075944

Han, L., Shi, S., Gong, T., Zhang, Z., & Sun, X. (2013). Cancer stem cells: Therapeutic implications and perspectives in cancer therapy. *Acta Pharmaceutica Sinica. B*, *3*(2), 65–75. doi:10.1016/j.apsb.2013.02.006

Holland, J. D., Klaus, A., Garratt, A. N., & Birchmeier, W. (2013). Wnt signaling in stem and cancer stem cells. *Current Opinion in Cell Biology*, *25*(2), 254–264. doi:10.1016/j.ceb.2013.01.004 PMID:23347562

Huang, E. H., Hynes, M. J., Zhang, T., Ginestier, C., Dontu, G., Appelman, H., Fields, J. Z., Wicha, M. S., & Boman, B. M. (2009). Aldehyde dehydrogenase 1 is a marker for normal and malignant human colonic stem cells (SC) and tracks SC overpopulation during colon tumorigenesis. *Cancer Research*, *69*(8), 3382–3389. doi:10.1158/0008-5472.CAN-08-4418 PMID:19336570

Hynes, M. J., Huang, K. M., & Huang, E. H. (2009). Review Paper: Implications of the "Cancer Stem Cell" Hypothesis on Murine Models of Colon Cancer and Colitis-associated Cancer. *Veterinary Pathology*, *46*(5), 819–835. doi:10.1354/vp.08-VP-0172-H-REV PMID:19429978

Isbell, G., & Levin, B. (1988). Ulcerative colitis and colon cancer. *Gastroenterology Clinics of North America*, *17*(4), 773–791. PMID:3068141

Ivanovich, J. L., Read, T. E., Ciske, D. J., Kodner, I. J., & Whelan, A. J. (1999). A practical approach to familial and hereditary colorectal cancer. *The American Journal of Medicine*, *107*(1), 68–77. doi:10.1016/S0002-9343(99)00168-0 PMID:10403355

Kavanagh, D. O., Carter, M. C., Keegan, D., Doherty, G., Smith, M. J., Hyland, J. M. P., Mulcahy, H., Sheahan, K., O' Connell, P. R., O' Donoghue, D. P., & Winter, D. C. (2014). Management of colorectal cancer in patients with inflammatory bowel disease. *Techniques in Coloproctology*, *18*(1), 23–28. doi:10.100710151-013-0981-3 PMID:23407916

Kheirelseid, E. A. H., Miller, N., & Kerin, M. J. (2013). Molecular biology of colorectal cancer: Review of the literature. *American Journal of Molecular Biology*, *03*(02), 72–80. doi:10.4236/ajmb.2013.32010

Koch, U., Krause, M., & Baumann, M. (2010). Cancer stem cells at the crossroads of current cancer therapy failures—Radiation oncology perspective. *Seminars in Cancer Biology*, *20*(2), 116–124. doi:10.1016/j.semcancer.2010.02.003 PMID:20219680

Lee, J. J., Rothenberg, M. E., Seeley, E. S., Zimdahl, B., Kawano, S., Lu, W.-J., Shin, K., Sakata-Kato, T., Chen, J. K., Diehn, M., Clarke, M. F., & Beachy, P. A. (2016). Control of inflammation by stromal Hedgehog pathway activation restrains colitis. *Proceedings of the National Academy of Sciences of the United States of America*, *113*(47), E7545–E7553. doi:10.1073/pnas.1616447113 PMID:27815529

Levine, J. S., & Ahnen, D. J. (2006). Clinical practice. Adenomatous polyps of the colon. *The New England Journal of Medicine*, *355*(24), 2551–2557. doi:10.1056/NEJMcp063038 PMID:17167138

Li, J., Mizukami, Y., Zhang, X., Jo, W.-S., & Chung, D. C. (2005). Oncogenic K-ras Stimulates Wnt Signaling in Colon Cancer Through Inhibition of GSK-3β. *Gastroenterology*, *128*(7), 1907–1918. doi:10.1053/j.gastro.2005.02.067 PMID:15940626

Loftus, E. V. Jr. (2004). Clinical epidemiology of inflammatory bowel disease: Incidence, prevalence, and environmental influences. *Gastroenterology*, *126*(6), 1504–1517. doi:10.1053/j.gastro.2004.01.063 PMID:15168363

Maitland, N. J., & Collins, A. T. (2008). Prostate cancer stem cells: A new target for therapy. *Journal of Clinical Oncology*, *26*(17), 2862–2870. doi:10.1200/JCO.2007.15.1472 PMID:18539965

Miyaki, M., Konishi, M., Kikuchi-Yanoshita, R., Enomoto, M., Igari, T., Tanaka, K., ... Fukayama, M. (1994). Characteristics of somatic mutation of the adenomatous polyposis coli gene in colorectal tumors. *Cancer Research*, *54*(11), 3011–3020. PMID:8187091

Munro, M. J., Wickremesekera, S. K., Peng, L., Tan, S. T., & Itinteang, T. (2018). Cancer stem cells in colorectal cancer: A review. *Journal of Clinical Pathology*, *71*(2), 110–116. doi:10.1136/jclinpath-2017-204739 PMID:28942428

Nawa, T., Kato, J., Kawamoto, H., Okada, H., Yamamoto, H., Kohno, H., Endo, H., & Shiratori, Y. (2008). Differences between right- and left-sided colon cancer in patient characteristics, cancer morphology and histology. *Journal of Gastroenterology and Hepatology*, *23*(3), 418–423. doi:10.1111/j.1440-1746.2007.04923.x PMID:17532785

Ng, S. C., Shi, H. Y., Hamidi, N., Underwood, F. E., Tang, W., Benchimol, E. I., Panaccione, R., Ghosh, S., Wu, J. C. Y., Chan, F. K. L., Sung, J. J. Y., & Kaplan, G. G. (2018). Worldwide incidence and prevalence of inflammatory bowel disease in the 21st century: A systematic review of population-based studies. *Lancet*, *390*(10114), 2769–2778. doi:10.1016/S0140-6736(17)32448-0 PMID:29050646

O'Connor, P. M., Lapointe, T. K., Beck, P. L., & Buret, A. G. (2010). Mechanisms by which inflammation may increase intestinal cancer risk in inflammatory bowel disease. *Inflammatory Bowel Diseases*, *16*(8), 1411–1420. doi:10.1002/ibd.21217 PMID:20155848

Okamoto, R., Tsuchiya, K., Nemoto, Y., Akiyama, J., Nakamura, T., Kanai, T., & Watanabe, M. (2009). Requirement of Notch activation during regeneration of the intestinal epithelia. *American Journal of Physiology. Gastrointestinal and Liver Physiology*, *296*(1), G23–G35. doi:10.1152/ajpgi.90225.2008 PMID:19023031

Pannuti, A., Foreman, K., Rizzo, P., Osipo, C., Golde, T., Osborne, B., & Miele, L. (2010). Targeting Notch to Target Cancer Stem Cells. *Clinical Cancer Research*, *16*(12), 3141–3152. doi:10.1158/1078-0432.CCR-09-2823 PMID:20530696

Papadopoulos, V., Tsapakidis, K., Riobo Del Galdo, N. A., Papandreou, C. N., Del Galdo, F., Anthoney, A., Sakellaridis, N., Dimas, K., & Kamposioras, K. (2016). The Prognostic Significance of the Hedgehog Signaling Pathway in Colorectal Cancer. *Clinical Colorectal Cancer*, *15*(2), 116–127. doi:10.1016/j.clcc.2016.02.010 PMID:27032873

Pinczowski, D., Ekbom, A., Baron, J., Yuen, J., & Adami, H. O. (1994). Risk factors for colorectal cancer in patients with ulcerative colitis: A case-control study. *Gastroenterology*, *107*(1), 117–120. doi:10.1016/0016-5085(94)90068-X PMID:7912678

Prince, M. E., Sivanandan, R., Kaczorowski, A., Wolf, G. T., Kaplan, M. J., Dalerba, P., Weissman, I. L., Clarke, M. F., & Ailles, L. E. (2007). Identification of a subpopulation of cells with cancer stem cell properties in head and neck squamous cell carcinoma. *Proceedings of the National Academy of Sciences of the United States of America*, *104*(3), 973–978. doi:10.1073/pnas.0610117104 PMID:17210912

Reya, T., Morrison, S. J., Clarke, M. F., & Weissman, I. L. (2001). Stem cells, cancer, and cancer stem cells. *Nature*, *414*(6859), 105–111. doi:10.1038/35102167 PMID:11689955

Ricci-Vitiani, L., Lombardi, D. G., Pilozzi, E., Biffoni, M., Todaro, M., Peschle, C., & De Maria, R. (2007). Identification and expansion of human colon-cancer-initiating cells. *Nature*, *445*(7123), 111–115. doi:10.1038/nature05384 PMID:17122771

Risio, M. (2010). Reprint of: The natural history of adenomas. *Best Practice & Research. Clinical Gastroenterology*, *24*(4), 397–406. doi:10.1016/j.bpg.2010.08.002 PMID:20833344

Romano, M., & Francesco, DE, F., Zarantonello, L., Ruffolo, C., Ferraro, G. A., Zanus, G., … Cillo, U. (2016). From Inflammation to Cancer in Inflammatory Bowel Disease: Molecular Perspectives. *Anticancer Research, 36*(4), 1447–1460. PMID:27069120

Segditsas, S., & Tomlinson, I. (2006). Colorectal cancer and genetic alterations in the Wnt pathway. *Oncogene, 25*(57), 7531–7537. doi:10.1038j.onc.1210059 PMID:17143297

Shacter, E., & Weitzman, S. A. (2002). Chronic inflammation and cancer. *Oncology (Williston Park, N.Y.), 16*(2), 217–226. PMID:11866137

Shenoy, A. K., Fisher, R. C., Butterworth, E. A., Pi, L., Chang, L.-J., Appelman, H. D., Chang, M., Scott, E. W., & Huang, E. H. (2012). Transition from colitis to cancer: High Wnt activity sustains the tumor-initiating potential of colon cancer stem cell precursors. *Cancer Research, 72*(19), 5091–5100. doi:10.1158/0008-5472.CAN-12-1806 PMID:22902411

Sikandar, S. S., Pate, K. T., Anderson, S., Dizon, D., Edwards, R. A., Waterman, M. L., & Lipkin, S. M. (2010). NOTCH signaling is required for formation and self-renewal of tumor-initiating cells and for repression of secretory cell differentiation in colon cancer. *Cancer Research, 70*(4), 1469–1478. doi:10.1158/0008-5472.CAN-09-2557 PMID:20145124

Singh, S. K., Hawkins, C., Clarke, I. D., Squire, J. A., Bayani, J., Hide, T., Henkelman, R. M., Cusimano, M. D., & Dirks, P. B. (2004). Identification of human brain tumour initiating cells. *Nature, 432*(7015), 396–401. doi:10.1038/nature03128 PMID:15549107

Somasundaram, K. (2000). Tumor suppressor p53: Regulation and function. *Frontiers in Bioscience: A Journal and Virtual Library, 5*, D424-437. doi:10.2741/Somasund

Takaishi, S., Okumura, T., & Wang, T. C. (2008). Gastric cancer stem cells. *Journal of Clinical Oncology, 26*(17), 2876–2882. doi:10.1200/JCO.2007.15.2603 PMID:18539967

Thorsteinsdottir, S., Gudjonsson, T., Nielsen, O. H., Vainer, B., & Seidelin, J. B. (2011). Pathogenesis and biomarkers of carcinogenesis in ulcerative colitis. *Nature Reviews. Gastroenterology & Hepatology, 8*(7), 395–404. doi:10.1038/nrgastro.2011.96 PMID:21647200

Torres, J., Billioud, V., Sachar, D. B., Peyrin-Biroulet, L., & Colombel, J.-F. (2012). Ulcerative colitis as a progressive disease: The forgotten evidence. *Inflammatory Bowel Diseases, 18*(7), 1356–1363. doi:10.1002/ibd.22839 PMID:22162423

Ungaro, R., Mehandru, S., Allen, P. B., Peyrin-Biroulet, L., & Colombel, J.-F. (2017). Ulcerative colitis. *Lancet*, *389*(10080), 1756–1770. doi:10.1016/S0140-6736(16)32126-2 PMID:27914657

Velayos, F. S., Loftus, E. V. Jr, Jess, T., Harmsen, W S., Bida, J., Zinsmeister, A. R., Tremaine, W. J., & Sandborn, W. J. (2006). Predictive and protective factors associated with colorectal cancer in ulcerative colitis: A case-control study. *Gastroenterology*, *130*(7), 1941–1949. doi:10.1053/j.gastro.2006.03.028 PMID:16762617

Vermeulen, L., De Sousa, E., Melo, F., van der Heijden, M., Cameron, K., de Jong, J. H., Borovski, T., ... Medema, J. P. (2010). Wnt activity defines colon cancer stem cells and is regulated by the microenvironment. *Nature Cell Biology*, *12*(5), 468–476. doi:10.1038/ncb2048 PMID:20418870

Vogelstein, B., Fearon, E. R., Hamilton, S. R., Kern, S. E., Preisinger, A. C., Leppert, M., Smits, A. M. M., & Bos, J. L. (1988). Genetic alterations during colorectal-tumor development. *The New England Journal of Medicine*, *319*(9), 525–532. doi:10.1056/NEJM198809013190901 PMID:2841597

Wang, Z., Li, Y., Banerjee, S., & Sarkar, F. H. (2009). Emerging role of Notch in stem cells and cancer. *Cancer Letters*, *279*(1), 8–12. doi:10.1016/j.canlet.2008.09.030 PMID:19022563

Yang, Z. F., Ngai, P., Ho, D. W., Yu, W. C., Ng, M. N. P., Lau, C. K., Li, M. L. Y., Tam, K. H., Lam, C. T., Poon, R. T. P., & Fan, S. T. (2008). Identification of local and circulating cancer stem cells in human liver cancer. *Hepatology (Baltimore, Md.)*, *47*(3), 919–928. doi:10.1002/hep.22082 PMID:18275073

Yashiro, M. (2014). Ulcerative colitis-associated colorectal cancer. *World Journal of Gastroenterology*, *20*(44), 16389–16397. doi:10.3748/wjg.v20.i44.16389 PMID:25469007

Zhou, Y., Xia, L., Wang, H., Oyang, L., Su, M., Liu, Q., Lin, J., Tan, S., Tian, Y., Liao, Q., & Cao, D. (2018). Cancer stem cells in progression of colorectal cancer. *Oncotarget*, *9*(70), 33403–33415. doi:10.18632/oncotarget.23607 PMID:30279970

Chapter 10
The Multifaceted Role of Natural Agents in Colitis-Associated Cancer Prevention and Therapy

Ashok Kumar Kumar Pandurangan
https://orcid.org/0000-0003-2824-1757
B. S. Abdur Rahman Crescent Institute of Science and Technology, India

Suresh Kumar Anandasadagopan
https://orcid.org/0000-0001-5178-005X
Central Leather Research Institute, India

Neesar Ahmed
B. S. Abdur Rahman Crescent Institute of Science and Technology, India

ABSTRACT

Inflammatory bowel disease (IBD) is comprised of ulcerative colitis (UC) and Crohn's disease (CD) that was recognized by the inflammation in the colon. There are no proper medications are available to control the IBD in patients. NASIDs such as Aspirin, diclofenac, and ibuprofen are widely used to control the inflammation. On the other hand, the untreated prolonged inflammation leads to the development of cancer in the colon termed as colitis-associated cancer or inflammation-driven colon cancer. Oxidative stress and inflammation play key roles in the pathogenesis of colitis-associated cancer. Single dose of azozymethane (AOM) and three cycles of 2% dextran sodium sulfate (DSS) induces colitis-associated cancer (CAC) in

DOI: 10.4018/978-1-7998-3580-6.ch010

mouse. Hence, many natural products were tested in the preclinical model of colitis-associated cancer. Each of these natural agents modulate important signaling pathway to control the colitis-associated cancer (CAC). In this review, the authors tabulated all the natural agents that culminate the colitis-associated cancer in the preclinical models.

INTRODUCTION

Inflammatory bowel disease (IBD) is sub categorized into two major diseases namely ulcerative colitis (UC) and Crohn's disease (CD). The incidence of UC worldwide is in a steady rise due to the intake of unbalanced diet. It has been reported that UC is associated with an increased levels of various inflammatory markers such as myeloperoxidase (MPO), interleukin (IL)-1β, IL-6, IL-17, IL-21, tumor necrosis factor-alpha (TNF-α), nuclear factor-kappa B (NF-κB), Inducible nitric oxide synthase (iNOS) and cyclooxygenase-2 (COX-2). It was also known that untreated chronic inflammation in the colon leads the development of colitis associated cancer (CAC) (Pandurangan and Esa, 2014). There several signalling pathways were identified in the transformation of UC to colitis associated cancer. Oxidative stress plays a vital role in the pathogenesis of UC. Hence, many natural products that possess antioxidant ability were used for the treatment of UC in the preclinical level (Pandurangan et al., 2015; Pandurangan et al., 2015a; Pandurangan et al., 2016). So far, Non-steroidal anti-inflammatory drugs such as 5-aminosalicylic acid (5-ASA), Balsalazide, mesalamine, olsalazine, and sulfasalazine were used in the treatment of UC. Still, the research is underway to find suitable drug to treat UC without any side effects.

The pathogenesis of CAC was explained in derail in many published reports (Figure 1). When a normal epithelium undergo injury by the production of reactive oxygen species by various environmental mutagens. This injury leads to the formation of aberrant crypt foci (ACF) which is considered as a pre-neoplastic lesion of Colorectal cancer. Several pro-inflammatory cytokines

NF-κB Pathway and Colitis Associated Cancer

The development of inflammation-related cancer is a long period of tumor promotion, and persistent inflammation facilitates tumor formation by activating the proliferation and antiapoptotic properties of premalignant cells. Moreover, the localized inflammatory microenvironment can promote accumulation mutations and genetic changes after tumor formation. Many reports have documented the critical link between inflammation and the development of CRC. Among the many signaling pathways that are involved in colonic inflammation, the NF-κB pathway is central. NF-κB proteins are involved in the control of many normal cellular and physiological processes, including immune and inflammatory responses, developmental processes, cellular growth and apoptosis.

Figure 1.

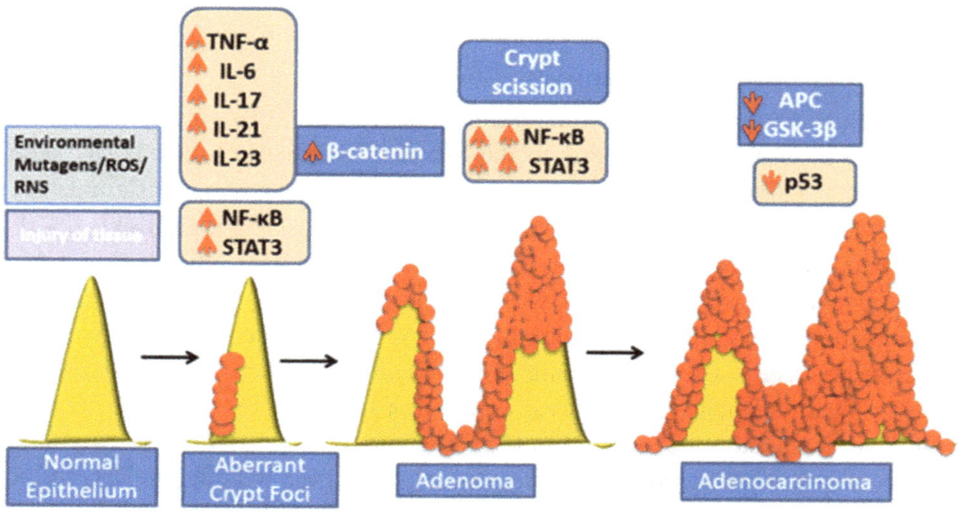

STAT3 Signaling and Colitis Associated Cancer

Signal transducer and activator of transcription (STAT) 3 protein is a member of the STAT family of transcription factors, which are initially located in the cytoplasm in their inactive form. After stimulation by extracellular signals, such as cytokines, growth factors and hormones, Janus kinases (AKs) are activated and then induce the phosphorylation of STAT3 at tyrosine residue 705 (Y705) . Phosphorylated STAT3 proteins dimerize via their Src-homology 2 (SH2) domains and translocate to the nucleus, where they regulate the expression of numerous critical genes involved in cell-cycle progression, proliferation, migration, invasion and survival. However, the constitutive activation of STAT3 is frequently detected in clinical samples from a wide range of human carcinoma, particularly CRC. Hence, STAT3 is considered the most important target of chemoprevention and therapy in CAC.

Nrf2 Pathway and Colitis Associated Cancer

The NF-E2-related factor 2 (Nrf2), a member of the Cap-N-Collar family of transcription factors, under normal conditions it is sequestered in the cytoplasm by the Kelch-like ECH associated protein 1 (Keap1), resulting in enhanced proteosomal degradation of Nrf2 (Dinkova-Kostova, 2005; Furukawa, 2005). During oxidative stress, Nrf2 is released from Keap1, either through oxidative modification of Keap1 or after phosphorylation by redox sensitive protein kinases. Nrf2 then translocates into the nucleus and in combination with other transcription factors, activates the gene transcription of genes containing an antioxidant response element (ARE), resulting in cytoprotective adaptive responses (Kobayashi, 2005). This adaptive response is characterized by the upregulation of antioxidative enzymes and decreased sensitivity to oxidative damage and cytotoxicity (Osburn, 2006; Zhu, 2005). Antioxidative enzymes also attenuate inflammatory damage and neutralize the ROS involved in inflammatory signaling pathways (Chen, 2004). Nrf2 plays a critical role in protecting against inflammation-associated CRC, supporting and extending a published report showing that Nrf2 knockout increases the susceptibility to inflammation-associated aberrant crypt foci (Osburn, 2007). Activation of Nrf2 signaling resulted in suppression of colitis associated CRC (Li, 2008; Chiou, 2012; Yang, 2014; Pandurangan, 2014). Nrf2 is activated by at least two mechanisms that include stabilization of Nrf2 via keap 1 cysteine thiol modification and phosphorylation of Nrf2 by upstream kinases (Surh, 2008). Many natural products had proven already, that activation of Nrf2 will protect from CAC.

Ziziphus Jujuba Fruit and Colitis Associated Cancer

Ziziphus jujuba fruit possess bioactive molecules (flavonoids, polysaccharides, oleamide and triterpenoids). Traditionally, Ziziphus jujuba fruit is most commonly used for the treatment of various ailments including digetive complications, diabetes mellitus, diarrhea, liver, kidney complications and skin infections. Periasamy et al., (2015) reported that administration of Ziziphus jujuba fruit at the dose of 5% and 10% reduced the aberrant crypt foci formation in colitis associated cancer mice model induced by AOM/DSS. Further, Ziziphus jujuba fruit significantly reduced circulating white blood cells, monocytes, lymphocytes, platelets, basophils, neutrophils, and eosinophils, when compared to CAC mice. The authors of thre article conclude that Ziziphus jujuba supplementation may delay the progression of CAC from hyperplasia to dysplasia and ultimately adenocarcinoma and cancer(Periasamy, 2015).

Cocoa and Colitis Associated Cancer

Cocoa is a rich source of polyphenols, and cocoa beans contain 6-8% total polyphenols. Over 8,000 phenolic structures are known, ranging from simple molecules, such as phenolic acids, to highly polymerized substances, such as flavonoids (Ali, 2014). In particular, cocoa beans possess major polyphenolic contents, such as anthocyanidins/ anthocyanins, catechins, flavonol, glycosides and proanthocyanidins (Kelm, 2006). Cocoa polyphenol has many beneficial effects, such as antioxidant (Rodriguez-Ramiro, 2011), antiinflammatory (Becker, 2013), hypoglycemic (Sarmadi, 2012), and antiproliferative properties (Martin, 2013). Cocoa induces apoptosis in HepG2 hepatic cancer cells by activating caspase 3 (Yang, 2012). Cocoa also inhibits tumor formation by interfering with cell cycle pathways in prostate cancer (Peng, 2010). Pandurangan et al., (2014) (Pandurangan, 2015) demonstrates that cocoa improves the colonic antioxidant anti-inflammatory potential *via* the induction of enzymatic and nonenzymatic antioxidant enzymes, such as SOD, CAT, GPx, GR, and GSH, and by suppressing the expression of iNOS and COX-2. They also showed that 10% cocoa diet administration activates Nrf2 and its downstream targets, NQO1 and UDP-GT in AOM/DSS-induced mice and cocoa was identified as a potent inducer of Nrf2 and its downstream targets. The reduced tumor number in 10% coco diet treated mice is correlated with the upregulated expression of Nrf2. Polyphenolic contents of cocoa, such as catechin, (-) epicatechin and procyanidins B2, were previously shown to activate and enhance the translocation of Nrf2 (Granado-Serrano, 2007; Cheng, 2013). A study from Saadatdoust et al (Saadatdoust, 2015) showed that cocoa intensely inhibits tumorigenesis in the AOM/DSS model of CAC. Their findings revealed that the antitumorigenic effect of cocoa is mediated, in part, by limiting IL-6/STAT3 signaling. Cocoa diet (5% and 10%) significantly reduces colonic *IL-6* expression and the subsequent inhibition of STAT3. Cocoa was shown to inhibit the expression of NF-κB. The potent anti-inflammatory effect of cocoa diet was further demonstrated by the finding that cocoa significantly decreases the expression levels of *TNF-α, IL-1β* and *IL-17* and the expression/activity levels of $CD68^+$ and Myeloperoxidase (MPO) in colonic tissues during CAC development.

Digitoflavone and Colitis Associated Cancer

Digitoflavone (3, 0, 4, 5, 7-tetrahydroxyflavone), a flavone subclass of flavonoids, vegetables and fruits such as celery, parsley, broccoli, onion leaves, carrots, peppers, cabbages, apple skins, and chrysanthemum flowers are digitoflavone rich (Neuhouser, 2004; Miean, 2001; Gates, 2007). Plants rich in digitoflavone have been used as Chinese traditional medicine for hypertension, inflammatory diseases, and cancer (Harborne, 2000). Also, it has been known to have chemopreventive effects against malignant tumors *in vivo* (Pandurangan, 2014; Pandurangan, 2014; Pandurangan, 2014; Pandurangan, 2014). Digitoflavone inhibits IκBα kinase and enhances apoptosis induced by TNF-α through downregulation of expression of nuclear factor κB-regulated gene products in PANC-1 human pancreatic cancer cells (Cai, 2013). The chemopreventive role of digitoflavone in AOM-DSS induced colorectal cancer model. Digitoflavone was post-treated after the initiation of stage of colorectal cancer. Compared with AOM group, digitoflavone group shown lower cancer incidents (50% compare with AMO group 100%), reduced numbers and size of macroscopical tumors and recovered colon length. General histological observation found that digitoflavone retained a better colonic histoarchitecture with less loss of crypts. Further protein and mRNA level Analysis indicated the chemopreventive role of digitoflavone may through the activation of Nrf2 and inhibition of inflammation (Yang, 2014).

Astaxanthin and Colitis Associated Cancer

Astaxanthin is a red-orange colored xanthophyll carotenoid with powerful biological antioxidant. This naturally occurred carotenoid is present in salmonid, shrimp, and crustacean aquaculture to provide the pink color characteristic of that species. Increasing evidence suggests that Astaxanthin is a potent anti-tumor agent in several experimental animal models. For example, Astaxanthin suppresses urinary bladder carcinogenesis in mice (Tanaka, 1994) and colon carcinogenesis in rats (Tanaka, 1995) and oral carcinogenesis in rats (Tanaka, 1995). Yasui et al (Yasui, 2011) revealed that, they evaluated the effects of Astaxanthin at three dose levels, 50, 100 and 200 ppm in diet, on CAC-induced mice. Also, immunohistochemical expressions of NF-κB, a proliferation marker of proliferating cell nuclear antigen (PCNA), an apoptosis marker of survivin, and certain inflammatory cytokines, including TNF-a and IL-1β, in colonic adenocarcinomas were analyzed. They found that dietary Astaxanthin inhibited the DSS-induced-inflammation and AOM/DSS-induced-CAC in mice through suppressing the expression of cytokines including NF-κB. They conclude that NF-κB signaling pathway may plays an important role and can be a potential target to treat CAC.

3,3'Diindolylmethane and Colitis Associated Cancer

3,3-Diindolylmethane (DIM) is a major dimer formed in acidic conditions from indole-3-carbinol, an autolysis product of the abundant glucobrassicin in cruciferous vegetables. DIM has antiproliferative effects against various cancers, including gastric, prostate, pancreatic, and breast cancer (Nachshon-Kedmi, 2003; Zhu, 2016; Goldberg, 2015; Nicastro, 2013). Moreover, a previous study showed that DIM inhibits lipopolysaccharide (LPS)-induced production of inflammatory mediators in murine macrophages via downregulation of NF-κB signaling (Cho, 2008). These previous observations led Kim et al., (Kim, 2009) to examine the therapeutic effects of DIM on intestinal inflammation and CAC. They investigate the effects of DIM, a dextran sodium sulfate (DSS)-induced mouse colitis model and an azoxymethane (AOM)/DSS-induced colon cancer model were selected as the subjects for this study. They showed that DIM administration dramatically attenuated weight loss, colon shortening, and severe clinical signs in a colitis model. Further, DIM dramatically suppressed tumor formation in AOM/DSS-induced BALB/c mice. They conclude that DIM suppressed inflammatory reactions in DSS-induced colonic inflammation by inhibiting NF-κB activation and indicate that suppressed production of NO, PGE_2, and proinflammatory cytokines such as IL-6, TNF-α, and IFN-γ in DIM-treated colons might be the result of inhibited NF-κB activation.

American Ginseng and Colitis Associated Cancer

American ginseng (*Panax quinquefolius*) (AG) is a perennial native of North America, and ginseng is one of the most popular medicinal herbs used in the world (O'Hara, 1998). American Ginsengs consists of saponins (generally called ginsenosides) and acidic polysaccharides have been the main focus of its pharmacologic activities (Wang, 2010; Kim, 1998; Park, 2011; Lee, 2006; Choi, 2008). Water-soluble polysaccharides also have medicinal properties, including immunomodulating and antiproliferative effects (Jia, 2009). A study from Poudyal et al., (Poudyal, 2012) revealed that, the hexane fractions of AG, inhibits the CAC tumors by inhibiting the expressions of iNOS and COX-2 and also induces apoptosis. Another study als revealed that AG inhibits the expression of c-Jun and other tumor promoting proteins along with the cell proliferation in CAC (Cui, 2010).

Juice of Sugar Beets and Colitis Associated Cancer

It was first discovered in the juice of sugar beets (*Beta vulgaris*) in the 19th century (Craig, 2004), and since then has been found in various microorganisms, plants and animals (Steenge, 2003; Kim, 2002). Betaine is an essential biochemical molecule of the methionine/homeocysteine cycle and is synthesized by conversion of choline. It plays central roles in choline-mediated one-carbon metabolism, structural integrity and signaling functions of cell membranes, and neurotransmitter synthesis (Zeisel, 1994). A recent report enumerates that administration of betaine effectively suppressed AOM/DSS-induced mouse colon tumor incidence with inflammation by suppressing the expression of cytokines, such as TNF-α, IL-6, COX-2 and iNOS. In addition, treatment with betaine decreased ROS generation and modulation of total glutathione concentration (Kim, 2014).

DA-6034 and Colitis Associated Cancer

DA-6034 (7-carboxymethyloxy-39,49,5-trimethoxyflavone), a synthetic derivative of eupatilin (flavonoid) prevents and improves acute murine colitis and inhibits inflammation-related colon carcinogenesis by the inhibition of COX-2 and phosphoIKKa and by the induction of apoptosis in AOM/DSS-induced CAC (Nam, 2008).

Canolol and Colitis Associated Cancer

Canolol (4-vinyl-2,6-dimethoxyphenol) is a phenolic compound found in crude canola oil and recently reported to be strong anti-oxidant and anti-mutagenic compound compared to flavonoids (Kuwahara, 2004). In the AOM/DSS-induced CAC model, mice receiving canolol had a reduced occurrence of cancer, to 60%, compared with control mice, 100% of which had colon cancer. The numbers of tumors in each mouse were also significantly reduced in mice receiving the canolol-containing diet (5.6±2.0) compared with azoxymethane/DSS control mice (10.8±4.2). No apparent toxicity of canolol was observed. Moreover, inflammatory cytokines (*i.e.* cyclooxygenase-2, inducible nitric oxide synthase and tumor necrosis factor-α) and oxidative responding molecules, i.e. heme oxygenase-1, in colon were suppressed during this treatment. In a mouse colon 26 solid tumor model, canolol significantly suppressed COX-2 expression; however, no significant tumor growth inhibition was observed, suggesting that canolol preferably shows chemopreventive effects during the stages of initiation/promotion. Canolol may, thus, be considered a potential cancer preventive agent or supplement (Fang, 2013).

Apple Oligogalactan and Colitis Associated Cancer

An apple oligogalactan composed of five galacturonic acids and evaluated the protective effects on colitis and colon carcinogenesis using a mouse model of CAC. Liu et al., the effect of apple oligogalactan at different dosese on LPS/TLR4/NF-κB signaling pathway by investigating the level and distribution of TLR4 and production of TNF-α at different stages of inflammation induced by 1,2-dimethylhydrazine (DMH)/DSS *in vivo* and the effect on the expression and localization of TLR4, phosphorylation of IκB and production of TNF-α induced by LPS *in vitro*. Apple oligogalactin, effectively controls the tumor formation as well as downregulates TLR4 and TNF-α expressions in CAC mice (Liu, 2010).

Curcumin and Colitis Associated Cancer

Curcumin (1,7-bis(4-hydroxy-3-methoxyphenyl)-1,6-heptadiene-3,5-dione) is a polyphenol found in this dietary spice, derived from dried rhizomes of the perennial herb *Curcuma longa Linn.*, a member of the ginger family. Interest in this dietary polyphenol has grown in recent years because of its vast array of beneficial pharmacological effects including chemosensitizing, radiosensitizing, wound healing activities, antimicrobial, antiviral, antifungical, cholekinetic, antioxidant, anti-inflammatory and immunomodulatory benefits. Villegas et al., (2011) demonstrated that the protective/preventive effect of curcumin in the progression of CAC, which was correlated with a lowered immunoreactivity of β-catenin, a non-modification of p53 expression, a reduction of proinflammatory cytokine levels and a decrease of inflammatory protein overexpression (Villegas, 2011).

O-1602 and Colitis Associated Cancer

Cannabis has been known for a long time to relieve symptoms of cachexia and pain associated with cancer therapy, but what has emerged is that cannabinoids themselves (natural, synthetic, and endocannabinoids) have the ability to inhibit cancer development and progression. Many of the antineoplastic effects of cannabinoids involve the activity of CB1 and CB2. O-1602, an atypical cannabinoid, inhibits tumor growth in CAC through multiple mechanisms. In the mouse model, treatment with O-1602 (3 mg/kg, i.p., 12×) reduced tumor area by 50% and tumor incidence by 30%. Histological scoring revealed a significant decrease in tumor load. In tumor tissue, O-1602 decreased levels of proliferating cell nuclear antigen (PCNA), activation of oncogenic transcription factors STAT3 and NFκB p65, and expression of TNF-α while levels for proapoptotic markers, such as p53 and BAX, increased. The in vivo effects of O-1602 on PCNA, BAX, and p53 were also observed in HT-29 and SW480 colon cancer cells (Kargl, 2013).

Diallyl Trisulfide and Colitis Associated Cancer

Diallyl trisulfide (DATS), was a organosulfur compound present in garlic and some of the other organosulfur compounds also derived from garlic, especially diallyl sulfide, diallyl disulfide, have been considered to contribute to its chemopreventive and cytoprotective activities (Wu, 2004). Among these three organosulfur compounds DATS is thought to be most potent in terms of anti-carcinogenic activities (Seki, 2008). From the published reports it is generally beleived that the anti-carcinogenic activities of DATS are associated with induction of cancer cell apoptosis, inhibition of aberrant cell cycle progression, and induction of phase 2 carcinogen detoxifying enzymes (Antony, 2011). DATS also inhibited capillary-like tube formation and migration of human umbilical vain endothelial cells *via* suppression of vascular endothelial growth factor secretion (Xiao, 2006) and invasion of COLO 205 human colon cancer cells by blocking expression of matrix metalloproteinase-2, -7, and -9 (Lai, 2012). DATS appears to exert its chemopreventive effects through modulation of multiple cellular signal transduction pathways involved in multi-stage carcinogenesis. Lee et al., (Lee, 2013) reported that DATS attenuated the DSS-induced colitis in mouse colon. DATS also inhibited overexpression of COX-2 and iNOS, which is attributable to its blockade of the nuclear transcription factor NF-κB signaling *via* suppression of phosphorylation of IκB-α. The inhibitory effect of NF-κB activity by garlic derived organosulfurs has also been reported. They also revealed that DATS suppressed the DNA binding activity and phosphorylation of STAT3 at Tyr 705 and expression of its target protein cyclin D1 (Lee, 2013).

Baicalein and Colitis Associated Cancer

Baicalein is a natural plant flavone originally isolated from the roots of *Scutellaria baicalensis*. This compound exhibits various biological effects, including anti-inflammatory and antitumor activity. PPARγ agonists can inhibit the activities of signal dependent transcription factors, such as NF-κB. This function could contribute to the anti-inflammatory actions of PPARγ. Baicalein suppresses the NF-κB activity through the PPARγ activation and reduces the inflammation as well as tumor formation in CAC (Kim, 2013).

CONCLUSION

Colitis associated cancer is a serious health problem in all over the world. Major researches are ongoing to develop new and novel drugs the cure colitis associated cancer. On the other hand, understanding the pathogenesis of colitis associated cancer is vital. Because, that will give the information on the moelcular targets to treat colitis associated cancer. In this chapter we summarized the natural agents that alleviate the colitis associated cancer by modulating the key signaling pathways. We found that natural agents such as cocoa, Bufalin, Diallyl trisulfide, Baicalein, curcumin and canalol are effective against colitis associated cancer at the preclinical level. These natural agents can be used as chemotherapeutic drugs when it will be proven in clinical trials.

REFERENCES

Ali, F., Ismail, A., & Kersten, S. (2014). Molecular mechanisms underlying the potential antiobesity-related diseases effect of cocoa polyphenols. *Molecular Nutrition & Food Research*, *58*(1), 33–48. doi:10.1002/mnfr.201300277 PMID:24259381

Antony, M. L., & Singh, S. V. (2011). Molecular mechanisms and targets of cancer chemoprevention by garlic-derived bioactive compound diallyl trisulfide. *Indian Journal of Experimental Biology*, *49*(11), 805. PMID:22126011

Becker, K., Geisler, S., Ueberall, F., Fuchs, D., & Gostner, J. M. (2013). Immunomodulatory properties of cacao extracts - potential consequences for medical applications. *Frontiers in Pharmacology*, *4*, 154. doi:10.3389/fphar.2013.00154 PMID:24376420

Cai, X., Lu, W., Yang, Y., Yang, J., Ye, J., Gu, Z., Hu, C., Wang, X., & Cao, P. (2013). Digitoflavone inhibits IkappaBalpha kinase and enhances apoptosis induced by TNFalpha through downregulation of expression of nuclear factor kappaB-regulated gene products in human pancreatic cancer cells. *PLoS One*, *8*(10), e77126. doi:10.1371/journal.pone.0077126 PMID:24146961

Chen, X. L., & Kunsch, C. (2004). Induction of cytoprotective genes through Nrf2/antioxidant response element pathway: A new therapeutic approach for the treatment of inflammatory diseases. *Current Pharmaceutical Design*, *10*(8), 879–891. doi:10.2174/1381612043452901 PMID:15032691

Cheng, Y. T., Wu, C. H., Ho, C. Y., & Yen, G. C. (2013). Catechin protects against ketoprofen-induced oxidative damage of the gastric mucosa by up-regulating Nrf2 in vitro and in vivo. *The Journal of Nutritional Biochemistry*, *24*(2), 475–483. doi:10.1016/j.jnutbio.2012.01.010 PMID:22704780

Chiou, Y.-S., Ma, N. J.-L., Sang, S., Ho, C.-T., Wang, Y.-J., & Pan, M.-H. (2012). Peracetylated (−)-epigallocatechin-3-gallate (AcEGCG) potently suppresses dextran sulfate sodium-induced colitis and colon tumorigenesis in mice. *Journal of Agricultural and Food Chemistry*, *60*(13), 3441–3451. doi:10.1021/jf300441p PMID:22409325

Cho, H. J., Seon, M. R., Lee, Y. M., Kim, J., Kim, J. K., Kim, S. G., & Park, J. H. (2008). 3,3′-Diindolylmethane suppresses the inflammatory response to lipopolysaccharide in murine macrophages. *The Journal of Nutrition*, *138*(1), 17–23. doi:10.1093/jn/138.1.17 PMID:18156398

Choi, H.-S., Kim, K.-H., Sohn, E., Park, J.-D., Kim, B.-O., Moon, E.-Y., Rhee, D.-K., & Pyo, S. (2008). Red ginseng acidic polysaccharide (RGAP) in combination with IFN-γ results in enhanced macrophage function through activation of the NF-κB pathway. *Bioscience, Biotechnology, and Biochemistry*, *72*(7), 1817–1825. doi:10.1271/bbb.80085 PMID:18603775

Craig, S. A. (2004). Betaine in human nutrition. *The American Journal of Clinical Nutrition*, *80*(3), 539–549. doi:10.1093/ajcn/80.3.539 PMID:15321791

Cui, X., Jin, Y., Poudyal, D., Chumanevich, A. A., Davis, T., Windust, A., Hofseth, A., Wu, W., Habiger, J., Pena, E., Wood, P., Nagarkatti, M., Nagarkatti, P. S., & Hofseth, L. (2010). Mechanistic insight into the ability of American ginseng to suppress colon cancer associated with colitis. *Carcinogenesis*, *31*(10), 1734–1741. doi:10.1093/carcin/bgq163 PMID:20729391

Dinkova-Kostova, A. T., Holtzclaw, W. D., & Kensler, T. W. (2005). The role of Keap1 in cellular protective responses. *Chemical Research in Toxicology*, *18*(12), 1779–1791. doi:10.1021/tx050217c PMID:16359168

Fang, J., Seki, T., Tsukamoto, T., Qin, H., Yin, H., Liao, L., Nakamura, H., & Maeda, H. (2013). Protection from inflammatory bowel disease and colitis-associated carcinogenesis with 4-vinyl-2,6-dimethoxyphenol (canolol) involves suppression of oxidative stress and inflammatory cytokines. *Carcinogenesis*, *34*(12), 2833–2841. doi:10.1093/carcin/bgt309 PMID:24064222

Furukawa, M., & Xiong, Y. (2005). BTB protein Keap1 targets antioxidant transcription factor Nrf2 for ubiquitination by the Cullin 3-Roc1 ligase. *Molecular and Cellular Biology*, *25*(1), 162–171. doi:10.1128/MCB.25.1 162-171.2005 PMID:15601839

Gates, M. A., Tworoger, S. S., Hecht, J. L., De Vivo, I., Rosner, B., & Hankinson, S. E. (2007). A prospective study of dietary flavonoid intake and incidence of epithelial ovarian cancer. *International Journal of Cancer*, *121*(10), 2225–2232. doi:10.1002/ijc.22790 PMID:17471564

Goldberg, A. A., Draz, H., Montes-Grajales, D, Olivero-Verbel, J., Safe, S. H., & Sanderson, J. T. (2015). 3,3′-Diindolylmethane (DIM) and its ring-substituted halogenated analogs (ring-DIMs) induce differential mechanisms of survival and death in androgen-dependent and -independent prostate cancer cells. *Genes & Cancer*, *6*(5-6), 265–280. doi:10.18632/genesandcancer.60 PMID:26124925

Granado-Serrano, A. B., Angeles Martín, M., Izquierdo-Pulido, M., Goya, L., Bravo, L., & Ramos, S. (2007). Molecular mechanisms of (-)-epicatechin and chlorogenic acid on the regulation of the apoptotic and survival/proliferation pathways in a human hepatoma cell line. *Journal of Agricultural and Food Chemistry*, *55*(5), 2020–2027. doi:10.1021/jf062556x PMID:17286412

Harborne, J. B., & Williams, C. A. (2000). Advances in flavonoid research since 1992. *Phytochemistry*, *55*(6), 481–504. doi:10.1016/S0031-9422(00)00235-1 PMID:11130659

Jia, L., & Zhao, Y. (2009). Current evaluation of the millennium phytomedicine-ginseng (I): Etymology, pharmacognosy, phytochemistry, market and regulations. *Current Medicinal Chemistry*, *16*(19), 2475–2484. doi:10.2174/092986709788682146 PMID:19601793

Kargl, J., Haybaeck, J., Stancic, A., Andersen, L., Marsche, G., Heinemann, A., & Schicho, R. (2013). O-1602, an atypical cannabinoid, inhibits tumor growth in colitis-associated colon cancer through multiple mechanisms. *Journal of Molecular Medicine (Berlin, Germany)*, *91*(4), 449–458. doi:10.100700109-012-0957-1 PMID:22965195

Kelm, M. A., Johnson, J. C., Robbins, R. J., Hammerstone, J. F., & Schmitz, H. H. (2006). High-performance liquid chromatography separation and purification of cacao (Theobroma cacao L.) procyanidins according to degree of polymerization using a diol stationary phase. *Journal of Agricultural and Food Chemistry*, *54*(5), 1571–1576. doi:10.1021/jf0525941 PMID:16506802

Kim, D. H., Hossain, M. A., Kang, Y. J., Jang, J. Y., Lee, Y. J., Im, E., Yoon, J.-H., Kim, H. S., Chung, H. Y., & Kim, N. D. (2013). Baicalein, an active component of Scutellaria baicalensis Georgi, induces apoptosis in human colon cancer cells and prevents AOM/DSS-induced colon cancer in mice. *International Journal of Oncology*, *43*(5), 1652–1658. doi:10.3892/ijo.2013.2086 PMID:24008356

Kim, D. H., Sung, B., Kang, Y. J., Jang, J. Y., Hwang, S. Y., Lee, Y., Kim, M., Im, E., Yoon, J.-H., Kim, C. M., Chung, H. Y., & Kim, N. D. (2014). Anti-inflammatory effects of betaine on AOM/DSSinduced colon tumorigenesis in ICR male mice. *International Journal of Oncology*, *45*(3), 1250–1256. doi:10.3892/ijo.2014.2515 PMID:24969167

Kim, K. H., Lee, Y. S., Jung, I. S., Park, S. Y., Chung, H. Y., Lee, I. R., & Yun, Y. S. (1998). Acidic polysaccharide from Panax ginseng, ginsan, induces Th1 cell and macrophage cytokines and generates LAK cells in synergy with rIL-2. *Planta Medica*, *64*(2), 110–115. doi:10.1055-2006-957385 PMID:9525101

Kim, S. K., & Kim, Y. C. (2002). Attenuation of bacterial lipopolysaccharide-induced hepatotoxicity by betaine or taurine in rats. *Food and Chemical Toxicology*, *40*(4), 545–549. doi:10.1016/S0278-6915(01)00102-8 PMID:11893413

Kim, Y. H., Kwon, H. S., Kim, D. H., Shin, E. K., Kang, Y. H., Park, J. H., ... Kim, J. K. (2009). 3,3′-diindolylmethane attenuates colonic inflammation and tumorigenesis in mice. *Inflammatory Bowel Diseases*, *15*(8), 1164–1173. doi:10.1002/ibd.20917 PMID:19334074

Kobayashi, M., & Yamamoto, M. (2005). Molecular mechanisms activating the Nrf2-Keap1 pathway of antioxidant gene regulation. *Antioxidants & Redox Signaling*, *7*(3-4), 385–394. doi:10.1089/ars.2005.7.385 PMID:15706085

Kuwahara, H., Kanazawa, A., Wakamatu, D., Morimura, S., Kida, K., Akaike, T., & Maeda, H. (2004). Antioxidative and antimutagenic activities of 4-vinyl-2,6-dimethoxyphenol (canolol) isolated from canola oil. *Journal of Agricultural and Food Chemistry*, *52*(14), 4380–4387. doi:10.1021/jf040045+ PMID:15237940

Lai, K.-C., Kuo, C.-L., Ho, H.-C., Yang, J.-S., Ma, C.-Y., Lu, H.-F., Huang, H.-Y., Chueh, F.-S., Yu, C.-C., & Chung, J.-G. (2012). Diallyl sulfide, diallyl disulfide and diallyl trisulfide affect drug resistant gene expression in colo 205 human colon cancer cells in vitro and in vivo. *Phytomedicine*, *19*(7), 625–630. doi:10.1016/j.phymed.2012.02.004 PMID:22397993

Lee, H. J., Lee, H. G., Choi, K. S., Surh, Y. J., & Na, H. K. (2013). Diallyl trisulfide suppresses dextran sodium sulfate-induced mouse colitis: NF-kappaB and STAT3 as potential targets. *Biochemical and Biophysical Research Communications*, *437*(2), 267–273. doi:10.1016/j.bbrc.2013.06.064 PMID:23811270

Lee, J. H., Shim, J. S., Lee, J. S., Kim, M. K., Chung, M. S., & Kim, K. H. (2006). Pectin-like acidic polysaccharide from Panax ginseng with selective antiadhesive activity against pathogenic bacteria. *Carbohydrate Research*, *341*(9), 1154–1163. doi:10.1016/j.carres.2006.03.032 PMID:16643869

Li, W., Khor, T. O., Xu, C., Shen, G., Jeong, W. S., Yu, S., & Kong, A. N. (2008). Activation of Nrf2-antioxidant signaling attenuates NFkappaB-inflammatory response and elicits apoptosis. *Biochemical Pharmacology*, *76*(11), 1485–1489. doi:10.1016/j.bcp.2008.07.017 PMID:18694732

Liu, L., Li, Y. H., Niu, Y. B., Sun, Y., Guo, Z. J., Li, Q., Li, C., Feng, J., Cao, S. S., & Mei, Q. B. (2010). An apple oligogalactan prevents against inflammation and carcinogenesis by targeting LPS/TLR4/NF-κB pathway in a mouse model of colitis-associated colon cancer. *Carcinogenesis*, *31*(10), 1822–1832. doi:10.1093/carcin/bgq070 PMID:20400476

Martin, M. A., Goya, L., & Ramos, S. (2013). Potential for preventive effects of cocoa and cocoa polyphenols in cancer. *Food and Chemical Toxicology*, *56*, 336–351. doi:10.1016/j.fct.2013.02.020 PMID:23439478

Miean, K. H., & Mohamed, S. (2001). Flavonoid (myricetin, quercetin, kaempferol, luteolin, and apigenin) content of edible tropical plants. *Journal of Agricultural and Food Chemistry*, *49*(6), 3106–3112. doi:10.1021/jf000892m PMID:11410016

Nachshon-Kedmi, M., Yannai, S., Haj, A., & Fares, F. A. (2003). Indole-3-carbinol and 3,3′-diindolylmethane induce apoptosis in human prostate cancer cells. *Food and Chemical Toxicology*, *41*(6), 745–752. doi:10.1016/S0278-6915(03)00004-8 PMID:12738179

Nam, S. Y., Kim, J. S., Kim, J. M., Lee, J. Y., Kim, N., Jung, H. C., & Song, I. S. (2008). DA-6034, a derivative of flavonoid, prevents and ameliorates dextran sulfate sodium-induced colitis and inhibits colon carcinogenesis. *Experimental Biology and Medicine (Maywood, N.J.)*, *233*(2), 180–191. doi:10.3181/0707-RM-186 PMID:18222973

Neuhouser, M. L. (2004). Dietary flavonoids and cancer risk: Evidence from human population studies. *Nutrition and Cancer*, *50*(1), 1–7. doi:10.120715327914nc5001_1 PMID:15572291

Nicastro, H. L., Firestone, G. L., & Bjeldanes, L. F. (2013). 3,3′-diindolylmethane rapidly and selectively inhibits hepatocyte growth factor/c-Met signaling in breast cancer cells. *The Journal of Nutritional Biochemistry*, *24*(11), 1882–1888. doi:10.1016/j.jnutbio.2013.05.004 PMID:23968581

O'Hara, M., Kiefer, D., Farrell, K., & Kemper, K. (1998). A review of 12 commonly used medicinal herbs. *Archives of Family Medicine*, *7*(6), 523–536. doi:10.1001/archfami.7.6.523 PMID:9821826

Osburn, W. O., Karim, B., Dolan, P. M., Liu, G., Yamamoto, M., Huso, D. L., & Kensler, T. W. (2007). Increased colonic inflammatory injury and formation of aberrant crypt foci in Nrf2-deficient mice upon dextran sulfate treatment. *International Journal of Cancer*, *121*(9), 1883–1891. doi:10.1002/ijc.22943 PMID:17631644

Osburn, W. O., Wakabayashi, N., Misra, V., Nilles, T., Biswal, S., Trush, M. A., & Kensler, T. W. (2006). Nrf2 regulates an adaptive response protecting against oxidative damage following diquat-mediated formation of superoxide anion. *Archives of Biochemistry and Biophysics*, *454*(1), 7–15. doi:10.1016/j.abb.2006.08.005 PMID:16962985

Pandurangan, A. K., Ananda Sadagopan, S. K., Dharmalingam, P., & Ganapasam, S. (2014). Luteolin, a bioflavonoid inhibits Azoxymethane-induced colorectal cancer through activation of Nrf2 signaling. *Toxicology Mechanisms and Methods*, *24*(1), 13–20. doi:10.3109/15376516.2013.843111 PMID 24024667

Pandurangan, A. K., Dharmalingam, P., Sadagopan, S. K., & Ganapasam, S. (2014). Luteolin inhibits matrix metalloproteinase 9 and 2 in azoxymethane-induced colon carcinogenesis. *Human and Experimental Toxicology*, *33*(11), 1176–1185. doi:10.1177/0960327114522502 PMID:24532706

Pandurangan, A. K., & Esa, N. M. (2014). Luteolin, a bioflavonoid inhibits colorectal cancer through modulation of multiple signaling pathways: A review. *Asian Pacific Journal of Cancer Prevention*, *15*(14), 5501–5508. doi:10.7314/APJCP.2014.15.14.5501 PMID:25081655

Pandurangan, A. K., Ismail, S., Saadatdoust, Z., & Esa, N. M. (2015). Allicin alleviates Dextran sodium sulfate (DSS)-induced ulcerative colitis in BALB/c mice. Oxidative Medicine and Cellular Longevity.

Pandurangan, A. K., Kumar, S. A. S., Dharmalingam, P., & Ganapasam, S. (2014). Luteolin, a bioflavonoid inhibits azoxymethane-induced colon carcinogenesis: Involvement of iNOS and COX-2. *Pharmacognosy Magazine*, *10*(38, Suppl 2), S306. doi:10.4103/0973-1296.133285 PMID:24991108

Pandurangan, A. K., Mohebali, N., Hasanpourghadi, M., Looi, C. Y., Mustafa, M. R., & Norhaizan, M. E. (2016). Boldine suppresses dextran sulfate sodium-induced mouse experimental colitis: NF-κB and IL-6/STAT3 as potential targets. *BioFactors (Oxford, England)*, *42*(3), 247–258. PMID:26891685

Pandurangan, A. K., Mohebali, N., Norhaizan, M. E., & Looi, C. Y. (2015a). Gallic acid attenuates dextran sodium sulfate (DSS)-induced experimental acute ulcerative colitis in BALB/c mice. *Drug Design, Development and Therapy*, *9*(1), 3932–3934.

Pandurangan, A. K., Mohebali, N., Norhaizan, M. E., Looi, C. Y., Salmiah, I., & Saadatdoust, Z. (2015). Gallic acid suppresses inflammation of dextran sodium sulfate-induced colitis in mice: Possible mechanisms. *International Immunopharmacology*, *28*(2), 1034–1043. doi:10.1016/j.intimp.2015.08.019 PMID:26319951

Pandurangan, A. K., & Norhaizan, M. E. (2014). Signal Transducer and Activator of Transcription 3: A Promising target in colitis associated cancer. *Asian Pacific Journal of Cancer Prevention*, *15*(2), 551–560. doi:10.7314/APJCP.2014.15.2.551 PMID:24568457

Pandurangan, A. K., Saadatdoust, Z., Esa, N. M., Hamzah, H., & Ismail, A. (2015). Dietary Cocoa protects against colitis-associated cancer by activating Nrf2/Keap1 pathway. *BioFactors (Oxford, England)*, *41*(1), 1–14. doi:10.1002/biof.1195 PMID:25545372

Pandurangan, A. K., Saadatdoust, Z., Hamzah, H., & Ismail, A. (2015). Dietary cocoa protects against colitis-associated cancer by activating the Nrf2/Keap1 pathway. *BioFactors (Oxford, England)*, *41*(1), 1–14. doi:10.1002/biof.1195 PMID:25545372

Park, E., Hwang, I., Song, J. Y., & Jee, Y. (2011). Acidic polysaccharide of Panax ginseng as a defense against small intestinal damage by whole-body gamma irradiation of mice. *Acta Histochemica*, *113*(1), 19–23. doi:10.1016/j.acthis.2009.07.003 PMID:19767060

Peng, L., Khan, N., Afaq, F., Ye, C., & Mukhtar, H. (2010). In vitro and in vivo effects of water extract of white cocoa tea (Camellia ptilophylla) against human prostate cancer. *Pharmaceutical Research*, *27*(6), 1128–1137. doi:10.100711095-010-0052-7 PMID:20224992

Poudyal, D., Le, P. M., Davis, T., Hofseth, A. B., Chumanevich, A., Chumanevich, A. A., ... Hofseth, L. J. (2012). A hexane fraction of American ginseng suppresses mouse colitis and associated colon cancer: Anti-inflammatory and proapoptotic mechanisms. *Cancer Prevention Research (Philadelphia, Pa.)*, *5*(4), 685–696. doi:10.1158/1940-6207.CAPR-11-0421 PMID:22293630

Rodriguez-Ramiro, I., Ramos, S., Lopez-Oliva, E., Agis-Torres, A., Gomez-Juaristi, M., Mateos, R., Bravo, L., Goya, L., & Martin, M. A. (2011). Cocoa-rich diet prevents azoxymethane-induced colonic preneoplastic lesions in rats by restraining oxidative stress and cell proliferation and inducing apoptosis. *Molecular Nutrition & Food Research*, *55*(12), 1895–1899. doi:10.1002/mnfr.201100363 PMID:21953728

Saadatdoust, Z., Pandurangan, A. K., Ananda Sadagopan, S. K., Esa, N. M., Ismail, A., & Mustafa, M. R. (2015). Dietary cocoa attenuates colitis associated cancer: Crucial involvement of IL/6/STAT3 pathway. *The Journal of Nutritional Biochemistry*, *26*(12), 1547–1558. doi:10.1016/j.jnutbio.2015.07.024 PMID:26355019

Saadatdoust, Z., Pandurangan, A. K., Ananda Sadagopan, S. K., Mohd Esa, N., Ismail, A., & Mustafa, M. R. (2015). Dietary cocoa inhibits colitis associated cancer: A crucial involvement of the IL-6/STAT3 pathway. *The Journal of Nutritional Biochemistry*. Advance online publication. doi:10.1016/j.jnutbio.2015.07.024 PMID:26355019

Sarmadi, B., Aminuddin, F., Hamid, M., Saari, N., Abdul-Hamid, A., & Ismail, A. (2012). Hypoglycemic effects of cocoa (Theobroma cacao L.) autolysates. *Food Chemistry*, *134*(2), 905–911. doi:10.1016/j.foodchem.2012.02.202 PMID:23107706

Seki, T., Hosono, T., Hosono-Fukao, T., Inada, K., Tanaka, R., Ogihara, J., & Ariga, T. (2008). Anticancer effects of diallyl trisulfide derived from garlic. *Asia Pacific Journal of Clinical Nutrition, 17*(Suppl 1), 249–252. PMID:18296348

Steenge, G. R., Verhoef, P., & Katan, M. B. (2003). Betaine supplementation lowers plasma homocysteine in healthy men and women. *The Journal of Nutrition, 133*(5), 1291–1295. doi:10.1093/jn/133.5.1291 PMID:12730412

Sun, X., Ng, T. T. H., Sham, K. W. Y., Zhang, L., Chan, M. T. V., Wu, W. K. K., & Cheng, C. H. K. (2019, October). Bufalin, a Traditional Chinese Medicine Compound, Prevents Tumor Formation in Two Murine Models of Colorectal Cancer. *Cancer Prevention Research (Philadelphia, Pa.), 12*(10), 653–666. doi:10.1158/1940-6207.CAPR-19-0134 PMID:31431500

Surh, Y.-J., Kundu, J. K., & Na, H.-K. (2008). Nrf2 as a master redox switch in turning on the cellular signaling involved in the induction of cytoprotective genes by some chemopreventive phytochemicals. *Planta Medica, 74*(13), 1526–1539. doi:10.1055-0028-1088302 PMID:18937164

Tanaka, T., Kawamori, T., Ohnishi, M., Makita, H., Mori, H., Satoh, K., & Hara, A. (1995). Suppression of azoxymethane-induced rat colon carcinogenesis by dietary administration of naturally occurring xanthophylls astaxanthin and canthaxanthin during the postinitiation phase. *Carcinogenesis, 16*(12), 2957–2963. doi:10.1093/carcin/16.12.2957 PMID:8603470

Tanaka, T., Makita, H., Ohnishi, M., Mori, H., Satoh, K., & Hara, A. (1995). Chemoprevention of rat oral carcinogenesis by naturally occurring xanthophylls, astaxanthin and canthaxanthin. *Cancer Research, 55*(18), 4059–4064. PMID:7664280

Tanaka, T., Morishita, Y., Suzui, M., Kojima, T., Okumura, A., & Mori, H. (1994). Chemoprevention of mouse urinary bladder carcinogenesis by the naturally occurring carotenoid astaxanthin. *Carcinogenesis, 15*(1), 15–19. doi:10.1093/carcin/15.1.15 PMID:8293542

Villegas, I., Sanchez-Fidalgo, S., & de la Lastra, C. A. (2011). Chemopreventive effect of dietary curcumin on inflammation-induced colorectal carcinogenesis in mice. *Molecular Nutrition & Food Research, 55*(2), 259–267. doi:10.1002/mnfr.201000225 PMID:20848615

Wang, J., Li, S., Fan, Y., Chen, Y., Liu, D., Cheng, H., Gao, X., & Zhou, Y. (2010). Anti-fatigue activity of the water-soluble polysaccharides isolated from Panax ginseng C. A. Meyer. *Journal of Ethnopharmacology, 130*(2), 421–423. doi:10.1016/j.jep.2010.05.027 PMID:20580802

Wu, C.-C., Chung, J., Tsai, S.-J., Yang, J., & Sheen, L. (2004). Differential effects of allyl sulfides from garlic essential oil on cell cycle regulation in human liver tumor cells. *Food and Chemical Toxicology*, *42*(12), 1937–1947. doi:10.1016/j.fct.2004.07.008 PMID:15500931

Xiao, D., Li, M., Herman-Antosiewicz, A., Antosiewicz, J., Xiao, H., Lew, K. L., Zeng, Y., Marynowski, S. W., & Singh, S. V. (2006). Diallyl trisulfide inhibits angiogenic features of human umbilical vein endothelial cells by causing Akt inactivation and down-regulation of VEGF and VEGF-R2. *Nutrition and Cancer*, *55*(1), 94–107. doi:10.120715327914nc5501_12 PMID:16965246

Yang, X. R., Wang, Y. Y., La, K. K., Peng, L., Song, X. H., Shi, X. G., Zhu, X., Leung, P., Ko, C., & Ye, C. X. (2012). Inhibitory effects of cocoa tea (Camellia ptilophylla) in human hepatocellular carcinoma HepG2 in vitro and in vivo through apoptosis. *The Journal of Nutritional Biochemistry*, *23*(9), 1051–1057. doi:10.1016/j.jnutbio.2011.05.010 PMID:22018604

Yang, Y., Cai, X., Yang, J., Sun, X., Hu, C., Yan, Z., Xu, X., Lu, W., Wang, X., & Cao, P. (2014). Chemoprevention of dietary digitoflavone on colitis-associated colon tumorigenesis through inducing Nrf2 signaling pathway and inhibition of inflammation. *Molecular Cancer*, *13*(1), 48. doi:10.1186/1476-4598-13-48 PMID:24602443

Yasui, Y., Hosokawa, M., Mikami, N., Miyashita, K., & Tanaka, T. (2011). Dietary astaxanthin inhibits colitis and colitis-associated colon carcinogenesis in mice via modulation of the inflammatory cytokines. *Chemico-Biological Interactions*, *193*(1), 79–87. doi:10.1016/j.cbi.2011.05.006 PMID:21621527

Zeisel, S. H., & Blusztajn, J. K. (1994). Choline and human nutrition. *Annual Review of Nutrition*, *14*(1), 269–296. doi:10.1146/annurev.nu.14.070194.001413 PMID:7946521

Zhu, H., Itoh, K., Yamamoto, M., Zweier, J. L., & Li, Y. (2005). Role of Nrf2 signaling in regulation of antioxidants and phase 2 enzymes in cardiac fibroblasts: Protection against reactive oxygen and nitrogen species-induced cell injury. *FEBS Letters*, *579*(14), 3029–3036. doi:10.1016/j.febslet.2005.04.058 PMID:15896789

Zhu, Y., Zhang, B., Gong, A., Fu, H., Zhang, X., Shi, H., Sun, Y., Wu, L., Pan, Z., Mao, F., Zhu, W., Qian, H., & Xu, W. (2016). Anti-cancer drug 3,3′-diindolylmethane activates Wnt4 signaling to enhance gastric cancer cell stemness and tumorigenesis. *Oncotarget*, *7*(13), 16311–16324. doi:10.18632/oncotarget.7684 PMID:26918831

APPENDIX

S.No	Natural products	Mechanistic action in CAC	Reference
1	American Gingseng	Decreased the expressions of iNOS, COX-2 and apoptosis. Increased the expression of p53.	(Poudyal, 2012; Cui, 2010)
2	Apple Oligogalectin	Decreased expressions of TLR4, TNF-α and IκB .	(Liu, 2010)
3	Astaxanthin	Decreased the expressions of PCNA, Survivin, NF-κB, TNF-α, IL-1β, COX-2 and iNOS.	(Yasui, 2011)
4	Baicalein	Increased the expressions of PPARγ, Procaspase 3, 8, 9 and PARP. Decreased the expressions of iNOS, p50-NF-κB and pIκB.	(Kim, 2013)
5	Betaine	Decreased the expressions of TNF-α, IL-6, p50-NF-κB, iNOS and COX-2.	(Kim, 2014)
6	O-1602	Decreased the expressions of PCNA, p-STAT3, NFκB p65 and TNF-α. Increased the expression of p53 and Bax	(Kargl, 2013)
7	Canolol	Decreased the expressions of TNF-α, iNOS, COX-2, HO-1 and IL-12	(Fang, 2013)
8	Curcumin	Decreased the expressions of COX-2, iNOS, PGES, TNF-α and β-catenin	(Villegas, 2011)
9	Cocoa	Decreased the cell proliferation evidenced by ki67 and PCNA. Decreased the expressions of, IL-6, TNF-α, iNOS, COX-2, p-STAT3, p65-NFκB, Bcl2 Increased the expressions of Nrf2, UDP-GT and Bax.	(Pandurangan, 2015; Saadatdoust, 2015)
10	DA-6034	Decreased the expressions of Ki-67, p-IKKa and COX-2	(Nam, 2008
11	Diallyl trisulfide	Decreased the expressions of p65-NFκB, p-IκB-α, iNOS, COX-2, p-STAT3, Cyclin D1 and p-ERK.	(Lee, 2013)
12	3,3-Diindolylmethane	Decreased the expressions of IL-6, TNF-α, iNOS, COX-2 and p65-NFκB.	(Kim, 2009) (Kim, 2009)

Compilation of References

Abdelmegid, A. M., Abdo, F. K., Ahmed, F. E., & Kattaia, A. A. A. (2019). Therapeutic effect of gold nanoparticles on DSS-induced ulcerative colitis in mice with reference to interleukin-17 expression. *Scientific Reports*, *9*(1), 10176. doi:10.103841598-019-46671-1 PMID:31308463

Abdulkhaleq, L. A., Assi, M. A., Abdullah, R., Zamri-Saad, M., Taufiq-Yap, Y. H., & Hezmee, M. N. M. (2018). The crucial roles of inflammatory mediators in inflammation: A review. *Veterinary World*, *11*(5), 627–635. doi:10.14202/vetworld.2018.627-635 PMID:29915501

Abron, J. D., Singh, N. P., Price, R. L., Nagarkatti, M., Nagarkatti, P. S., & Singh, U. P. (2018). Genistein induces macrophage polarization and systemic cytokine to ameliorate experimental colitis. *PLoS One*, *13*(7), e0199631. doi:10.1371/journal.pone.0199631 PMID:30024891

Adil, A.A.M., Bommanabonia, A.K., Vaithy, A., Kumar, S., Waseem, M., & Jamal, S. (2019). Differential expression of Helios, Neuropilin-1 and FoxP3 in head and neck squamous cell carcinoma (HNSCC) patients. *Biotech.*, *9*(5), 178.

Adil, A.A.M., Vallinayagam, L., Chitra, K., Jamal, S., Pandurangan, A.K., & Ahmed, N. (2019). Increased Expression of TGF-β and IFN-γ in Peripheral Blood Mononuclear Cells (PBMCs) Cultured in Conditioned Medium (CM) of K562. *Cell Culture, 38*(2), 173-83.

Afzali, A. (2019). The Impact of Racial and Ethnic Differences in Inflammatory Bowel Disease Phenotype in the United States. *e-WGN Expert Point of View Articles Collection.* https://www.worldgastroenterology.org/publications/e-wgn/e-wgn-expert-point-of-view-articles-collection/the-impact-of-racial-and-ethnic-differences-in-ibd-phenotype-in-the-us

Aggarwal, B. B., Kunnumakkara, A. B., Harikumar, K. B., Gupta, S. R., Tharakan, S. T., Koca, C., & Sung, B. (2009). Signal transducer and activator of transcription-3, inflammation, and cancer: How intimate is the relationship? *Annals of the New York Academy of Sciences*, *1171*(1), 59–76. Advance online publication. doi:10.1111/j.1749-6632.2009.04911.x PMID:19723038

Aggeletopoulou, I., Konstantakis, C., Assimakopoulos, S. F., & Triantos, C. (2019). The role of the gut microbiota in the treatment of inflammatory bowel diseases. *Microbial Pathogenesis*, *137*, 103774. doi:10.1016/j.micpath.2019.103774 PMID:31586663

Ahmad, I., Mehmood, Z., & Mohammad, F. (1998). Screening of some Indian medicinal plants for their antimicrobial properties. *Journal of Ethnopharmacology*, *62*(2), 183–193. doi:10.1016/S0378-8741(98)00055-5 PMID:9741890

Ahmed, N., Mohamed Adil, A. A., Lavanya, V., & Jamal, S. (2014). Cancer immunotherapy: Targeting immunosuppressive tumor microenvironment. *Oncobiology and Targets.*, *1*(1), 16–21. doi:10.4103/2395-4469.145382

Al Bakir, I., Curtius, K., & Graham, T. A. (2018). From colitis to cancer: An evolutionary trajectory that merges maths and biology. *Frontiers in Immunology*, *9*, 2368. doi:10.3389/fimmu.2018.02368 PMID:30386335

Alatab, S., Sepanlou, S. G., Ikuta, K., Vahedi, H., Bisignano, C., Safiri, S., Sadeghi, A., Nixon, M. R., Abdoli, A., Abolhassani, H., Alipour, V., Almadi, M. A. H., Almasi-Hashiani, A., Anushiravani, A., Arabloo, J., Atique, S., Awasthi, A., Badawi, A., Baig, A. A. A., ... Naghavi, M. (2020). The global, regional, and national burden of inflammatory bowel disease in 195 countries and territories, 1990-2017: A systematic analysis for the Global Burden of Disease Study 2017. *The Lancet. Gastroenterology & Hepatology*, *5*(1), 17–30. doi:10.1016/S2468-1253(19)30333-4 PMID:31648971

Alberts, B. (1994). Cell junctions, cell adhesion and the extracellular matrix. *Molecular Biology of the Cell*, 949–1009.

Al-Hajj, M., Wicha, M. S., Benito-Hernandez, A., Morrison, S. J., & Clarke, M. F. (2003). Prospective identification of tumorigenic breast cancer cells. *Proceedings of the National Academy of Sciences of the United States of America*, *100*(7), 3983–3988. doi:10.1073/pnas.0530291100 PMID:12629218

Ali, F., Ismail, A., & Kersten, S. (2014). Molecular mechanisms underlying the potential antiobesity-related diseases effect of cocoa polyphenols. *Molecular Nutrition & Food Research*, *58*(1), 33–48. doi:10.1002/mnfr.201300277 PMID:24259381

Aljubran, A., Elshenawy, M. A., Kandil, M., Zahir, M. N., Shaheen, A., Gad, A., Alshaer, O., Alzahrani, A., Eldali, A., & Bazarbashi, S. (2019). Efficacy of Regorafenib in Metastatic Colorectal Cancer: A Multi-institutional Retrospective Study. *Clinical Medicine Insights. Oncology*, *13*, 1179554918825447. doi:10.1177/1179554918825447 PMID:30728734

Al-Rehaily, A. J., Al-Howiriny, T. S., Al-Sohaibanib, M. O., & Rafatullah, S. (2002). Gastroprotective effects of 'Amla' Emblica officinalis on in vivo test models in rats. *Phytomedicine*, *9*(6), 515–522. doi:10.1078/09447110260573146 PMID:12403160

Al-Rejaie, S. S., Abuohashish, H. M., Al-Enazi, M. M., Al-Assaf, A. H., Parmar, M. Y., & Ahmed, M. M. (2013). Protective effect of naringenin on acetic acid-induced ulcerative colitis in rats. *World Journal of Gastroenterology*, *19*(34), 5633–5644. doi:10.3748/wjg.v19.i34.5633 PMID:24039355

Anand, K. K., Singh, B., Saxena, A. K., Chandan, B. K., Gupta, V. N., & Bhardwaj, V. (1997). 3,4,5,-Trihydroxy benzoic acid (gallic acid), the hepatoprotective principle in the fruits of Terminalia belerica-bioassay guided activity. *Pharmacological Research*, *36*(4), 315–321. doi:10.1006/phrs.1997.0236 PMID:9425622

Ananthakrishnan, A. N. (2015). Epidemiology and risk factors for IBD. *Nature Reviews. Gastroenterology & Hepatology*, *12*(4), 205–217. doi:10.1038/nrgastro.2015.34 PMID:25732745

Andrews, A. L., Holloway, J. W., Puddicombe, S. M., Holgate, S. T., & Davies, D. E. (2002). Kinetic analysis of the interleukin-13 receptor complex. *The Journal of Biological Chemistry*, *277*(48), 46073–46078. doi:10.1074/jbc.M209560200 PMID:12354755

Antony, M. L., & Singh, S. V. (2011). Molecular mechanisms and targets of cancer chemoprevention by garlic-derived bioactive compound diallyl trisulfide. *Indian Journal of Experimental Biology*, *49*(11), 805. PMID:22126011

Aqil, F., Khan, M. S., Owais, M., & Ahmad, I. (2005). Effect of certain bioactive plant extracts on clinical isolates of beta-lactamase producing methicillin resistant Staphylococcus aureus. *Journal of Basic Microbiology*, *45*(2), 106–114. doi:10.1002/jobm.200410355 PMID:15812867

Arap, M. A., Lahdenranta, J., Mintz, P. J., Hajitou, A., Sarkis, Á. S., Arap, W., & Pasqualini, R. (2004). Cell surface expression of the stress response chaperone GRP78 enables tumor targeting by circulating ligands. *Cancer Cell*, *6*(3), 275–284. doi:10.1016/j.ccr.2004.08.018 PMID:15380518

Arber, N., Shapira, I., Ratan, J., Stern, B., Hibshoosh, H., Moshkowitz, M., Gammon, M., Fabian, I., & Halpern, Z. (2000). Activation of c-K-ras mutations in human gastrointestinal tumors. *Gastroenterology*, *118*(6), 1045–1050. doi:10.1016/S0016-5085(00)70357-X PMID:10833479

Arijs, I., De Hertogh, G., Lemmens, B., Van Lommel, L., de Bruyn, M., Vanhove, W., Cleynen, I., Machiels, K., Ferrante, M., Schuit, F., Van Assche, G., Rutgeerts, P., & Vermeire, S. (2018). Effect of vedolizumab (anti-α4β7-integrin) therapy on histological healing and mucosal gene expression in patients with UC. *Gut*, *67*(1), 43–52. doi:10.1136/gutjnl-2016-312293 PMID:27802155

Arora, Z., & Shen, B. (2015). Biological therapy for ulcerative colitis. *Gastroenterology Report*, *3*(2), 103–109. doi:10.1093/gastro/gou070 PMID:25344680

Arruda, J. M., Bogetza, A. L., Vellankia, S., Wrenb, A., & Yehb, A. M. (2018). Yoga as adjunct therapy for adolescents with inflammatory bowel disease: A pilot clinical trial. *Complementary Therapies in Medicine*, *41*, 99–104. doi:10.1016/j.ctim.2018.09.007 PMID:30477870

Artchoudane, S., Bhavanani, A. B., Ramanathan, M., & Mariangela, A. (2019). Yoga as a therapeutic tool in autism: A detailed review. *Yoga Mimamsa*, *51*(1), 3–16. doi:10.4103/ym.ym_3_19

Artchoudane, S., Ranganadin, P., Bhavanani, A. B., Ramanathan, M., & Madanmohan, T. (2018). Effect of adjuvant yoga therapy on pulmonary function and quality of life among patients with Chronic Obstructive Pulmonary Disease: A randomized control trial. *SBV J Basic. Cli and Appl Health Science*, *2*, 117–122.

Atherton, H. C., Jones, G., & Danahay, H. (2003). IL-13-induced changes in the goblet cell density of human bronchial epithelial cell cultures: MAP kinase and phosphatidylinositol 3-kinase regulation. *American Journal of Physiology. Lung Cellular and Molecular Physiology*, *285*(3), L730–L739. doi:10.1152/ajplung.00089.2003 PMID:12794003

Atreya, I., Atreya, R., & Neurath, M. F. (2008). NF-κB in inflammatory bowel disease. *Journal of Internal Medicine*, *263*(6), 591–596. doi:10.1111/j.1365-2796.2008.01953.x PMID:18479258

Atreya, R., & Neurath, M. F. (2005). Involvement of IL-6 in the pathogenesis of inflammatory bowel disease and colon cancer. *Clinical Reviews in Allergy & Immunology*, *28*(3), 187–195. doi:10.1385/CRIAI:28:3:187 PMID:16129903

Avdagić, N., Zaćiragić, A., Babić, N., Hukić, M., Šeremet, M., Lepara, O., & Nakaš-Ićindić, E. (2013). Nitric oxide as a potential biomarker in inflammatory bowel disease. *Bosnian Journal of Basic Medical Sciences*, *13*(1), 5. doi:10.17305/bjbms.2013.2402 PMID:23448603

Axelrad, J. E., Lichtiger, S., & Yajnik, V. (2016). Inflammatory bowel disease and cancer: The role of inflammation, immunosuppression, and cancer treatment. *World Journal of Gastroenterology*, *22*(20), 4794–4801. doi:10.3748/wjg.v22.i20.4794 PMID:27239106

Azuma, T., Shigeshiro, M., Kodama, M., Tanabe, S., & Suzuki, T. (2013). Supplemental naringenin prevents intestinal barrier defects and inflammation in colitic mice. *The Journal of Nutrition*, *143*(6), 827–834. doi:10.3945/jn.113.174508 PMID:23596159

Baars, J. E., Looman, C. W. N., Steyerberg, E. W., Beukers, R., Tan, A. C. I. T. L., Weusten, B. L. A. M., Kuipers, E. J., & van der Woude, C. J. (2011). The risk of inflammatory bowel disease-related colorectal carcinoma is limited: Results from a nationwide nested case-control study. *The American Journal of Gastroenterology*, *106*(2), 319–328. doi:10.1038/ajg.2010.428 PMID:21045815

Bäckhed, F., Roswall, J., Peng, Y., Feng, Q., Jia, H., Kovatcheva-Datchary, P., ... Khan, M. T. (2015). Dynamics and stabilization of the human gut microbiome during the first year of life. *Cell Host & Microbe*, *17*(5), 690–703. doi:10.1016/j.chom.2015.04.004 PMID:25974306

Badamaranahalli, S. S., Kopparam, M., Bhagawati, S. T., & Durg, S. (2015). Embelin lipid nanospheres for enhanced treatment of ulcerative colitis - Preparation, characterization and in vivo evaluation. *European Journal of Pharmaceutical Sciences*, *76*, 73–82. doi:10.1016/j.ejps.2015.05.003 PMID:25957524

Bager, P., Simonsen, J., Nielsen, N. M., & Frisch, M. (2012). Cesarean section and offspring's risk of inflammatory bowel disease: A national cohort study. *Inflammatory Bowel Diseases*, *18*(5), 857–862. Advance online publication. doi:10.1002/ibd.21805 PMID:21739532

Bajpai, V. K., Rahman, A., Shukla, S., Shukla, S., Arafat, S. M., Hossain, M. A., & ... . (2010). In vitro kinetics and antifungal activity of various extracts of Terminalia chebula seeds against plant pathogenic fungi. *Archiv für Phytopathologie und Pflanzenschutz*, *43*(8), 801–809. doi:10.1080/03235400802246887

Baker, A.-M., Cross, W., Curtius, K., Al Bakir, I., Choi, C.-H. R., Davis, H. L., Temko, D., Biswas, S., Martinez, P., Williams, M. J., Lindsay, J. O., Feakins, R., Vega, R., Hayes, S. J., Tomlinson, I. P. M., McDonald, S. A. C., Moorghen, M., Silver, A., East, J. E., ... Graham, T. A. (2019). Evolutionary history of human colitis-associated colorectal cancer. *Gut*, *68*(6), 985–995. doi:10.1136/gutjnl-2018-316191 PMID:29991641

Bandyopadhyay, S. K., Pakrashi, S. C., & Pakrashi, A. (2000). The role of antioxidant activity of Phyllanthus emblica fruits on prevention from indomethacin induced gastric ulcer. *Journal of Ethnopharmacology*, *70*(2), 171–176. doi:10.1016/S0378-8741(99)00146-4 PMID:10771207

Bang, B., & Lichtenberger, L. M. (2016). Methods of inducing inflammatory bowel disease in mice. *Current Protocols in Pharmacology, 72*(5), 51-42.

Bannaga, A. S., & Selinger, C. P. (2015). Inflammatory bowel disease and anxiety: Links, risks, and challenges faced. *Clinical and Experimental Gastroenterology*, *8*, 111–117. doi:10.2147/CEG.S57982 PMID:25848313

Barmeyer, C., Fromm, M., & Schulzke, J. D. (2017). Active and passive involvement of claudins in the pathophysiology of intestinal inflammatory diseases. *Pflügers Archiv*, *469*(1), 15–26. doi:10.100700424-016-1914-6 PMID:27904960

Baskol, M., Baskol, G., Koçer, D., Ozbakir, O., & Yucesoy, M. (2008). Advanced oxidation protein products: A novel marker of oxidative stress in ulcerative colitis. *Journal of Clinical Gastroenterology*, *42*(6), 687–691. doi:10.1097/MCG.0b013e318074f91f PMID:18574392

Basso, P. J., Fonseca, M. T. C., Bonfá, G., Alves, V. B. F., Sales-Campos, H., Nardini, V., & Cardoso, C. R. B. (2014). Association among genetic predisposition, gut microbiota, and host immune response in the etiopathogenesis of inflammatory bowel disease. *Brazilian Journal of Medical and Biological Research*, *47*(9), 727–737. doi:10.1590/1414-431X20143932 PMID:25075576

Baumgart, D. C., & Carding, S. R. (2007). Inflammatory bowel disease: Cause and immunobiology. *Lancet*, *369*(9573), 1627–1640. doi:10.1016/S0140-6736(07)60750-8 PMID:17499605

Baumgart, D. C., & Sandborn, W. J. (2012). Crohn's disease. *Lancet*, *380*(9853), 1590–1605. doi:10.1016/S0140-6736(12)60026-9 PMID:22914295

Baxter, N. T., Zackular, J. P., Chen, G. Y., & Schloss, P. D. (2014). Structure of the gut microbiome following colonization with human feces determines colonic tumor burden. *Microbiome*, *2*(1), 20. doi:10.1186/2049-2618-2-20 PMID:24967088

Beaugerie, L., & Itzkowitz, S. H. (2015). Cancers Complicating Inflammatory Bowel Disease. *The New England Journal of Medicine*, *373*(2), 195. doi:10.1056/NEJMc1505689 PMID:26154801

Becattini, S., Taur, Y., & Pamer, E. G. (2016). Antibiotic-induced changes in the intestinal microbiota and disease. *Trends in Molecular Medicine*, *22*(6), 458–478. doi:10.1016/j.molmed.2016.04.003 PMID:27178527

Becker, C., Fantini, M. C., & Neurath, M. F. (2006). TGF-beta as a T cell regulator in colitis and colon cancer. *Cytokine & Growth Factor Reviews*, *17*(1-2), 97–106. doi:10.1016/j.cytogfr.2005.09.004 PMID:16298544

Becker, C., Fantini, M. C., Schramm, C., Lehr, H. A., Wirtz, S., Nikolaev, A., & Neurath, M. F. (2004). TGF-β suppresses tumor progression in colon cancer by inhibition of IL-6 trans-signaling. *Immunity*, *21*(4), 491–501. doi:10.1016/j.immuni.2004.07.020 PMID:15485627

Becker, K., Geisler, S., Ueberall, F., Fuchs, D., & Gostner, J. M. (2013). Immunomodulatory properties of cacao extracts - potential consequences for medical applications. *Frontiers in Pharmacology*, *4*, 154. doi:10.3389/fphar.2013.00154 PMID:24376420

Belapurkar, P., Goyal, P., & Tiwari-Barua, P. (2014). Immunomodulatory effects of triphala and its individual constituents: A review. *Indian Journal of Pharmaceutical Sciences*, *76*(6), 467–475. PMID:25593379

Betancur-Galvis, L. A., Morales, G. E., Forero, J. E., & Roldan, J. (2002). Cytotocxic and antiviral activties of Colombian medicinal plant exatracts of the Euphorbia genus. *Memorias do Instituto Oswaldo Cruz*. Advance online publication. doi:10.1590/S0074-02762002000400017

Bhattacharya, N., Yuan, R., Prestwood, T. R., Penny, H. L., DiMaio, M. A., Reticker-Flynn, N. E., ... Tolentino, L. (2016). Normalizing microbiota-induced retinoic acid deficiency stimulates protective CD8+ T cell-mediated immunity in colorectal cancer. *Immunity*, *45*(3), 641–655. doi:10.1016/j.immuni.2016.08.008 PMID:27590114

Bhattacharya, S. K., Bhattacharya, A., Sairam, K., & Ghosa, S. (2002). Effect of bioactive tannoid principles of Emblica officinalis on ischemia-reperfusion-induced oxidative stress in rat heart. *Phytomedicine*, *9*(2), 171–174. doi:10.1078/0944-7113-00090 PMID:11995952

Bhattacharyya, S., Dudeja, P. K., & Tobacman, J. K. (2009). ROS, Hsp27, and IKKβ mediate dextran sodium sulfate (DSS) activation of IκBa, NFκB, and IL-8. *Inflammatory Bowel Diseases*, *15*(5), 673–683. doi:10.1002/ibd.20821 PMID:19085995

Bhavanani, A. B. (2013). A closing word. In A. B. Bhavanani (Ed.), *Yoga Chikitsa: Application of yoga as a therapy* (1st ed.). Dhivyananda Creations.

Bhavanani, A. B., Sanjay, Z., & Madanmohan, T. (2011). Immediate Effect of Sukha Pranayama on Cardiovascular Variables in Patients of Hypertension. *International Journal of Yoga Therapy*, *21*(1), 73–76. doi:10.17761/ijyt.21.1.y007g513416341 72 PMID:22398346

Bhol, K. C., & Schechter, P. J. (2007). Effects of nanocrystalline silver (NPI 32101) in a rat model of ulcerative colitis. *Digestive Diseases and Sciences*, *52*(10), 2732–2742. doi:10.100710620-006-9738-4 PMID:17436088

Björkholm, B., Bok, C. M., Lundin, A., Rafter, J., Hibberd, M. L., & Pettersson, S. (2009). Intestinal microbiota regulate xenobiotic metabolism in the liver. *PLoS One*, *4*(9), e6958. doi:10.1371/journal.pone.0006958 PMID:19742318

Blanco Calvo, M., Bolós Fernández, V., Medina Villaamil, V., Aparicio Gallego, G., Díaz Prado, S., & Grande Pulido, E. (2009). Biology of BMP signaling and cancer. *Clinical & Translational Oncology*, *11*(3), 126–137. doi:10.1007/S12094-009-0328-8 PMID:19293049

Bodai, B. I., Nakata, T. E., Wong, W. T., Clark, D. R., Lawenda, S., Tsou, C., & ... . (2018). Lifestyle Medicine: A Brief Review of Its Dramatic Impact on Health and Survival. *The Permanente Journal*, *22*, 17–025. doi:10.7812/TPP/17-025 PMID:29035175

Boismenu, R., & Chen, Y. P. (2000). Insights from mouse models of colitis. *Journal of Leukocyte Biology*, *67*(3), 267–278. doi:10.1002/jlb.67.3.267 PMID:10733087

Boleij, A., Hechenbleikner, E. M., Goodwin, A. C., Badani, R., Stein, E. M., Lazarev, M. G., ... Platz, E. A. (2015). The Bacteroides fragilis toxin gene is prevalent in the colon mucosa of colorectal cancer patients. *Clinical Infectious Diseases*, *60*(2), 208–215. doi:10.1093/cid/ciu787 PMID:25305284

Bollrath, J., Phesse, T. J., von Burstin, V. A., Putoczki, T., Bennecke, M., Bateman, T., & Greten, F. R. (2009). gp130-mediated Stat3 activation in enterocytes regulates cell survival and cell-cycle progression during colitis-associated tumorigenesis. *Cancer Cell*, *15*(2), 91–102. doi:10.1016/j.ccr.2009.01.002 PMID:19185844

Bonnet, D., & Dick, J. E. (1997). Human acute myeloid leukemia is organized as a hierarchy that originates from a primitive hematopoietic cell. *Nature Medicine*, *3*(7), 730–737. doi:10.1038/nm0797-730 PMID:9212098

Bos, J. L., Fearon, E. R., Hamilton, S. R., Verlaan-de Vries, M., van Boom, J. H., van der Eb, A. J., & Vogelstein, B. (1987). Prevalence of ras gene mutations in human colorectal cancers. *Nature*, *327*(6120), 293–297. doi:10.1038/327293a0 PMID:3587348

Bramhall, M., Florez-Vargas, O., Stevens, R., Brass, A., & Cruickshank, S. (2015). Quality of methods reporting in animal models of colitis. *Inflammatory Bowel Diseases*, *21*(6), 1248–1259. doi:10.1097/MIB.0000000000000369 PMID:25989337

Bray, F., Ferlay, J., Soerjomataram, I., Siegel, R. L., Torre, L. A., & Jemal, A. (2018). Global cancer statistics 2018: GLOBOCAN estimates of incidence and mortality worldwide for 36 cancers in 185 countries. *CA: a Cancer Journal for Clinicians*, *68*(6), 394–424. doi:10.3322/caac.21492 PMID:30207593

Bruni, D., Angell, H. K., & Galon, J. (2020). The immune contexture and Immunoscore in cancer prognosis and therapeutic efficacy. *Nature Reviews. Cancer*, *20*(11), 662–680. doi:10.103841568-020-0285-7 PMID:32753728

Buckley, J. P., Cook, S. F., Allen, J. K., & Kappelman, M. D. (2015). Prevalence of chronic narcotic use among children with inflammatory bowel disease. *Clinical Gastroenterology and Hepatology*, *13*(2), 310–315. doi:10.1016/j.cgh.2014.07.057 PMID:25117776

Buettner, R., Corzano, R., Rashid, R., Lin, J., Senthil, M., Hedvat, M., Schroeder, A., Mao, A., Herrmann, A., Yim, J., Li, H., Yuan, Y.-C., Yakushijin, K., Yakushijin, F., Vaidehi, N., Moore, R., Gugiu, G., Lee, T. D., Yip, R., ... Williams, J. C. (2011). Alkylation of cysteine 468 in stat3 defines a novel site for therapeutic development. *ACS Chemical Biology*, *6*(5), 432–443. Advance online publication. doi:10.1021/cb100253e PMID:21226522

Bu, Y., & Cao, D. (2012). The origin of cancer stem cells. *Frontiers in Bioscience (Scholar Edition)*, *4*, 819–830. PMID:22202093

Cai, X., Lu, W., Yang, Y., Yang, J., Ye, J., Gu, Z., Hu, C., Wang, X., & Cao, P. (2013). Digitoflavone inhibits IkappaBalpha kinase and enhances apoptosis induced by TNFalpha through downregulation of expression of nuclear factor kappaB-regulated gene products in human pancreatic cancer cells. *PLoS One*, *8*(10), e77126. doi:10.1371/journal.pone.0077126 PMID:24146961

Camuesco, D., Comalada, M., Rodriguez-Cabezas, M. E., Nieto, A., Lorente, M. D., Concha, A., Zarzuelo, A., & Gálvez, J. (2004). The intestinal anti-inflammatory effect of quercitrin is associated with an inhibition in iNOS expression. *British Journal of Pharmacology*, *143*(7), 908–918. doi:10.1038j.bjp.0705941 PMID:15533892

Camus, M., Tosolini, M., Mlecnik, B., Pagès, F., Kirilovsky, A., Berger, A., Costes, A., Bindea, G., Charoentong, P., Bruneval, P., Trajanoski, Z., Fridman, W.-H., & Galon, J. (2009). Coordination of intratumoral immune reaction and human colorectal cancer recurrence. *Cancer Research*, *69*(6), 2685–2693. doi:10.1158/0008-5472.CAN-08-2654 PMID:19258510

Carbonero, F., Benefiel, A. C., Alizadeh-Ghamsari, A. H., & Gaskins, H. R. (2012). Microbial pathways in colonic sulfur metabolism and links with health and disease. *Frontiers in Physiology*, *3*, 448. doi:10.3389/fphys.2012.00448 PMID:23226130

Carmody, R. N., & Turnbaugh, P. J. (2014). Host-microbial interactions in the metabolism of therapeutic and diet-derived xenobiotics. *The Journal of Clinical Investigation*, *124*(10), 4173–4181. doi:10.1172/JCI72335 PMID:25105361

Carpentino, J. E., Hynes, M. J., Appelman, H. D., Zheng, T., Steindler, D. A., Scott, E. W., & Huang, E. H. (2009). Aldehyde dehydrogenase-expressing colon stem cells contribute to tumorigenesis in the transition from colitis to cancer. *Cancer Research*, *69*(20), 8208–8215. doi:10.1158/0008-5472.CAN-09-1132 PMID:19808966

Castangia, I., Nacher, A., Caddeo, C., Merino, V., Diez-Sales, O., Catalan-Latorre, A., Fernàndez-Busquets, X., Fadda, A. M., & Manconi, M. (2015). Therapeutic efficacy of quercetin enzyme-responsive nanovesicles for the treatment of experimental colitis in rats. *Acta Biomaterialia*, *13*, 216–227. doi:10.1016/j.actbio.2014.11.017 PMID:25463498

Castro-Dopico, T., Dennison, T. W., Ferdinand, J. R., Mathews, R. J., Fleming, A., Clift, D., Stewart, B. J., Jing, C., Strongili, K., Labzin, L. I., Monk, E. J. M., Saeb-Parsy, K., Bryant, C. E., Clare, S., Parkes, M., & Clatworthy, M. R. (2019). Anti-commensal IgG Drives Intestinal Inflammation and Type 17 Immunity in Ulcerative Colitis. *Immunity*, *50*(4), 1099–1114 e1010. doi:10.1016/j.immuni.2019.02.006 PMID:30876876

Chalaris, A., Schmidt-Arras, D., Yamamoto, K., & Rose-John, S. (2012). Interleukin-6 trans-signaling and colonic cancer associated with inflammatory bowel disease. *Digestive Diseases (Basel, Switzerland)*, *30*(5), 492–499. doi:10.1159/000341698 PMID:23108305

Chambers, W. M., Warren, B. F., Jewell, D. P., & Mortensen, N. J. M. (2005). Cancer surveillance in ulcerative colitis. *British Journal of Surgery*, *92*(8), 928–936. doi:10.1002/bjs.5106 PMID:16034807

Chami, B., Martin, N. J. J., Dennis, J. M., & Witting, P. K. (2018). Myeloperoxidase in the inflamed colon: A novel target for treating inflammatory bowel disease. *Archives of Biochemistry and Biophysics*, *645*, 61–71. doi:10.1016/j.abb.2018.03.012 PMID:29548776

Chandra-Kuntal, K., & Singh, S. V. (2010). Diallyl trisulfide inhibits activation of signal transducer and activator of transcription 3 in prostate cancer cells in culture and In vivo. *Cancer Prevention Research (Philadelphia, Pa.)*, *3*(11), 1473–1483. Advance online publication. doi:10.1158/1940-6207.CAPR-10-0123 PMID:20959517

Chandrasekar, V. T., & Venu, N. (2015). So What Is Crohn's Disease and Ulcerative Colitis? Pathophysiology of Crohn's Disease and Ulcerative Colitis. In *Inflammatory Bowel Disease* (pp. 15–23). Springer.

Chang, C. S., & Lin, C. S. (2010). Development of antioxidant activity and pattern recognition of Terminalia chebula Retzius extracts and its fermented products. *Hung Kuang J*, *61*, 115–129.

Chavan, S., Sava, L., Saxena, V., Pillai, S., Sontakke, A., & Ingole, D. (2005). Reduced glutathione: Importance of specimen collection. *Indian Journal of Clinical Biochemistry*, *20*(1), 150–152. Advance online publication. doi:10.1007/BF02893062 PMID:23105514

Cheng, Y. T., Wu, C. H., Ho, C. Y., & Yen, G. C. (2013). Catechin protects against ketoprofen-induced oxidative damage of the gastric mucosa by up-regulating Nrf2 in vitro and in vivo. *The Journal of Nutritional Biochemistry*, *24*(2), 475–483. doi:10.1016/j.jnutbio.2012.01.010 PMID:22704780

Chen, Q., Gou, S., Ma, P., Song, H., Zhou, X., Huang, Y., Kwon Han, M., Wan, Y., Kang, Y., & Xiao, B. (2019). Oral administration of colitis tissue-accumulating porous nanoparticles for ulcerative colitis therapy. *International Journal of Pharmaceutics*, *557*, 135–144. doi:10.1016/j.ijpharm.2018.12.046 PMID:30594685

Chen, Q., Si, X., Ma, L., Ma, P., Hou, M., Bai, S., Wu, X., Wan, Y., Xiao, B., & Merlin, D. (2017). Oral delivery of curcumin via porous polymeric nanoparticles for effective ulcerative colitis therapy. *Journal of Materials Chemistry. B, Materials for Biology and Medicine*, *5*(29), 5881–5891. doi:10.1039/C7TB00328E PMID:29081976

Chen, X. L., & Kunsch, C. (2004). Induction of cytoprotective genes through Nrf2/antioxidant response element pathway: A new therapeutic approach for the treatment of inflammatory diseases. *Current Pharmaceutical Design*, *10*(8), 879–891. doi:10.2174/1381612043452901 PMID:15032691

Chen, Y., Segarini, P., Raoufi, F., Bradham, D., & Leask, A. (2001). Connective tissue growth factor is secreted through the Golgi and is degraded in the endosome. *Experimental Cell Research*, *271*(1), 109–117. doi:10.1006/excr.2001.5364 PMID:11697887

Chiba, M., Abe, T., Tsuda, H., Sugawara, T., Tsuda, S., Tozawa, H., & ... . (2010). Lifestyle-related disease in Crohn's disease: Relapse prevention by a semi-vegetarian diet. *World Journal of Gastroenterology*, *16*(20), 2484–2495. doi:10.3748/wjg.v16.i20.2484 PMID:20503448

Chiba, M., Nakane, K., Takayama, Y., Sugawara, K., Ohno, H , Ishii, H., & .... (2016). Development and Application of a Plant-Based Diet Scoring System for Japanese Patients with Inflammatory Bowel Disease. *The Permanente Journal*, *20*(4), 16–019. doi:10.7812/TPP/16-019 PMID:27768566

Chiou, Y. S., Ma, N. J., Sang, S., Ho, C. T., Wang, Y. J., & Pan, M. H. (2012). Peracetylated (-)-epigallocatechin-3-gallate (AcEGCG) potently suppresses dextran sulfate sodium-induced colitis and colon tumorigenesis in mice. *Journal of Agricultural and Food Chemistry*, *60*(13), 3441–3451. doi:10.1021/jf300441p PMID:22409325

Cho, H. J., Seon, M. R., Lee, Y. M., Kim, J., Kim, J. K., Kim, S. G., & Park, J. H. (2008). 3,3′-Diindolylmethane suppresses the inflammatory response to lipopolysaccharide in murine macrophages. *The Journal of Nutrition*, *138*(1), 17–23. doi:10.1093/jn/138.1.17 PMID:18156398

Choi, H.-S., Kim, K.-H., Sohn, E., Park, J.-D., Kim, B.-O., Moon, E.-Y., Rhee, D.-K., & Pyo, S. (2008). Red ginseng acidic polysaccharide (RGAP) in combination with IFN-γ results in enhanced macrophage function through activation of the NF-κB pathway. *Bioscience, Biotechnology, and Biochemistry*, *72*(7), 1817–1825. doi:10.1271/bbb.80085 PMID:18603775

Choudhary, G. P. (2011). Wound healing activity of ethanolic extract of Terminalia chebula Retz. *International Journal of Pharma and Bio Sciences*, *2*, 48–52.

Chung, D. C. (2000). The genetic basis of colorectal cancer: Insights into critical pathways of tumorigenesis. *Gastroenterology*, *119*(3), 854–865. doi:10.1053/gast.2000.16507 PMID:10982779

Cibicek, N., Roubalova, L., Vrba, J., Zatloukalova, M., Ehrmann, J., Zapletalova, J., Večeřa, R., Křen, V., & Ulrichová, J. (2016). Protective effect of isoquercitrin against acute dextran sulfate sodium-induced rat colitis depends on the severity of tissue damage. *Pharmacological Reports*, *68*(6), 1197–1204. doi:10.1016/j.pharep.2016.07.007 PMID:27657482

Clarke, M. F., Dick, J. E., Dirks, P. B., Eaves, C. J., Jamieson, C. H. M., Jones, D. L., Visvader, J., Weissman, I. L., & Wahl, G. M. (2006). Cancer stem cells—perspectives on current status and future directions: AACR Workshop on cancer stem cells. *Cancer Research*, *66*(19), 9339–9344. doi:10.1158/0008-5472.CAN-06-3126 PMID:16990346

Clevers, H. (2006). Wnt/beta-catenin signaling in development and disease. *Cell*, *127*(3), 469–480. doi:10.1016/j.cell.2006.10.018 PMID:17081971

Cochrane, C. R., Szczepny, A., Watkins, D. N., & Cain, J. E. (2015). Hedgehog Signaling in the Maintenance of Cancer Stem Cells. *Cancers (Basel)*, *7*(3), 1554–1585. doi:10.3390/cancers7030851 PMID:26270676

Cohen, A. B., Lee, D., Long, M. D., Kappelman, M. D., Martin, C. F., Sandler, R. S., & Lewis, J. D. (2013). Dietary patterns and self-reported associations of diet with symptoms of inflammatory bowel disease. *Digestive Diseases and Sciences*, *58*(5), 1322–1328. doi:10.100710620-012-2373-3 PMID:22923336

Cohn, H. M., Dave, M., & Loftus, E. V. Jr. (2017). Understanding the Cautions and Contraindications of Immunomodulator and Biologic Therapies for Use in Inflammatory Bowel Disease. *Inflammatory Bowel Diseases*, *23*(8), 1301–1315. doi:10.1097/MIB.0000000000001199 PMID:28708806

Colitis-Associated Cancer. (2016). Overview. Springer.

Comalada, M., Camuesco, D., Sierra, S., Ballester, I., Xaus, J., Galvez, J., & Zarzuelo, A. (2005). In vivo quercitrin anti-inflammatory effect involves release of quercetin, which inhibits inflammation through down-regulation of the NF-kappaB pathway. *European Journal of Nutrition*, *35*(2), 584–592. PMID:15668926

Conforti, F., Sosa, S., Marrelli, M., Menichini, F., Statti, G. A., Uzunov, D., Tubaro, A., & Menichini, F. (2009). The protective ability of Mediterranean dietary plants against the oxidative damage: The role of radical oxygen species in inflammation and the polyphenol, flavonoid and sterol contents. *Food Chemistry*, *112*(3), 587–594. doi:10.1016/j.foodchem.2008.06.013

Cosnes, J., Gower–Rousseau, C., Seksik, P., & Cortot, A. (2011). Epidemiology and Natural History of Inflammatory Bowel Diseases. *Gastroenterology*, *140*(6), 1785–1794.e4. doi:10.1053/j.gastro.2011.01.055 PMID:21530745

Courthion, H., Mugnier, T., Rousseaux, C., Moller, M., Gurny, R., & Gabriel, D. (2018). Self-assembling polymeric nanocarriers to target inflammatory lesions in ulcerative colitis. *Journal of Controlled Release*, *275*, 32–39. doi:10.1016/j.jconrel.2017.07.044 PMID:28774843

Coussens, L. M., & Werb, Z. (2002). Inflammation and cancer. *Nature*, *420*(6917), 860–867. doi:10.1038/nature01322 PMID:12490959

Craig, S. A. (2004). Betaine in human nutrition. *The American Journal of Clinical Nutrition*, *80*(3), 539–549. doi:10.1093/ajcn/80.3.539 PMID:15321791

Crespo, M. E., Galvez, J., Cruz, T., Ocete, M. A., & Zarzuelo, A. (1999). Anti-inflammatory activity of diosmin and hesperidin in rat colitis induced by TNBS. *Planta Medica*, *65*(7), 651–653. doi:10.1055-2006-960838 PMID:10575379

Cruz, T., Galvez, J., Ocete, M. A., Crespo, M. E., de Medina, F. S., & Zarzuelo, A. (1998). Oral administration of rutoside can ameliorate inflammatory bowel disease in rats. *Life Sciences*, *62*(7), 687–695. doi:10.1016/S0024-3205(97)01164-8 PMID:9472728

Cui, L., Feng, L., Zhang, Z. H., & Jia, X. B. (2014). The anti-inflammation effect of baicalin on experimental colitis through inhibiting TLR4/NF-kappaB pathway activation. *International Immunopharmacology*, *23*(1), 294–303. doi:10.1016/j.intimp.2014.09.005 PMID:25239813

Cui, X., Jin, Y., Poudyal, D., Chumanevich, A. A., Davis, T., Windust, A., Hofseth, A., Wu, W., Habiger, J., Pena, E., Wood, P., Nagarkatti, M., Nagarkatti, P. S., & Hofseth, L. (2010). Mechanistic insight into the ability of American ginseng to suppress colon cancer associated with colitis. *Carcinogenesis*, *31*(10), 1734–1741. doi:10.1093/carcin/bgq163 PMID:20729391

Cunningham, K. E., & Turner, J. R. (2012). Myosin light chain kinase: Pulling the strings of epithelial tight junction function. *Annals of the New York Academy of Sciences*, *1258*(1), 34–42. doi:10.1111/j.1749-6632.2012.06526.x PMID:22731713

da Silva, B. C., Lyra, A. C., Mendes, C. M. C., Ribeiro, C. P. O., Lisboa, S. R. O., de Souza, M. T. L., Portela, R. C., & Santana, G. O. (2015). The demographic and clinical characteristics of ulcerative colitis in a northeast Brazilian population. *BioMed Research International*, *2015*, 2015. doi:10.1155/2015/359130 PMID:26509150

da Silva, B. C., Lyra, A. C., Rocha, R., & Santana, G. O. (2014). Epidemiology, demographic characteristics and prognostic predictors of ulcerative colitis. *World Journal of Gastroenterology*, *20*(28), 9458–9467. doi:10.3748/wjg.v20.i28.9458 PMID:25071340

Daines, M. O., & Hershey, G. K. K. (2002). A novel mechanism by which interferon-γ can regulate interleukin (IL)-13 responses: Evidence for intracellular stores of IL-13 receptor α-2 and their rapid mobilization by interferon-γ. *The Journal of Biological Chemistry*, *277*(12), 10387–10393. doi:10.1074/jbc.M108109200 PMID:11786536

Dai, S. X., Zou, Y., Feng, Y. L., Liu, H. B., & Zheng, X. B. (2012). Baicalin down-regulates the expression of macrophage migration inhibitory factor (MIF) effectively for rats with ulcerative colitis. *Phytotherapy Research*, *26*(4), 498–504. doi:10.1002/ptr.3581 PMID:21887805

Dame, M. K., Bhagavathula, N., Mankey, C., DaSilva, M., Paruchuri, T., Aslam, M. N., & Varani, J. (2010). Human colon tissue in organ culture: Preservation of normal and neoplastic characteristics. *In Vitro Cellular & Developmental Biology. Animal*, *46*(2), 114–122. doi:10.100711626-009-9247-9 PMID:19915935

Danese, S., & Fiocchi, C. (2006). Etiopathogenesis of inflammatory bowel diseases. *World Journal of Gastroenterology*, *12*(30), 4807. Advance online publication. doi:10.3748/wjg.v12.i30.4807 PMID:16937461

Danese, S., Sans, M., de la Motte, C., Graziani, C., West, G., Phillips, M. H., Pola, R., Rutella, S., Willis, J., Gasbarrini, A., & Fiocchi, C. (2006). Angiogenesis as a Novel Component of Inflammatory Bowel Disease Pathogenesis. *Gastroenterology*, *130*(7), 2060–2073. Advance online publication. doi:10.1053/j.gastro.2006.03.054 PMID:16762629

Davidson, L. A., Callaway, E. S., Kim, E., Weeks, B. R., Fan, Y.-Y., Allred, C. D., & Chapkin, R. S. (2015). Targeted Deletion of p53 in Lgr5-Expressing Intestinal Stem Cells Promotes Colon Tumorigenesis in a Preclinical Model of Colitis-Associated Cancer. *Cancer Research*, *75*(24), 5392–5397. doi:10.1158/0008-5472.CAN-15-1706 PMID:26631266 de Souza, H. S., & Fiocchi, C. (2016). Immunopathogenesis of IBD: Current state of the art. *Nature Reviews. Gastroenterology & Hepatology*, *13*(1), 13–27. doi:10.1038/nrgastro.2015.186 PMID:26627550

Deng, Z., Rong, Y., Teng, Y., Mu, J., Zhuang, X., Tseng, M., Samykutty, A., Zhang, L., Yan, J., Miller, D., Suttles, J., & Zhang, H. G. (2017). Broccoli-Derived Nanoparticle Inhibits Mouse Colitis by Activating Dendritic Cell AMP-Activated Protein Kinase. *Molecular Therapy*, *25*(7), 1641–1654. doi:10.1016/j.ymthe.2017.01.025 PMID:28274798

Desai, H. G., & Gupte, P. A. (2005). Increasing incidence of Crohn's disease in India: Is it related to improved sanitation? *Indian Journal of Gastroenterology*. PMID:15778522

Dhawan, P., Ahmad, R., Srivastava, A. S., & Singh, A. B. (2011). Cancer stem cells and colorectal cancer: An overview. *Current Topics in Medicinal Chemistry*, *11*(13), 1592–1598. doi:10.2174/156802611796117694 PMID:21446911

di Mola, F. F., Di Sebastiano, P., Gardini, A., Innocenti, P., Zimmermann, A., Büchler, M. W., & Friess, H. (2004). Differential expression of connective tissue growth factor in inflammatory bowel disease. *Digestion*, *69*(4), 245–253. doi:10.1159/000079845 PMID:15256831

DiDonato, J. A., Mercurio, F., & Karin, M. (2012). NF-κB and the link between inflammation and cancer. *Immunological Reviews*, *246*(1), 379–400. doi:10.1111/j.1600-065X.2012.01099.x PMID:22435567

Ding, Y., Liang, Y., Deng, B., Qiao, A., Wu, K., Xiao, W., & Gong, W. (2014). Induction of TGF-beta and IL-10 production in dendritic cells using astilbin to inhibit dextran sulfate sodium-induced colitis. *Biochemical and Biophysical Research Communications*, *446*(2), 529–534. doi:10.1016/j.bbrc.2014.02.136 PMID:24613838

Dinkova-Kostova, A. T., Holtzclaw, W. D., & Kensler, T. W. (2005). The role of Keap1 in cellular protective responses. *Chemical Research in Toxicology*, *18*(12), 1779–1791. doi:10.1021/tx050217c PMID:16359168

Ditto, B., Eclache, M., & Goldman, N. (2006). Short-term autonomic and cardiovascular effects of mindfulness body scan meditation. *Annals of Behavioral Medicine*, *32*(3), 227–234. doi:10.120715324796abm3203_9 PMID:17107296

Dobbins, W. O. III. (1984). Dysplasia and malignancy in inflammatory bowel disease. *Annual Review of Medicine*, *35*(1), 33–48. doi:10.1146/annurev.me.35.020184.000341 PMID:6372661

Dodda, D., Chhajed, R., & Mishra, J. (2014). Protective effect of quercetin against acetic acid induced inflammatory bowel disease (IBD) like symptoms in rats: Possible morphological and biochemical alterations. *Pharmacological Reports*, *66*(1), 169–173. doi:10.1016/j.pharep.2013.08.013 PMID:24905324

Douillard, J. Y., Siena, S., Cassidy, J., Tabernero, J., Burkes, R., Barugel, M., Humblet, Y., Bodoky, G., Cunningham, D., Jassem, J., Rivera, F., Kocákova, I., Ruff, P., Błasińska-Morawiec, M., Šmakal, M., Canon, J. L., Rother, M., Oliner, K. S., Tian, Y., ... Sidhu, R. (2014). Final results from PRIME: Randomized phase III study of panitumumab with FOLFOX4 for first-line treatment of metastatic colorectal cancer. *Annals of Oncology: Official Journal of the European Society for Medical Oncology*, *25*(7), 1346–1355. doi:10.1093/annonc/mdu141 PMID:24718886

Douillard, J. Y., Siena, S., Cassidy, J., Tabernero, J., Burkes, R., Barugel, M., Humblet, Y., Bodoky, G., Cunningham, D., Jassem, J., Rivera, F., Kocákova, I., Ruff, P., Błasińska-Morawiec, M., Šmakal, M., Canon, J.-L., Rother, M., Oliner, K. S., Wolf, M., & Gansert, J. (2010). Randomized, phase III trial of panitumumab with infusional fluorouracil, leucovorin, and oxaliplatin (FOLFOX4) versus FOLFOX4 alone as first-line treatment in patients with previously untreated metastatic colorectal cancer: The PRIME study. *Journal of Clinical Oncology*, *28*(31), 4697–4705. doi:10.1200/JCO.2009.27.4860 PMID:20921465

Dou, W., Mukherjee, S., Li, H., Venkatesh, M., Wang, H., Kortagere, S., Peleg, A., Chilimuri, S. S., Wang, Z.-T., Feng, Y., Fearon, E. R., & Mani, S. (2012). Alleviation of gut inflammation by Cdx2/Pxr pathway in a mouse model of chemical colitis. *PLoS One*, *7*(7), e36075. doi:10.1371/journal.pone.0036075 PMID:22815676

Dou, W., Zhang, J. J., Zhang, E. Y., Sun, A. N., Ding, L. L., Chou, G. X., Wang, Z., & Mani, S. (2013). Chrysin Ameliorates chemically induced colitis in the mouse through modulation of a PXR/NF-kappa B signaling pathway. *The Journal of Pharmacology and Experimental Therapeutics*, *345*(3), 473–482. doi:10.1124/jpet.112.201863 PMID:23536316

Dou, W., Zhang, J., Li, H., Kortagere, S., Sun, K., Ding, L., Ren, G., Wang, Z., & Mani, S. (2014). Plant flavonol isorhamnetin attenuates chemically induced inflammatory bowel disease via a PXR-dependent pathway. *The Journal of Nutritional Biochemistry*, *25*(9), 923–933. doi:10.1016/j.jnutbio.2014.04.006 PMID:24913217

Dou, W., Zhang, J., Sun, A., Zhang, E., Ding, L., Mukherjee, S., Wei, X., Chou, G., Wang, Z.-T., & Mani, S. (2013). Protective effect of naringenin against experimental colitis via suppression of Toll-like receptor 4/NF-kappaB signalling. *British Journal of Nutrition*, *110*(4), 599–608. doi:10.1017/S0007114512005594 PMID:23506745

Dou, Y. X., Zhou, J. T., Wang, T. T., Huang, Y. F., Chen, V. P., Xie, Y. L., Lin, Z.-X., Gao, J.-S., Su, Z.-R., & Zeng, H. F. (2018). Self-nanoemulsifying drug delivery system of bruceine D: A new approach for anti-ulcerative colitis. *International Journal of Nanomedicine*, *13*, 5887–5907. doi:10.2147/IJN.S174146 PMID:30319255

Duan, W., Yu, Y., & Zhang, L. (2005). Antiatherogenic effects of Phyllanthus emblica associated with corilagin and it analogue. *Yakugaku Zasshi*, *125*(7), 587–591. doi:10.1248/yakushi.125.587 PMID:15997216

Dubuquoy, L., Rousseaux, C., Thuru, X., Peyrin, L., Romano, O., Chavatte, P., & ... . (2006). PPARg as a new therapeutic in inflammatory bowel diseases. *Gut*, *55*(9), 1341–1349. doi:10.1136/gut.2006.093484 PMID:16905700

Duricova, D., Burisch, J., Jess, T., Gower-Rousseau, C., & Lakatos, P. L. (2014). Age-related differences in presentation and course of inflammatory bowel disease: An update on the population-based literature. *Journal of Crohn's and Colitis*, *8*(11), 1351–1361. doi:10.1016/j.crohns.2014.05.006 PMID:24951261

Dutta, B. K., Rahman, I., & Das, T. K. (1998). Antifungal activity of Indian plant extracts. *Mycoses*, *41*(11-12), 535–536. doi:10.1111/j.1439-0507.1998.tb00718.x PMID:9919899

Du, W., Hong, J., Wang, Y. C., Zhang, Y. J., Wang, P., Su, W. Y., & Fang, J. Y. (2012). Inhibition of JAK2/STAT3 signalling induces colorectal cancer cell apoptosis via mitochondrial pathway. *Journal of Cellular and Molecular Medicine*, *16*(8), 1878–1888. doi:10.1111/j.1582-4934.2011.01483.x PMID:22050790

Eaden, J. A., Abrams, K. R., & Mayberry, J. F. (2001). The risk of colorectal cancer in ulcerative colitis: A meta-analysis. *Gut*, *48*(4), 526–535. doi:10.1136/gut.48.4.526 PMID:11247898

Edwards, J. T., Radford-Smith, G. L., & Florin, T. H. (2001). Chronic narcotic use in inflammatory bowel disease patients: Prevalence and clinical characteristics. *Journal of Gastroenterology and Hepatology*, *16*(11), 1235–1238. doi:10.1046/j.1440-1746.2001.02468.x PMID:11903741

Eisenach, J. C., Curry, R., Rauck, R., Pan, P., & Yaksh, T. L. (2010). Role of spinal cyclooxygenase in human postoperative and chronic pain. *Anesthesiology*, *112*(5), 1225–1233. Advance online publication. doi:10.1097/ALN.0b013e3181d94dc0 PMID:20395820

Ellerby, H. M., Arap, W., Ellerby, L. M., Kain, R., Andrusiak, R., Del Rio, G., ... Bredesen, D. E. (1999). Anti-cancer activity of targeted pro-apoptotic peptides. *Nature Medicine*, *5*(9), 1032–1038. doi:10.1038/12469 PMID:10470080

Empey, L. R., Jewell, L. D., Garg, M. L., Thomson, A. B. R., Clandinin, M. T., & Fedorak, R. N. (1991). Fish oil-enriched diet is mucosal protective against acetic acid-induced colitis in rats. *Canadian Journal of Physiology and Pharmacology*, *69*(4), 480–487. Advance online publication. doi:10.1139/y91-072 PMID:1647851

Eramo, A., Lotti, F., Sette, G., Pilozzi, E., Biffoni, M., Di Virgilio, A., Conticello, C., Ruco, L., Peschle, C., & De Maria, R. (2008). Identification and expansion of the tumorigenic lung cancer stem cell population. *Cell Death and Differentiation*, *15*(3), 504–514. doi:10.1038j.cdd.4402283 PMID:18049477

Eun, S. H., Woo, J. T., & Kim, D. H. (2017). Tangeretin Inhibits IL-12 Expression and NF-kappaB Activation in Dendritic Cells and Attenuates Colitis in Mice. *Planta Medica*, *83*(6), 527–533. PMID:27806407

Fang, J., Seki, T., Tsukamoto, T., Qin, H., Yin, H., Liao, L., Nakamura, H., & Maeda, H. (2013). Protection from inflammatory bowel disease and colitis-associated carcinogenesis with 4-vinyl-2,6-dimethoxyphenol (canolol) involves suppression of oxidative stress and inflammatory cytokines. *Carcinogenesis*, *34*(12), 2833–2841. doi:10.1093/carcin/bgt309 PMID:24064222

Feagan, B. G., Sandborn, W. J., Gasink, C., Jacobstein, D., Lang, Y., Friedman, J. R., Blank, M. A., Johanns, J., Gao, L.-L., Miao, Y., Adedokun, O. J., Sands B. E., Hanauer, S. B., Vermeire, S., Targan, S., Ghosh, S., de Villiers, W. J., Colombel, J.-F., Tulassay, Z., ... Rutgeerts, P. (2016). Ustekinumab as Induction and Maintenance Therapy for Crohn's Disease. *The New England Journal of Medicine*, *375*(20), 1946–1960. doi:10.1056/NEJMoa1602773 PMID:27959607

Feakins, R. M. (2013). Inflammatory bowel disease biopsies: Updated British Society of Gastroenterology reporting guidelines. *Journal of Clinical Pathology*, *66*(12), 1005–1026. doi:10.1136/jclinpath-2013-201885 PMID:23999270

Fearon, E. R., & Vogelstein, B. (1990). A genetic model for colorectal tumorigenesis. *Cell, 61*(5), 759-767.

Fearon, E. R., & Vogelstein, B. (1990). A genetic model for colorectal tumorigenesis. *Cell*, *61*(5), 759–767. doi:10.1016/0092-8674(90)90186-I PMID:2188735

Feng, J., Guo, C., Zhu, Y., Pang, L., Yang, Z., Zou, Y., & Zheng, X. (2014). Baicalin down regulates the expression of TLR4 and NFkB-p65 in colon tissue in mice with colitis induced by dextran sulfate sodium. *International Journal of Clinical and Experimental Medicine*, *7*(11), 4063–4072. PMID:25550915

Feuerstein, J. D., & Cheifetz, A. S. (2014). Ulcerative colitis: Epidemiology, diagnosis, and management. *Mayo Clinic Proceedings*, *89*(11), 1553–1563 doi:10.1016/j.mayocp.2014.07.002 PMID:25199861

Fierer, N., Bradford, M. A., & Jackson, R. B. (2007). Toward an ecological classification of soil bacteria. *Ecology*, *88*(6), 1354–1364. doi:10.1890/05-1839 PMID:17601128

Flamant, M., & Roblin, X. (2018). Inflammatory bowel disease: Towards a personalized medicine. *Therapeutic Advances in Gastroenterology*, *11*, 1–15. doi:10.1177/1756283X17745029 PMID:29383027

Fohlinger, M., Palamides, P., Mansmann, U., Beigel, F. Siebeck, M., & Gropp, R. (2016). Immunological profiling of patients with ulcerative colitis leads to identification of two inflammatory conditions and CD1a as a disease marker *Journal of Translational Medicine*, *14*(1), 310. doi:10.118612967-016-1048-9 PMID:27809916

Frank, D. N., Robertson, C. E., Hamm, C. M., Kpadeh, Z., Zhang, T., Chen, H., ... Pace, N. R. (2011). Disease phenotype and genotype are associated with shifts in intestinal-associated microbiota in inflammatory bowel diseases. *Inflammatory Bowel Diseases*, *17*(1), 179–184. doi:10.1002/ibd.21339 PMID:20839241

Fre, S., Huyghe, M., Mourikis, P., Robine, S., Louvard, D., & Artavanis-Tsakonas, S. (2005). Notch signals control the fate of immature progenitor cells in the intestine. *Nature*, *435*(7044), 964–968. doi:10.1038/nature03589 PMID:15959516

Fujita, K. I., & Sparreboom, A. (2010). Pharmacogenetics of irinotecan disposition and toxicity: A review. *Current Clinical Pharmacology*, *5*(3), 209–217. doi:10.2174/157488410791498806 PMID:20406168

Furukawa, M., & Xiong, Y. (2005). BTB protein Keap1 targets antioxidant transcription factor Nrf2 for ubiquitination by the Cullin 3-Roc1 ligase. *Molecular and Cellular Biology*, *25*(1), 162–171. doi:10.1128/MCB.25.1.162-171.2005 PMID:15601839

Fu, X. Y. (2006). STAT3 in immune responses and inflammatory bowel diseases. *Cell Research*, *16*(2), 214–219. doi:10.1038j.cr.7310029 PMID:16474436

G., P., G., S., I., G., L., A., E., M., G., C., … R., T. (2014). Growing-up with an ileal-pouch: Adult-patient controlled and coetaneous population-based long-term evaluation of patients operated on in the developmental age in two Italian referral Centres. *Colorectal Disease*.

Gabriela Pop, M. (2019). Stem Cell Markers in Colon Cancer. In M. Gabriela Pop (Ed.), *Basic Principles and Practice in Surgery*. doi:10.5772/intechopen.84315

Gallinger, Z. R., Rumman, A., Pivovarov, K., Fortinsky, K. J., Steinhart, A. H., & Weizman, A. V. (2017). Frequency and Variables Associated with Fasting Orders in Inpatients with Ulcerative Colitis: The Audit of Diet Orders-Ulcerative Colitis (ADORE-UC) Study. *Inflammatory Bowel Diseases*, *23*(10), 1790–1795. doi:10.1097/MIB.0000000000001244 PMID:28906293

Galluzzi, L., Vitale, I., Michels, J., Brenner, C., Szabadkai, G., Harel-Bellan, A., Castedo, M., & Kroemer, G. J. C. D. (2014). Systems biology of cisplatin resistance: Past, present and future. *Cell Death & Disease*, *5*(5), e1257–e1257. doi:10.1038/cddis.2013.428 PMID:24874729

Galon, J., Angell, H. K., Bedognetti, D., & Marincola, F. M. (2013). The continuum of cancer immunosurveillance: Prognostic, predictive, and mechanistic signatures. *Immunity*, *39*(1), 11–26. doi:10.1016/j.immuni.2013.07.008 PMID:23890060

Galon, J., & Bruni, D. (2019). Approaches to treat immune hot, altered and cold tumours with combination immunotherapies. *Nature Reviews. Drug Discovery*, *18*(3), 197–218. doi:10.103841573-018-0007-y PMID:30610226

Galon, J., Fridman, W. H., & Pagès, F. (2007). The adaptive immunologic microenvironment in colorectal cancer: A novel perspective. *Cancer Research*, *67*(5), 1883–1886. doi:10.1158/0008-5472.CAN-06-4806 PMID:17332313

Galon, J., Pagès, F., Marincola, F. M., Thurin, M., Trinchieri, G., Fox, B. A., Gajewski, T. F., & Ascierto, P. A. (2012). The immune score as a new possible approach for the classification of cancer. *Journal of Translational Medicine*, *10*(1), 1. doi:10.1186/1479-5876-10-1 PMID:22214470

Galvez, J., Coelho, G., Crespo, M. E., Cruz, T., Rodriguez-Cabezas, M. E., Concha, A., Gonzalez, M., & Zarzuelo, A. (2001). Intestinal anti-inflammatory activity of morin on chronic experimental colitis in the rat. *Alimentary Pharmacology & Therapeutics*, *15*(12), 2027–2039. doi:10.1046/j.1365-2036.2001.01133.x PMID:11736735

Gao, W., Zhang, L., Wang, X., Yu, L., Wang, C., & Gong, Y. (2018). The combination of indirubin and isatin attenuates dextran sodium sulfate induced ulcerative colitis in mice. *Biochemistry and Cell Biology*, *96*(5), 636–645. Advance online publication. doi:10.1139/bcb-2018-0041 PMID:29671340

Gasparetto, M., & Guariso, G. (2014). Crohn's disease and growth deficiency in children and adolescents. *World Journal of Gastroenterology: WJG*, *20*(37), 13219. doi:10.3748/wjg.v20.i37.13219 PMID:25309059

Gates, M. A., Tworoger, S. S., Hecht, J. L., De Vivo, I., Rosner, B., & Hankinson, S. E. (2007). A prospective study of dietary flavonoid intake and incidence of epithelial ovarian cancer. *International Journal of Cancer*, *121*(10), 2225–2232. doi:10.1002/ijc.22790 PMID:17471564

Geagea, A. G., Rizzo, M., Eid, A., Hussein, I. H., Zgheib, Z., Zeenny, M. N., & … . (2017). Tea catechins induce crosstalk between signaling pathways and stabilize mast cells in ulcerative colitis. *Journal of Biological Regulators and Homeostatic Agents*, *31*(4), 865–877. PMID:29254289

Geboes, K. (2001). Crohn's disease, ulcerative colitis or indeterminate colitis—how important is it to differentiate? *Acta Gastro-Enterologica Belgica*, *64*(2), 197–200. PMID:11475135

Ghosh, A., Das, B. K., Roy, A., Mandal, B., & Chandra, G. (2008). Antibacterial activity of some medicinal plant extracts. *Journal of Natural Medicines*, *62*(2), 259–262. doi:10.100711418-007-0216-x PMID:18404337

Ghosh, A., Sharma, A., & Talukder, G. (1992). Relative protection given by extract of Phyllanthus emblica fruit and an equivalent amount of vitamin C against a known clastogen-caesium chloride. *Food and Chemical Toxicology*, *30*(10), 865–869. doi:10.1016/0278-6915(92)90052-M PMID:1427509

Ghosh, S., & Hayden, M. S. (2008). New regulators of NF-κB in inflammation. *Nature Reviews. Immunology*, *8*(11), 837–848. Advance online publication. doi:10.1038/nri2423 PMID:18927578

Giehl, K. (2005). Oncogenic Ras in tumour progression and metastasis. *Biological Chemistry*, *386*(3), 193–205. doi:10.1515/BC.2005.025 PMID:15843165

Gillen, C. D., Walmsley, R. S., Prior, P., Andrews, H. A., & Allan, R. N. (1994). Ulcerative colitis and Crohn's disease: A comparison of the colorectal cancer risk in extensive colitis. *Gut*, *35*(11), 1590–1592. doi:10.1136/gut.35.11.1590 PMID:7828978

Giuffrida, P., Caprioli, F., Facciotti, F., & Di Sabatino, A. (2019). The role of interleukin-13 in chronic inflammatory intestinal disorders. *Autoimmunity Reviews*, *18*(5), 549–555. doi:10.1016/j.autrev.2019.03.012 PMID:30844559

Gokhale, S. B., Kokate, C. K., & Purohit, A. P. (2003). Tannins. In Pharmacognosy (pp. 258–9). Pune, India: Nirali Prakashan.

Goldberg, A. A., Draz, H., Montes-Grajales, D., Olivero-Verbel, J., Safe, S. H., & Sanderson, J. T. (2015). 3,3′-Diindolylmethane (DIM) and its ring-substituted halogenated analogs (ring-DIMs) induce differential mechanisms of survival and death in androgen-dependent and -independent prostate cancer cells. *Genes & Cancer*, *6*(5-6), 265–280. doi:10.18632/genesandcancer.60 PMID:26124925

Gorrini, C., Harris, I. S., & Mak, T. W. (2013). Modulation of oxidative stress as an anticancer strategy. *Nature Reviews. Drug Discovery*, *12*(12), 931–947. doi:10.1038/nrd4002 PMID:24287781

Gou, S., Huang, Y., Wan, Y., Ma, Y., Zhou, X., Tong, X., Huang, J., Kang, Y., Pan, G., Dai, F., & Xiao, B. (2019). Multi-bioresponsive silk fibroin-based nanoparticles with on-demand cytoplasmic drug release capacity for CD44-targeted alleviation of ulcerative colitis. *Biomaterials*, *212*, 39–54. doi:10.1016/j.biomaterials.2019.05.012 PMID:31103945

Granado-Serrano, A. B., Angeles Martín, M., Izquierdo-Pulido, M., Goya, L., Bravo, L., & Ramos, S. (2007). Molecular mechanisms of (-)-epicatechin and chlorogenic acid on the regulation of the apoptotic and survival/proliferation pathways in a human hepatoma cell line. *Journal of Agricultural and Food Chemistry*, *55*(5), 2020–2027. doi:10.1021/jf062556x PMID:17286412

Greten, F. R., Eckmann, L., Greten, T. F., Park, J. M., Li, Z. W., Egan, L. J., & Karin, M. (2004). IKKβ links inflammation and tumorigenesis in a mouse model of colitis-associated cancer. *Cell*, *118*(3), 285–296. doi:10.1016/j.cell.2004.07.013 PMID:15294155

Grivennikov, S. I. (2013). Inflammation and colorectal cancer: Colitis-associated neoplasia. *Seminars in Immunopathology*, *35*(2), 229–244. doi:10.100700281-012-0352-6 PMID:23161445

Grivennikov, S., Karin, E., Terzic, J., Mucida, D., Yu, G. Y., Vallabhapurapu, S., Scheller, J., Rose-John, S., Cheroutre, H., Eckmann, L., & Karin, M. (2009). IL-6 and Stat3 are required for survival of intestinal epithelial cells and development of colitis-associated cancer. *Cancer Cell*, *15*(2), 103–113. doi:10.1016/j.ccr.2009.01.001 PMID:19185845

Grover, I. S., & Bala, S. (1992). Antimutagenic activity of Terminalia chebula (myrobalan) in Salmonella typhimurium. *Indian Journal of Experimental Biology*, *30*, 339–341. PMID:1459604

Guada, M., Beloqui, A., Alhouayek, M., Muccioli, G. G., Dios-Vieitez Mdel, C., Preat, V., & Blanco-Prieto, M. J. (2016). Cyclosporine A-loaded lipid nanoparticles in inflammatory bowel disease. *International Journal of Pharmaceutics*, *503*(1-2), 196–198. doi:10.1016/j.ijpharm.2016.03.012 PMID:26972380

Guan, F., Liu, A. B., Li, G., Yang, Z., Sun, Y., Yang, C. S., & Ju, J. (2012). Deleterious effects of high concentrations of (-)-epigallocatechin-3-gallate and atorvastatin in mice with colon inflammation. *Nutrition and Cancer*, *64*(6), 847–855. doi:10.1080/01635581.2012.695424 PMID:22716294

Guan, Q. (2019). A Comprehensive Review and Update on the Pathogenesis of Inflammatory Bowel Disease. *Journal of Immunology Research*, *2019*, 7247238. doi:10.1155/2019/7247238 PMID:31886308

Guazelli, C. F., Fattori, V., Colombo, B. B., Georgetti, S. R., Vicentini, F. T., Casagrande, R., Baracat, M. M., & Verri, W. A. Jr. (2013). Quercetin-loaded microcapsules ameliorate experimental colitis in mice by anti-inflammatory and antioxidant mechanisms. *Journal of Natural Products*, *76*(2), 200–208. doi:10.1021/np300670w PMID:23347547

Guerrouahen, B. S., Maccalli, C., Cugno, C., Rutella, S., & Akporiaye, E. T. (2019). Reverting Immune Suppression to Enhance Cancer Immunotherapy. *Frontiers in Oncology*, *9*, 1554. doi:10.3389/fonc.2019.01554 PMID:32039024

Gugulothu, D., Kulkarni, A., Patravale, V., & Dandekar, P. (2014). pH-sensitive nanoparticles of curcumin-celecoxib combination: Evaluating drug synergy in ulcerative colitis model. *Journal of Pharmaceutical Sciences*, *103*(2), 687–696. doi:10.1002/jps.23828 PMID:24375287

Günther, U., Bateman, A. C., Beattie, R. M., Bauer, M., MacDonald, T. T., & Kaskas, B. A. (2010). Connective tissue growth factor expression is increased in collagenous colitis and coeliac disease. *Histopathology*, *57*(3), 427–435. doi:10.1111/j.1365-2559.2010.03652.x PMID:20840672

Guo, A., He, D. M., Xu, H. B., Geng, C. A., & Zhao, J. (2015). Promotion of regulatory T cell induction by immunomodulatory herbal medicine licorice and its two constituents. *Scientific Reports*, *5*(1), 14046. doi:10.1038rep14046 PMID:26370586

Gupta, R. A., & DuBois, R. N. (2001). Colorectal cancer prevention and treatment by inhibition of cyclooxygenase-2. *Nature Reviews. Cancer*, *1*(1), 11–21. doi:10.1038/35094017 PMID:11900248

Gustaw, W., Kordowska-Wiater, M., & Kozioł, J. (2011). The influence of selected prebiotics on the growth of lactic acid bacteria for bio-yoghurt production. *Acta Scientiarum Polonorum. Technologia Alimentaria*, *10*(4), 455–466. PMID:22230927

Gutiérrez-Díaz, I., Fernández-Navarro, T., Sánchez, B., Margolles, A., & González, S. (2016). Mediterranean diet and faecal microbiota: A transversal study. *Food & Function*, *7*(5), 2347–2356. doi:10.1039/C6FO00105J PMID:27137178

Gyde, S., Prior, P., Dew, M. J., Saunders, V., Waterhouse, J. A., & Allan, R. N. (1982). Mortality in ulcerative colitis. *Gastroenterology*, *83*(1 Pt 1), 36–43. doi:10.1016/S0016-5085(82)80281-3 PMID:7075944

Hagenlocher, Y., Gommeringer, S., Held, A., Feilhauer, K., Köninger, J., Bischoff, S. C., & Lorentz, A. (2018). Nobiletin acts anti-inflammatory on murine IL-10$^{-/-}$ colitis and human intestinal fibroblasts. *European Journal of Nutrition*, 1391–1401. PMID:29525889

Haiser, H. J., & Turnbaugh, P. J. (2013). Developing a metagenomic view of xenobiotic metabolism. *Pharmacological Research*, *69*(1), 21–31. doi:10.1016/j.phrs.2012.07.009 PMID:22902524

Han, L., Shi, S., Gong, T., Zhang, Z., & Sun, X. (2013). Cancer stem cells: Therapeutic implications and perspectives in cancer therapy. *Acta Pharmaceutica Sinica. B*, *3*(2), 65–75. doi:10.1016/j.apsb.2013.02.006

Han, Y. W., Shi, W., Huang, G. T. J., Haake, S. K., Park, N. H., Kuramitsu, H., & Genco, R. J. (2000). Interactions between periodontal bacteria and human oral epithelial cells: Fusobacterium nucleatum adheres to and invades epithelial cells. *Infection and Immunity*, *68*(6), 3140–3146. doi:10.1128/IAI.68.6.3140-3146.2000 PMID:10816455

Hanyang, L., Xuanzhe, L., Xuyang, C., Yujia, Q., Jiarong, F., Jun, S., & Zhihua, R. (2017). Application of zebrafish models in inflammatory bowel disease. *Frontiers in Immunology*, *8*, 501. doi:10.3389/fimmu.2017.00501 PMID:28515725

Haque, R., Bin-Hafeez, B., Ahmad, I., Parvez, S., Panday, S., & Raisuddin, S. (2001). Protective effects of Emblica officinalis Gaertn. in cyclophosphamide-treated mice. *Human and Experimental Toxicology*, *20*(12), 643–650. doi:10.1191/096032701718890568 PMID:11936579

Haratani, K., Hayashi, H., Takahama, T., Nakamura, Y., Tomida, S., Yoshida, T., Chiba, Y., Sawada, T., Sakai, K., Fujita, Y., Togashi, Y., Tanizaki, J., Kawakami, H., Ito, A., Nishio, K., & Nakagawa, K. (2019). Clinical and immune profiling for cancer of unknown primary site. *Journal for Immunotherapy of Cancer*, *7*(1), 251. doi:10.118640425-019-0720-z PMID:31519206

Harborne, J. B., & Williams, C. A. (2000). Advances in flavonoid research since 1992. *Phytochemistry*, *55*(6), 481–504. doi:10.1016/S0031-9422(00)00235-1 PMID:11130659

Harikumar, K. B., Sabu, M. C., Lima, P. S., & Kuttan, R. (2004). Modulation of haematopoetic system and antioxidant enzymes by Emblica officinalis Gaertn. and its protective role against gamma radiation induced damages in mice. *Journal of Radiation Research*, *45*(4), 549–554. doi:10.1269/jrr.45.549 PMID:15635265

Harris, M. S., Hartman, D., Lemos, B. R., Erlich, E. C., Spence, S., Kennedy, S., Ptak, T., Pruitt, R., Vermeire, S., & Fox, B. S. (2016). AVX-470, an Orally Delivered Anti-Tumour Necrosis Factor Antibody for Treatment of Active Ulcerative Colitis: Results of a First-in-Human Trial. *Journal of Crohn's and Colitis*, *10*(6), 631–640. doi:10.1093/ecco-jcc/jjw036 PMID:26822613

Hartman, D. S., Tracey, D. E., Lemos, B. R., Erlich, E. C., Burton, R. E., Keane, D. M., Patel, R., Kim, S., Bhol, K. C., Harris, M. S., & Fox, B. S. (2016). Effects of AVX-470, an Oral, Locally Acting Anti-Tumour Necrosis Factor Antibody, on Tissue Biomarkers in Patients with Active Ulcerative Colitis. *Journal of Crohn's and Colitis*, *10*(6), 641–649. doi:10.1093/ecco-jcc/jjw026 PMID:26802087

Havel, J.J., Chowell, D., & Chan, T.A. (2019). *The evolving landscape of biomarkers for checkpoint inhibitor immunotherapy*. Academic Press.

Hecker, M., Zasłona, Z., Kwapiszewska, G., Niess, G., Zakrzewicz, A., Hergenreider, E., & Morty, R. E. (2010). *Dysregulation of the Interleukin 13 Receptor System: A Novel Pathomechanism in Pulmonary Arterial Hypertension*. Academic Press.

Hecker, E. (1968). Cocarcinogenic Principles from the Seed Oil of Croton tiglium and from Other Euphorbiaceae. *Cancer Research*. PMID:5723975

He, F., Wu, C., Li, P., Li, N., Zhang, D., Zhu, Q., Ren, W., & Peng, Y. (2018). Functions and signaling pathways of amino acids in intestinal inflammation. *BioMed Research International*, *2018*, 9171905. doi:10.1155/2018/9171905 PMID:29682569

Hendrickson, B. A., Gokhale, R., & Cho, J. H. (2002). Clinical aspects and pathophysiology of inflammatory bowel disease. *Clinical Microbiology Reviews*, *15*(1), 79–94. doi:10.1128/CMR.15.1.79-94.2002 PMID:11781268

Hersh, A. L., Shapiro, D. J., Pavia, A. T., & Shah, S. S. (2011). Antibiotic prescribing in ambulatory pediatrics in the United States. *Pediatrics*, *128*(6), 1053–1061. Advance online publication. doi:10.1542/peds.2011-1337 PMID:22065263

Holland, J. D., Klaus, A., Garratt, A. N., & Birchmeier, W. (2013). Wnt signaling in stem and cancer stem cells. *Current Opinion in Cell Biology*, *25*(2), 254–264. doi:10.1016/j.ceb.2013.01.004 PMID:23347562

Holmberg, F. E. O., Pedersen, J., Jorgensen, P., Soendergaard, C., Jensen, K. B., & Nielsen, O. H. (2018). Intestinal barrier integrity and inflammatory bowel disease: Stem cell-based approaches to regenerate the barrier. *Journal of Tissue Engineering and Regenerative Medicine*, *12*(4), 923–935. doi:10.1002/term.2506 PMID:28636192

Hooper, L. V., & Macpherson, A. J. (2010). Immune adaptations that maintain homeostasis with the intestinal microbiota. *Nature Reviews. Immunology*, *10*(3), 159–169. doi:10.1038/nri2710 PMID:20182457

Hou, J. K., Abraham, B., & El-Serag, H. (2011). Dietary intake and risk of developing inflammatory bowel disease: A systematic review of the literature. *The American Journal of Gastroenterology*, *106*(4), 563–573. Advance online publication. doi:10.1038/ajg.2011.44 PMID:21468064

Huang, E. H., Hynes, M. J., Zhang, T., Ginestier, C., Dontu, G., Appelman, H., Fields, J. Z., Wicha, M. S., & Boman, B. M. (2009). Aldehyde dehydrogenase 1 is a marker for normal and malignant human colonic stem cells (SC) and tracks SC overpopulation during colon tumorigenesis. *Cancer Research*, *69*(8), 3382–3389. doi:10.1158/0008-5472.CAN-08-4418 PMID:19336570

Huang, Y., Guo, J., & Gui, S. (2018). Orally targeted galactosylated chitosan poly(lactic-co-glycolic acid) nanoparticles loaded with TNF-a siRNA provide a novel strategy for the experimental treatment of ulcerative colitis. *European Journal of Pharmaceutical Sciences*, *125*, 232–243. doi:10.1016/j.ejps.2018.10.009 PMID:30315858

Hung, Y. L., Fang, S. H., Wang, S. C., Cheng, W. C., Liu, P. L., Su, C. C., Chen, C.-S., Huang, M.-Y., Hua, K.-F., Shen, K.-H., Wang, Y.-T., Suzuki, K., & Li, C. Y. (2017). Corylin protects LPS-induced sepsis and attenuates LPS-induced inflammatory response. *Scientific Reports*, *7*(1), 46299. Advance online publication. doi:10.1038/srep46299 PMID:28397806

Hussein, I. A. H., Tohme, R., Kassem Barada, M. H. M., Freund, J. N., Jurjus, R. A., Karam, W., & Jurjus, A. (2008). Inflammatory bowel disease in rats: Bacterial and chemical interaction. *World Journal of Gastroenterology: WJG*, *14*(25), 4028. doi:10.3748/wjg.14.4028 PMID:18609687

Hynes, M. J., Huang, K. M., & Huang, E. H. (2009). Review Paper: Implications of the "Cancer Stem Cell" Hypothesis on Murine Models of Colon Cancer and Colitis-associated Cancer. *Veterinary Pathology*, *46*(5), 819–835. doi:10.1354/vp.08-VP-0172-H-REV PMID:19429978

Iglesias, N., Galbis, E., Diaz-Blanco, M. J., Lucas, R., Benito, E., & de-Paz, M. V. (2019). Nanostructured Chitosan-Based Biomaterials for Sustained and Colon-Specific Resveratrol Release. *International Journal of Molecular Sciences*, *20*(2), 398. Advance online publication. doi:10.3390/ijms20020398 PMID:30669264

Isbell, G., & Levin, B. (1988). Ulcerative colitis and colon cancer. *Gastroenterology Clinics of North America*, *17*(4), 773–791. PMID:3068141

Ishihara, J., & Ishihara, A. (2019). *Targeted antibody and cytokine cancer immunotherapies through collagen affinity*. Academic Press.

Itzkowitz, S. H., & Yio, X. (2004). Inflammation and cancer IV. Colorectal cancer in inflammatory bowel disease: The role of inflammation. *American Journal of Physiology. Gastrointestinal and Liver Physiology*, *287*(1), G7–G17. doi:10.1152/ajpgi.00079.2004 PMID:15194558

Ivanovich, J. L., Read, T. E., Ciske, D. J., Kodner, I. J., & Whelan, A. J. (1999). A practical approach to familial and hereditary colorectal cancer. *The American Journal of Medicine*, *107*(1), 68–77. doi:10.1016/S0002-9343(99)00168-0 PMID:10403355

Ivanov, K., Kolev, N., Tonev, A., Nikolova, G., Krasnaliev, I., Softova, E., & Tonchev, A. (2009). Comparative analysis of prognostic significance of molecular markers of apoptosis with clinical stage and tumor differentiation in patients with colorectal cancer: A single institute experience. *Hepato-Gastroenterology*, *56*(89), 94–98. PMID:19453036

Iwao, Y., Tomiguchi, I., Domura, A., Mantaira, Y., Minami, A., Suzuki, T., Ikawa, T., Kimura, S., & Itai, S. (2018). Inflamed site-specific drug delivery system based on the interaction of human serum albumin nanoparticles with myeloperoxidase in a murine model of experimental colitis. *European Journal of Pharmaceutics and Biopharmaceutics*, *125*, 141–147. doi:10.1016/j.ejpb.2018.01.016 PMID:29407223

Iwashita, J., Sato, Y., Sugaya, H., Takahashi, N., Sasaki, H., & Abe, T. (2003). mRNA of MUC2 is stimulated by IL-4, IL-13 or TNF-α through a mitogen-activated protein kinase pathway in human colon cancer cells. *Immunology and Cell Biology*, *81*(4), 275–282. doi:10.1046/j.1440-1711.2003.t01-1-01163.x PMID:12848848

Jackson, A. L., & Loeb, L. A. (2001). The contribution of endogenous sources of DNA damage to the multiple mutations in cancer. *Mutation Research. Fundamental and Molecular Mechanisms of Mutagenesis*, *477*(1-2), 7–21. doi:10.1016/S0027-5107(01)00091-4 PMID:11376682

Jain, S., Garg, T., Kushwah, V., Thanki, K., Agrawal, A. K., & Dora, C. P. (2017). alpha-Tocopherol as functional excipient for resveratrol and coenzyme Q10-loaded SNEDDS for improved bioavailability and prophylaxis of breast cancer. *Journal of Drug Targeting*, *25*(6), 554–565. doi:10.1080/1061186X.2017.1298603 PMID:28274130

Jain, S., Shapiro, S. L., Swanick, S., Roesch, S. C., Mills, P. J., Bell, I., & Schwartz, G. E. R. (2007). A randomized controlled trial of mindfulness meditation versus relaxation training: Effects on distress, positive states of mind, rumination, and distraction. *Annals of Behavioral Medicine*, *33*(1), 11–21. doi:10.120715324796abm3301_2 PMID:17291166

Jan, G. B. A. S., Belzacq, A. S., Haouzi, D., Rouault, A., Metivier, D., Kroemer, G., & Brenner, C. (2002). Propionibacteria induce apoptosis of colorectal carcinoma cells via short-chain fatty acids acting on mitochondria. *Cell Death and Differentiation*, *9*(2), 179–188. doi:10.1038j.cdd.4400935 PMID:11840168

Jeena, K. J., Joy, K. L., & Kuttan, R. (1999). Effect of Emblica officinalis, Phyllanthus amarus and Picrorrhiza kurroa on N-nitrosodiethylamine induced hepatocarcinogenesis. *Cancer Letters*, *136*(1), 11–16. doi:10.1016/S0304-3835(98)00294-8 PMID:10211933

Jia, L., & Zhao, Y. (2009). Current evaluation of the millennium phytomedicine-ginseng (I): Etymology, pharmacognosy, phytochemistry, market and regulations. *Current Medicinal Chemistry*, *16*(19), 2475–2484. doi:10.2174/092986709788682146 PMID:19601793

Johnson, A. C., & Greenwood-Van Meerveld, B. (2017). Critical evaluation of animal models of gastrointestinal disorders. *Handbook of Experimental Pharmacology*, *239*, 289–317. doi:10.1007/164_2016_120 PMID:28176046

Jones, G. W., McLoughlin, R. M., Hammond, V. J., Parker, C. R., Williams, J. D., Malhotra, R., & Jones, S. A. (2010). Loss of CD4+ T cell IL-6R expression during inflammation underlines a role for IL-6 trans signaling in the local maintenance of Th17 cells. *Journal of Immunology (Baltimore, Md.: 1950)*, *184*(4), 2130–2139. doi:10.4049/jimmunol.0901528 PMID:20083667

Jonker, D. J., O'Callaghan, C. J., Karapetis, C. S., Zalcberg, J. R., Tu, D., Au, H.-J., Berry, S. R., Krahn, M., Price, T., Simes, R. J., Tebbutt, N. C., van Hazel, G., Wierzbicki, R., Langer, C., & Moore, M. J. (2007). Cetuximab for the Treatment of Colorectal Cancer. *The New England Journal of Medicine*, *357*(20), 2040–2048. doi:10 1056/NEJMoa071834 PMID:18003960

Jose, J. K., & Kuttan, R. (2000). Hepatoprotective activity of Emblica officinalis and chyavanprash. *Journal of Ethnopharmacology*, *72*(1-2), 135–140. doi:10.1016/S0378-8741(00)00219-1 PMID:10967464

Jostins, L., Ripke, S., Weersma, R. K., Duerr, R. H., McGovern, D. P., Hui, K. Y., Lee, J. C., Philip Schumm, L., Sharma, Y., Anderson, C. A., Essers, J., Mitrovic, M., Ning, K., Cleynen, I., Theatre, E., Spain, S. L., Raychaudhuri, S., Goyette, P., Wei, Z., ... Cho, J. H. (2012). Host-microbe interactions have shaped the genetic architecture of inflammatory bowel disease. *Nature*, *491*(7422), 119–124. doi:10.1038/nature11582 PMID:23128233

Jowett, S. L., Seal, C. J., Pearce, M. S., Phillips, E., Gregory, W., Barton, J. R., & ... . (2004). Influence of dietary factors on the clinical course of ulcerative colitis: A prospective cohort study. *Gut*, *53*(10), 1479–1484. doi:10.1136/gut.2003.024828 PMID:15361498

Juang, L. J., & Sheu, S. J. (2005). Chemical identification of the sources of commercial Fructus chebulae. *Phytochemical Analysis*, *16*(4), 246–251. doi:10.1002/pca.823 PMID:16042149

Jung, O. B., Dong, Y. Y., Koan, S. W., Tae, M. K., Ung, S. L., Jeong, H. S., ... Jin, T. H. (2007). Inhibition of cell growth and induction of apoptosis via inactivation of NF-κB by a sulfurcompound isolated from garlic in human colon cancer cells. *Journal of Pharmacological Sciences*, *104*(4), 374–383. Advance online publication. doi:10.1254/jphs.FP0070789

Kamdar, K., Khakpour, S., Chen, J., Leone, V., Brulc, J., Mangatu, T., ... Young, G. (2016). Genetic and metabolic signals during acute enteric bacterial infection alter the microbiota and drive progression to chronic inflammatory disease. *Cell Host & Microbe*, *19*(1), 21–31. doi:10.1016/j.chom.2015.12.006 PMID:26764594

Kanazawa, K., Konishi, F., Mitsuoka, T., Terada, A., Itoh, K., Narushima, S., Kumemura, M., & Kimura, H. (1996). Factors influencing the development of sigmoid colon cancer: Bacteriologic and biochemical studies. *Cancer: Interdisciplinary International Journal of the American Cancer Society*, *77*(8), 1701–1706. doi:10.1002/(SICI)1097-0142(19960415)77:8<1701::AID-CNCR42>3.0.CO;2-0 PMID:8608565

Kang, T. H., & Kim, H. J. (2016). Farewell to animal testing: Innovations on human intestinal microphysiological systems. *Micromachines*, *7*(7), 107. doi:10.3390/mi7070107 PMID:30404281

Kannan, P., Ramadevi, S. R., & Waheeta, H. (2009). Antibacterial activity of Terminalia chebula fruit extract. *African Journal of Microbiological Research*, *3*, 180–184.

Kaplan, G. G., & Ng, S. C. (2017). Understanding and preventing the global increase of inflammatory bowel disease. *Gastroenterology*, *152*(2), 313–321. doi:10.1053/j.gastro.2016.10.020 PMID:27793607

Kaplan, M. A., & Korelitz, B. I. (1988). Narcotic dependence in inflammatory bowel disease. *Journal of Clinical Gastroenterology*, *10*(3), 275–278. doi:10.1097/00004836-198806000-00010 PMID:2980762

Kappelman, M. D., Rifas–Shiman, S. L., Kleinman, K., Ollendorf, D., Bousvaros, A., Grand, R. J., & Finkelstein, J. A. (2007). The prevalence and geographic distribution of Crohn's disease and ulcerative colitis in the United States. *Clinical Gastroenterology and Hepatology*, *5*(12), 1424–1429. doi:10.1016/j.cgh.2007.07.012 PMID:17904915

Kargl, J., Haybaeck, J., Stancic, A., Andersen, L., Marsche, G., Heinemann, A., & Schicho, R. (2013). O-1602, an atypical cannabinoid, inhibits tumor growth in colitis-associated colon cancer through multiple mechanisms. *Journal of Molecular Medicine (Berlin, Germany)*, *91*(4), 449–458. doi:10.100700109-012-0957-1 PMID:22965195

Karin, M., & Greten, F. R. (2005). NF-κB: Linking inflammation and immunity to cancer development and progression. *Nature Reviews. Immunology*, *5*(10), 749–759. doi:10.1038/nri1703 PMID:16175180

Karrasch, T., Kim, J. S., Jang, B. I., & Jobin, C. (2007). The flavonoid luteolin worsens chemical-induced colitis in NF-kappaB(EGFP) transgenic mice through blockade of NF-kappaB-dependent protective molecules. *PLoS One*, *2*(7), e596. doi:10.1371/journal.pone.0000596 PMID:17611628

Kasaian, M. T., Raible, D., Marquette, K., Cook, T. A., Zhou, S., Tan, X. Y., & Tchistiakova, L. (2011). IL-13 antibodies influence IL-13 clearance in humans by modulating scavenger activity of IL-13Rα2. *Journal of Immunology (Baltimore, Md.: 1950), 187*(1), 561–569. doi:10.4049/jimmunol.1100467 PMID:21622864

Kaser, A., Molnar, C., & Tilg, H. (1998). Differential regulation of interleukin 4 and interleukin 13 production by interferon α. *Cytokine, 10*(2), 75–81. doi:10.1006/cyto.1997.0270 PMID:9512896

Kashyap, P. C., Marcobal, A., Ursell, L. K., Smits, S. A., Sonnenburg, E. D., Costello, E. K., ... Knight, R. (2013). Genetically dictated change in host mucus carbohydrate landscape exerts a diet-dependent effect on the gut microbiota. *Proceedings of the National Academy of Sciences of the United States of America, 110*(42), 17059–17064. doi:10.1073/pnas.1306070110 PMID:24062455

Katsanos, K. H., & Papadakis, K. A. (2017). Inflammatory bowel disease: Updates on molecular targets for biologics. *Gut and Liver, 11*(4), 455–463. doi:10.5009/gnl16308 PMID:28486793

Kaur, S., Arora, S., Kaur, K., & Kumar, S. (2002). The in vitro antimutagenic activity of Triphala an Indian herbal drug. *Food and Chemical Toxicology, 40*(4), 527–534. doi:10.1016/S0278-6915(01)00101-6 PMID:11893411

Kaur, S., & Jaggi, R. K. (2010). Antinociceptive activity of chronic administration of different extracts of Terminalia bellerica Roxb. and Terminalia chebula Retz. fruits. *Indian Journal of Experimental Biology, 48*(9), 925–930. PMID:21506501

Kavanagh, D. O., Carter, M. C., Keegan, D., Doherty, G., Smith, M. J., Hyland, J. M. P., Mulcahy, H., Sheahan, K., O' Connell, P. R., O' Donoghue, D. P., & Winter, D. C. (2014). Management of colorectal cancer in patients with inflammatory bowel disease. *Techniques in Coloproctology, 18*(1), 23–28. doi:10.100710151-013-0981-3 PMID:23407916

Kedia, S., & Ahuja, V. (2017). Epidemiology of Inflammatory Bowel Disease in India: The Great Shift East. *Inflammatory Intestinal Diseases, 2*(2), 102–115. doi:10.1159/000465522 PMID:30018961

Kelm, M. A., Johnson, J. C., Robbins, R. J., Hammerstone, J. F., & Schmitz, H. H. (2006). High-performance liquid chromatography separation and purification of cacao (Theobroma cacao L.) procyanidins according to degree of polymerization using a diol stationary phase. *Journal of Agricultural and Food Chemistry, 54*(5), 1571–1576. doi:10.1021/jf0525941 PMID:16506802

Kerlin, M., Long, M., Kappelman, M., Martin, C., & Sandler, R. S. (2018). Profiles of patients who use marijuana for inflammatory bowel disease. *Digestive Diseases and Sciences, 63*(6), 1600–1604. doi:10.100710620-018-5040-5 PMID:29594968

Kheirelseid, E. A. H., Miller, N., & Kerin, M. J. (2013). Molecular biology of colorectal cancer: Review of the literature. *American Journal of Molecular Biology, 03*(02), 72–80. doi:10.4236/ajmb.2013.32010

Kiesler, P., Fuss, I. J., & Strober, W. (2015). Experimental models of inflammatory bowel diseases. *Cellular and Molecular Gastroenterology and Hepatology*, *1*(2), 154–170. doi:10.1016/j.jcmgh.2015.01.006 PMID:26000334

Kim, D. H., Hossain, M. A., Kang, Y. J., Jang, J. Y., Lee, Y. J., Im, E., Yoon, J.-H., Kim, H. S., Chung, H. Y., & Kim, N. D. (2013). Baicalein, an active component of Scutellaria baicalensis Georgi, induces apoptosis in human colon cancer cells and prevents AOM/DSS-induced colon cancer in mice. *International Journal of Oncology*, *43*(5), 1652–1658. doi:10.3892/ijo.2013.2086 PMID:24008356

Kim, D. H., Sung, B., Kang, Y. J., Jang, J. Y., Hwang, S. Y., Lee, Y., Kim, M., Im, E., Yoon, J.-H., Kim, C. M., Chung, H. Y., & Kim, N. D. (2014). Anti-inflammatory effects of betaine on AOM/DSSinduced colon tumorigenesis in ICR male mice. *International Journal of Oncology*, *45*(3), 1250–1256. doi:10.3892/ijo.2014.2515 PMID:24969167

Kim, D. S., Kim, S. J., Kim, M. C., Jeon, Y. D., Um, J. Y., & Hong, S. H. (2012). The therapeutic effect of chelidonic acid on ulcerative colitis. *Biological & Pharmaceutical Bulletin*, *35*(5), 666–671. Advance online publication. doi:10.1248/bpb.35.666 PMID:22687399

Kim, H. J., Yokozawa, T., Kim, H. Y., Tohda, C., Rao, T. P., & Juneja, L. R. (2005). Influence of amla (Emblica officinalis Gaertn.) on hypercholesterolemia and lipid peroxidation in cholesterol-fed rats. *Journal of Nutritional Science and Vitaminology*, *51*(6), 413–418. doi:10.3177/jnsv.51.413 PMID:16521700

Kim, H., Kong, H., Choi, B., Yang, Y., Kim, Y., Lim, M. J., Neckers, L., & Jung, Y. (2005). Metabolic and pharmacological properties of rutin, a dietary quercetin glycoside, for treatment of inflammatory bowel disease. *Pharmaceutical Research*, *22*(9), 1499–1509. doi:10.100711095-005-6250-z PMID:16132362

Kim, K. H., Lee, Y. S., Jung, I. S., Park, S. Y., Chung, H. Y., Lee, I. R., & Yun, Y. S. (1998). Acidic polysaccharide from Panax ginseng, ginsan, induces Th1 cell and macrophage cytokines and generates LAK cells in synergy with rIL-2. *Planta Medica*, *64*(2), 110–115. doi:10.1055-2006-957385 PMID:9525101

Kim, S. K., & Kim, Y. C. (2002). Attenuation of bacterial lipopolysaccharide-induced hepatotoxicity by betaine or taurine in rats. *Food and Chemical Toxicology*, *40*(4), 545–549. doi:10.1016/S0278-6915(01)00102-8 PMID:11893413

Kim, T. G., Kang, S. Y., Jung, K. K., Kang, J. H., Lee, E., Han, H. M., & Kim, S. H. (2001). Antiviral activities of extracts isolated from Terminalis chebula Retz., Sanguisorba officinalis L., Rubus coreanus Miq. and Rheum palmatum L. against hepatitis B virus. *Phytotherapy Research*, *15*(8), 718–720. doi:10.1002/ptr.832 PMID:11746867

Kim, Y. H., Kwon, H. S., Kim, D. H., Shin, E. K., Kang, Y. H., Park, J. H., ... Kim, J. K. (2009). 3,3′-diindolylmethane attenuates colonic inflammation and tumorigenesis in mice. *Inflammatory Bowel Diseases*, *15*(8), 1164–1173. doi:10.1002/ibd.20917 PMID:19334074

Kim, Y. S., Son, M., Ko, J. I., Cho, H., Yoo, M., Kim, W. B., Song, I. S., & Kim, C. Y. (1999). Effect of DA-6034, a derivative of flavonoid, on experimental animal models of inflammatory bowel disease. *Archives of Pharmacal Research, 22*(4), 354–360. doi:10.1007/BF02979057 PMID:10489873

Kirsner, J. B. (2001). Historical origins of current IBD concepts. *World Journal of Gastroenterology, 7*(2), 175. Advance online publication. doi:10.3748/wjg.v7.i2.175 PMID:11819757

Klampfer, L. (2008). The role of signal transducers and activators of transcription in colon cancer. *Frontiers in Bioscience, 13*(1), 2888–2899. doi:10.2741/2893 PMID:17981761

Knights, D., Lassen, K. G., & Xavier, R. J. (2013). Advances in inflammatory bowel disease pathogenesis: Linking host genetics and the microbiome. *Gut, 62*(10), 1505–1510. Advance online publication. doi:10.1136/gutjnl-2012-303954 PMID:24037875

Knight-Sepulveda, K., Kais, S., Santaolalla, R., & Abreu, M. T. (2015). Diet and Inflammatory Bowel Disease. *Gastroenterology & Hepatology, 11*(8), 511–520. PMID:27118948

Kobayashi, M., & Yamamoto, M. (2005). Molecular mechanisms activating the Nrf2-Keap1 pathway of antioxidant gene regulation. *Antioxidants & Redox Signaling, 7*(3-4), 385–394. doi:10.1089/ars.2005.7.385 PMID:15706085

Koch, U., Krause, M., & Baumann, M. (2010). Cancer stem cells at the crossroads of current cancer therapy failures—Radiation oncology perspective. *Seminars in Cancer Biology, 20*(2), 116–124. doi:10.1016/j.semcancer.2010.02.003 PMID:20219680

Kolios, G. (2016). Animal models of inflammatory bowel disease: How useful are they really? *Current Opinion in Gastroenterology, 32*(4), 251–257. doi:10.1097/MOG.0000000000000287 PMID:27206158

Konstantinidis, A. K., Puddicombe, S. M., Mochizuki, A., Sheth, P. D., Yang, I. A., Yoshisue, H., ... Holloway, J. W. (2008). Cellular localization of interleukin 13 receptor alpha2 in human primary bronchial epithelial cells and fibroblasts. *Journal of Investigational Allergology & Clinical Immunology, 18*(3), 174–180. PMID:18564628

Kook, S.-H., Choi, K. C., Cho, S.-W., Cho, H.-K., Lee, K. D., & Lee, J.-C. (2015). Catechin-7-*O*-β-D-glucopyranoside isolated from the seed of Phaseolus calcaratus Roxburgh ameliorates experimental colitis in rats. *International Immunopharmacology, 29*(2), 521–527. doi:10.1016/j.intimp.2015.10.003 PMID:26453508

Kopetz, S., Grothey, A., Yaeger, R., Van Cutsem, E., & Desai, J. (2019). Encorafenib, Binimetinib, and Cetuximab in BRAF V600E-Mutated. *Colorectal Cancer, 381*(17), 1632–1643. PMID:31566309

Kornbluth, A., & Sachar, D. B. (2010). Ulcerative colitis practice guidelines in adults: American college of gastroenterology, practice parameters committee. *The American Journal of Gastroenterology, 105*(3), 501–523. Advance online publication. doi:10.1038/ajg.2009.727 PMID:20068560

Krishnamurthy, N., & Kurzrock, R. (2018). Targeting the Wnt/beta-catenin pathway in cancer: Update on effectors and inhibitors. *Cancer Treatment Reviews*, *62*, 50–60. doi:10.1016/j.ctrv.2017.11.002 PMID:29169144

Kroemer, G., Galluzzi, L., Kepp, O., & Zitvogel, L. (2013). Immunogenic cell death in cancer therapy. *Annual Review of Immunology*, *31*(1), 51–72. doi:10.1146/annurev-immunol-032712-100008 PMID:23157435

Kuwahara, H., Kanazawa, A., Wakamatu, D., Morimura, S., Kida, K., Akaike, T., & Maeda, H. (2004). Antioxidative and antimutagenic activities of 4-vinyl-2,6-dimethoxyphenol (canolol) isolated from canola oil. *Journal of Agricultural and Food Chemistry*, *52*(14), 4380–4387. doi:10.1021/jf040045+ PMID:15237940

Kwang, S. A., Sethi, G., & Aggarwal, B. B. (2007). Embelin, an inhibitor of X chromosome-linked inhibitor-of-apoptosis protein, blocks nuclear factor-κB (NF-κB) signaling pathway leading to suppression of NF-κB-regulated antiapoptotic and metastatic gene products. *Molecular Pharmacology*, *71*(1), 209–219. Advance online publication. doi:10.1124/mol.106.028787

Kwon, K. H., Murakami, A., Tanaka, T., & Ohigashi, H. (2005). Dietary rutin, but not its aglycone quercetin, ameliorates dextran sulfate sodium-induced experimental colitis in mice: Attenuation of pro-inflammatory gene expression. *Biochemical Pharmacology*, *69*(3), 395–406. doi:10.1016/j.bcp.2004.10.015 PMID:15652231

Lai, K.-C., Kuo, C.-L., Ho, H.-C., Yang, J.-S., Ma, C.-Y., Lu, H.-F., Huang, H.-Y., Chueh, F.-S., Yu, C.-C., & Chung, J.-G. (2012). Diallyl sulfide, diallyl disulfide and diallyl trisulfide affect drug resistant gene expression in colo 205 human colon cancer cells in vitro and in vivo. *Phytomedicine*, *19*(7), 625–630. doi:10.1016/j.phymed.2012.02.004 PMID:22397993

Lai, X., & Friedman, A. (2017). Exosomal microRNA concentrations in colorectal cancer: A mathematical model. *Journal of Theoretical Biology*, *415*, 70–83. doi:10.1016/j.jtbi.2016.12.006 PMID:27993628

Landy, J., Ronde, E., English, N., Clark, S. K., Hart, A. L., Knight, S. C., Ciclitira, P. J., & Al-Hassi, H. O. (2016). Tight junctions in inflammatory bowel diseases and inflammatory bowel disease associated colorectal cancer. *World Journal of Gastroenterology*, *22*(11), 3117–3126. doi:10.3748/wjg.v22.i11.3117 PMID:27003989

Lee, H. J., Lee, H. G., Choi, K. S., Surh, Y. J., & Na, H. K. (2013). Diallyl trisulfide suppresses dextran sodium sulfate-induced mouse colitis: NF-kappaB and STAT3 as potential targets. *Biochemical and Biophysical Research Communications*, *437*(2), 267–273. doi:10.1016/j.bbrc.2013.06.064 PMID:23811270

Lee, H. S., Koo, Y. C., Suh, H. J., Kim, K. Y., & Lee, K. W. (2010). Preventive effects of chebulic acid isolated from Terminalia chebula on advanced glycation end product-induced endothelial cell dysfunction. *Journal of Ethnopharmacology*, *131*(3), 567–574. doi:10.1016/j.jep.2010.07.039 PMID:20659546

Lee, J. H., Shim, J. S., Lee, J. S., Kim, M. K., Chung, M. S., & Kim, K. H. (2006). Pectin-like acidic polysaccharide from Panax ginseng with selective antiadhesive activity against pathogenic bacteria. *Carbohydrate Research*, *341*(9), 1154–1163. doi:10.1016/j.carres.2006.03.032 PMID:16643869

Lee, J. J., Rothenberg, M. E., Seeley, E. S., Zimdahl, B., Kawano, S., Lu, W.-J., Shin, K., Sakata-Kato, T., Chen, J. K., Diehn, M., Clarke, M. F., & Beachy, P. A. (2016). Control of inflammation by stromal Hedgehog pathway activation restrains colitis. *Proceedings of the National Academy of Sciences of the United States of America*, *113*(47), E7545–E7553. doi:10.1073/pnas.1616447113 PMID:27815529

Lee, K. H., Ahn, B. S., Cha, D., Jang, W. W., Choi, E., Park, S., Park, J. H., Oh, J., Jung, D. E., Park, H., Park, J. H., Suh, Y., Jin, D., Lee, S., Jang, Y.-H., Yoon, T., Park, M.-K., Seong, Y., Pyo, J., ... Kronbichler, A. (2020). Understanding the immunopathogenesis of autoimmune diseases by animal studies using gene modulation: A comprehensive review. *Autoimmunity Reviews*, *19*(3), 102469. doi:10.1016/j.autrev.2020.102469 PMID:31918027

Lee, S. H., Kwon, J., & Cho, M.-L. (2018). Immunological pathogenesis of inflammatory bowel disease. *Intestinal Research*, *16*(1), 26. doi:10.5217/ir.2018.16.1.26 PMID:29422795

Lehouritis, P., Cummins, J., Stanton, M., Murphy, C. T., McCarthy, F. O., Reid, G., Urbaniak, C., Byrne, W. L., & Tangney, M. (2015). Local bacteria affect the efficacy of chemotherapeutic drugs. *Scientific Reports*, *5*(1), 14554. doi:10.1038rep14554 PMID:26416623

Leonardi, C. L., Kimball, A. B., Papp, K. A., Yeilding, N., Guzzo, C., Wang, Y., Li, S., Dooley, L. T., & Gordon, K. B. (2008). Efficacy and safety of ustekinumab, a human interleukin-12/23 monoclonal antibody, in patients with psoriasis: 76-week results from a randomised, double-blind, placebo-controlled trial (PHOENIX 1). *Lancet*, *371*(9625), 1665–1674. doi:10.1016/S0140-6736(08)60725-4 PMID:18486739

Levine, J. S., & Ahnen, D. J. (2006). Clinical practice. Adenomatous polyps of the colon. *The New England Journal of Medicine*, *355*(24), 2551–2557. doi:10.1056/NEJMcp063038 PMID:17167138

Lichtenstein, G. R., Feagan, B. G., Cohen, R. D., Salzberg, B. A., Diamond, R. H., Price, S., Langholff, W., Londhe, A., & Sandborn, W. J. (2012). Serious infection and mortality in patients with Crohn's disease: More than 5 years of follow-up in the TREAT™ registry. *The American Journal of Gastroenterology*, *107*(9), 1409–1422. doi:10.1038/ajg.2012.218 PMID:22890223

Lichtenstern, C.R., Ngu, R.K., & Shalapour, S. (2020). *Immunotherapy, Inflammation and Colorectal Cancer*. Academic Press.

Lida, N., Dzutsev, A., Stewart, C. A., Smith, L., Bouladoux, N., Weingarten, R. A., ... Dai, R. M. (2013). Commensal bacteria control cancer response to therapy by modulating the tumor microenvironment. *Science*, *342*(6161), 967–970. doi:10.1126cience.1240527 PMID:24264989

Li, H., & Jia, W. (2013). Cometabolism of microbes and host: Implications for drug metabolism and drug-induced toxicity. *Clinical Pharmacology and Therapeutics*, *94*(5), 574–581. doi:10.1038/clpt.2013.157 PMID:23933971

Li, J., Chen, H., Wang, B., Cai, C., Yang, X., Chai, Z., & Feng, W. (2017). ZnO nanoparticles act as supportive therapy in DSS-induced ulcerative colitis in mice by maintaining gut homeostasis and activating Nrf2 signaling. *Scientific Reports*, *7*(1), 43126. doi:10.1038rep43126 PMID:28233796

Li, J., Mizukami, Y., Zhang, X., Jo, W.-S., & Chung, D. C. (2005). Oncogenic K-ras Stimulates Wnt Signaling in Colon Cancer Through Inhibition of GSK-3β. *Gastroenterology*, *128*(7), 1907–1918. doi:10.1053/j.gastro.2005.02.067 PMID:15940626

Lim, B. O. (2004). Efficacy of wogonin in the production of immunoglobulins and cytokines by mesenteric lymph node lymphocytes in mouse colitis induced with dextran sulfate sodium. *Bioscience, Biotechnology, and Biochemistry*, *68*(12), 2505–2511. doi:10.1271/bbb.68.2505 PMID:15618621

Lin, X. B., Dieleman, L. A., Ketabi, A., Bibova, I., Sawyer, M. B., Xue, H., Field, C. J., Baracos, V. E., & Gänzle, M. G. (2012). Irinotecan (CPT-11) chemotherapy alters intestinal microbiota in tumour bearing rats. *PLoS One*, *7*(7), e39764. doi:10.1371/journal.pone.0039764 PMID:22844397

Liu, L., Li, Y. H., Niu, Y. B., Sun, Y., Guo, Z. J., Li, Q., Li, C., Feng, J., Cao, S. S., & Mei, Q. B. (2010). An apple oligogalactan prevents against inflammation and carcinogenesis by targeting LPS/TLR4/NF-κB pathway in a mouse model of colitis-associated colon cancer. *Carcinogenesis*, *31*(10), 1822–1832. doi:10.1093/carcin/bgq070 PMID:20400476

Li, W., Khor, T. O., Xu, C., Shen, G., Jeong, W. S., Yu, S., & Kong, A. N. (2008). Activation of Nrf2-antioxidant signaling attenuates NFkappaB-inflammatory response and elicits apoptosis. *Biochemical Pharmacology*, *76*(11), 1485–1489. doi:10.1016/j.bcp.2008.07.017 PMID:18694732

Li, Y., Shen, L., & Luo, H. (2016). Luteolin ameliorates dextran sulfate sodium-induced colitis in mice possibly through activation of the Nrf2 signaling pathway. *International Immunopharmacology*, *40*, 24–31. doi:10.1016/j.intimp.2016.08.020 PMID:27569028

Loftus, E. V. Jr. (2004). Clinical epidemiology of inflammatory bowel disease: Incidence, prevalence, and environmental influences. *Gastroenterology*, *126*(6), 1504–1517. doi:10.1053/j.gastro.2004.01.063 PMID:15168363

Lopez, J., & Grinspan, A. (2016). Fecal microbiota transplantation for inflammatory bowel disease. *Gastroenterology & Hepatology*, *12*(6), 374. PMID:27493597

Losh, M., Martin, G. E., Lee, M., Klusek, J., Sideris, J., Barron, S., & Wassink, T. (2017). Developmental Markers of Genetic Liability to Autism in Parents: A Longitudinal, Multigenerational Study. *Journal of Autism and Developmental Disorders*, *47*(3), 834–845. doi:10.100710803-016-2996-x PMID:28070788

Lo, W. C., Martin, E. W. Jr, Hitchcock, C. L., & Friedman, A. (2013). Mathematical model of colitis-associated colon cancer. *Journal of Theoretical Biology*, *317*, 20–29. doi:10.1016/j.jtbi.2012.09.025 PMID:23026764

Luo, C., & Zhang, H. (2017). The role of proinflammatory pathways in the pathogenesis of colitis-associated colorectal cancer. *Mediators of Inflammation*, *2017*, 2017. doi:10.1155/2017/5126048 PMID:28852270

Luo, X., Yu, Z., Deng, C., Zhang, J., Ren, G., Sun, A., Mani, S., Wang, Z., & Dou, W. (2017). Baicalein ameliorates TNBS-induced colitis by suppressing TLR4/MyD88 signaling cascade and NLRP3 inflammasome activation in mice. *Scientific Reports*, *7*(1), 16374. doi:10.103841598-017-12562-6 PMID:29180692

Lu, R., Wu, S., Zhang, Y. G., Xia, Y., Liu, X., Zheng, Y., ... Li, L. (2014). Enteric bacterial protein AvrA promotes colonic tumorigenesis and activates colonic beta-catenin signaling pathway. *Oncogenesis*, *3*(6), e105. doi:10.1038/oncsis.2014.20 PMID:24911876

Lyons, Y.A., Wu, S.Y., Overwijk, W.W., Baggerly, K.A., & Sood, A.K. (2017). Immune cell profiling in cancer: molecular approaches to cell-specific identification. *NPJ Precision Oncology, 1*(1), 26.

Macfarlane, G. T., & Cummings, J. H. (1999). Probiotics and prebiotics: Can regulating the activities of intestinal bacteria benefit health? *BMJ (Clinical Research Ed.)*, *318*(7189), 999–1003. doi:10.1136/bmj.318.7189.999 PMID:10195977

Magee, E. A., Edmond, L. M., Tasker, S. M., Kong, S. C., Curno, R., & Cummings, J. H. (2005). Associations between diet and disease activity in ulcerative colitis patients using a novel method of data analysis. *Nutrition Journal*, *4*(1), 7. doi:10.1186/1475-2891-4-7 PMID:15705205

Ma, H., Diao, Y., Zhao, D., Li, K., & Kang, T. (2010). A new alternative to treat swine influenza A virus infection: Extracts from Terminalia chebula Retz. *African Journal of Microbiological Research*, *4*, 497–499.

Mahdi, B. M. (2018). Introductory Chapter: Inflammatory Bowel Disease. In New Concepts in Inflammatory Bowel Disease. IntechOpen.

Mahlich, J., Matsuoka, K., Nakamura, Y., & Sruamsiri, R. (2017). The relationship between socio-demographic factors, health status, treatment type, and employment outcome in patients with inflammatory bowel disease in Japan. *BMC Public Health*, *17*(1), 1–7. doi:10.118612889-017-4516-0 PMID:28676039

Maitland, N. J., & Collins, A. T. (2008). Prostate cancer stem cells: A new target for therapy. *Journal of Clinical Oncology*, *26*(17), 2862–2870. doi:10.1200/JCO.2007.15.1472 PMID:18539965

Ma, J., Liu, J., Wang, Z., Gu, X., Fan, Y., Zhang, W., & Cai, D. (2014). NF-kappaB-dependent microRNA-425 upregulation promotes gastric cancer cell growth by targeting PTEN upon IL-1β induction. *Molecular Cancer*, *13*(1), 1–11. doi:10.1186/1476-4598-13-40

Ma, K. W., Cheung, T. T., Leung, B., She, B. W. H., Chok, K. S. H., Chan, A. C. Y., Dai, W. C., & Lo, C. M. (2019). Adjuvant chemotherapy improves oncological outcomes of resectable intrahepatic cholangiocarcinoma: A meta-analysis. *Medicine*, *98*(5), e14013. doi:10.1097/MD.0000000000014013 PMID:30702559

Malekzadeh, F., Ehsanifar, H., Shahamat, M., Levin, M., & Colwell, R. R. (2001). Antibacterial activity of black myrobalan (Terminalia chebula Retz) against Helicobacter pylori. *International Journal of Antimicrobial Agents*, *18*(1), 85–88. doi:10.1016/S0924-8579(01)00352-1 PMID:11463533

Malik, A., Sharma, D., Zhu, Q., Karki, R., Guy, C. S., Vogel, P., & Kanneganti, T. D. (2016). IL-33 regulates the IgA-microbiota axis to restrain IL-1α–dependent Colitis and tumorigenesis. *The Journal of Clinical Investigation*, *126*(12), 4469–4481. doi:10.1172/JCI88625 PMID:27775548

Manach, C., & Donovan, J. L. (2004). Pharmacokinetics and metabolism of dietary flavonoids in humans. *Free Radical Research*, *38*(8), 771–785. doi:10.1080/10715760410001727858 PMID:15493450

Manna, S., Bhattacharrya, D., Basak, D. K., & Mandal, T. K. (2004). Single oral dose toxicity study of α-cypermethrin in rats. *Indian Journal of Pharmacology*.

Mantzouranis, G., Fafliora, E., Saridi, M., Tatsioni, A., Glanztounis, G., Albani, E., & … . (2018). Alcohol and narcotics use in inflammatory bowel disease. *Annals of Gastroenterology*, *31*(6), 649–658. doi:10.20524/aog.2018.0302 PMID:30386114

Marchesi, J. R., Adams, D. H., Fava, F., Hermes, G. D., Hirschfield, G. M., Hold, G., ... Thomas, L. V. (2016). The gut microbiota and host health: A new clinical frontier. *Gut*, *65*(2), 330–339. doi:10.1136/gutjnl-2015-309990 PMID:26338727

Marchesi, J. R., Dutilh, B. E., Hall, N., Peters, W. H., Roelofs, R., Boleij, A., & Tjalsma, H. (2011). Towards the human colorectal cancer microbiome. *PLoS One*, *6*(5), e20447. doi:10.1371/journal.pone.0020447 PMID:21647227

Marco, E. J., Hinkley, L. B. N., Hill, S. S., & Nagarajan, S. S. (2011). Sensory processing in autism: A review of neurophysiologic findings. *Pediatric Research*, *69*(5 Pt 2), 48R–54R. doi:10.1203/PDR.0b013e3182130c54 PMID:21289533

Martin, M. A., Goya, L., & Ramos, S. (2013). Potential for preventive effects of cocoa and cocoa polyphenols in cancer. *Food and Chemical Toxicology*, *56*, 336–351. doi:10.1016/j.fct.2013.02.020 PMID:23439478

Martin, R., Chain, F., Miquel, S., Motta, J. P., Vergnolle, N., Sokol, H., & Langella, P. (2017). Using murine colitis models to analyze probiotics-host interactions. *FEMS Microbiology Reviews*, *41*(Supp_1), S49–S70. doi:10.1093/femsre/fux035 PMID:28830096

Mascaraque, C., Gonzalez, R., Suarez, M. D., Zarzuelo, A., Sanchez de Medina, F., & Martinez-Augustin, O. (2015). Intestinal anti-inflammatory activity of apigenin K in two rat colitis models induced by trinitrobenzenesulfonic acid and dextran sulphate sodium. *British Journal of Nutrition*, *113*(4), 618–626. doi:10.1017/S0007114514004292 PMID:25654996

Mathur, R., Sharma, A., Dixit, V. P., & Varma, M. (1996). Hypolipidaemic effect of fruit juice of Emblica officinalis in cholesterol-fed rabbits. *Journal of Ethnopharmacology*, *50*(2), 61–68. doi:10.1016/0378-8741(95)01308-3 PMID:8866725

Maxwell, J. R., Brown, W. A., Smith, C. L., Byrne, F. R., & Viney, J. L. (2009). Methods of inducing inflammatory bowel disease in mice. Current Protocols in Pharmacology.

Maynard, C. L., & Weaver, C. T. (2009). Intestinal effector T Cells in health and disease. *Immunity*, *31*(3), 389–400. doi:10.1016/j.immuni.2009.08.012 PMID:19766082

Mayne, C. G., & Williams, C. B. (2013). Induced and natural regulatory T cells in the development of inflammatory bowel disease. *Inflammatory Bowel Diseases*, *19*(8), 1772–1788. Advance online publication. doi:10.1097/MIB.0b013e318281f5a3 PMID:23656897

McCoy, A. N., Araujo-Perez, F., Azcarate-Peril, A., Yeh, J. J., Sandler, R. S., & Keku, T. O. (2013). Fusobacterium is associated with colorectal adenomas. *PLoS One*, *8*(1), e53653. doi:10.1371/journal.pone.0053653 PMID:23335968

McKenzie, A. N., Li, X., Largaespada, D. A., Sato, A., Kaneda, A., Zurawski, S. M., & Copeland, N. G. (1993). Structural comparison and chromosomal localization of the human and mouse IL-13 genes. *Journal of Immunology (Baltimore, Md.: 1950)*, *150*(12), 5436–5444. PMID:8099936

Medina, M. Á. (2018). Mathematical modeling of cancer metabolism. *Critical Reviews in Oncology/Hematology*, *124*, 37–40. doi:10.1016/j.critrevonc.2018.02.004 PMID:29548484

Meeusen, E., Lim, E., & Mathivanan, S. (2017). Secreted Tumor Antigens - Immune Biomarkers for Diagnosis and Therapy. *Proteomics*, *17*(23-24), 1600442. doi:10.1002/pmic.201600442 PMID:28714192

Mentella, M. C., Scaldaferri, F., Pizzoferrato, M., Gasbarrini, A., & Miggiano, G. A. D. (2020). Nutrition, IBD and gut Microbiota: A review. *Nutrients*, *12*(4), 944. doi:10.3390/nu12040944 PMID:32235316

Metcalf, C. (2002). Crohn's disease: an overview. *Nursing Standard, 16*(31), 45.

Miean, K. H., & Mohamed, S. (2001). Flavonoid (myricetin, quercetin, kaempferol, luteolin, and apigenin) content of edible tropical plants. *Journal of Agricultural and Food Chemistry*, *49*(6), 3106–3112. doi:10.1021/jf000892m PMID:11410016

Milackova, I., Prnova, M. S., Majekova, M., Sotnikova, R., Stasko, M., Kovacikova, L., Banerjee, S., Veverka, M., & Stefek, M. (2015). 2-Chloro-1,4-naphthoquinone derivative of quercetin as an inhibitor of aldose reductase and anti-inflammatory agent. *Journal of Enzyme Inhibition and Medicinal Chemistry*, *30*(1), 107–113. doi:10.3109/14756366.2014.892935 PMID:24666303

Miłkowska, P., Popko, K., Demkow, U., & Wolańczyk, T. (2017). Pro-inflammatory Cytokines in Psychiatric Disorders in Children and Adolescents: A Review. *Advances in Experimental Medicine and Biology*, *1021*, 73–80. doi:10.1007/5584_2017_32 PMID:28405892

Mira-Pascual, L., Cabrera-Rubio, R., Ocon, S., Costales, P., Parra, A., Suarez, A., Moris, F., Rodrigo, L., Mira, A., & Collado, M. C. (2015). Microbial mucosal colonic shifts associated with the development of colorectal cancer reveal the presence of different bacterial and archaeal biomarkers. *Journal of Gastroenterology*, *50*(2), 167–179. doi:10.100700535-014-0963-x PMID:24811328

Mirsepasi-Lauridsen, H. C., Du, Z., Struve, C., Charbon, G., Karczewski, J., Krogfelt, K. A., & Wells, J. M. (2016). Secretion of alpha-hemolysin by Escherichia coli disrupts tight junctions in ulcerative colitis patients. *Clinical and Translational Gastroenterology*, *7*(3), e149. doi:10.1038/ctg.2016.3 PMID:26938480

Mishra, M., Pathak, U. N., & Khan, A. B. (1981). Emblica officinalis Gaertn and serum cholesterol level in experimental rabbits. *British Journal of Experimental Pathology*, *62*, 526–528. PMID:7295546

Mitchell, J. P., & Carmody, R. J. (2018). NF-kappa B and the transcriptional control of inflammation. *International Review of Cell and Molecular Biology*, *335*, 41–84. doi:10.1016/bs.ircmb.2017.07.007 PMID:29305014

Miyaki, M., Konishi, M., Kikuchi-Yanoshita, R., Enomoto, M., Igari, T., Tanaka, K., ... Fukayama, M. (1994). Characteristics of somatic mutation of the adenomatous polyposis coli gene in colorectal tumors. *Cancer Research*, *54*(11), 3011–3020. PMID:8187091

Miyoshi, J., Bobe, A. M., Miyoshi, S., Huang, Y., Hubert, N., Delmont, T. O., Eren, A. M., Leone, V., & Chang, E. B. (2017). Peripartum Antibiotics Promote Gut Dysbiosis, Loss of Immune Tolerance, and Inflammatory Bowel Disease in Genetically Prone Offspring. *Cell Reports*, *20*(2), 491–504. Advance online publication. doi:10.1016/j.celrep.2017.06.060 PMID:28700948

Mizoguchi, A. (2012). Animal models of inflammatory bowel disease. *Progress in Molecular Biology and Translational Science*, *105*, 263–320. doi:10.1016/B978-0-12-394596-9.00009-3 PMID:22137435

Moayyedi, P., Surette, M. G., Kim, P. T., Libertucci, J., Wolfe, M., Onischi, C., Armstrong, D., Marshall, J. K., Kassam, Z., Reinisch, W., & Lee, C. H. (2015). Fecal microbiota transplantation induces remission in patients with active ulcerative Colitis in a randomized controlled trial. *Gastroenterology*, *149*(1), 102–109. doi:10.1053/j.gastro.2015.04.001 PMID:25857665

Mochizuki, M., & Hasegawa, N. (2005). Protective effect of (-)-epigallocatechin gallate on acute experimental colitis. *Journal of Health Science*, *51*(3), 362–364. doi:10.1248/jhs.51.362

Mochizuki, M., & Hasegawa, N. (2010). (-)-Epigallocatechin-3-gallate reduces experimental colon injury in rats by regulating macrophage and mast cell. *Phytotherapy Research*, *24*(S1), S120–S122. doi:10.1002/ptr.2862 PMID:19548282

Mohan, K., Paramasivam, R., Chandran, P., Veerasami, V., Gnanasekaran, A., Shanmugam, A., & … . (2011). Inhibition of Hepatitis B virus DNA polymerase and modulation of TH1 and TH2 cytokine secretion by three Indian medicinal plants and its correlation with antiviral properties. *Journal of Pharmacy Research*, *4*, 1044–1046.

Molodecky, N. A., & Kaplan, G. G. (2010). Environmental risk factors for inflammatory bowel disease. *Gastroenterology & Hepatology*, *6*(5), 339. PMID:20567592

Molodecky, N. A., Soon, I. S., Rabi, D. M., Ghali, W. A., Ferris, M., Chernoff, G., Benchimol, E. I., Panaccione, R., Ghosh, S., Barkema, H. W., & Kaplan, G. G. (2012). Increasing incidence and prevalence of the inflammatory bowel diseases with time, based on systematic review. *Gastroenterology*, *142*(1), 46–54.e42. Advance online publication. doi:10.1053/j.gastro.2011.10.001 PMID:22001864

Moore, M., Gill, S., Asmis, T., Berry, S., Burkes, R., Zbuk, K., Alcindor, T., Jeyakumar, A., Chan, T., Rao, S., Spratlin, J., Tang, P. A., Rothenstein, J., Chan, E., Bendell, J., Kudrik, F., Kauh, J., Tang, S., Gao, L., ... Strevel, E. (2016). Randomized phase II study of modified FOLFOX-6 in combination with ramucirumab or icrucumab as second-line therapy in patients with metastatic colorectal cancer after disease progression on first-line irinotecan-based therapy. *Annals of Oncology: Official Journal of the European Society for Medical Oncology*, *27*(12), 2216–2224. doi:10.1093/annonc/mdw412 PMID:27733377

Morampudi, V., Dalwadi, U., Bhinder, G., Sham, H. P., Gill, S. K., Chan, J., ... Gibson, D. L. (2016). The goblet cell-derived mediator RELM-β drives spontaneous Colitis in Muc2-deficient mice by promoting commensal microbial dysbiosis. *Mucosal Immunology*, *9*(5), 1218–1233. doi:10.1038/mi.2015.140 PMID:26813339

Moreno, J. J. (2017). Eicosanoid receptors: Targets for the treatment of disrupted intestinal epithelial homeostasis. *European Journal of Pharmacology*, *796*, 7–19. doi:10.1016/j.ejphar.2016.12.004 PMID:27940058

Mukhopadhya, I., Hansen, R., Nicholl, C. E., Alhaidan, Y. A., Thomson, J. M., Berry, S. H., Pattinson, C., Stead, D. A., Russell, R. K., El-Omar, E. M., & Hold, G. L. (2011). A comprehensive evaluation of colonic mucosal isolates of Sutterella wadsworthensis from inflammatory bowel disease. *PLoS One*, *6*(10), e27076. doi:10.1371/journal.pone.0027076 PMID:22073125

Mullie, P., Clarys, P., Deriemaeker, P., & Hebbelinck, M. (2007). Estimation of daily human intake of food flavonoids. *Plant Foods for Human Nutrition (Dordrecht, Netherlands)*, *62*(3), 93–98. doi:10.100711130-007-0047-7 PMID:17597415

Munro, M. J., Wickremesekera, S. K., Peng, L., Tan, S. T., & Itinteang, T. (2018). Cancer stem cells in colorectal cancer: A review. *Journal of Clinical Pathology*, *71*(2), 110–116. doi:10.1136/jclinpath-2017-204739 PMID:28942428

Mutoh, M., Watanabe, K., Kitamura, T., Shoji, Y., Takahashi, M., Kawamori, T., ... Wakabayashi, K. (2002). Involvement of prostaglandin E receptor subtype EP4 in colon carcinogenesis. *Cancer Research*, *62*(1), 28–32. PMID:11782353

Nachshon-Kedmi, M., Yannai, S., Haj, A., & Fares, F. A. (2003). Indole-3-carbinol and 3,3′-diindolylmethane induce apoptosis in human prostate cancer cells. *Food and Chemical Toxicology*, *41*(6), 745–752. doi:10.1016/S0278-6915(03)00004-8 PMID:12738179

Naeem, M., Bae, J., Oshi, M. A., Kim, M. S., Moon, H. R., Lee, B. L., ... Yoo, J. W. (2018). Colon-targeted delivery of cyclosporine A using dual-functional Eudragit((R)) FS30D/PLGA nanoparticles ameliorates murine experimental colitis. *International Journal of Nanomedicine*, *13*, 1225–1240. doi:10.2147/IJN.S157566 PMID:29535519

Naeem, M., Oshi, M. A., Kim, J., Lee, J., Cao, J., Nurhasni, H., Im, E., Jung, Y., & Yoo, J. W. (2018). pH-triggered surface charge-reversal nanoparticles alleviate experimental murine colitis via selective accumulation in inflamed colon regions. *Nanomedicine (London)*, *14*(3), 823–834. doi:10.1016/j.nano.2018.01.003 PMID:29353017

Nagar, S., Belapurkar, P., Barua, P. T., & Goyal, P. (2011). Antimicrobial and phytochemical analysis of Triphala and comparison with its individual constituents. *National Journal of Life Sciences*, *8*, 101–103.

Nam, S. Y., Kim, J. S., Kim, J. M., Lee, J. Y., Kim, N., Jung, H. C., & Song, I. S. (2008). DA-6034, a derivative of flavonoid, prevents and ameliorates dextran sulfate sodium-induced colitis and inhibits colon carcinogenesis. *Experimental Biology and Medicine (Maywood, N.J.)*, *233*(2), 180–191. doi:10.3181/0707-RM-186 PMID:18222973

Nawa, T., Kato, J., Kawamoto, H., Okada, H., Yamamoto, H., Kohno, H., Endo, H., & Shiratori, Y. (2008). Differences between right- and left-sided colon cancer in patient characteristics, cancer morphology and histology. *Journal of Gastroenterology and Hepatology*, *23*(3), 418–423. doi:10.1111/j.1440-1746.2007.04923.x PMID:17532785

Neuhouser, M. L. (2004). Dietary flavonoids and cancer risk: Evidence from human population studies. *Nutrition and Cancer*, *50*(1), 1–7. doi:10.120715327914nc5001_1 PMID:15572291

Ng, S. C., Shi, H. Y., Hamidi, N., Underwood, F. E., Tang, W., Benchimol, E. I., Panaccione, R., Ghosh, S., Wu, J. C. Y., Chan, F. K. L., Sung, J. J. Y., & Kaplan, G. G. (2018). Worldwide incidence and prevalence of inflammatory bowel disease in the 21st century: A systematic review of population-based studies. *Lancet*, *390*(10114), 2769–2778. doi:10.1016/S0140-6736(17)32448-0 PMID:29050646

Ng, S. C., Tang, W., Ching, J. Y., Wong, M., Chow, C. M., Hui, A. J., Wong, T. C., Leung, V. K., Tsang, S. W., Yu, H. H., Li, M. F., Ng, K. K., Kamm, M. A., Studd, C., Bell, S., Leong, R., de Silva, H. J., Kasturiratne, A., Mufeena, M. N. F., ... Chan, F. K. L. (2013). Incidence and phenotype of inflammatory bowel disease based on results from the Asia-pacific Crohn's and colitis epidemiology study. *Gastroenterology*, *145*(1), 158–165 e152. doi:10.1053/j.gastro.2013.04.007 PMID:23583432

Nicastro, H. L., Firestone, G. L., & Bjeldanes, L. F. (2013). 3,3′-diindolylmethane rapidly and selectively inhibits hepatocyte growth factor/c-Met signaling in breast cancer cells. *The Journal of Nutritional Biochemistry*, *24*(11), 1882–1888. doi:10.1016/j.jnutbio.2013.05.004 PMID:23968581

Nidhi, D., Dadwal, A., Hallan, S. S., Sharma, S., & Mishra, N. (2017, August 18). A., Hallan, S. S., Sharma, S., & Mishra, N. (2017). Development of enteric-coated microspheres of embelin for their beneficial pharmacological potential in ulcerative colitis. *Artificial Cells, Nanomedicine, and Biotechnology*, *45*(6), 1092–1100. Advance online publication. doi:10.1080/21691401.2016.1202258 PMID:27388946

Nieman, D. C., Kay, C. D., Rathore, A. S., Grace, M. H., Strauch, R. C., Stephan, E. H., Sakaguchi, C., & Lila, M. (2018). Increased plasma levels of gut-derived phenolics linked to walking and running following two weeks of flavonoid supplementation. *Nutrients*, *10*(11), 1718. doi:10.3390/nu10111718 PMID:30423955

Nishitani, Y., Yamamoto, K., Yoshida, M., Azuma, T., Kanazawa, K., Hashimoto, T., & Mizuno, M. (2013). Intestinal anti-inflammatory activity of luteolin: Role of the aglycone in NF-kappa B inactivation in macrophages co-cultured with intestinal epithelial cells. *BioFactors (Oxford, England)*, *39*(5), 522–533. doi:10.1002/biof.1091 PMID:23460110

O'Connor, P. M., Lapointe, T. K., Beck, P. L., & Buret, A. G. (2010). Mechanisms by which inflammation may increase intestinal cancer risk in inflammatory bowel disease. *Inflammatory Bowel Diseases*, *16*(8), 1411–1420. doi:10.1002/ibd.21217 PMID:20155848

O'Hara, M., Kiefer, D., Farrell, K., & Kemper, K. (1998). A review of 12 commonly used medicinal herbs. *Archives of Family Medicine*, *7*(6), 523–536. doi:10.1001/archfami.7.6.523 PMID:9821826

Ocete, M. A., Galvez, J., Crespo, M. E., Cruz, T., Gonzalez, M., Torres, M. I., & Zarzuelo, A. (1998). Effects of morin on an experimental model of acute colitis in rats. *Pharmacology*, *57*(5), 261–270. doi:10.1159/000028250 PMID:9742291

Ohhara, Y., Fukuda, N., Takeuchi, S., Honma, R., Shimizu, Y., Kinoshita, I., & Dosaka-Akita, H. (2016). Role of targeted therapy in metastatic colorectal cancer. *World Journal of Gastrointestinal Oncology*, *8*(9), 642–655. doi:10.4251/wjgo.v8.i9.642 PMID:27672422

Okamoto, R., Tsuchiya, K., Nemoto, Y., Akiyama, J., Nakamura, T., Kanai, T., & Watanabe, M. (2009). Requirement of Notch activation during regeneration of the intestinal epithelia. *American Journal of Physiology. Gastrointestinal and Liver Physiology*, *296*(1), G23–G35. doi:10.1152/ajpgi.90225.2008 PMID:19023031

Olejarz, W., Dominiak, A., Żołnierzak, A., Kubiak-Tomaszewska, G., & Lorenc, T. (2020). Tumor-Derived Exosomes in Immunosuppression and Immunotherapy. *Journal of Immunology Research*, *2020*, 6272498. doi:10.1155/2020/6272498 PMID:32537468

Olivera, P., Danese, S., Jay, N., Natoli, G., & Peyrin-Biroulet, L. (2019). Big data in IBD: A look into the future. *Nature Reviews. Gastroenterology & Hepatology*, *16*(5), 312–321. doi:10.103841575-019-0102-5 PMID:30659247

Ordas, I., Eckmann, L., Talamini, M., Baumgart, D. C., & Sandborn, W. J. (2012). Ulcerative colitis. *Lancet*, *380*(9853), 1606–1619. doi:10.1016/S0140-6736(12)60150-0 PMID:22914296

Osburn, W. O., Karim, B., Dolan, P. M., Liu, G., Yamamoto, M., Huso, D. L., & Kensler, T. W. (2007). Increased colonic inflammatory injury and formation of aberrant crypt foci in Nrf2-deficient mice upon dextran sulfate treatment. *International Journal of Cancer*, *121*(9), 1883–1891. doi:10.1002/ijc.22943 PMID:17631644

Osburn, W. O., Wakabayashi, N., Misra, V., Nilles, T., Biswal, S., Trush, M. A., & Kensler, T. W. (2006). Nrf2 regulates an adaptive response protecting against oxidative damage following diquat-mediated formation of superoxide anion. *Archives of Biochemistry and Biophysics*, *454*(1), 7–15. doi:10.1016/j.abb.2006.08.005 PMID:16962985

Osmani, L., Askin, F., Gabrielson, E., & Li, Q. K. (2018). Current WHO guidelines and the critical role of immunohistochemical markers in the subclassification of non-small cell lung carcinoma (NSCLC): Moving from targeted therapy to immunotherapy. *Seminars in Cancer Biology*, *52*, 103–109. doi:10.1016/j.semcancer.2017.11.019 PMID:29183778

Ou, J., Carbonero, F., Zoetendal, E. G., DeLany, J. P., Wang, M., Newton, K., Gaskins, H. R., & O'Keefe, S. J. (2013). Diet, microbiota, and microbial metabolites in colon cancer risk in rural Africans and African Americans. *The American Journal of Clinical Nutrition*, *98*(1), 111–120. doi:10.3945/ajcn.112.056689 PMID:23719549

Owczarek, D., Rodacki, T., Domagala-Rodacka, R., Cibor, D., & Mach, T. (2016). Diet and nutritional factors in inflammatory bowel diseases. *World Journal of Gastroenterology*, *22*(3), 895–905. doi:10.3748/wjg.v22.i3.895 PMID:26811635

Panda, S., & Kar, A. (2003). Fruit extract of Emblica officinalis ameliorates hyperthyroidism and hepatic lipid peroxidation in mice. *Die Pharmazie*, *58*, 753–755. PMID:14609291

Pandurangan, A. K., Ismail, S., Saadatdoust, Z., & Esa, N. M. (2015). Allicin alleviates Dextran sodium sulfate (DSS)-induced ulcerative colitis in BALB/c mice. Oxidative Medicine and Cellular Longevity.

Pandurangan, A. K., Ananda Sadagopan, S. K., Dharmalingam, P., & Ganapasam, S. (2014). Luteolin, a bioflavonoid inhibits Azoxymethane-induced colorectal cancer through activation of Nrf2 signaling. *Toxicology Mechanisms and Methods*, *24*(1), 13–20. doi:10.3109/15376516.2013.843111 PMID:24024667

Pandurangan, A. K., Dharmalingam, P., Sadagopan, S. K., & Ganapasam, S. (2014). Luteolin inhibits matrix metalloproteinase 9 and 2 in azoxymethane-induced colon carcinogenesis. *Human and Experimental Toxicology*, *33*(11), 1176–1185. doi:10.1177/0960327114522502 PMID:24532706

Pandurangan, A. K., & Esa, N. M. (2014). Luteolin, a bioflavonoid inhibits colorectal cancer through modulation of multiple signaling pathways: A review. *Asian Pacific Journal of Cancer Prevention*, *15*(14), 5501–5508. doi:10.7314/APJCP.2014.15.14.5501 PMID:25081655

Pandurangan, A. K., Kumar, S. A. S., Dharmalingam, P., & Ganapasam, S. (2014). Luteolin, a bioflavonoid inhibits azoxymethane-induced colon carcinogenesis: Involvement of iNOS and COX-2. *Pharmacognosy Magazine*, *10*(38, Suppl 2), S306. doi:10.4103/0973-1296.133285 PMID:24991108

Pandurangan, A. K., Mohebali, N., Hasanpourghadi, M., Looi, C. Y., Mustafa, M. R., & Norhaizan, M. E. (2016). Boldine suppresses dextran sulfate sodium-induced mouse experimental colitis: NF-κB and IL-6/STAT3 as potential targets. *BioFactors (Oxford, England)*, *42*(3), 247–258. PMID:26891685

Pandurangan, A. K., Mohebali, N., Norhaizan, M. E., & Looi, C. Y. (2015a). Gallic acid attenuates dextran sodium sulfate (DSS)-induced experimental acute ulcerative colitis in BALB/c mice. *Drug Design, Development and Therapy*, *9*(1), 3932–3934.

Pandurangan, A. K., Mohebali, N., Norhaizan, M. E., Looi, C. Y., Salmiah, I., & Saadatdoust, Z. (2015). Gallic acid suppresses inflammation of dextran sodium sulfate-induced colitis in mice: Possible mechanisms. *International Immunopharmacology*, *28*(2), 1034–1043. doi:10.1016/j.intimp.2015.08.019 PMID:26319951

Pandurangan, A. K., & Norhaizan, M. E. (2014). Signal Transducer and Activator of Transcription 3: A Promising target in colitis associated cancer. *Asian Pacific Journal of Cancer Prevention*, *15*(2), 551–560. doi:10.7314/APJCP.2014.15.2.551 PMID:24568457

Pandurangan, A. K., Saadatdoust, Z., Esa, N. M., Hamzah, H., & Ismail, A. (2015). Dietary Cocoa protects against colitis-associated cancer by activating Nrf2/Keap1 pathway. *BioFactors (Oxford, England)*, *41*(1), 1–14. doi:10.1002/biof.1195 PMID:25545372

Panes, J., & Salas, A. (2018). Past, present and future of therapeutic interventions targeting leukocyte trafficking in inflammatory bowel disease. *Journal of Crohn's and Colitis*, *12*(suppl_2), S633–S640. doi:10.1093/ecco-jcc/jjy011 PMID:30137311

Panizza, P. S. B., Viana, P. C. C., Horvat, N., dos Santos, V. R., de Araújo, D. A. P., Yamanari, T. R., & Cerri, G. G. (2017). Inflammatory bowel disease: current role of imaging in diagnosis and detection of complications: gastrointestinal imaging. *Radiographics*, *37*(2), 701–702. doi:10.1148/rg.2017160050 PMID:28287943

Pannuti, A., Foreman, K., Rizzo, P., Osipo, C., Golde, T., Osborne, B., & Miele, L. (2010). Targeting Notch to Target Cancer Stem Cells. *Clinical Cancer Research*, *16*(12), 3141–3152. doi:10.1158/1078-0432.CCR-09-2823 PMID:20530696

Papadopoulos, V., Tsapakidis, K., Riobo Del Galdo, N. A., Papandreou, C. N., Del Galdo, F., Anthoney, A., Sakellaridis, N., Dimas, K., & Kamposioras, K. (2016). The Prognostic Significance of the Hedgehog Signaling Pathway in Colorectal Cancer. *Clinical Colorectal Cancer*, *15*(2), 116–127. doi:10.1016/j.clcc.2016.02.010 PMID:27032873

Papaioannou, N. E., Beniata, O. V., Vitsos, P., Tsitsilonis, O., & Samara, P. (2016). Harnessing the immune system to improve cancer therapy. *Annals of Translational Medicine*, *4*(14), 261. doi:10.21037/atm.2016.04.01 PMID:27563648

Park, E., Hwang, I., Song, J. Y., & Jee, Y. (2011). Acidic polysaccharide of Panax ginseng as a defense against small intestinal damage by whole-body gamma irradiation of mice. *Acta Histochemica*, *113*(1), 19–23. doi:10.1016/j.acthis.2009 07.003 PMID:19767060

Park, M. Y., Ji, G. E., & Sung, M. K. (2012). Dietary kaempferol suppresses inflammation of dextran sulfate sodium-induced colitis in mice. *Digestive Diseases and Sciences*, *57*(2), 355–363. doi:10.100710620-011-1883-8 PMID:21901258

Patterson, H., Nibbs, R., Mcinnes, I., & Siebert, S. (2014). Protein kinase inhibitors in the treatment of inflammatory and autoimmune diseases. *Clinical and Experimental Immunology*, *176*(1), 1–10. Advance online publication. doi:10.1111/cei.12248 PMID:24313320

Pei, L. Y., Ke, Y. S., Zhao, H. H., Wang, L., Jia, C., Liu, W. Z., Fu, Q., Shi, M., Cui, J., & Li, S. C. (2019). Role of colonic microbiota in the pathogenesis of ulcerative colitis. *BMC Gastroenterology*, *19*(1), 10. doi:10.118612876-019-0930-3 PMID:30642266

Peng, L., Khan, N., Afaq, F., Ye, C., & Mukhtar, H. (2010). In vitro and in vivo effects of water extract of white cocoa tea (Camellia ptilophylla) against human prostate cancer. *Pharmaceutical Research*, *27*(6), 1128–1137. doi:10.100711095-010-0052-7 PMID:20224992

Perianayagam, J. B., Sharma, S. K., Joseph, A., & Christina, A. J. (2004). Evaluation of anti-pyretic and analgesic activity of Emblica officinalis Gaertn. *Journal of Ethnopharmacology*, *95*(1), 83–85. doi:10.1016/j.jep.2004.06.020 PMID:15374611

Permpoon, V., Pongpirul, K., & Anuras, S. (2016). Ethnic variations in ulcerative colitis: Experience of an international hospital in Thailand. *World Journal of Gastrointestinal Pharmacology and Therapeutics*, *7*(3), 428–433. doi:10.4292/wjgpt.v7.i3.428 PMID:27602244

Petersen, I., Gilbert, R., Evans, S., Ridolfi, A., & Nazareth, I. (2010). Oral antibiotic prescribing during pregnancy in primary care: UK population-based study. *The Journal of Antimicrobial Chemotherapy*, *65*(10), 2238–2246. Advance online publication. doi:10.1093/jac/dkq307 PMID:20716554

Pickert, G., Neufert, C., Leppkes, M., Zheng, Y., Wittkopf, N., Warntjen, M., Lehr, H.-A., Hirth, S., Weigmann, B., Wirtz, S., Ouyang, W., Neurath, M. F., & Becker, C. (2009). STAT3 links IL-22 signaling in intestinal epithelial cells to mucosal wound healing. *The Journal of Experimental Medicine*, *206*(7), 1465–1472. Advance online publication. doi:10.1084/jem.20082683 PMID:19564350

Pinczowski, D., Ekbom, A., Baron, J., Yuen, J., & Adami, H. O. (1994). Risk factors for colorectal cancer in patients with ulcerative colitis: A case-control study. *Gastroenterology*, *107*(1), 117–120. doi:10.1016/0016-5085(94)90068-X PMID:7912678

Pithadia, A. B., & Jain, S. (2011). Treatment of inflammatory bowel disease (IBD). *Pharmacological Reports*, *63*(3), 629–642. doi:10.1016/S1734-1140(11)70575-8 PMID:21857074

Podolsky, D. K. (1991). Inflammatory bowel disease. *The New England Journal of Medicine*, *325*(13), 928–937. doi:10.1056/NEJM199109263251306 PMID:1881418

Poh, S., Putt, K. S., & Low, P. S. (2017). Folate-Targeted Dendrimers Selectively Accumulate at Sites of Inflammation in Mouse Models of Ulcerative Colitis and Atherosclerosis. *Biomacromolecules*, *18*(10), 3082–3088. doi:10.1021/acs.biomac.7b00728 PMID:28863264

Polat, F. R., & Karaboga, I. (2018). Immunohistochemical examination of anti-inflammatory and anti-apoptotic effects of hesperetin on trinitrobenzene sulfonic acid induced colitis in rats. *Biotechnic & Histochemistry*, 1–8. PMID:30383440

Popivanova, B. K., Kitamura, K., Wu, Y., Kondo, T., Kagaya, T., Kaneko, S., & Mukaida, N. (2008). Blocking TNF-α in mice reduces colorectal carcinogenesis associated with chronic colitis. *The Journal of Clinical Investigation*, *118*(2), 560–570. doi:10.1172/JCI32453 PMID:18219394

Poudyal, D., Le, P. M., Davis, T., Hofseth, A. B., Chumanevich, A., Chumanevich, A. A., ... Hofseth, L. J. (2012). A hexane fraction of American ginseng suppresses mouse colitis and associated colon cancer: Anti-inflammatory and proapoptotic mechanisms. *Cancer Prevention Research (Philadelphia, Pa.)*, *5*(4), 685–696. doi:10.1158/1940-6207.CAPR-11-0421 PMID:22293630

Power, K. A., Lu, J. T., Monk, J. M., Lepp, D., Wu, W. Q., Zhang, C., Liu, R., Tsao, R., Robinson, L. E., Wood, G. A., & Wolyn, D. J. (2016). Purified rutin and rutin-rich asparagus attenuates disease severity and tissue damage following dextran sodium sulfate-induced colitis. *Molecular Nutrition & Food Research*, *60*(11), 2396–2412. doi:10.1002/mnfr.201500890 PMID:27349947

Price, T. J., Peeters, M., Kim, T. W., Li, J., Cascinu, S., Ruff, P., Suresh, A. S., Thomas, A., Tjulandin, S., Zhang, K., Murugappan, S., & Sidhu, R. (2014). Panitumumab versus cetuximab in patients with chemotherapy-refractory wild-type KRAS exon 2 metastatic colorectal cancer (ASPECCT): A randomised, multicentre, open-label, non-inferiority phase 3 study. *The Lancet. Oncology*, *15*(6), 569–579. doi:10.1016/S1470-2045(14)70118-4 PMID:24739896

Prince, M. E., Sivanandan, R., Kaczorowski, A., Wolf, G. T., Kaplan, M. J., Dalerba, P., Weissman, I. L., Clarke, M. F., & Ailles, L. E. (2007). Identification of a subpopulation of cells with cancer stem cell properties in head and neck squamous cell carcinoma. *Proceedings of the National Academy of Sciences of the United States of America*, *104*(3), 973–978. doi:10.1073/pnas.0610117104 PMID:17210912

Prorok-Hamon, M., Friswell, M. K., Alswied, A., Roberts, C. L., Song, F., Flanagan, P. K., ... Hall, N. (2014). Colonic mucosa-associated diffusely adherent afaC+ Escherichia coli expressing lpfA and pks are increased in inflammatory bowel disease and colon cancer. *Gut*, *63*(5), 761–770. doi:10.1136/gutjnl-2013-304739 PMID:23846483

Qin, H. Y., Wu, J. C., Tong, X. D., Sung, J. J., Xu, H. X., & Bian, Z. X. (2011). Systematic review of animal models of post-infectious/post-inflammatory irritable bowel syndrome. *Journal of Gastroenterology and Hepatology*, *46*(2), 164–174. PMID:20848144

Quezada, S. M., & Cross, R. K. (2012). Association of age at diagnosis and ulcerative colitis phenotype. *Digestive Diseases and Sciences*, *57*(9), 2402–2407. doi:10.100710620-012-2081-z PMID:22370916

Rabe, B., Chalaris, A., May, U., Waetzig, G. H., Seegert, D., Williams, A. S., & Scheller, J. (2008). Transgenic blockade of interleukin 6 transsignaling abrogates inflammation. *Blood*, *111*(3), 1021–1028. doi:10.1182/blood-2007-07-102137 PMID:17989316

Rachmawati, H., Pradana, A. T., Safitri, D., & Adnyana, I. K. (2017). Multiple Functions of D-alpha-Tocopherol Polyethylene Glycol 1000 Succinate (TPGS) as Curcumin Nanoparticle Stabilizer: In Vivo Kinetic Profile and Anti-Ulcerative Colitis Analysis in Animal Model. *Pharmaceutics, 9*(3), 24. Advance online publication. doi:10.3390/pharmaceutics9030024 PMID:28754010

Radulovic, K., Normand, S., Rehman, A., Delanoye-Crespin, A., Chatagnon, J., Delacre, M., Waldschmitt, N., Poulin, L. F., Iovanna, J., Ryffel, B., Rosenstiel, P., & Chamaillard, M. (2018). A dietary flavone confers communicable protection against colitis through NLRP6 signaling independently of inflammasome activation. *Mucosal Immunology, 11*(3), 811–819. doi:10.1038/mi.2017.87 PMID:29139477

Rajak, S., Banerjee, S. K., Sood, S., Dinda, K. A., Gupta, Y. K., & Maulik, S. K. (2004). Emblica officinalis causes myocardial adaptation and protects against oxidative stress in ischemic-reperfusion injury in rats. *Phytotherapy Research, 18*(1), 54–60. doi:10.1002/ptr.1367 PMID:14750202

Rajilić-Stojanović, M., & de Vos, W. M. (2014). The first 1000 cultured species of the human gastrointestinal microbiota. *FEMS Microbiology Reviews, 38*(5), 996–1047. doi:10.1111/1574-6976.12075 PMID:24861948

Ramos, G. P., & Papadakis, K. A. (2019). Mechanisms of disease: Inflammatory bowel diseases. *Mayo Clinic Proceedings, 94*(1), 155–165. doi:10.1016/j.mayocp.2018.09.013 PMID:30611442

Randhawa, P. K., Singh, K., Singh, N., & Jaggi, A. S. (2014). A review on chemical-induced inflammatory bowel disease models in rodents. *The Korean Journal of Physiology & Pharmacology; Official Journal of the Korean Physiological Society and the Korean Society of Pharmacology, 18*(4), 279–288. doi:10.4196/kjpp.2014.18.4.279 PMID:25177159

Ran, X., Li, Y. H., Chen, G. X., Fu, S. P., He, D. W., Huang, B. X., Wei, L., Lin, Y., Guo, Y., & Hu, G. (2018). Farrerol ameliorates TNBS-induced colonic inflammation by inhibiting ERK1/2, JNK1/2, and NF-kappa B signaling pathway. *International Journal of Molecular Sciences, 19*(7), 2037. doi:10.3390/ijms19072037 PMID:30011811

Ran, Z. H., Chen, C., & Xiao, S. D. (2008). Epigallocatechin-3-gallate ameliorates rats colitis induced by acetic acid. *Biomedicine and Pharmacotherapy, 62*(3), 189–196. doi:10.1016/j.biopha.2008.02.002 PMID:18325726

Rastogi, R. P., & Mehrotra, B. N. (1991). Indian Medicinal Plants. In Compendium of Indian Medicinal plants - vol 1, (pp.1960-69). Central Drug Research Institute (CDRI), Lucknow and Publication and Information Directorate, Council of Scientific and Industrial Research (CSIR), New Delhi.

Rastogi, R. P., & Mehrotra, B. N. (1993). Indian Medicinal Plants. In Compendium of Indian Medicinal Plants - vol III, (pp.1985-89). Central Drug Research Institute (CDRI), Lucknow and Publication and Information Directorate, Council of Scientific and Industrial Research (CSIR), New Delhi.

Rastogi, R. P., & Mehrotra, B. N. (1995). Indian Medicinal Plants. In Compendium of Indian Medicinal Plants - vol IV, (pp.1985-89). Central Drug Research Institute (CDRI), Lucknow and Publication and Information Directorate, Council of Scientific and Industrial Research (CSIR), New Delhi.

Ravishankar, B., & Shukla, V. J. (2007). Indian systems of medicine: A brief profile. *AJTCAM*, *4*(3), 319–337. doi:10.4314/ajtcam.v4i3.31226 PMID:20161896

Ray, G. (2016). Inflammatory bowel disease in India-Past, present and future. *World Journal of Gastroenterology*, *22*(36), 8123. doi:10.3748/wjg.v22.i36.8123 PMID:27688654

Reddy, D. B., Reddy, T. C., Jyotsna, G., Sharan, S., Priya, N., Lakshmipathi, V., & Reddanna, P. (2009). Chebulagic acid, a COX-LOX dual inhibitor isolated from the fruits of Terminalia chebula Retz., induces apoptosis in COLO-205 cell line. *Journal of Ethnopharmacology*, *124*(3), 506–512. doi:10.1016/j.jep.2009.05.022 PMID:19481594

Reddy, T. C., Aparoy, P., Babu, N. K., Kumar, K. A., Kalangi, S. K., & Reddanna, P. (2010). Kinetics and docking studies of a COX-2 inhibitor isolated from Terminalia bellerica fruits. *Protein and Peptide Letters*, *17*(10), 1251–1257. doi:10.2174/092986610792231537 PMID:20441561

Reinisch, W., Hung, K., Hassan-Zahraee, M., & Cataldi, F. (2018). Targeting endothelial ligands: ICAM-1/alicaforsen, MAdCAM-1. *Journal of Crohn's and Colitis*, *12*(suppl_2), S669–S677. doi:10.1093/ecco-jcc/jjy059 PMID:29757363

Reya, T., Morrison, S. J., Clarke, M. F., & Weissman, I. L. (2001). Stem cells, cancer, and cancer stem cells. *Nature*, *414*(6859), 105–111. doi:10.1038/35102167 PMID:11689955

Ribeiro, D., Freitas, M., Lima, J. L. F. C., & Fernandes, E. (2015). Proinflammatory pathways: The modulation by flavonoids. *Medicinal Research Reviews*, *35*(5), 877–936. doi:10.1002/med.21347 PMID:25926332

Ribeiro, D., Proenca, C., Rocha, S., Lima, J. L. F. C., Carvalho, F., Fernandes, E., & Freitas, M. (2018). Immunomodulatory effects of flavonoids in the prophylaxis and treatment of inflammatory bowel diseases: A comprehensive review. *Current Medicinal Chemistry*, *25*(28), 3374–3412. doi:10.2174/0929867325666180214121734 PMID:29446723

Ricci-Vitiani, L., Lombardi, D. G., Pilozzi, E., Biffoni, M., Todaro, M., Peschle, C., & De Maria, R. (2007). Identification and expansion of human colon-cancer-initiating cells. *Nature*, *445*(7123), 111–115. doi:10.1038/nature05384 PMID:17122771

Risio, M. (2010). Reprint of: The natural history of adenomas. *Best Practice & Research. Clinical Gastroenterology*, *24*(4), 397–406. doi:10.1016/j.bpg.2010.08.002 PMID:20833344

Rivlin, R. S. (2001). Historical Perspective on the Use of Garlic. *The Journal of Nutrition*, *131*(3), 951S–954S. Advance online publication. doi:10.1093/jn/131.3.951S PMID:11238795

Rodriguez-Ramiro, I., Ramos, S., Lopez-Oliva, E., Agis-Torres, A., Gomez-Juaristi, M., Mateos, R., Bravo, L., Goya, L., & Martin, M. A. (2011). Cocoa-rich diet prevents azoxymethane-induced colonic preneoplastic lesions in rats by restraining oxidative stress and cell proliferation and inducing apoptosis. *Molecular Nutrition & Food Research*, *55*(12), 1895–1899. doi:10.1002/mnfr.201100363 PMID:21953728

Rogan, D. F., Cousins, D. J., Santangelo, S., Ioannou, P. A., Antoniou, M., Lee, T. H., & Staynov, D. Z. (2004). Analysis of intergenic transcription in the human IL-4/IL-13 gene cluster. *Proceedings of the National Academy of Sciences of the United States of America*, *101*(8), 2446–2451. doi:10.1073/pnas.0308327100 PMID:14983029

Rohr, M., Narasimhulu, C. A., Sharma, D., Doomra, M., Riad, A., Naser, S., & Parthasarathy, S. (2018). Inflammatory diseases of the gut. *Journal of Medicinal Food*, *21*(2), 113–126. doi:10.1089/jmf.2017.0138 PMID:29389238

Romano, M., & Francesco, DE, F., Zarantonello, L., Ruffolo, C., Ferraro, G. A., Zanus, G., … Cillo, U. (2016). From Inflammation to Cancer in Inflammatory Bowel Disease: Molecular Perspectives. *Anticancer Research*, *36*(4), 1447–1460. PMID:27069120

Romano, M., Sironi, M., Toniatti, C., Polentarutti, N., Fruscella, P., Ghezzi, P., & Mantovani, A. (1997). Role of IL-6 and its soluble receptor in induction of chemokines and leukocyte recruitment. *Immunity*, *6*(3), 315–325. doi:10.1016/S1074-7613(00)80334-9 PMID:9075932

Romero, M., Vera, B., Galisteo, M., Toral, M., Galvez, J., Perez-Vizcaino, F., & Duarte, J. (2017). Protective vascular effects of quercitrin in acute TNBS-colitis in rats: The role of nitric oxide. *Food & Function*, *8*(8), 2702–2711. doi:10.1039/C7FO00755H PMID:28703832

Rosen, L. S., Jacobs, I. A., & Burkes, R. L. (2017). Bevacizumab in Colorectal Cancer: Current Role in Treatment and the Potential of Biosimilars. *Targeted Oncology*, *12*(5), 599–610. doi:10.100711523-017-0518-1 PMID:28801849

Rossen, N. G., MacDonald, J. K., de Vries, E. M., D'Haens, G. R., de Vos, W. M., Zoetendal, E. G., & Ponsioen, C. Y. (2015). Fecal microbiota transplantation as novel therapy in gastroenterology: A systematic review. *World journal of gastroenterology. WJG*, *21*(17), 5359. doi:10.3748/wjg.v21.i17.5359 PMID:25954111

Rossetti, S., Actis, G. C., Fadda, M., Rizzetto, M., & Palmo, A. (2004). The use of the anti-tumour necrosis factor monoclonal antibody-infliximab-to treat ulcerative colitis: Implications and trends beyond the available data. *Digestive and Liver Disease*, *36*(6), 426–431. Advance online publication. doi:10.1016/S1590-8658(04)00088-X PMID:15248385

Roth, M. P., Petersen, G. M., McElree, C., Feldman, E., & Rotter, J. I. (1989). Geographic origins of Jewish patients with inflammatory bowel disease. *Gastroenterology*, *97*(4), 900–904. doi:10.1016/0016-5085(89)91495-9 PMID:2777043

Roy, P. K., Rashid, F., Bragg, J., Ibdah, J. A., Hepatology, D. G., Medicine, U. M. S., Columbia, Missouri, & States, U. (2008). Role of the JNK signal transduction pathway in inflammatory bowel disease. *World Journal of Gastroenterology*, *14*(2), 200–202. doi:10.3748/wjg.14.200 PMID:18186555

Rubin, D. C., Shaker, A., & Levin, M. S. (2012). Chronic intestinal inflammation: Inflammatory bowel disease and colitis-associated colon cancer. *Frontiers in Immunology*, *3*, 107. doi:10.3389/fimmu.2012.00107 PMID:22586430

Saadatdoust, Z., Pandurangan, A. K., Ananda Sadagopan, S. K., Esa, N. M., Ismail, A., & Mustafa, M. R. (2015). Dietary cocoa attenuates colitis associated cancer: Crucial involvement of IL/6/STAT3 pathway. *The Journal of Nutritional Biochemistry*, *26*(12), 1547–1558. doi:10.1016/j.jnutbio.2015.07.024 PMID:26355019

Saadati, H. R., Wittig, M., Helbig, I., Hasler, R., Anderson, C. A., Mathew, C. G., Kupcinskas, L., Parkes, M., Karlsen, T. H., Rosenstiel, P., Schreiber, S., & Franke, A. (2016). Genome-wide rare copy number variation screening in ulcerative colitis identifies potential susceptibility loci. *BMC Medical Genetics*, *17*(1), 26. doi:10.118612881-016-0289-z PMID:27037036

Sabiu, S., & Ashafa, O. T. A. (2016). Toxicological implications and laxative potential of ethanol root extract of Morella serrata in loperamide-induced constipated Wistar rats. *Pharmaceutical Biology*, *54*(12), 2901–2908. Advance online publication. doi:10.1080/13880209.2016.1193885 PMID:27267728

Sadra, A., Kweon, H. S., Huh, S. O., & Cho, J. (2017). Gastroprotective and gastric motility benefits of AD-lico/Healthy Gut™ Glycyrrhiza inflata extract. *Animal Cells and Systems*, *21*(4), 255–262. Advance online publication. doi:10.1080/19768354.2017.1357660 PMID:30460076

Sahu, B. D., Kumar, J. M., & Sistla, R. (2016). Fisetin, a dietary flavonoid, ameliorates experimental colitis in mice: Relevance of NF-kappaB signaling. *The Journal of Nutritional Biochemistry*, *28*, 171–182. doi:10.1016/j.jnutbio.2015.10.004 PMID:26878795

Sairam, M., Neetu, D., Yogesh, B., Anju, B., Dipti, P., Pauline, T., Sharma, S. K., Sarada, S. K. S., Ilavazhagan, G., Kumar, D., & Selvamurthy, W. (2002). Cyto-protective and immunomodulating properties of Amla (Emblica officinalis) on lymphocytes: An in vitro study. *Journal of Ethnopharmacology*, *81*(1), 5–10. doi:10.1016/S0378-8741(01)00421-4 PMID:12020921

Sairenji, T., Collins, K. L., & Evans, D. V. (2017). An update on inflammatory bowel disease. *Primary Care*, *44*(4), 673–692. doi:10.1016/j.pop.2017.07.010 PMID:29132528

Sakai, T., Furoku, S., Nakamoto, M., Shuto, E., Hosaka, T., Nishioka, Y., & Sone, S. (2011). Soy isoflavone equol perpetuates dextran sulfate sodium-induced acute colitis in mice. *Bioscience, Biotechnology, and Biochemistry*, *75*(3), 593–595. doi:10.1271/bbb.100710 PMID:21389602

Saleem, A., Husheem, M., Harkonen, P., & Pihlaja, K. (2002). Inhibition of cancer cell growth by crude extract and the phenolics of Terminalia chebula Retz fruit. *Journal of Ethnopharmacology*, *81*(3), 327–336. doi:10.1016/S0378-8741(02)00099-5 PMID:12127233

Salmaninejad, A., Zamani, M. R., Pourvahedi, M., Golchehre, Z., Hosseini Bereshneh, A., & Rezaei, N. (2016). Cancer/Testis Antigens: Expression, Regulation, Tumor Invasion, and Use in Immunotherapy of Cancers. *Immunological Investigations*, *45*(7), 619–640. doi:10.1080/08820139.2016.1197241 PMID:27603913

Sancheti, G., Jindal, A., Kumari, R., & Goyal, P. K. (2005). Chemopreventive action of Emblica officinalis on skin carcinogenesis in mice. *Asian Pacific Journal of Cancer Prevention*, *6*, 197–201. PMID:16101333

Sanchez de Medina, F., Vera, B., Galvez, J., & Zarzuelo, A. (2002). Effect of quercitrin on the early stages of hapten induced colonic inflammation in the rat. *Life Sciences*, *70*(26), 3097–3108. doi:10.1016/S0024-3205(02)01568-0 PMID:12008093

Sandborn, W. J., Feagan, B. G., Fedorak, R. N., Scherl, E., Fleisher, M. R., Katz, S., Johanns, J., Blank, M., & Rutgeerts, P. (2008). A randomized trial of Ustekinumab, a human interleukin-12/23 monoclonal antibody, in patients with moderate-to-severe Crohn's disease. *Gastroenterology*, *135*(4), 1130–1141. doi:10.1053/j.gastro.2008.07.014 PMID:18706417

Sandborn, W. J., & Hanauer, S. B. (1999). Antitumor necrosis factor therapy for Inflammatory Bowel Disease: A review of agents, pharmacology, clinical results, and safety. *Inflammatory Bowel Diseases*, *5*(2), 119–133. Advance online publication. doi:10.1097/00054725-199905000-00008 PMID:10338381

Sandborn, W. J., Lee, S. D., Tarabar, D., Louis, E., Klopocka, M., Klaus, J., Reinisch, W., Hébuterne, X., Park, D.-I., Schreiber, S., Nayak, S., Ahmad, A., Banerjee, A., Brown, L. S., Cataldi, F., Gorelick, K. J., Cheng, J. B., Hassan-Zahraee, M., Clare, R., & D'Haens, G. R. (2018). Phase II evaluation of anti-MAdCAM antibody PF-00547659 in the treatment of Crohn's disease: Report of the OPERA study. *Gut*, *67*(10), 1824–1835. doi:10.1136/gutjnl-2016-313457 PMID:28982740

Sanford, D., Thornley, P., Teriaky, A., Chande, N., & Gregor, J. (2014). Opioid use is associated with decreased quality of life in patients with Crohn's disease. *Saudi Journal of Gastroenterology*, *20*(3), 182–187. doi:10.4103/1319-3767.133020 PMID:24976282

Santoft, F., Hedman-Lagerlof, E., Salomonsson, S., Lindsater, E., Ljotsson, B., & Kecklund, G. (2020). Inflammatory cytokines in patients with common mental disorders treated with cognitive behavior therapy. *Brain, Behavior, & Immunity – Health*. (in press)

Sarmadi, B., Aminuddin, F., Hamid, M., Saari, N., Abdul-Hamid, A., & Ismail, A. (2012). Hypoglycemic effects of cocoa (Theobroma cacao L.) autolysates. *Food Chemistry*, *134*(2), 905–911. doi:10.1016/j.foodchem.2012.02.202 PMID:23107706

Sartore-Bianchi, A., Trusolino, L., Martino, C., Bencardino, K., Lonardi, S., Bergamo, F., Zagonel, V., Leone, F., Depetris, I., Martinelli, E., Troiani, T., Ciardiello, F., Racca, P., Bertotti, A., Siravegna, G., Torri, V., Amatu, A., Ghezzi, S., Marrapese, G., ... Siena, S. (2016). Dual-targeted therapy with trastuzumab and lapatinib in treatment-refractory, KRAS codon 12/13 wild-type, HER2-positive metastatic colorectal cancer (HERACLES): A proof-of-concept, multicentre, open-label, phase 2 trial. *The Lancet. Oncology*, *17*(6), 738–746. doi:10.1016/S1470-2045(16)00150-9 PMID:27108243

Sartor, R. B. (2006). Mechanisms of disease: Pathogenesis of Crohn's disease and ulcerative colitis. *Nature Clinical Practice. Gastroenterology & Hepatology*, *3*(7), 390–407. doi:10.1038/ncpgasthep0528 PMID:16819502

Sartor, R. B. (2008). Microbial influences in inflammatory bowel diseases. *Gastroenterology*, *134*(2), 577–594. doi:10.1053/j.gastro.2007.11.059 PMID:18242222

Sasaki, M., & Klapproth, J. M. (2012). The role of bacteria in the pathogenesis of ulcerative colitis. *Journal of Signal Transduction*, *704953*, 1–6. Advance online publication. doi:10.1155/2012/704953 PMID:22619714

Scanlan, P. D., Shanahan, F., Clune, Y., Collins, J. K., O'Sullivan, G. C., O'Riordan, M., Holmes, E., Wang, Y., & Marchesi, J. R. (2008). Culture-independent analysis of the gut microbiota in colorectal cancer and polyposis. *Environmental Microbiology*, *10*(3), 789–798. doi:10.1111/j.1462-2920.2007.01503.x PMID:18237311

Schett, G., & Neurath, M. F. (2018). Resolution of chronic inflammatory disease: Universal and tissue-specific concepts. *Nature Communications*, *9*(1), 9. doi:10.103841467-018-05800-6 PMID:30111884

Schmoll, H. J., Cunningham, D., Sobrero, A., Karapetis, C. S., Rougier, P., Koski, S. L., Kocakova, I., Bondarenko, I., Bodoky, G., Mainwaring, P., Salazar, R., Barker, P., Mookerjee, B., Robertson, J., & Van Cutsem, E. (2012). Cediranib with mFOLFOX6 versus bevacizumab with mFOLFOX6 as first-line treatment for patients with advanced colorectal cancer: A double-blind, randomized phase III study (HORIZON III). *Journal of Clinical Oncology*, *30*(29), 3588–3595. doi:10.1200/JCO.2012.42.5355 PMID:22965961

Schwanke, R. C., Marcon, R., Meotti, F. C., Bento, A. F., Dutra, R. C., Pizzollatti, M. G., & Calixto, J. B. (2013). Oral administration of the flavonoid myricitrin prevents dextran sulfate sodium-induced experimental colitis in mice through modulation of PI3K/Akt signaling pathway. *Molecular Nutrition & Food Research*, *57*(11), 1938–1949. doi:10.1002/mnfr.201300134 PMID:23861337

Sears, C. L., & Pardoll, D. M. (2011). Perspective: Alpha-bugs, their microbial partners, and the link to colon cancer. *The Journal of Infectious Diseases*, *203*(3), 306–311. doi:10.1093/jinfdis/jiq061 PMID:21208921

Segal, A. W. (2016). Making sense of the cause of Crohn's–a new look at an old disease. *F1000 Research*, 5. PMID:28105308

Segditsas, S., & Tomlinson, I. (2006). Colorectal cancer and genetic alterations in the Wnt pathway. *Oncogene*, *25*(57), 7531–7537. doi:10.1038j.onc.1210059 PMID:17143297

Seher, A., Nickel, J., Mueller, T. D., Kneitz, S., Gebhardt, S., ter Vehn, T. M., & Sebald, W. (2011). Gene expression profiling of connective tissue growth factor (CTGF) stimulated primary human tenon fibroblasts reveals an inflammatory and wound healing response in vitro. *Molecular Vision*, *17*, 53. PMID:21245951

Seibel, J., Molzberger, A. F., Hertrampf, T., Laudenbach-Leschowski, U., & Diel, P. (2009). Oral treatment with genistein reduces the expression of molecular and biochemical markers of inflammation in a rat model of chronic TNBS-induced colitis. *European Journal of Nutrition*, *48*(4), 213–220. doi:10.100700394-009-0004-3 PMID:19234664

Seito, L. N., Sforcin, J. M., Bastos, J. K., & Di Stasi, L. C. (2015). Zeyheria montana Mart. (Bignoniaceae) as source of antioxidant and immunomodulatory compounds with beneficial effects on intestinal inflammation. *The Journal of Pharmacy and Pharmacology*, *67*(4), 597–604. doi:10.1111/jphp.12354 PMID:25556766

Seki, T., Hosono, T., Hosono-Fukao, T., Inada, K., Tanaka, R., Ogihara, J., & Ariga, T. (2008). Anticancer effects of diallyl trisulfide derived from garlic. *Asia Pacific Journal of Clinical Nutrition*, *17*(Suppl 1), 249–252. PMID:18296348

Seo, G. S., & Chae, S. C. (2014). Biological therapy for ulcerative colitis: An update. *World Journal of Gastroenterology*, *20*(37), 13234–13238. doi:10.3748/wjg.v20.i37.13234 PMID:25309060

Shacter, E., & Weitzman, S. A. (2002). Chronic inflammation and cancer. *Oncology (Williston Park, N.Y.)*, *16*(2), 217–226. PMID:11866137

Shaila, H. P., Udupa, A. L., & Udupa, S. L. (1995). Preventive actions of Terminalia belerica in experimentally induced atherosclerosis. *International Journal of Cardiology*, *49*(2), 101–106. doi:10.1016/0167-5273(95)02285-5 PMID:7628881

Shalkami, A. S., Hassan, M., & Bakr, A. G. (2018). Anti-inflammatory, antioxidant and anti-apoptotic activity of diosmin in acetic acid-induced ulcerative colitis. *Human and Experimental Toxicology*, *37*(1), 78–86. doi:10.1177/0960327117694075 PMID:29187079

Sharma, M. P., & Ahuja, V. (2009). Abdominal (gastrointestinal tract) tuberculosis in adult. In H. S. Schaaf, A. Zumla, & J. M. Grange (Eds.), *Tuberculosis: A comprehensive clinical reference (pp* (pp. 424–431). Saunders/Elsevier. doi:10.1016/B978-1-4160-3988-4.00039-1

Sharma, M., Kaur, R., Kaushik, K., & Kaushal, N. (2019). Redox modulatory protective effects of ω-3 fatty acids rich fish oil against experimental colitis. *Toxicology Mechanisms and Methods*, *29*(4), 244–254. Advance online publication. doi:10.1080/15376516.2018.1553220 PMID:30489199

Sharma, P., Poojary, G., Dwivedi, S. N., & Deepak, K. K. (2015). Effect of Yoga-Based Intervention in Patients with Inflammatory Bowel Disease. *International Journal of Yoga Therapy*, *25*(1), 101–112. doi:10.17761/1531-2054-25.1.101 PMID:26667293

Sharma, S. K., & Mohan, A. (2004). Extrapulmonary tuberculosis. *The Indian Journal of Medical Research*, *120*, 316–353. PMID:15520485

Sheibanie, A. F., Yen, J. H., Khayrullina, T., Emig, F., Zhang, M., Tuma, R., & Ganea, D. (2007). The proinflammatory effect of prostaglandin E2 in experimental inflammatory bowel disease is mediated through the IL-23 IL-17 axis. *Journal of Immunology (Baltimore, Md.: 1950)*, *178*(12), 8138–8147. doi:10.4049/jimmunol.178.12.8138 PMID:17548652

Sheng, H., Shao, J., Morrow, J. D., Beauchamp, R. D., & DuBois, R. N. (1998). Modulation of apoptosis and Bcl-2 expression by prostaglandin E2 in human colon cancer cells. *Cancer Research*, *58*(2), 362–366. PMID:9443418

Shenoy, A. K., Fisher, R. C., Butterworth, E. A., Pi, L., Chang, L.-J., Appelman, H. D., Chang, M., Scott, E. W., & Huang, E. H. (2012). Transition from colitis to cancer: High Wnt activity sustains the tumor-initiating potential of colon cancer stem cell precursors. *Cancer Research*, *72*(19), 5091–5100. doi:10.1158/0008-5472.CAN-12-1806 PMID:22902411

Shen, X. J., Rawls, J. F., Randall, T. A., Burcall, L., Mpande, C., Jenkins, N., Jovov, B., Abdo, Z., Sandler, R. S., & Keku, T. O. (2010). Molecular characterization of mucosal adherent bacteria and associations with colorectal adenomas. *Gut Microbes*, *1*(3), 138–147. doi:10.4161/gmic.1.3.12360 PMID:20740058

Shinde, L., More, S. M., Junne, S. B., & Wadje, S. S. (2011). The antifungal activity of five Terminalia species checked by paper disk method. *Int J Pharma Res Dev*, *3*, 36–40.

Shin, E. K., Kwon, H. S., Kim, Y. H., Shin, H. K., & Kim, J. K. (2009). Chrysin, a natural flavone, improves murine inflammatory bowel diseases. *Biochemical and Biophysical Research Communications*, *381*(4), 502–507. doi:10.1016/j.bbrc.2009.02.071 PMID:19233127

Shirwaikar Thomas, A., Schwartz, M., & Quigley, E. (2019). Gastrointestinal lymphoma: The new mimic. *BMJ Open Gastroenterology*, *6*(1), e000320. doi:10.1136/bmjgast-2019-000320 PMID:31645987

Shivashankara, K. S., & Acharya, S. N. (2010). Bioavailability of dietary polyphenols and the cardiovascular diseases. *The Open Nutraceuticals Journal*, *3*(1), 227–241. doi:10.2174/1876396001003010227

Siczek, K., Zatorski, H., Chmielowiec-Korzeniowska, A., Pulit-Prociak, J., Smiech, M., Kordek, R., Tymczyna, L., Banach, M., & Fichna, J. (2017). Synthesis and evaluation of anti-inflammatory properties of silver nanoparticle suspensions in experimental colitis in mice. *Chemical Biology & Drug Design*, *89*(4), 538–547. doi:10.1111/cbdd.12876 PMID:27696734

Sigel, J. E., Petras, R. E., Lashner, B. A., Fazio, V. W., & Goldblum, J. R. (1999). Intestinal adenocarcinoma in Crohn's disease: A report of 30 cases with a focus on coexisting dysplasia. *The American Journal of Surgical Pathology*, *23*(6), 651–655. doi:10.1097/00000478-199906000-00003 PMID:10366146

Sikandar, S. S., Pate, K. T., Anderson, S., Dizon, D., Edwards, R. A., Waterman, M. L., & Lipkin, S. M. (2010). NOTCH signaling is required for formation and self-renewal of tumor-initiating cells and for repression of secretory cell differentiation in colon cancer. *Cancer Research*, *70*(4), 1469–1478. doi:10.1158/0008-5472.CAN-09-2557 PMID:20145124

Silverberg, M. S., Satsangi, J., Ahmad, T., Arnott, I. D., Bernstein, C. N., Brant, S. R., . . . Warren, B. F. (2005). Toward an integrated clinical, molecular and serological classification of inflammatory bowel disease: report of a Working Party of the 2005 Montreal World Congress of Gastroenterology. *Can J Gastroenterol, 19 Suppl A*, 5A-36A. 10.1155/2005/269076

Singh, I., Sharma, A., Nunia, V., & Goyal, P. K. (2005). Radioprotection of Swiss albino mice by Emblica officinalis. *Phytotherapy Research*, *19*(5), 444–446. doi:10.1002/ptr.1600 PMID:16106381

Singh, M. P., & Sharma, C. S. (2009). Wound healing activity of Terminalia chebula in experimentally induced diabetic rats. *International Journal of Pharm Tech Research*, *1*, 1267–1270.

Singh, S. K., Hawkins, C., Clarke, I. D., Squire, J. A., Bayani, J., Hide, T., Henkelman, R. M., Cusimano, M. D., & Dirks, P. B. (2004). Identification of human brain tumour initiating cells. *Nature*, *432*(7015), 396–401. doi:10.1038/nature03128 PMID:15549107

Sobhani, I., Tap, J., Roudot-Thoraval, F., Roperch, J. P., Letulle, S., Langella, P., Corthier, G., Van Nhieu, J. T., & Furet, J. P. (2011). Microbial dysbiosis in colorectal cancer (CRC) patients. *PLoS One*, *6*(1), e16393. doi:10.1371/journal.pone.0016393 PMID:21297998

Soccalingam, A., Ramanathan, M., & Bhavanani, A. B. (2020). Yoga therapy on Cognitive function in Neurodevelopmental disorders. In T. Wadhera & D. Kakkara (Eds.), *Interdisciplinary Approaches to Altering Neurodevelopmental Disorders* (pp. 143–161). IGI-Global. doi:10.4018/978-1-7998-3069-6.ch009

Soh, J. S., Jo, S. I., Lee, H., Do, E., Hwang, S. W., Park, S. H., Ye, B. D., Byeon, J.-S., Yang, S.-K., Kim, J. H., Yang, D.-H., Kim, S.-Y., & Myung, S.-J. (2019). Immunoprofiling of Colitis-associated and Sporadic Colorectal Cancer and its Clinical Significance. *Scientific Reports*, *9*(1), 6833. doi:10.103841598-019-42986-1 PMID:31048714

Sokol, H., Beaugerie, L., Maynadié, M., Laharie, D., Dupas, J. L., Flourié, B., Lerebours, E., Peyrin-Biroulet, L., Allez, M., Simon, T., Carrat, F., & Brousse, N. (2012). Excess primary intestinal lymphoproliferative disorders in patients with inflammatory bowel disease. *Inflammatory Bowel Diseases*, *18*(11), 2063–2071. doi:10.1002/ibd.22889 PMID:22271569

Somasundaram, K. (2000). Tumor suppressor p53: Regulation and function. *Frontiers in Bioscience: A Journal and Virtual Library, 5*, D424-437. doi:10.2741/Somasund

Song, R., Li, Y., Hao, W., Wang, B., Yang, L., & Xu, F. (2018). Identification and analysis of key genes associated with ulcerative colitis based on DNA microarray data. *Medicine*, *97*(21), e10658. doi:10.1097/MD.0000000000010658 PMID:29794741

Song, Z. M., Liu, F., Chen, Y. M., Liu, Y. J., Wang, X. D., & Du, S. Y. (2019). CTGF-mediated ERK signaling pathway influences the inflammatory factors and intestinal flora in ulcerative colitis. *Biomedicine and Pharmacotherapy*, *111*, 1429–1437. doi:10.1016/j.biopha.2018.12.063 PMID:30841458

Sonnenberg, A., McCarty, D. J., & Jacobsen, S. J. (1991). Geographic variation of inflammatory bowel disease within the United States. *Gastroenterology*, *100*(1), 143–149. doi:10.1016/0016-5085(91)90594-B PMID:1983816

Sotnikova, R., Nosalova, V., & Navarova, J. (2013). Efficacy of quercetin derivatives in prevention of ulcerative colitis in rats. *Interdisciplinary Toxicology*, *6*(1), 9–12. doi:10.2478/intox-2013-0002 PMID:24170973

Soufli, I., Toumi, R., Rafa, H., & Touil-Boukoffa, C. (2016). Overview of cytokines and nitric oxide involvement in immuno-pathogenesis of inflammatory bowel diseases. *World Journal of Gastrointestinal Pharmacology and Therapeutics*, *7*(3), 353–360. doi:10.4292/wjgpt.v7.i3.353 PMID:27602236

Souza, R. F., Lei, J., Yin, J., Appel, R., Zou, T. T., Zhou, X., & Meltzer, S. J. (1997). A transforming growth factor beta 1 receptor type II mutation in ulcerative colitis-associated neoplasms. *Gastroenterology*, *112*(1), 40–45. doi:10.1016/S0016-5085(97)70217-8 PMID:8978341

Spanogiannopoulos, P., & Turnbaugh, P. J. (2018). Broad collateral damage of drugs against the gut microbiome. *Nature Reviews. Gastroenterology & Hepatology*, *15*(8), 457–458. doi:10.103841575-018-0028-3 PMID:29752457

Spano, J. P., Milano, G., Rixe, C., & Fagard, R. (2006). JAK/STAT signalling pathway in colorectal cancer: A new biological target with therapeutic implications. *European Journal of Cancer*, *42*(16), 2668–2670. Advance online publication. doi:10.1016/j.ejca.2006.07.006 PMID:16963263

Spiik, A. K., Ridderstad, A., Axelsson, L. G., Midtvedt, T., Björk, L., & Pettersson, S. (2002). Abrogated lymphocyte infiltration and lowered CD14 in dextran sulfate induced colitis in mice treated with p65 antisense oligonucleotides. *International Journal of Colorectal Disease*, *17*(4), 223–232. Advance online publication. doi:10.100700384-001-0366-3 PMID:12073070

Stallmach, A., Hagel, S., & Bruns, T. (2010). Adverse effects of biologics used for treating IBD. *Best Practice & Research. Clinical Gastroenterology*, *24*(2), 167–182. doi:10.1016/j.bpg.2010.01.002 PMID:20227030

Steenge, G. R., Verhoef, P., & Katan, M. B. (2003). Betaine supplementation lowers plasma homocysteine in healthy men and women. *The Journal of Nutrition*, *133*(5), 1291–1295. doi:10.1093/jn/133.5.1291 PMID:12730412

Stenson, W. F. (2014). The universe of arachidonic acid metabolites in inflammatory bowel disease: Can we tell the good from the bad? *Current Opinion in Gastroenterology*, *30*(4), 347–351. doi:10.1097/MOG.0000000000000075 PMID:24837228

Suchalatha, S., Srinivasulu, C., & Devi, S. C. (2005). Antioxidant activity of ethanolic extract of Terminalia chebula fruit against isoproterenol-induced oxidative stress in rats. *Indian Journal of Biochemistry & Biophysics*, *42*, 246–249. PMID:23923550

Sun, A. N., Ren, G. Y., Deng, C., Zhang, J. L., Luo, X. P., Wu, X. J., Mani, S., Dou, W., & Wang, Z. (2016). C-glycosyl flavonoid orientin improves chemically induced inflammatory bowel disease in mice. *Journal of Functional Foods*, *21*, 418–430. doi:10.1016/j.jff.2015.12.029

Sun, X., Ng, T. T. H., Sham, K. W. Y., Zhang, L., Chan, M. T. V., Wu, W. K. K., & Cheng, C. H. K. (2019, October). Bufalin, a Traditional Chinese Medicine Compound, Prevents Tumor Formation in Two Murine Models of Colorectal Cancer. *Cancer Prevention Research (Philadelphia, Pa.)*, *12*(10), 653–666. doi:10.1158/1940-6207.CAPR-19-0134 PMID:31431500

Sun, Y., Li, L., Xie, R., Wang, B., Jiang, K., & Cao, H. (2019). Stress Triggers Flare of Inflammatory Bowel Disease in Children and Adults. *Frontiers in Pediatrics*, *7*, 432. doi:10.3389/fped.2019.00432 PMID:31709203

Sun, Y., Wu, X. X., Yin, Y., Gong, F. Y., Shen, Y., Cai, T. T., Zhou, X.-B., Wu, X.-F., & Xu, Q. (2010). Novel immunomodulatory properties of cirsilineol through selective inhibition of IFN-gamma signaling in a murine model of inflammatory bowel disease. *Biochemical Pharmacology*, *79*(2), 229–238. doi:10.1016/j.bcp.2009.08.014 PMID:19698701

Sun, Y., Zhao, Y., Yao, J., Zhao, L., Wu, Z., Wang, Y., Pan, D., Miao, H., Guo, Q., & Lu, N. (2015). Wogonoside protects against dextran sulfate sodium-induced experimental colitis in mice by inhibiting NF-kappaB and NLRP3 inflammasome activation. *Biochemical Pharmacology*, *94*(2), 142–154. doi:10.1016/j.bcp.2015.02.002 PMID:25677765

Surh, Y.-J., Kundu, J. K., & Na, H.-K. (2008). Nrf2 as a master redox switch in turning on the cellular signaling involved in the induction of cytoprotective genes by some chemopreventive phytochemicals. *Planta Medica*, *74*(13), 1526–1539. doi:10.1055-0028-1088302 PMID:18937164

Suryanarayana, P., Kumar, P. A., Saraswat, M., Petrash, J. M., & Reddy, G. B. (2004). Inhibition of aldose reductase by tannoid principles of Emblica officinalis: Implications for the prevention of sugar cataract. *Molecular Vision*, *10*, 148–154. PMID:15031705

SuryaPrakash, D.V., Satya, N.S., Avanigadda, S., & Vanglapati, M. (2012). Pharmacological review on Terminalia chebula. *International Journal of Research in Pharmaceutical and Biomedical Sciences*, *3*, 679–683.

Suthienkul, O., Miyazaki, O., Chulasiri, M., Kositanont, U., & Oishi, K. (1993). Retroviral reverse transcriptase inhibitory activity in Thai herbs and spices: Screening with Moloney murine leukemia viral enzyme. *The Southeast Asian Journal of Tropical Medicine and Public Health*, *24*, 751–755. PMID:7524165

Suzuki, K., Sugimura, K., Hasegawa, K., Yoshida, K., Suzuki, A., Ishizuka, K., ... Asakura, H. (2001). Activated platelets in ulcerative colitis enhance the production of reactive oxygen species by polymorphonuclear leukocytes. *Scandinavian Journal of Gastroenterology*. Advance online publication. doi:10.1080/003655201317097164 PMID:11761021

Syn, W. K., Witek, R. P., Curbishley, S. M., Jung, Y., Choi, S. S., Enrich, B., Omenetti, A., Agboola, K. M., Fearing, C. M., Tilg, H., Adams, D. H., & Diehl, A. M. (2009). Role for hedgehog pathway in regulating growth and function of invariant NKT cells. *European Journal of Immunology*, *39*(7), 1879–1892. doi:10.1002/eji.200838890 PMID:19544307

Takada, Y., Hisamatsu, T., Kamada, N., Kitazume, M. T., Honda, H., Oshima, Y., Saito, R., Takayama, T., Kobayashi, T., Chinen, H., Mikami, Y., Kanai, T., Okamoto, S., & Hibi, T. (2010). Monocyte chemoattractant protein-1 contributes to gut homeostasis and intestinal inflammation by composition of IL-10-producing regulatory macrophage subset. *Journal of Immunology (Baltimore, Md.: 1950)*, *184*(5), 2671–2676. doi:10.4049/jimmunol.0804012 PMID:20107182

Takaishi, S., Okumura, T., & Wang, T. C. (2008). Gastric cancer stem cells. *Journal of Clinical Oncology*, *26*(17), 2876–2882. doi:10.1200/JCO.2007.15.2603 PMID:18539967

Takiishi, T., Fenero, C. I. M., & Câmara, N. O. S. (2017). Intestinal barrier and gut microbiota: Shaping our immune responses throughout life. *Tissue Barriers*, *5*(4), e1373208. doi:10.1080/21688370.2017.1373208 PMID:28956703

Tanaka, T., Kawamori, T., Ohnishi, M., Makita, H., Mori, H., Satoh, K., & Hara, A. (1995). Suppression of azoxymethane-induced rat colon carcinogenesis by dietary administration of naturally occurring xanthophylls astaxanthin and canthaxanthin during the postinitiation phase. *Carcinogenesis*, *16*(12), 2957–2963. doi:10.1093/carcin/16.12.2957 PMID:8603470

Tanaka, T., Makita, H., Ohnishi, M., Mori, H., Satoh, K., & Hara, A. (1995). Chemoprevention of rat oral carcinogenesis by naturally occurring xanthophylls, astaxanthin and canthaxanthin. *Cancer Research*, *55*(18), 4059–4064. PMID:7664280

Tanaka, T., Morishita, Y., Suzui, M., Kojima, T., Okumura, A., & Mori, H. (1994). Chemoprevention of mouse urinary bladder carcinogenesis by the naturally occurring carotenoid astaxanthin. *Carcinogenesis*, *15*(1), 15–19. doi:10.1093/carcin/15.1.15 PMID:8293542

Tandon, H. D., & Prakash, A. (1972). Pathology of intestinal tuberculosis and its distinction from Crohn's disease. *Gut*, *13*(4), 260–269. doi:10.1136/gut.13.4.260 PMID:5033841

Tandon, R. K., Sarin, S. K., Bose, S. L., Berry, M., & Tandon, B. N. (1986). A clinic-radiological reappraisal of intestinal tuberculosis–Changing profile? *Gastroenterologia Japonica*, *21*(1), 17–22. doi:10.1007/BF02775935 PMID:3699397

Tang, H., Xiang, D., Wang, F., Mao, J., Tan, X., & Wang, Y. (2017). 5-ASA-loaded SiO2 nanoparticles-a novel drug delivery system targeting therapy on ulcerative colitis in mice. *Molecular Medicine Reports*, *15*(3), 1117–1122. doi:10.3892/mmr.2017.6153 PMID:28138699

Tan, Y., & Zheng, C. (2018). Effects of alpinetin on intestinal barrier function, inflammation and oxidative stress in dextran sulfate sodium-induced ulcerative colitis mice. *The American Journal of the Medical Sciences*, *355*(4), 377–386. doi:10.1016/j.amjms.2018.01.002 PMID:29661352

Tao, F., Qian, C., Guo, W., Luo, Q., Xu, Q., & Sun, Y. (2013). Inhibition of Th1/Th17 responses via suppression of STAT1 and STAT3 activation contributes to the amelioration of murine experimental colitis by a natural flavonoid glucoside icariin. *Biochemical Pharmacology*, *85*(6), 798–807. doi:10.1016/j.bcp.2012.12.002 PMID:23261528

Tariq, M., Hussain, S. J., Asif, M., & Jahan, M. (1977). Protective effect of fruit extracts of Emblica officinalis (Gaertn.) and Terminalia belerica (Roxb.) in experimental myocardial necrosis in rats. *Indian Journal of Experimental Biology*, *15*, 485–486. PMID:598885

Tatar, E. L., & Das, K. M. (2007). Improvement in ulcerative colitis symptoms after use of fish oil enemas. *Gastroenterology & Hepatology*. PMID:21960787

Tatiya-Aphiradee, N., Chatuphonprasert, W., & Jarukamjorn, K. (2018). Immune response and inflammatory pathway of ulcerative colitis. *Journal of Basic and Clinical Physiology and Pharmacology*, *30*(1), 1–10. doi:10.1515/jbcpp-2018-0036 PMID:30063466

Teng, M. W., Bowman, E. P., McElwee, J. J., Smyth, M. J., Casanova, J. L., Cooper, A. M., & Cua, D. J. (2015). IL-12 and IL-23 cytokines: From discovery to targeted therapies for immune-mediated inflammatory diseases. *Nature Medicine*, *21*(7), 719–729. doi:10.1038/nm.3895 PMID:26121196

Thakur, C. P., Thakur, B., Singh, S., Sinha, P. K., & Sinha, S. K. (1988). The Ayurvedic medicines Haritaki, Amala and Bahira reduce cholesterol induced atherosclerosis in rabbits. *International Journal of Cardiology*, *21*(2), 167–175. doi:10.1016/0167-5273(88)90219-7 PMID:3225068

Thomas, S., & Baumgart, D. C. (2012). Targeting leukocyte migration and adhesion in Crohn's disease and ulcerative colitis. *Inflammopharmacology*, *20*(1), 1–18. doi:10.100710787-011-0104-6 PMID:22205271

Thorsteinsdottir, S., Gudjonsson, T., Nielsen, O. H., Vainer, B., & Seidelin, J. B. (2011). Pathogenesis and biomarkers of carcinogenesis in ulcerative colitis. *Nature Reviews. Gastroenterology & Hepatology*, *8*(7), 395–404. doi:10.1038/nrgastro.2011.96 PMID:21647200

Tian, J., Lin, X., Zhou, W., & Xu, J. (2003). Hydroxyethyl starch inhibits NF-κB activation and prevents the expression of inflammatory mediators in endotoxic rats. *Annals of Clinical and Laboratory Science*, *33*(4), 451–458. PMID:14584760

Tiwari, A., Saraf, S., Verma, A., Panda, P. K., & Jain, S. K. (2018). Novel targeting approaches and signaling pathways of colorectal cancer: An insight. *World Journal of Gastroenterology*, *24*(39), 4428–4435. doi:10.3748/wjg.v24.i39.4428 PMID:30357011

Tjalsma, H., Boleij, A., Marchesi, J. R., & Dutilh, B. E. (2012). A bacterial driver–passenger model for colorectal cancer: Beyond the usual suspects. *Nature Reviews. Microbiology*, *10*(8), 575–582. doi:10.1038/nrmicro2819 PMID:22728587

Tomasello, G., Tralongo, P., Damiani, P., Sinagra, E., Di Trapani, B., Zeenny, M. N., ... Leone, A. (2014). Dismicrobism in inflammatory bowel disease and colorectal cancer: Changes in response of colocytes. *World Journal of Gastroenterology: WJG*, *20*(48), 18121. doi:10.3748/wjg.v20.i48.18121 PMID:25561781

Torres, J., Billioud, V., Sachar, D. B., Peyrin-Biroulet, L., & Colombel, J.-F. (2012). Ulcerative colitis as a progressive disease: The forgotten evidence. *Inflammatory Bowel Diseases*, *18*(7), 1356–1363. doi:10.1002/ibd.22839 PMID:22162423

Trivedi, P. J., & Adams, D. H. (2018). Chemokines and chemokine receptors as therapeutic targets in inflammatory bowel disease; pitfalls and promise. *Journal of Crohn's and Colitis*, *12*(12), 1508–1508. doi:10.1093/ecco-jcc/jjy130 PMID:30272117

Tulchinsky, H., Hawley, P. R., & Nicholls, R. J. (2003). Long-Term Failure after Restorative Proctocolectomy for Ulcerative Colitis. *Annals of Surgery*, *238*(2), 229–234. Advance online publication. doi:10.1097/01.sla.0000082121.84763.4c PMID:12894016

Ullman, T. A., & Itzkowitz, S. H. (2011). Intestinal inflammation and cancer. *Gastroenterology*, *140*(6), 1807–1816. doi:10.1053/j.gastro.2011.01.057 PMID 21530747

Undseth, R., Berstad, A., Kløw, N. E., Arnljot, K., Moi, K. S., & Valeur, J. (2014). Abnormal accumulation of intestinal fluid following ingestion of an unabsorbable carbohydrate in patients with irritable bowel syndrome: An MRI study. *Neurogastroenterology and Motility*, *26*(12), 1686–1693. doi:10.1111/nmo.12449 PMID:25271767

Ungaro, R., Colombel, J. F., Lissoos, T., & Peyrin-Biroulet, L. (2019). A treat-to-target update in ulcerative colitis: A systematic review. *The American Journal of Gastroenterology*, *114*(6), 874–883. doi:10.14309/ajg.0000000000000183 PMID:30908297

Van Der Kraak, L., Gros, P., & Beauchemin, N. (2015). Colitis-associated colon cancer: Is it in your genes? *World Journal of Gastroenterology*, *21*(41), 11688–11699. doi:10.3748/wjg.v21.i41.11688 PMID:26556996

Vaniquotes. (2018). Chapter 02.48. *Bhagavad Gita*. Retrieved 10 March 2020, from https://vaniquotes.org/wiki/BG_02.48_yoga-sthah_kuru_karmani .._cited

Velayos, F. S., Loftus, E. V. Jr, Jess, T., Harmsen, W. S., Bida, J., Zinsmeister, A. R., Tremaine, W. J., & Sandborn, W. J. (2006). Predictive and protective factors associated with colorectal cancer in ulcerative colitis: A case-control study. *Gastroenterology*, *130*(7), 1941–1949. doi:10.1053/j.gastro.2006.03.028 PMID:16762617

Venegas, D. P., Fuente, M. K. D., Landskron, G., González, M. J., Quera, R., Dijkstra, G., & ... . (2019). Short Chain Fatty Acids (SCFAs)-Mediated Gut Epithelial and Immune Regulation and its relevance for Inflammatory Bowel Diseases. *Frontiers in Immunology*, *10*, 277. doi:10.3389/fimmu.2019.00277 PMID:30915065

Vermeire, S., Ghosh, S., Panes, J., Dahlerup, J. F., Luegering, A., Sirotiakova, J., Strauch, U., Burgess, G., Spanton, J., Martin, S. W., & Niezychowski, W. (2011). The mucosal addressin cell adhesion molecule antibody PF-00547,659 in ulcerative colitis: A randomised study. *Gut*, *60*(8), 1068–1075. doi:10.1136/gut.2010.226548 PMID:21317177

Vermeire, S., Sandborn, W. J., Danese, S., Hébuterne, X., Salzberg, B. A., Klopocka, M., Tarabar, D., Vanasek, T., Greguš, M., Hellstern, P. A., Kim, J. S., Sparrow, M. P., Gorelick, K. J., Hinz, M., Ahmad, A., Pradhan, V., Hassan-Zahraee, M., Clare, R., Cataldi, F., & Reinisch, W. (2017). Anti-MAdCAM antibody (PF-00547659) for ulcerative colitis (TURANDOT): A phase 2, randomised, double-blind, placebo-controlled trial. *Lancet*, *390*(10090), 135–144. doi:10.1016/S0140-6736(17)30930-3 PMID:28527704

Vermeulen, L., De Sousa, E., Melo, F., van der Heijden, M., Cameron, K., de Jong, J. H., Borovski, T., ... Medema, J. P. (2010). Wnt activity defines colon cancer stem cells and is regulated by the microenvironment. *Nature Cell Biology*, *12*(5), 468–476. doi:10.1038/ncb2048 PMID:20418870

Vétizou, M., Pitt, J. M., Daillère, R., Lepage, P., Waldschmitt, N., Flament, C., ... Poirier-Colame, V. (2015). Anticancer immunotherapy by CTLA-4 blockade relies on the gut microbiota. *Science*, *350*(6264), 1079–1084. doi:10.1126cience.aad1329 PMID:26541610

Vezza, T., Rodriguez-Nogales, A., Algieri, F., Utrilla, M. P., Rodriguez-Cabezas, M. E., & Galvez, J. (2016). Flavonoids in inflammatory bowel disease: A review. *Nutrients*, *8*(4), 211. doi:10.3390/nu8040211 PMID:27070642

Viennois, E., Chen, F., & Merlin, D. (2013). NF-κB pathway in colitis-associated cancers. *Translational Gastrointestinal Cancer*, *2*(1), 21. PMID:23626930

Vilela, E. G., da Gama Torres, H. O., Martins, F. P., de Abreu Ferrari, M. D. L., Andrade, M. M., & da Cunha, A. S. (2012). Evaluation of inflammatory activity in Crohn's disease and ulcerative colitis. *World journal of gastroenterology. WJG*, *18*(9), 872. doi:10.3748/wjg.v18.i9.872 PMID:22408345

Villegas, I., Alarcon de la Lastra, C., Orjales, A., & La Casa, C. (2003). A new flavonoid derivative, dosmalfate, attenuates the development of dextran sulphate sodium-induced colitis in mice. *International Immunopharmacology*, *3*(13-14), 1731–1741. doi:10.1016/j.intimp.2003.07.002 PMID:14636824

Villegas, I., La Casa, C., Orjales, A., & Alarcon de la Lastra, C. (2003). Effects of dosmalfate, a new cytoprotective agent, on acute and chronic trinitrobenzene sulphonic acid-induced colitis in rats. *European Journal of Pharmacology*, *460*(2-3), 209–218. doi:10.1016/S0014-2999(02)02949-7 PMID:12559383

Villegas, I., Sanchez-Fidalgo, S., & de la Lastra, C. A. (2011). Chemopreventive effect of dietary curcumin on inflammation-induced colorectal carcinogenesis in mice. *Molecular Nutrition & Food Research*, *55*(2), 259–267. doi:10.1002/mnfr.201000225 PMID:20848615

Vine, K. L., Locke, J. M., Ranson, M., Benkendorff, K., Pyne, S. G., & Bremner, J. B. (2007). In vitro cytotoxicity evaluation of some substituted isatin derivatives. *Bioorganic & Medicinal Chemistry*, *15*(2), 931–938. Advance online publication. doi:10.1016/j.bmc.2006.10.035 PMID:17088067

Vinolo, M. A., Rodrigues, H. G., Nachbar, R. T., & Curi, R. (2011). Regulation of inflammation by short chain fatty acids. *Nutrients*, *3*(10), 858–876. doi:10.3390/nu3100858 PMID:22254083

Vitor, C. E., Figueiredo, C. P., Hara, D. B., Bento, A. F., Mazzuco, T. L., & Calixto, J. B. (2009). Therapeutic action and underlying mechanisms of a combination of two pentacyclic triterpenes, aand B-amyrin, in a mouse model of colitis. *British Journal of Pharmacology*, *157*(6), 1034–1044. Advance online publication. doi:10.1111/j.1476-5381.2009.00271.x PMID:19508397

Vochyanova, Z., Bartosova, L., Bujdakova, V., Fictum, P., Husnik, R., Suchy, P., Šmejkal, K., & Hošek, J. (2015). Diplacone and mimulone ameliorate dextran sulfate sodium-induced colitis in rats. *Fitoterapia*, *101*, 201–207. doi:10.1016/j.fitote.2015.01.012 PMID:25623260

Vogelstein, B., Fearon, E. R., Hamilton, S. R., Kern, S. E., Preisinger, A. C., Leppert, M., Smits, A. M. M., & Bos, J. L. (1988). Genetic alterations during colorectal-tumor development. *The New England Journal of Medicine*, *319*(9), 525–532. doi:10.1056/NEJM198809013190901 PMID:2841597

Waldner, M. J., & Neurath, M. F. (2012). Potential avenues for immunotherapy of colitis-associated neoplasia. *Immunotherapy*, *4*(4), 397–405. doi:10.2217/imt.12.15 PMID:22512634

Wang, D., Wang, H., Brown, J., Daikoku, T., Ning, W., Shi, Q., Richmond, A., Strieter, R., Dey, S. K., & DuBois, R. N. (2006). CXCL1 induced by prostaglandin E2 promotes angiogenesis in colorectal cancer. *The Journal of Experimental Medicine*, *203*(4), 941–951. doi:10.1084/jem.20052124 PMID:16567391

Wang, F., Song, Z. Y., Qu, X. J., Li, F., Zhang, L., Li, W. B , & Cui, S. X. (2018). M10, a novel derivative of myricetin, prevents ulcerative colitis and colorectal tumor through attenuating robust endoplasmic reticulum stress. *Carcinogenesis*, *39*(7), 889–899. doi:10.1093/carcin/bgy057 PMID:29757351

Wang, J. L., Gan, Y. J., Iqbal, S., Jiang, W., Yuan, Y. Y., & Wang, J. (2018). Delivery of tacrolimus with cationic lipid-assisted nanoparticles for ulcerative colitis therapy. *Biomaterials Science*, *6*(7), 1916–1922. doi:10.1039/C8BM00463C PMID:29850666

Wang, J., Li, S., Fan, Y., Chen, Y., Liu, D., Cheng, H., Gao, X., & Zhou, Y. (2010). Anti-fatigue activity of the water-soluble polysaccharides isolated from Panax ginseng C. A. Meyer. *Journal of Ethnopharmacology*, *130*(2), 421–423. doi:10.1016/j.jep.2010.05.027 PMID:20580802

Wang, T., Cai, G., Qiu, Y., Fei, N., Zhang, M., Pang, X., Jia, W., Cai, S., & Zhao, L. (2012). Structural segregation of gut microbiota between colorectal cancer patients and healthy volunteers. *The ISME Journal*, *6*(2), 320–329. doi:10.1038/ismej.2011.109 PMID:21850056

Wang, X., Sun, Y., Zhao, Y., Ding, Y., Zhang, X., Kong, L., Li, Z., Guo, Q., & Zhao, L. (2016). Oroxyloside prevents dextran sulfate sodium-induced experimental colitis in mice by inhibiting NF-kappaB pathway through PPARgamma activation. *Biochemical Pharmacology*, *106*, 70–81. doi:10.1016/j.bcp.2016.02.019 PMID:26947454

Wang, Y., Shen, W., Shi, X., Fu, F., Fan, Y., Shen, W., Cao, Y., Zhang, Q., & Qi, R. (2017). Alpha-Tocopheryl Succinate-Conjugated G5 PAMAM Dendrimer Enables Effective Inhibition of Ulcerative Colitis. *Advanced Healthcare Materials*, *6*(14), 1700276. Advance online publication. doi:10.1002/adhm.201700276 PMID:28474434

Wang, Z., Li, Y., Banerjee, S., & Sarkar, F. H. (2009). Emerging role of Notch in stem cells and cancer. *Cancer Letters*, *279*(1), 8–12. doi:10.1016/j.canlet.2008.09.030 PMID:19022563

Warren, R. L., Freeman, D. J., Pleasance, S., Watson, P., Moore, R. A., Cochrane, K., & Holt, R. A. (2013). Co-occurrence of anaerobic bacteria in colorectal carcinomas. *Microbiome*, *1*(1), 16. doi:10.1186/2049-2618-1-16 PMID:24450771

Watanabe, K., Kawamori, T., Nakatsugi, S., Ohta, T., Ohuchida, S., Yamamoto, H., ... Wakabayashi, K. (1999). Role of the prostaglandin E receptor subtype EP1 in colon carcinogenesis. *Cancer Research*, *59*(20), 5093–5096. PMID:10537280

Weisshof, R., El Jurdi, K., Zmeter, N., & Rubin, D. T. (2018). Emerging therapies for inflammatory bowel disease. *Advances in Therapy*, *35*(11), 1746–1762. doi:10.100712325-018-0795-9 PMID:30374806

Weitkunat, K., Schumann, S., Petzke, K. J., Blaut, M., Loh, G., & Klaus, S. (2015). Effects of dietary inulin on bacterial growth, short-chain fatty acid production and hepatic lipid metabolism in gnotobiotic mice. *The Journal of Nutritional Biochemistry*, *26*(9), 929–937. doi:10.1016/j.jnutbio.2015.03.010 PMID:26033744

Willett, C. G., Duda, D. G., Czito, B. G., Bendell, J. C., Clark, J. W., & Jain, R. K. (2007). Targeted therapy in rectal cancer. *Oncology (Williston Park, N.Y.)*, *21*(9), 1055. PMID:17910311

Wolf, A. J., Reyes, C. N., Liang, W., Becker, C., Shimada, K., Wheeler, M. L., Cho, H. C., Popescu, N. I., Coggeshall, K. M., Arditi, M., & Underhill, D. M. (2016). Hexokinase is an innate immune receptor for the detection of bacterial peptidoglycan. *Cell*, *166*(3), 624–636. doi:10.1016/j.cell.2016.05.076 PMID:27374331

Wright, K., Kolios, G., Westwick, J., & Ward, S. G. (1999). Cytokine-induced apoptosis in epithelial HT-29 cells is independent of nitric oxide formation: Evidence for an interleukin-13-driven phosphatidylinositol 3-kinase-dependent survival mechanism. *The Journal of Biological Chemistry*, *274*(24), 17193–17201. doi:10.1074/jbc.274.24.17193 PMID:10358077

Wu, C.-C., Chung, J., Tsai, S.-J., Yang, J., & Sheen, L. (2004). Differential effects of allyl sulfides from garlic essential oil on cell cycle regulation in human liver tumor cells. *Food and Chemical Toxicology*, *42*(12), 1937–1947. doi:10.1016/j.fct.2004.07.008 PMID:15500931

Wu, N., Yang, X., Zhang, R., Li, J., Xiao, X., Hu, Y., & Luan, C. (2013). Dysbiosis signature of fecal microbiota in colorectal cancer patients. *Microbial Ecology*, *66*(2), 462–470. doi:10.100700248-013-0245-9 PMID:23733170

Wu, Y., Sun, M., Wang, D., Li, G., Huang, J., Tan, S., Bao, L., Li, Q., Li, G., & Si, L. (2019). A PepT1 mediated medicinal nano-system for targeted delivery of cyclosporine A to alleviate acute severe ulcerative colitis. *Biomaterials Science*, *7*(10), 4299–4309. doi:10.1039/C9BM00925F PMID:31408067

Xavier, R. J., & Podolsky, D. K. (2007). Unravelling the pathogenesis of inflammatory bowel disease. *Nature*, *448*(7152), 427–434. doi:10.1038/nature06005 PMID:17653185

Xiao, B., Chen, Q., Zhang, Z., Wang, L., Kang, Y., Denning, T., & Merlin, D. (2018). TNFalpha gene silencing mediated by orally targeted nanoparticles combined with interleukin-22 for synergistic combination therapy of ulcerative colitis. *Journal of Controlled Release*, *287*, 235–246. doi:10.1016/j.jconrel.2018.08.021 PMID:30107214

Xiao, B., Xu, Z., Viennois, E., Zhang, Y., Zhang, Z., Zhang, M., Han, M. K., Kang, Y., & Merlin, D. (2017). Orally Targeted Delivery of Tripeptide KPV via Hyaluronic Acid-Functionalized Nanoparticles Efficiently Alleviates Ulcerative Colitis. *Molecular Therapy*, *25*(7), 1628–1640. doi:10.1016/j.ymthe.2016.11.020 PMID:28143741

Xiao, B., Zhang, Z., Viennois, E., Kang, Y., Zhang, M., Han, M. K., Chen, J., & Merlin, D. (2016). Combination Therapy for Ulcerative Colitis: Orally Targeted Nanoparticles Prevent Mucosal Damage and Relieve Inflammation. *Theranostics*, *6*(12), 2250–2266. doi:10.7150/thno.15710 PMID:27924161

Xiao, D., Li, M., Herman-Antosiewicz, A., Antosiewicz, J., Xiao, H., Lew, K. L., Zeng, Y., Marynowski, S. W., & Singh, S. V. (2006). Diallyl trisulfide inhibits angiogenic features of human umbilical vein endothelial cells by causing Akt inactivation and down-regulation of VEGF and VEGF-R2. *Nutrition and Cancer*, *55*(1), 94–107. doi:10.120715327914nc5501_12 PMID:16965246

Xia, Q., Xiao, P., Wan, L., & Kong, J. (1997). Ethnopharmacology of Phyllanthus emblica L. *Zhongguo Zhongyao Zazhi*, *22*, 515–574. PMID:11038937

Xie, Y.-H., Chen, Y.-X., & Fang, J.-Y. (2020). Comprehensive review of targeted therapy for colorectal cancer. *Signal Transduction and Targeted Therapy*, *5*(1), 22. doi:10.103841392-020-0116-z PMID:32296018

Xiong, Y., Chen, D., Yu, C., Lv, B., Peng, J., Wang, J., & Lin, Y. (2015). Citrus nobiletin ameliorates experimental colitis by reducing inflammation and restoring impaired intestinal barrier function. *Molecular Nutrition & Food Research*, *59*(5), 829–842. doi:10.1002/mnfr.201400614 PMID:25655748

Xu, L., Yang, Z. L., Li, P., & Zhou, Y. Q. (2009). Modulating effect of hesperidin on experimental murine colitis induced by dextran sulfate sodium. *Phytomedicine*, *16*(10), 989–995. doi:10.1016/j.phymed.2009.02.021 PMID:19386481

Yamashiro, T., Fukunaga, T., Kobashi, N., Kamioka, H., Nakanishi, T., Takigawa, M., & Takano-Yamamoto, T. (2001). Mechanical stimulation induces CTGF expression in rat osteocytes. *Journal of Dental Research*, *80*(2), 461–465. doi:10.1177/00220345010800021201 PMID:11332533

Yang, L., Shen, L., Li, Y., Li, Y., Yu, S., & Wang, S. (2017). Hyperoside attenuates dextran sulfate sodium-induced colitis in mice possibly via activation of the Nrf2 signalling pathway. *Journal of Inflammation*, *14*(1), 25. doi:10.118612950-017-0172-5 PMID:29162986

Yang, X. R., Wang, Y. Y., La, K. K., Peng, L., Song, X. H., Shi, X. G., Zhu, X., Leung, P., Ko, C., & Ye, C. X. (2012). Inhibitory effects of cocoa tea (Camellia ptilophylla) in human hepatocellular carcinoma HepG2 in vitro and in vivo through apoptosis. *The Journal of Nutritional Biochemistry*, *23*(9), 1051–1057. doi:10.1016/j.jnutbio.2011.05.010 PMID:22018604

Yang, Y., Cai, X., Yang, J., Sun, X., Hu, C., Yan, Z., Xu, X., Lu, W., Wang, X., & Cao, P. (2014). Chemoprevention of dietary digitoflavone on colitis-associated colon tumorigenesis through inducing Nrf2 signaling pathway and inhibition of inflammation. *Molecular Cancer*, *13*(1), 48. doi:10.1186/1476-4598-13-48 PMID:24602443

Yang, Y., & Jobin, C. (2017). Novel insights into microbiome in Colitis and colorectal cancer. *Current Opinion in Gastroenterology*, *33*(6), 422–427. doi:10.1097/MOG.0000000000000399 PMID:28877044

Yang, Z. F., Ngai, P., Ho, D. W., Yu, W. C., Ng, M. N. P., Lau, C. K., Li, M. L. Y., Tam, K. H., Lam, C. T., Poon, R. T. P., & Fan, S. T. (2008). Identification of local and circulating cancer stem cells in human liver cancer. *Hepatology (Baltimore, Md.)*, *47*(3), 919–928. doi:10.1002/hep.22082 PMID:18275073

Yashiro, M. (2014). Ulcerative colitis-associated colorectal cancer. *World Journal of Gastroenterology*, *20*(44), 16389–16397. doi:10.3748/wjg.v20.i44.16389 PMID:25469007

Yasui, Y., Hosokawa, M., Mikami, N., Miyashita, K., & Tanaka, T. (2011). Dietary astaxanthin inhibits colitis and colitis-associated colon carcinogenesis in mice via modulation of the inflammatory cytokines. *Chemico-Biological Interactions*, *193*(1), 79–87. doi:10.1016/j.cbi.2011.05.006 PMID:21621527

Yazeji, T., Moulari, B., Beduneau, A., Stein, V., Dietrich, D., Pellequer, Y., & Lamprecht, A. (2017). Nanoparticle-based delivery enhances anti-inflammatory effect of low molecular weight heparin in experimental ulcerative colitis. *Drug Delivery*, *24*(1), 811–817. doi:10.1080/10717544.2017.1324530 PMID:28509629

Ye, Z., Liu, Z. P., Henderson, A., Lee, K., Hostetter, J., Wannemuehler, M., & Hendrich, S. (2009). Increased CYP4B1 mRNA is associated with the inhibition of dextran sulfate sodium-induced colitis by caffeic acid in mice. *Experimental Biology and Medicine*, *234*(6), 605–616. doi:10.3181/0901-RM-1 PMID:19307459

Yorulmaz, E., Yorulmaz, H., Gökmen, E. S., Altınay, S., Küçük, S. H., Zengi, O., Çelik, D. S., & Şit, D. (2019). Therapeutic effectiveness of rectally administered fish oil and mesalazine in trinitrobenzenesulfonic acid-induced colitis. *Biomedicine and Pharmacotherapy*, *118*, 109247. Advance online publication. doi:10.1016/j.biopha.2019.109247 PMID:31351432

Young, A. R. D. J., Coulson, R., O'Brien, M., Deb, S., Lopata, A., Behren, A., Mathivanan, S., Lim, E., & Meeusen, E. (2019). Immunoprofiling of Breast Cancer Antigens Using Antibodies Derived from Local Lymph Nodes. *Cancers (Basel)*, *11*(5), 682. doi:10.3390/cancers11050682 PMID:31100936

Yue, G., Lai, P. S., Yin, K., Sun, F. F., Nagele, R. G., Liu, X., … Wong, P. Y. K. (2001). Colon epithelial cell death in 2,4,6-trinitrobenzenesulfonic acid-induced colitis is associated with increased inducible nitric-oxide synthase expression and peroxynitrite production. *Journal of Pharmacology and Experimental Therapeutics*.

Yu, H., Kortylewski, M., & Pardoll, D. (2007). Crosstalk between cancer and immune cells: Role of STAT3 in the tumour microenvironment. *Nature Reviews. Immunology*, *7*(1), 41–51. doi:10.1038/nri1995 PMID:17186030

Yukawa, T. A., Kurokawa, M., Sato, H., Yoshida, Y., Kageyama, S., Hasegawa, T., Namba, T., Imakita, M., Hozumi, T., & Shiraki, K. (1996). Prophylactic treatment of cytomegalovirus infection with traditional herbs. *Antiviral Research*, *32*(2), 63–70. doi:10.1016/0166-3542(95)00978-7 PMID:8891165

Zeisel, S. H., & Blusztajn, J. K. (1994). Choline and human nutrition. *Annual Review of Nutrition*, *14*(1), 269–296. doi:10.1146/annurev.nu.14.070194.001413 PMID:7946521

Zhang, H., Deng, A., Zhang, Z., Yu, Z., Liu, Y., Peng, S., Wu, L. Q., Qin, H. L., & Wang, W. J. (2016). The protective effect of epicatechin on experimental ulcerative colitis in mice is mediated by increasing antioxidation and by the inhibition of NF-κB pathway. *Pharmacological Reports*, *68*(3), 514–520. doi:10.1016/j.pharep.2015.12.011 PMID:26878122

Zhang, M., Viennois, E., Prasad, M., Zhang, Y., Wang, L., Zhang, Z., Han, M. K., Xiao, B., Xu, C., Srinivasan, S., & Merlin, D. (2016). Edible ginger-derived nanoparticles: A novel therapeutic approach for the prevention and treatment of inflammatory bowel disease and colitis-associated cancer. *Biomaterials*, *101*, 321–340. doi:10.1016/j.biomaterials.2016.06.018 PMID:27318094

Zhang, M., Xu, C., Liu, D., Han, M. K., Wang, L., & Merlin, D. (2018). Oral Delivery of Nanoparticles Loaded With Ginger Active Compound, 6-Shogaol, Attenuates Ulcerative Colitis and Promotes Wound Healing in a Murine Model of Ulcerative Colitis. *Journal of Crohn's and Colitis*, *12*(2), 217–229. doi:10.1093/ecco-jcc/jjx115 PMID:28961808

Zhang, X., Ma, Y., Ma, L., Zu, M., Song, H., & Xiao, B. (2019). Oral administration of chondroitin sulfate-functionalized nanoparticles for colonic macrophage-targeted drug delivery. *Carbohydrate Polymers*, *223*, 115126. doi:10.1016/j.carbpol.2019.115126 PMID:31426992

Zhao, J., Hong, T., Dong, M., Meng, Y., & Mu, J. (2013). Protective effect of myricetin in dextran sulphate sodium-induced murine ulcerative colitis. *Molecular Medicine Reports*, *7*(2), 565–570. doi:10.3892/mmr.2012.1225 PMID:23232835

Zhou, H., & Qian, H. (2018). Preparation and characterization of pH-sensitive nanoparticles of budesonide for the treatment of ulcerative colitis. *Drug Design, Development and Therapy*, *12*, 2601–2609. doi:10.2147/DDDT.S170676 PMID:30174414

Zhou, Y., Xia, L., Wang, H., Oyang, L., Su, M., Liu, Q., Lin, J., Tan, S., Tian, Y., Liao, Q., & Cao, D. (2018). Cancer stem cells in progression of colorectal cancer. *Oncotarget*, *9*(70), 33403–33415. doi:10.18632/oncotarget.23607 PMID:30279970

Zhu, H., Itoh, K., Yamamoto, M., Zweier, J. L., & Li, Y. (2005). Role of Nrf2 signaling in regulation of antioxidants and phase 2 enzymes in cardiac fibroblasts: Protection against reactive oxygen and nitrogen species-induced cell injury. *FEBS Letters*, *579*(14), 3029–3036. doi:10.1016/j.febslet.2005.04.058 PMID:15896789

Zhu, Q., Jin, Z., Wu, W., Gao, R., Guo, B., Gao, Z., & Qin, H. (2014). Analysis of the intestinal lumen microbiota in an animal model of colorectal cancer. *PLoS One*, *9*(3), e90849. doi:10.1371/journal.pone.0090849 PMID:24603888

Zhu, S., Jiang, X., Boudreau, M. D., Feng, G., Miao, Y., Dong, S., Wu, H., Zeng, M., & Yin, J. J. (2018). Orally administered gold nanoparticles protect against colitis by attenuating Toll-like receptor 4- and reactive oxygen/nitrogen species-mediated inflammatory responses but could induce gut dysbiosis in mice. *Journal of Nanobiotechnology*, *16*(1), 86. doi:10.118612951-018-0415-5 PMID:30384844

Zhu, W., Jin, Z. S., Yu, J. B., Liang, J., Yang, Q. D., Li, F. J., Shi, X., Zhu, X., & Zhang, X. (2016). Baicalin ameliorates experimental inflammatory bowel disease through polarization of macrophages to an M2 phenotype. *International Immunopharmacology*, *35*, 119–126. doi:10.1016/j.intimp.2016.03.030 PMID:27039210

Zhu, Y., Zhang, B., Gong, A., Fu, H., Zhang, X., Shi, H., Sun, Y., Wu, L., Pan, Z., Mao, F., Zhu, W., Qian, H., & Xu, W. (2016). Anti-cancer drug 3,3′-diindolylmethane activates Wnt4 signaling to enhance gastric cancer cell stemness and tumorigenesis. *Oncotarget*, *7*(13), 16311–16324. doi:10.18632/oncotarget.7684 PMID:26918831

Zingarelli, B., Hake, P. W., Burroughs, T. J., Piraino, G., O'Connor, M., & Denenberg, A. (2004). Activator protein-1 signalling pathway and apoptosis are modulated by poly(ADP-ribose) polymerase-1 in experimental colitis. *Immunology*, *113*(4), 509–517. doi:10.1111/j.1365-2567.2004.01991.x PMID:15554929

Zisman, T. L., & Rubin, D. T. (2008). Colorectal cancer and dysplasia in inflammatory bowel disease. *World journal of gastroenterology. WJG*, *14*(17), 2662. doi:10.3748/wjg.14.2662 PMID:18461651

Zou, Y., Dai, S. X., Chi, H. G., Li, T., He, Z. W., Wang, J., Ye, C.-G., Huang, G.-L., Zhao, B., Li, W.-Y., Wan, Z., Feng, J.-S., & Zheng, X.-B. (2015). Baicalin attenuates TNBS-induced colitis in rats by modulating the Th17/Treg paradigm. *Archives of Pharmacal Research*, *38*(10), 1873–1887. doi:10.100712272-014-0486-2 PMID:25269538

About the Contributors

Ashok Kumar Pandurangan is an associate professor in School of Life Sciences, B.S. Abdur Rahman Crescent Institute of Science and Technology, Vandalur, Chennai, India. He pursued his PhD in the prestigious University of Madras, Guindy campus, Chennai, India in the area of natural products as a therapeutic agent for colorectal cancer. Later, he was postdoctoral researcher in Center for Cancer research, Children's Hospital Oakland Research Institute, Oakland, California, USA. Further he completed two postdoctoral research programs in Department of Nutrition and Dietetics, Universiti of Putra Malaysia and Department of Pharmacology, University of Malaya, Malaysia. He is currently interested to work in the area of colitis associated cancer (CAC) in murine model. Colitis associated cancer is very common nowadays in developing countries. Ulcerative Colitis (UC) is a type of Inflammatory Bowel Disease (IBD), if untreated can be a risk of developing as colitis associated cancer. Numerous studies are underway to identify drugs that control both inflammation and cell proliferation. So, he is interested in identify some novel drugs from natural source and elucidate the molecular mechanisms involved in the process of curing colitis associated cancer. He published several articles on the effects of natural agents in these areas of interest.

* * *

Neesar Ahmed is Assistant Professor, School of Life Sciences, BSA Crescent Institute of Science & Technology, Chennai, India. He finished his Ph.D in National Centre for Cell Sciences, University of Pune-Pune Maharashtra, India. Later, he finished his postdoctoral Research at Wayne State University, USA (2011-2013). His research group is focused on inflammatory disorders in various human diseases and Immunotherapy. He is interested in investigating the mechanisms engaged by tumors to evade cancer immunosurveillance with special interest in the role and function of immunosuppressive cells. Our group is involved in studying the Ubiquitin mediated regulation of the inflammatory Tumor Microenvironment and Targeting E3 ligases involved in inflammation.

Suresh Kumar Anandasadagopan is currently working as a senior scientist in the Department of Biochemistry and Biotechnology, CSIR-Central Leather Research Institute, Adyar, Chennai, India. Previously he completed his PhD. in the prestigious University of Madras, Guindy campus, Chennai in the year 2010. Later, he moved to University of Pennsylvania (UPENN), Philadelphia, USA for his postdoctoral studies. Apart from that he worked as postdoctoral fellow in Department of Pharmacology, University of Malaya, Kuala Lumpur, Malaysia. He published several research and review articles in reputed peer-reviewed journals. He also received grants for his research work .

Soccalingam Artchoudane is Yoga Therapist, Center for Yogic Sciences (CYS), Aarupadai Veedu Medical College and Hospital (AVMC & H), Vinayaka Mission's Research Foundation (VMRF), Puducherry, India. He has completed MSc, MPhil, and is currently pursuing PhD in Yoga Therapy. He has published several research articles and conference proceedings on Yoga therapy for pulmonary and neuromuscular functions and neurodevelopmental disabilities. He has authored book chapters on yoga therapy for cognitive and digestive functions. He recently received the Achiever's Award for "Best Yoga Teacher" and 'Yuva Bharati'. He has designed several value added courses and yoga protocols on yoga therapy for medical and paramedical curriculum, and obtained copyright for the same. He is a professional member of Indian Yoga Association and member of the jury board, Pondicherry Yogasana Association.

Subhamoy Banerjee is an Assistant Professor in School of Life Science, B S Abdur Rahman Crescent Institute of Science and Technology, Chennai. He has done PhD from IIT Guwahati in nanobiotechnology and postdoc from IIT Delhi. He has authored 9 international publications and 2 book chapters. He works in the field of polymeric nanoparticle mediated drug delivery and computational biology with interest in computational virology and pathway analysis in disease cross-talk.

Félix Carvalho, PharmD (1990), PhD (1998), is Full Professor of Toxicology, at the Laboratory of Toxicology, Department of Biological Sciences, Faculty of Pharmacy at the University of Porto (FFUP), and researcher of the Research Unit on Applied Molecular Biosciences (UCIBIO) at REQUIMTE, Portugal. He is presently Head of the Toxicology Laboratory and President of the Scientific Council at FFUP, President of the Portuguese Society of Pharmacology, President-Elect of EUROTOX, and Vice-Director of UCIBIO. Félix Carvalho is also European Expert of the European Medicines Agency (EMA), and Member of the Committee for Evaluation of Medicines at the National Authority of Medicines and Health Products, I.P. (INFARMED), and participates in the editorial board of several scientific journals. During the past 29 years, Félix Carvalho published over 400 scientific articles / book chapters and is co-editor of two Books.

M. Luísa Corvo has been working on the development of drug carrier systems for the delivery anti-inflammatory drugs. Systems developed were liposomes (attractive delivery systems) for the treatment of Rheumatoid Arthritis and different type of nanoparticles, SOD Enzymosomes, to treat and visualize Ischaemia/Reperfusion Injury (following organ transplantation). Corvo has also been studying mechanisms of action of developed formulation and their correlation with biomarkers, tissue disposition and pharmacokinetics.

Eduarda Fernandes, PharmD (1991), PhD (1996), is Associate Professor at the Laboratory of Applied Chemistry, Department of Chemical Sciences, Faculty of Pharmacy at University of Porto (FFUP), and researcher of the Portuguese Research Centre for Sustainable Chemistry (LAQV) at REQUIMTE, Portugal. In 2002, she created a research unit within LAQV-REQUIMTE focused on the development and application of methodologies for the in vitro study of antioxidant, anti-inflammatory and antidiabetic properties of natural and synthetic compounds, in non-cellular and cellular models, (Free Radicals and Antioxidants Unit - FRAU), which she has been coordinating to the present (https://gabaiunitfra.wixsite.com/frau). Eduarda Fernandes has a vast supervision experience and holds 195+ publications, with 9.500+ citations and a h-index of 49 (Scopus).

Marisa Freitas (MF) completed her PhD degree in Pharmaceutical Sciences in 2010, in Faculty of Pharmacy of University of Porto. In 2012, MF was awarded with a post-Doc FCT fellowship and in 2016 she was hired Assistant Researcher from the project "New Technologies for three Health Challenges of Modern Societies: Diabetes, Drug Abuse and Kidney Diseases" (NORTE-01-0145-FEDER-000024). In April of 2019, MF was hired as Assistant Researcher in the project "Use of flavonoids in the prophylaxis of intestinal pro-inflammatory effects of silver nanoparticles (POCI-01-0145-FEDER-029248). Her high scientific competence is supported by the 75 publications in international journals, (70% in Q1 journals), 5 book chapters, 40 oral communications (6 as invited speaker) and 100+ poster communications in national and international conferences. Her h-index is 26 (Scopus) and she has 1900+ citations.

Pervaiz Iqbal is currently working as a Assistant Professor in the Department of Mathematics and Actuarial Science at B.S.A.R. Crescent Institute of Science & Technology Vandalur, Chennai, 600048 since July 2017. He has completed his Doctor's Degree from B.S. Abdur Rahman University, Vadalur, Chennai in 2017. He has published 8 papers in reputed International and National Journals. And he has presented 7 papers in International Conferences and 2 papers in National Journals.

Rubeena Khaliq is currently a research scholar in the Department of Mathematics at B.S.A.R Crescent Institute of Science and Technology since 2018.She has completed her masters in Mathematics from Baba Gulamshah Badshah Unversty Rajouri Jammu in 2016.

José Miguel Pimenta Ferreira de Oliveira graduated in Biochemistry, with specialization in Applied Biochemistry, Faculty of Sciences, University of Porto in 2000 and completed a PhD degree in Nutrition and Health Sciences from Wageningen University (VLAG Graduate School PhD Programme). In 2010, he was awarded the doctorate degree. Between 2000 and 2003 he investigated new genetic predictive biomarkers for stroke, myocardial infarction, and deep vein thrombosis. During this period as a volunteer researcher at Hospital Geral de Santo Antonio, he was introduced to techniques of DNA sequencing, quantitative real-time PCR and DNA polymorphism analyses, among others. From 2004 to 2010 he developed research in fungal genomics and biotechnology, Wageningen University, first as a fellow researcher and later on enrolled in a doctoral programme supported by VLAG Graduate School. The major areas covered were oxidative stress and protein secretion stress, which were investigated by functional genomics (including cloning, transformation, mutant screening), transcriptomics and shotgun proteomics. From 2011 he started studying the cytotoxic effects of phytochemicals as combined agents for osteosarcoma therapy in CESAM, University of Aveiro. The focus is on the cellular and molecular damages caused by phytochemicals, particularly flavonoids, in osteosarcoma in vitro cell models. Another topic of strong interest has been the response to phytochemicals at RNA transcripts level. Between 2012 and 2014 he additionally exercised consultancy activity in cloning and genotyping technologies in KLÓN – Innovative Technologies from Cloning, S.A., aiming to genetically charaterise plants with increased productivity for sustainable production. Currently, he studies the cytotoxic and inhibitory actions of phytochemicals in osteosarcoma in vitro and ex ovo cell models, as a contracted researcher at LAQV - REQUIMTE - Associate Laboratory for Green Chemistry, Technology and Clean Processes, University of Porto.

Daniela Ribeiro has a Master in Pharmaceutical Sciences (2010) and a PhD in Pharmaceutical Sciences - specialty of Pharmaceutical and Medicinal Chemistry (2014), by Faculty of Pharmacy of University of Porto (FFUP). From 2016 to 2018 she worked as a post-doctoral researcher at Institute of Sciences, Technologies and Agro-environment of the University of Porto (ICETA), within the scope of funded scientific research projects. She has been conducting her research activity focused on the study of antioxidant and anti-inflammatory activities of polyphenols and carotenoids. Of the Scientific Performance, stand out the co-authorship of 3 book chapters, the publication of 47 articles in indexed international journals (h-index of 18, by Scopus) and the presentation of a total of 91 oral and poster communications in national and international scientific meetings, with 3 attributed awards. She is Editor and reviewer of several indexed international journals. She currently is the responsible researcher of a funded scientific project, at Associated Laboratory for Green Chemistry (LAQV) of the Network of Chemistry and Technology (REQUI-MTE), being the work developed in the Laboratory of Applied Chemistry of FFUP.

Aadil Rashid Sheergojri is currently a Research Scholar in the Department of Mathematics B.S.A.R. Crescent Institute of Science & Technology Vandalur Chennai, 600048 since July 2019. He has completed his Master's degree from Lovely Professional University Jalandhar Punjab in 2018.

Mohammad Waseem is a currently a Professor at the School of Life Sciences, BS Abdur Rahman Crescent Institute of Science and Technology, India. He earned his BS program from MJP Rohilhnad University, India, and his MS and PhD program from Jamia Hamdard, New Delhi India. In his thesis, he has screened several anticancer drugs induced toxicity in mitochondria under in vitro and in vivo systems. And also, he has worked on the role of mitochondrial permeability transition in neuroprotection. After completing his Ph.D., he accepted a postdoctoral position at University of Alabama, USA. During this time, he has worked and investigated the action of novel anti-inflammatory drugs in inflammation mediates cancer in transgenic mice. Professor Waseem has more then 35 peer reviewed publications at impacted Journals. He is also a Life Member of American Association of Cancer Research, USA and other International Societies.

Index

A

C

D

E

F

G

I

L

M

N

S

U

W

www.ingramcontent.com/pod-product-compliance
Lightning Source LLC
LaVergne TN
LVHW081528300926
849161LV00006B/1348

turned out that the older tanks did well in difficult terrain and challenging climate. (Interestingly, the last delivery of T-34-85s from the USSR took place in 1973). The Vietnamese 'eighty-fives' from the 273rd Armoured Regiment took part in the final act of the war – the capture of Saigon in April 1975. The North Vietnamese also operated anti-aircraft vehicles developed in China, with twin 37 mm Type 63 cannons mounted on T-34-85 hulls (one such vehicle is preserved at the Aberdeen museum). Vietnamese T-34-85s took also part in the invasion of Cambodia and in 1979 they probably saw combat in the border conflict with China.

The last instance of combat use of T-34-85s in Asia was the war in Afghanistan in the 1980s. They were operated by Afghan Army units and according to some sources, also by Mujahedeen.

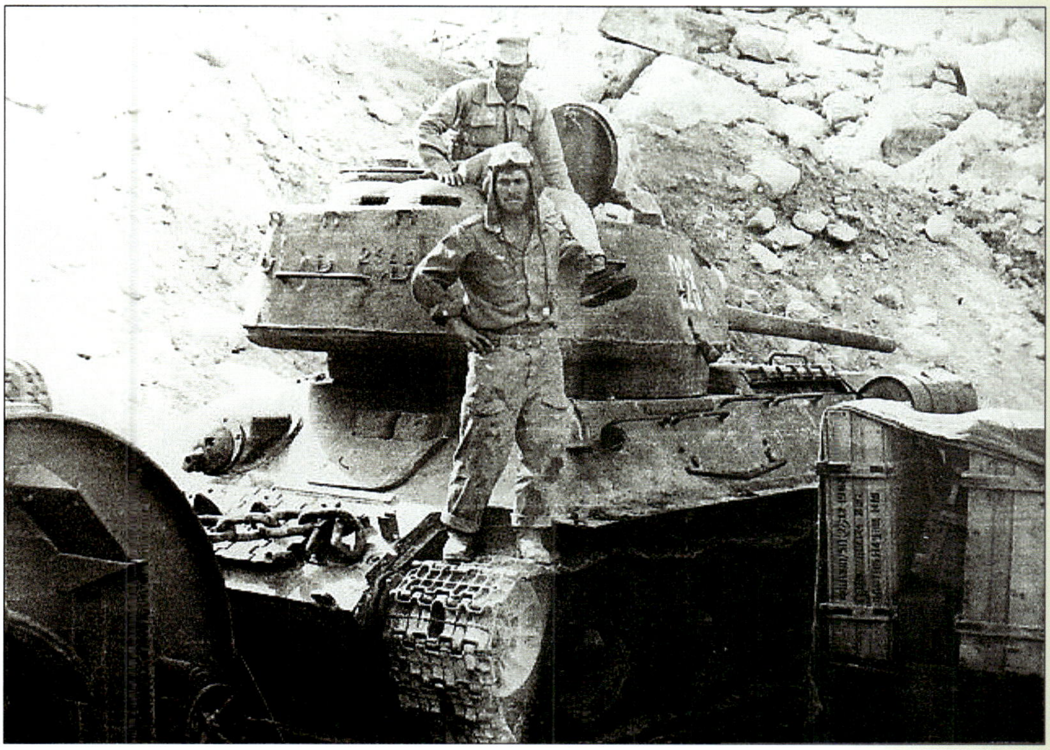

A T-34-85 of Afghan government forces on CHMZAP-5247 tank trailer, early 1980s.

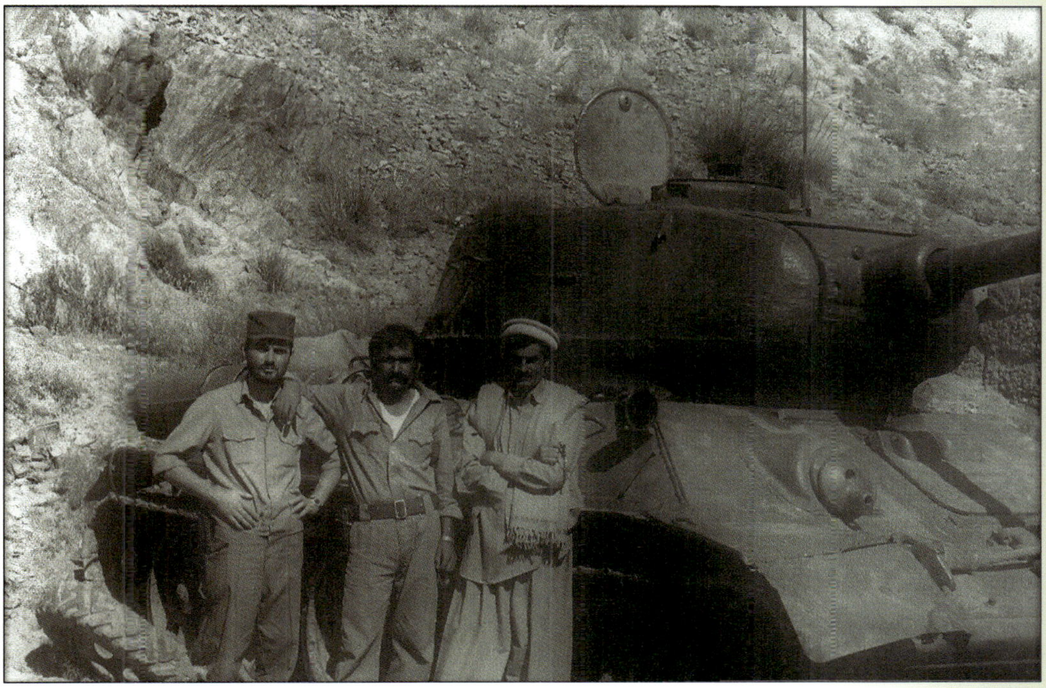

Afghan soldiers with a T-34-85 (probably of Plant No. 183 production), modernized to Model 1969 standard, 1980s. The tank has no markings or tactical number.

In the Middle East

Another region, where 'eighty-fives' saw combat was the Middle East. The first tanks of this type in the region (mostly of Czechoslovak production) arrived in Egypt in 1956, and were assigned to the 1st Armoured Brigade and probably the 2nd Armoured Brigade. Another unit was the 85th Tank Battalion, based in Cairo. It seems that by autumn 1956, only the 1st Armoured Brigade, called the "Soviet" brigade due to its equipment, had attained operational status. However, the combat debut of Egyptian T-34-85s was not impressive. During Operation 'Kadesh', Israeli units destroyed or captured at least 27 of the tanks (although other figures have also been published – e.g. 27 tanks captured and a dozen or so destroyed). It turned out that against Israeli Shermans and AMX-13s these tanks had almost no chance, but to great extent this was due to the difference in crew training level – excellent on the Israeli side and very poor on the Arab side.

In the late 1950s/early 1960s Syria also received T-34-85 tanks (deliveries from the USSR and Czechoslovakia). During the Six Day War in 1967 war the Arabs already used more modern T-54/55 tanks, but the T-34-85s were still in first line units, both Syrian and Egyptian. They mostly equipped armoured battalions assigned to infantry units. In June 1967 the T-34-85s were assigned, among others, to the Egyptian 2nd, 3rd and 7th Infantry Divisions. In case of the Syrian forces the situation was somewhat different. The T-34-85s also equipped battalions assigned to infantry units, but two armoured units as well – the 14th and 44th Armoured Brigades. Encounters with Israeli tanks (M50 and M51 Sherman, Centurion, M48 and M60 Patton) revealed that the T-34-85 was an obsolete weapon; in the Sinai, Egypt lost as many as 250 of these vehicles. The outcome of the fighting in the Golan Heights was more favourable for the Arabs – in combat in difficult terrain, Zahal lost about 160 tanks, while losses in the Syrian units amounted to 73 tanks (T-34-85, Panzer IV and T-54) and a dozen or so self-propelled guns (Su-100 and StuG III).

In another Arab-Israeli conflict – the Yom Kippur war of 1973 – the T-34-85s were used on a limited scale for auxiliary tasks. The obsolete tanks also found another application. After the Six Day war the Syrians placed numerous T-34-85s as stationary firing and observation points along the Israeli border and on in the Golan Heights. Also, self-propelled guns based on the T-34 chassis, designated T-34/122 were operated by the Syrian Army. These were Soviet D-30 howitzers mounted

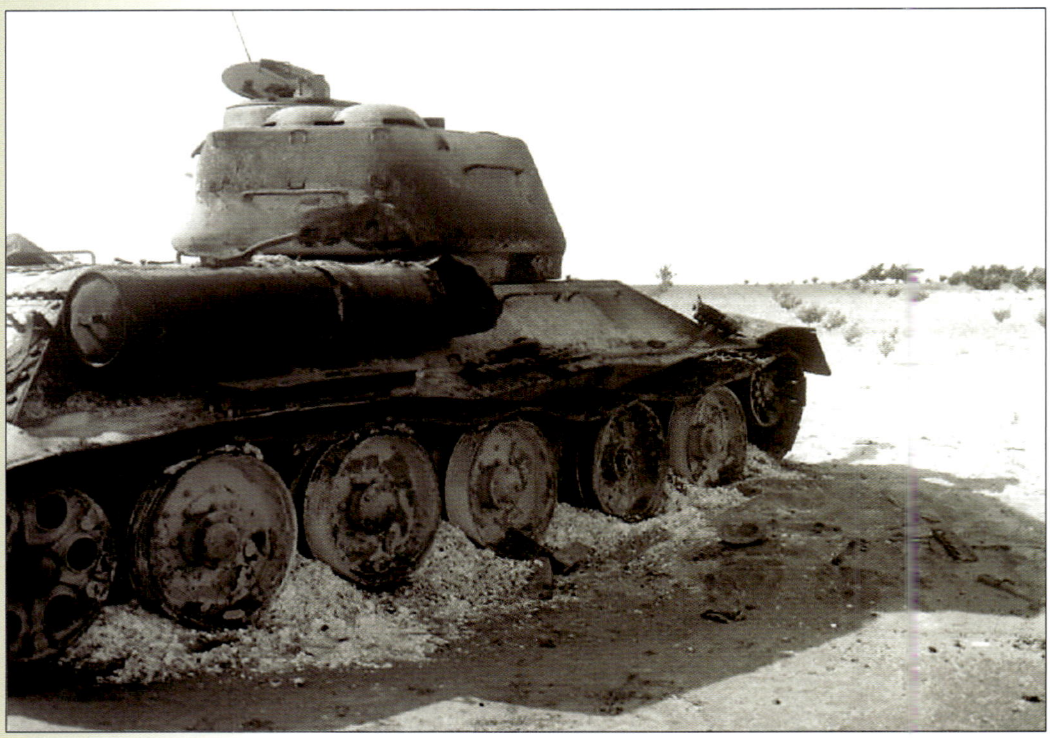

A burnt-out wreck of an Egyptian T-34-85 in the desert. The photograph was probably taken during the Six Day War in 1967.

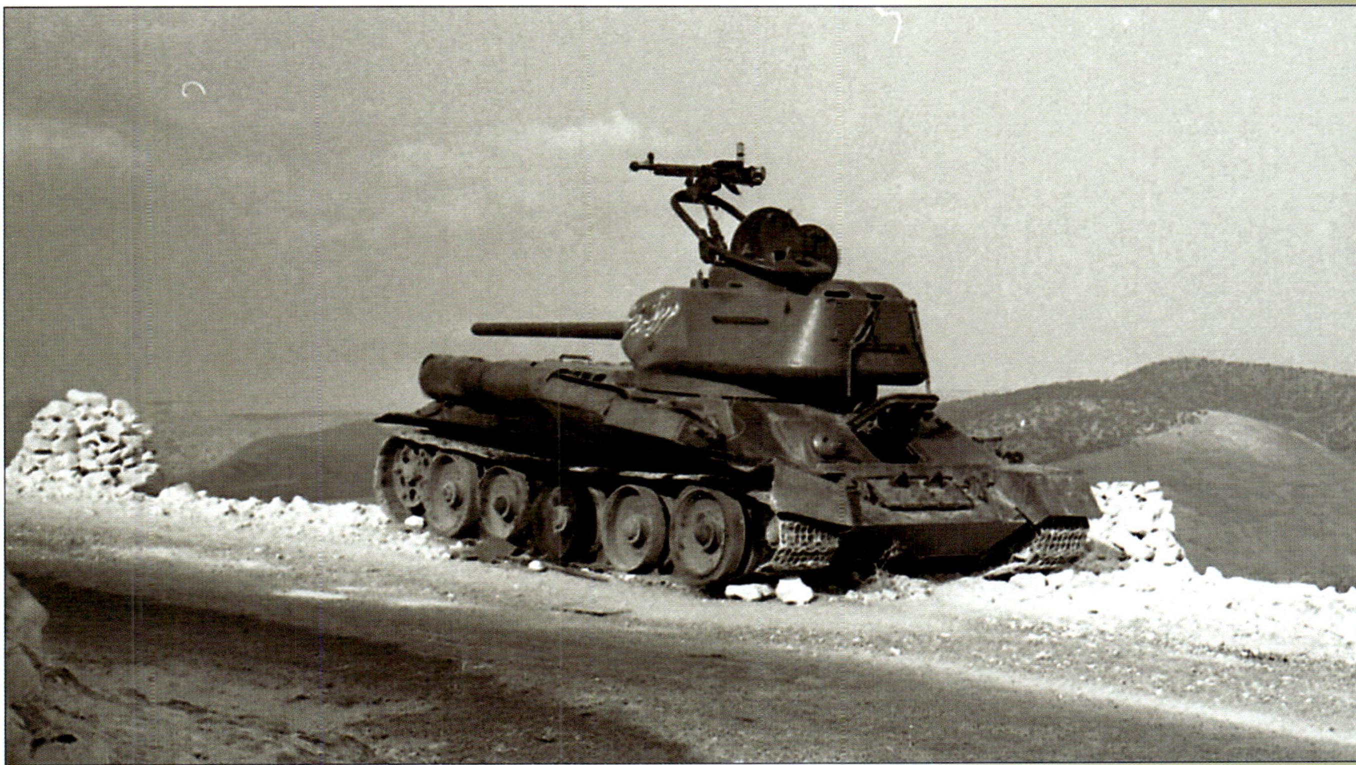

A Syrian T-34-85 (Czechoslovak production) lost during the Six Day War in 1967. The rail with grip for 12.7 mm DShK machine gun, characteristic for the Syrian tanks is well visible. The condition of the wheels indicates that the tank was burnt.

A group of Israeli citizens taking a trip to the battlefield after the end of the Six Day War in 1967. The T-34-85 tank has an identification triangle (probably red) painted on the forward fender.

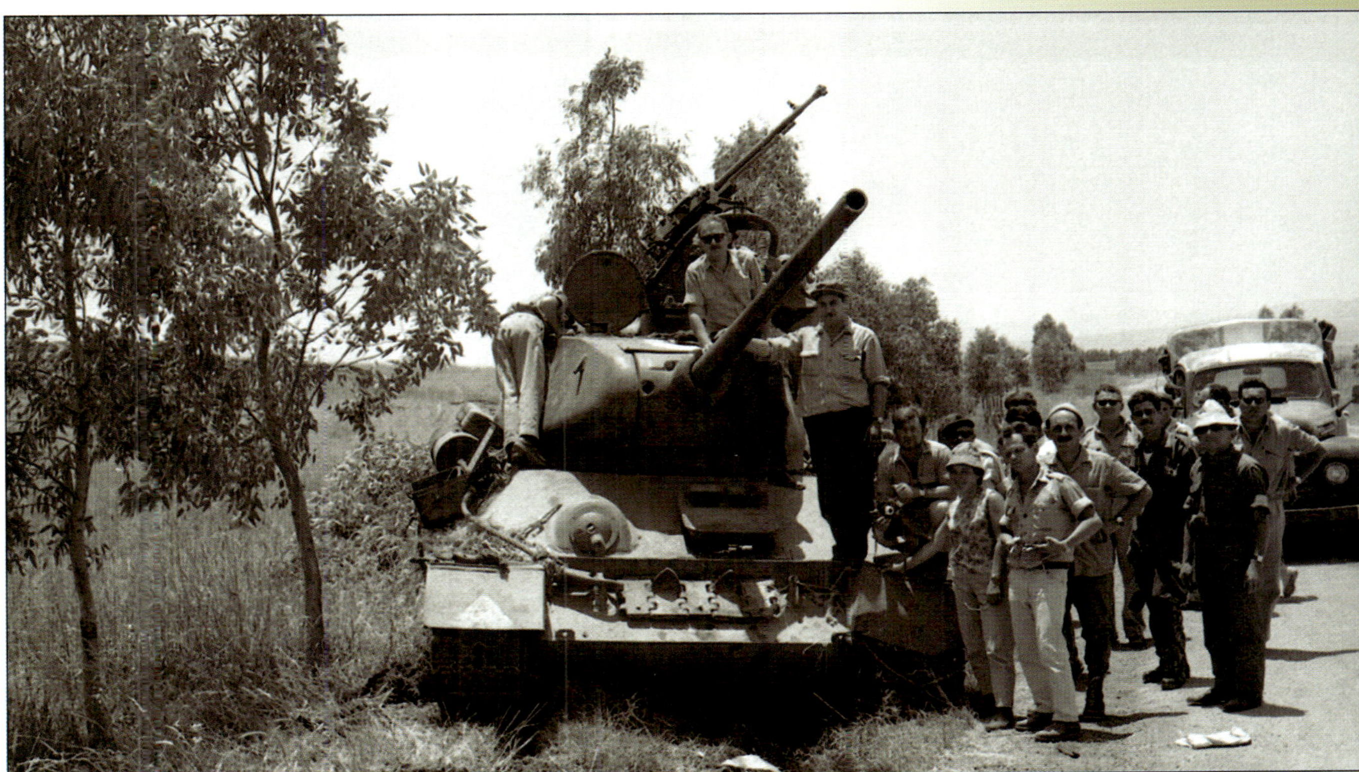

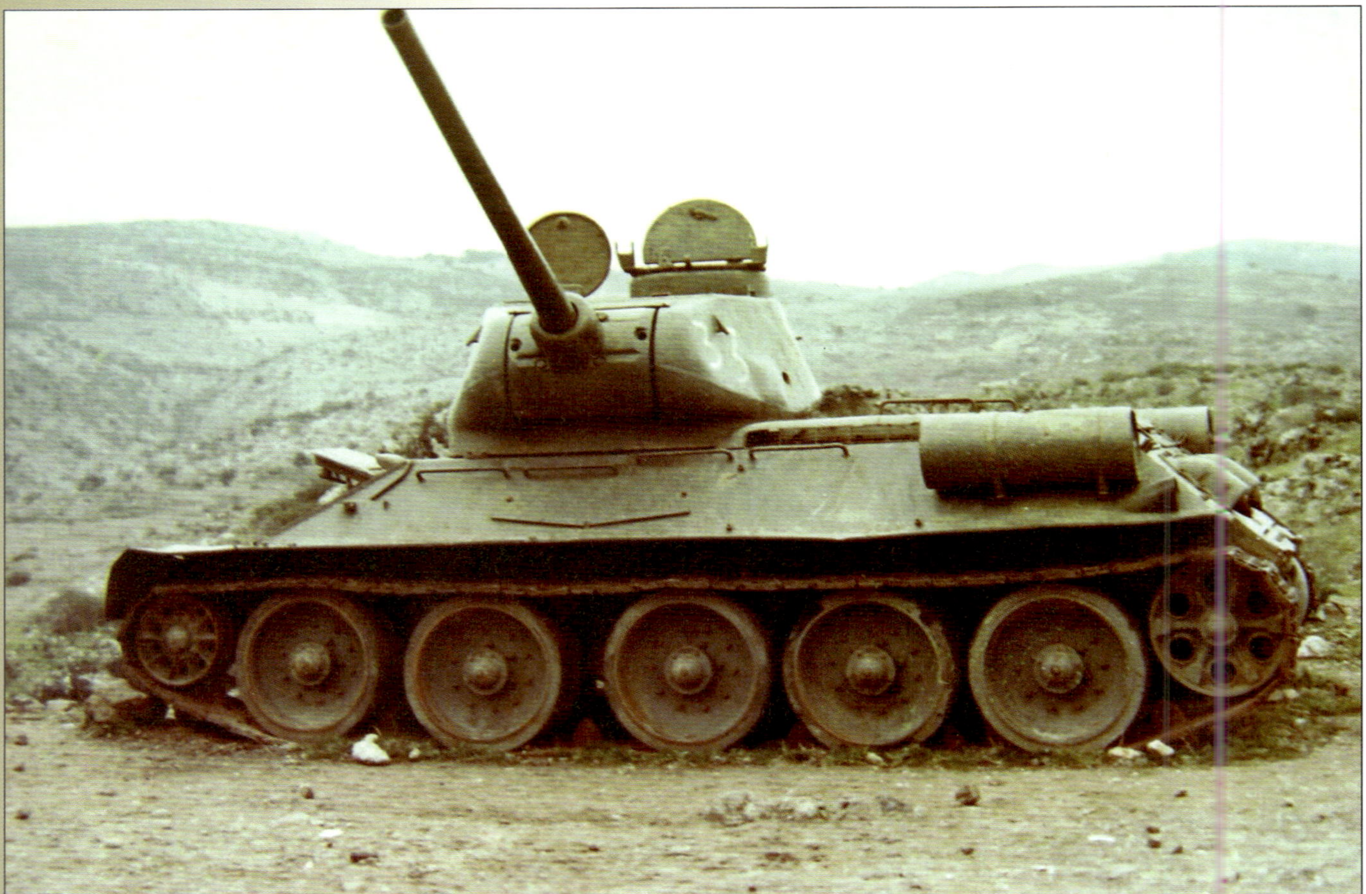

A Syrian T-34-85 of Czechoslovak production captured by Israeli forces during the Six Day War in 1967. The rail with machine gun mount had been dismantled. The number 33 on the turret was probably painted by the new owners during inventorying of the captured materiel. Remains of the red identification triangle are visible on the turret.

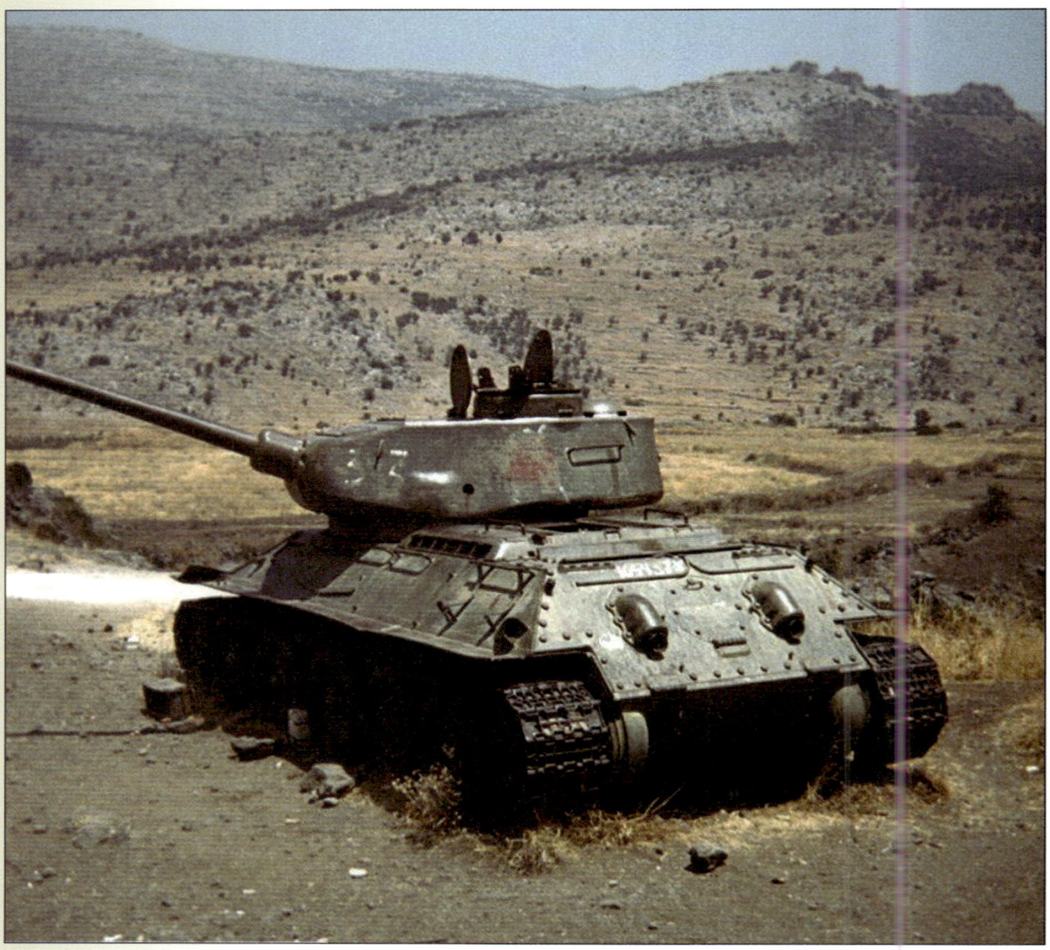

Another Syrian T-34-85 of Czechoslovak production lost during the Six Day War. A white lettering– the name of an Arab hero of the war with Israel is visible on the turret.

on a T-34-85 hull. In 1973 such vehicles equipped battalions assigned to the 1st and 3rd Armoured Divisions. Probably only the vehicles of the 1st Armoured Divisions saw combat (these were battalions of the 4th and 91st Armoured Brigades). Similar modifications were made by the Egyptians, with 100 mm BS-3 guns (and, according to some sources, the D-10) installed in some vehicles as well as examples with the D-30 howitzer. These were far more sophisticated designs than the Syrian howitzers, as the new armament was partially built into the standard T-34-85 turret. It is not known exactly when these vehicles were built, but it is most likely that they were created at the end of the 1960s and beginning of the 1970s. These vehicles probably saw combat in the Yom Kippur war, indicated by the fact that some were captured by Israel.

Other Middle East conflicts in which the T-34-85s saw combat were the 1962-70 civil war in North Yemen (in which Egyptian units equipped with T-34-85 tanks were involved in the fighting, supporting Republican forces, until 1967) and fighting in Lebanon (involving tanks used by units of pro-Syrian militia). According to some sources the T-34s were used in limited numbers by Iraq during the early period of the war with Iran (1980-1988). The Israelis also operated captured T-34-85s, but it seems that this was restricted to training units. The tanks were also displayed on parades, but never used in combat. Some captured tanks were used as observation points on the Syrian border and according to some sources tanks-bunkers were also placed near some kibbutzes.

The 21st century did not bring the combat career of the T-34 to an end. Known photographs depict T-34-85s during the rebellion in Libya in 2014, although it is not known whether or not they were used in combat. Photographs taken in 2015 show T-34-85s used in the fighting in Yemen. There are also photographs and film showing T-34s used in the civil war in Syria. These vehicles are probably not roadworthy, and used as static firing points. However, information is fragmentary and it is difficult to generalise or draw conclusions from the available reports.

A T-34-85 tank (Plant No. 183), operated by units of pro-Syrian militia in Lebanon in the early 1980. Also interesting is the tank in the background, particularly the inscription on its turret.

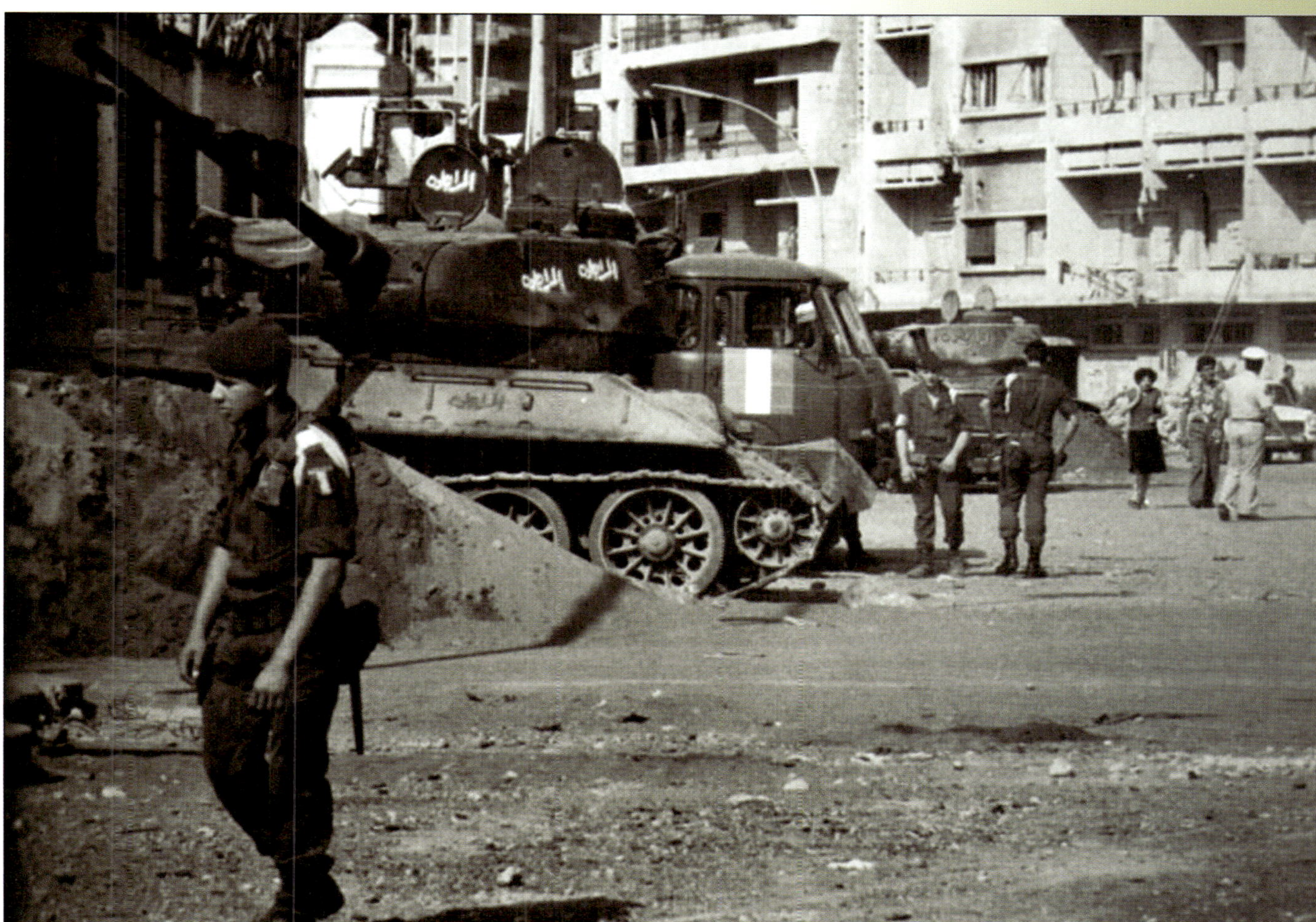

In Africa

The T-34-85 was used with success in African conflicts during the 1970s and 1980s (including in Egypt, Somalia, and West Sahara). On the largest scale these tanks were used by Ethiopian forces against the rebellion in Eritrea and in the war with Somalia during 1977–78. (The Somalis also used the T-34-85).

Angolan 'eighty-fives' fought against UNITA troops and subsequently supported Namibian units in combat against the RSA (Operation 'Protea', 1981). From 1975, Cuban T-34-85s with crews sent by Fidel Castro as "fraternal aid" participated in the fighting in Angola. They saw combat both against UNITA and South African forces. The experience of fighting in Angola revealed that in combat against infantry, particularly when they were poorly trained, the T-34-85 could still be effective. However the T-34 revealed its obsolete nature in engagements with advanced armoured cars such as the Panhard, AML-90 and Ratel-90. Advanced anti-tank guns and missiles were also deadly for the T-34-85.

South African soldiers with an Angolan T-34-85 of Plant No. 112 with two single ventilators, modernized to Model 1969 standard, captured during Operation "Protea" in 1981.

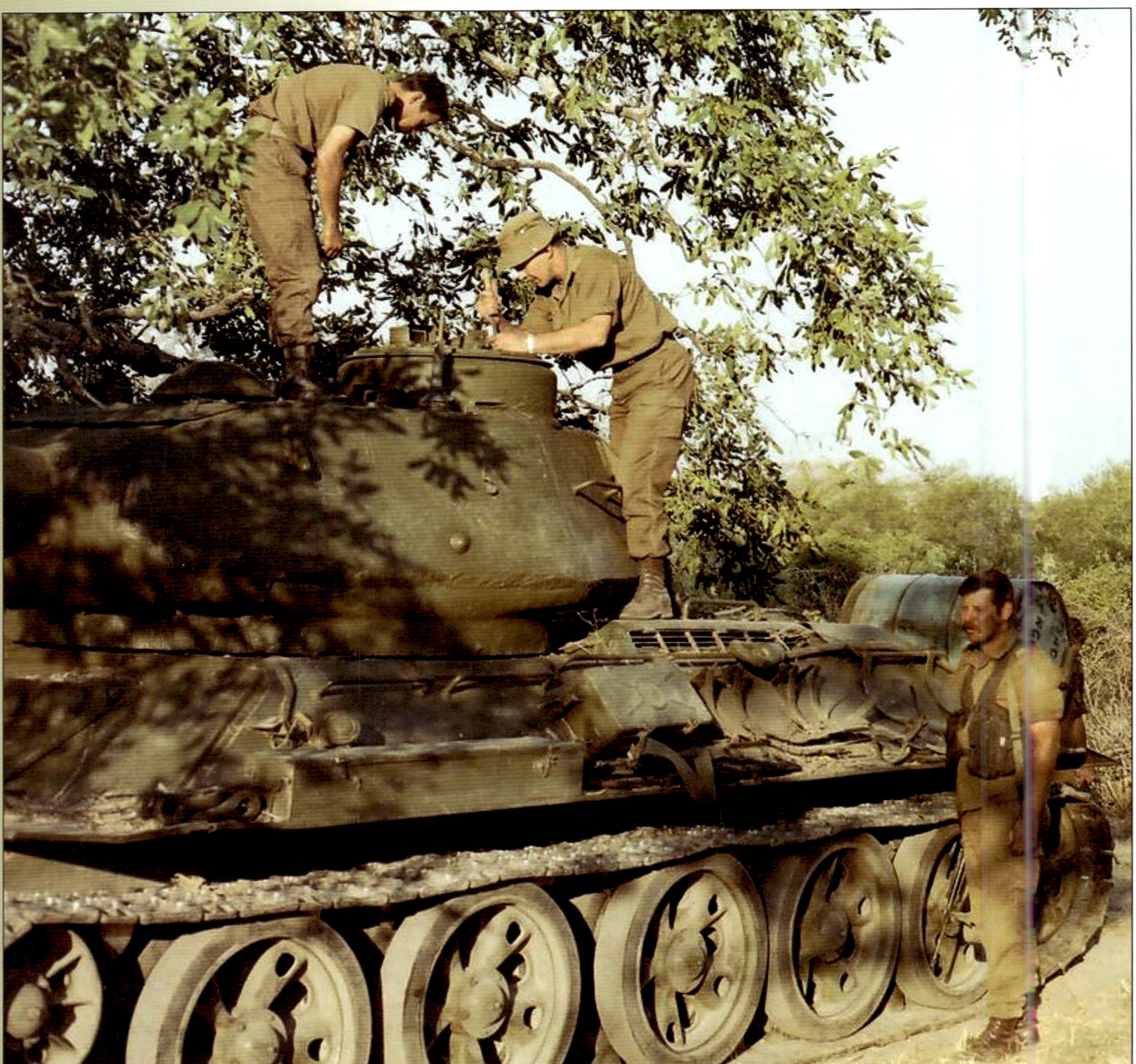

Post-war Europe

Europe was also the scene for use of the T-34-85 after 1945. In numerous countries these tanks were used to suppress anti-communist riots, including Polish T-34-85s on the streets of Poznań in June 1956. At least two of these tanks (including one sporting the tactical number 203) were captured by the insurgents and used to shell the Public Security Office's building. The T-34-85 tanks were used by the units of the Soviet Army Group in Germany for suppressing riots in East German cities in June 1953 (chiefly in Berlin). Soviet and East German T-34s were used for guarding the construction of the Berlin Wall in 1961. Polish and East German units participated in Operation 'Danube', using T-34-85 tanks during the intervention of Warsaw Pact nations in Czechoslovakia in 1968.

The 'eighty-fives' saw combat on the largest scale in Hungary in October and November 1956. During the fighting in October some Hungarian army troops took the side of the insurgents, who

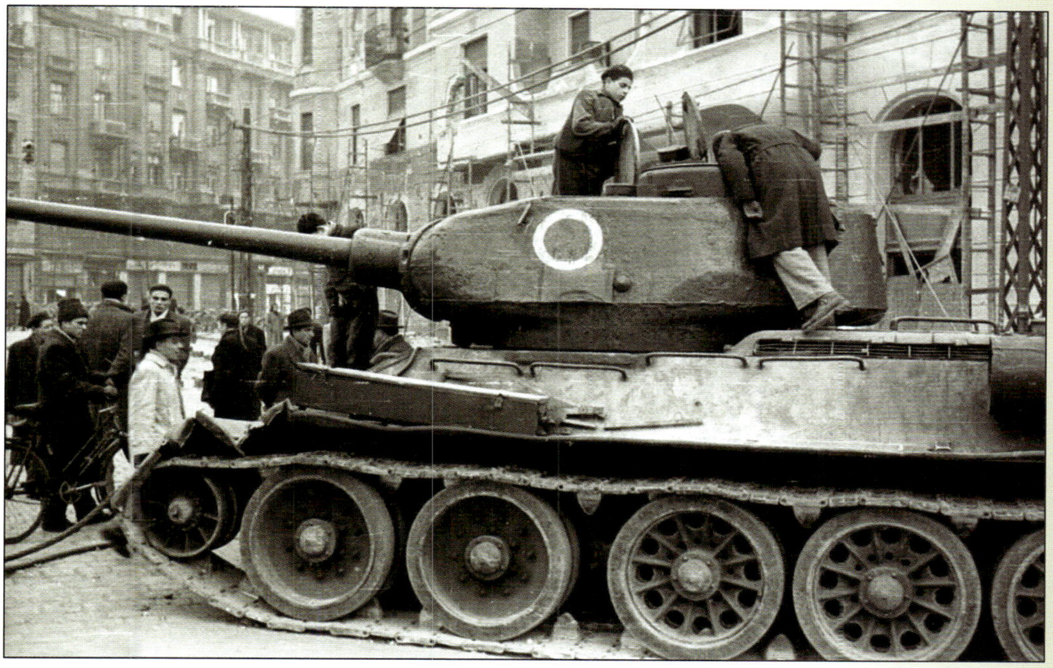

A T-34-85 (Plant No. 183) captured by Hungarian insurgents in Budapest in autumn of 1956. Note the white circle on the turret, in place, where usually the Hungarian government forces insignia was painted.

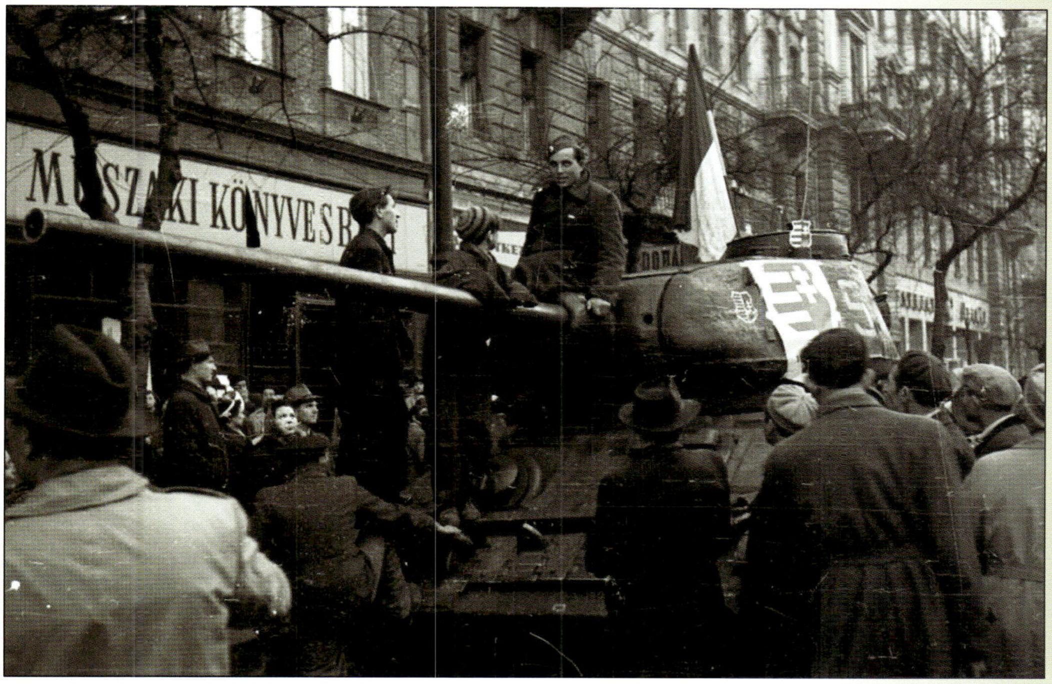

A T-34-85 (Plant No. 183) captured by Hungarian insurgents in Budapest in autumn of 1956. Markings of the revolutionary forces painted on the turret are visible.

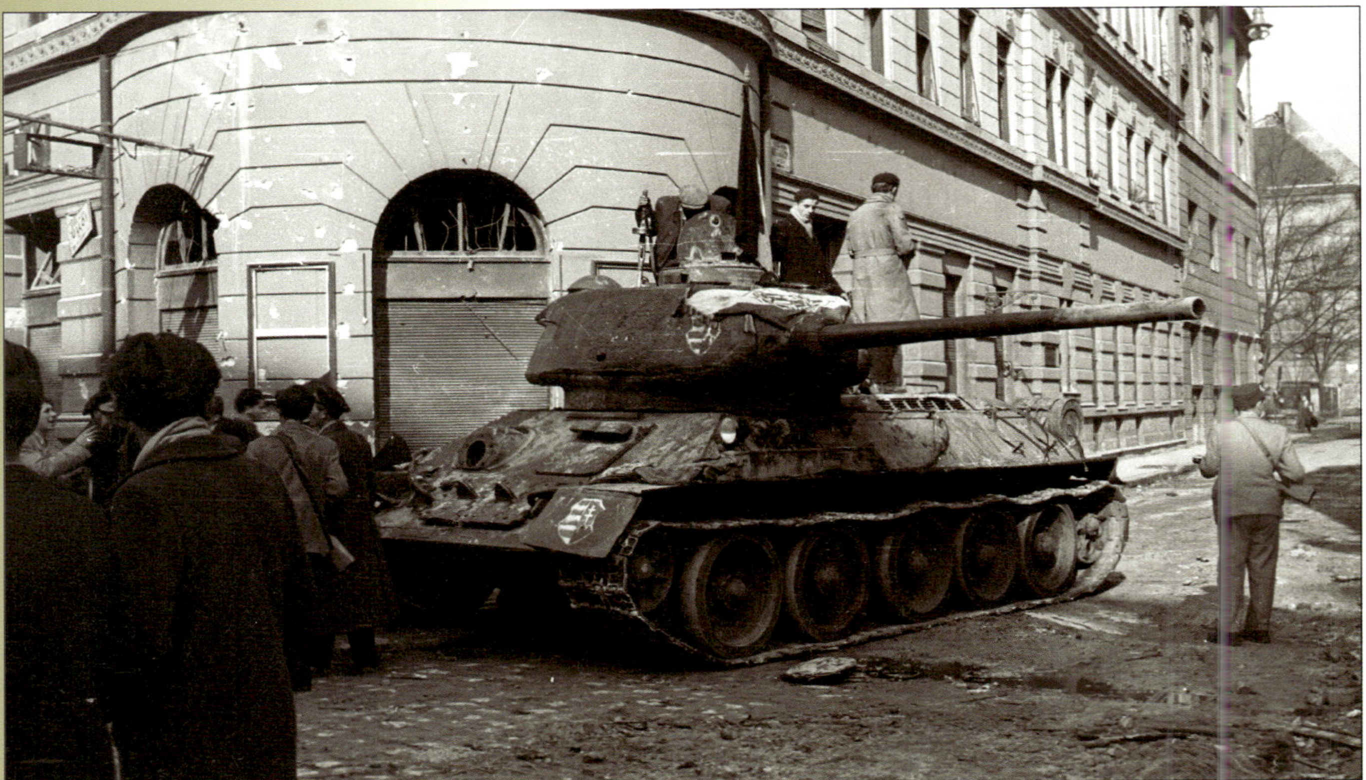

An insurrectionary T-34-85 (Plant No.112, with two single ventilators) with markings on the turret and fender.

thus obtained several T-34-85 tanks. However, the largest numbers of these vehicles were operated by three Soviet units which played a major role in suppressing the rebellion, the 2nd, 17th and 33rd Guards Mechanised Divisions. Several T-34-85s were burnt out in street fighting in Budapest. To destroy Soviet tanks and self-propelled guns the Hungarians used antitank and antiaircraft guns, grenades and Molotov cocktails.

In 1974 Cypriot Greeks attempted to repel the Turkish invasion (operations 'Attila I' and 'Attila II'). Thirty-two T-34-85s, delivered from the USSR via Egypt equipped two companies of the 23 Epilarhia Meson Armaton (Medium Tank Battalion). These were tanks from various factories, of wartime production but which had probably undergone modernisation patterned on the Model 1969 tank before delivery. In Cyprus, 12.7 mm Browning M2/M2HB machine gun mounts were installed on the turrets. At the outbreak of the hostilities the tanks stayed near the towns of Keryneia and Famagusta. Due to their poor technical condition and weak leadership, the tanks were not

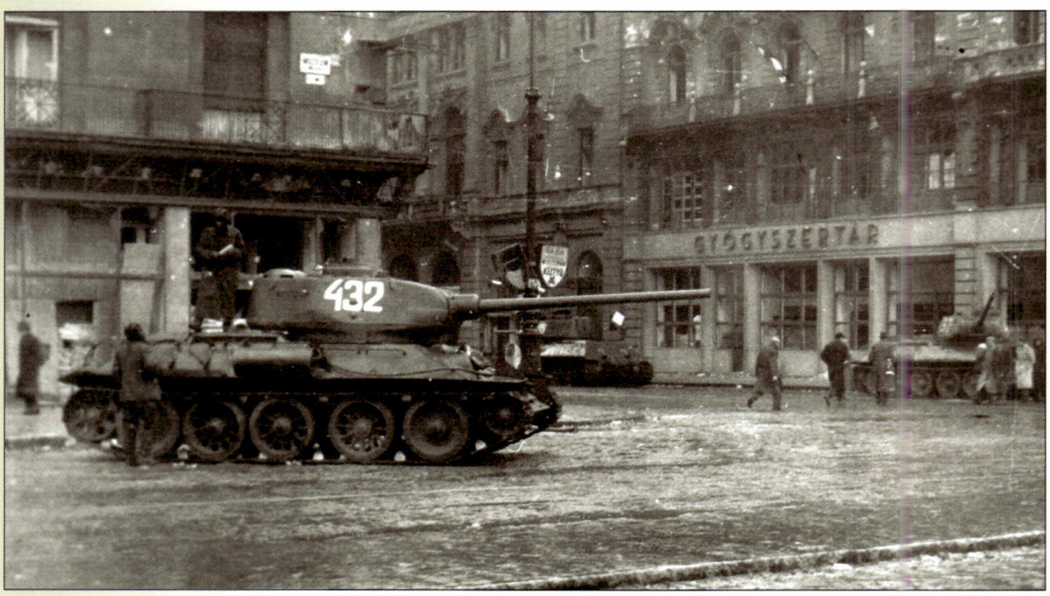

Soviet T-34-85s on the streets of Budapest, autumn of 1956. A tank with tactical number 432 (of Plant No. 183 production) is visible in the foreground.

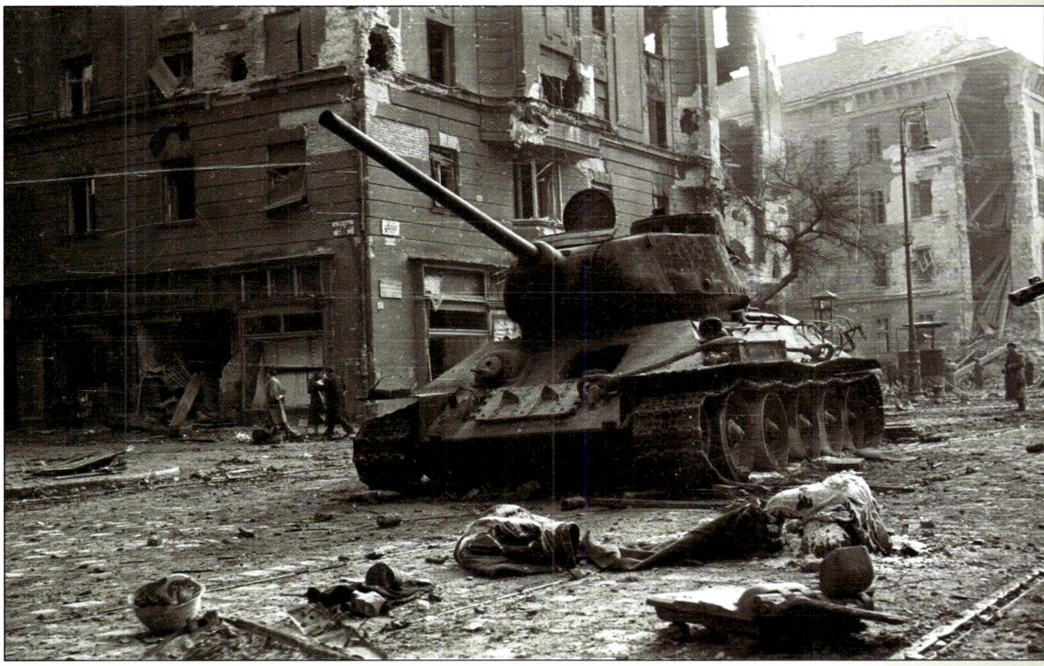

A burnt-out T-34-85 (Plant No. 183) on a Budapest street in autumn of 1956. The fighting in the city proved costly and hard for the Soviets, but their overwhelming superiority led to suppression of the Hungarian Revolution.

able to stop the Turkish invasion. In encounters with M113 armoured personnel carriers the crews of the T-34-85s scored some successes, but had little chance against M47 and M48 Patton tanks. Eleven tanks survived the war and in the autumn of 1974 they were assigned to a new unit – the 21st Reconnaissance Battalion (21. EAN). The T-34-85s remained in the inventory of the Cypriot units until 1984.

During the fighting in Cyprus in the summer of 1974 around 10-11 'eighty-fives' fell into Turkish hands. At least one of them was used against the Cypriot Greeks. After the war the Turks formed a special unit for operations in the enemy's rear using the captured T-34-85s.

In the 1990s the T-34 saw action again in the conflicts caused by the break-up of Yugoslavia. Although the Yugoslavian army (JNA) operated modern tanks (T-55 and T-72/M84) in 1991, T-34-85s were still in the inventory of reserve and training units. A large number of these tanks (several hundred) were also in JNA's storage depots. The 'eighty-fives' were used on various scales in virtually all Balkan conflicts of that time: the 'Ten Day War' in Slovenia, fighting in Croatia (1991–95) and the war in Bosnia (1992–95). During the first period of the conflict with the Croatians (1991–92) the Serbian units used the T-34s during the fighting in Krajina and in the southern sector of the front, near Dubrovnik. During the hostilities a number of these tanks fell into Croatian hands. One of the most famous Croatian T-34-85s was the tank named "Malo Bijelo" (Little White), operating near Dubrovnik as part of the 163rd Brigade 'Dubrovnik'. Reportedly this vehicle survived two antitank missile hits and its crew destroyed several enemy vehicles. Having driven out the Serbs the Croatians captured a dozen or so T-34-85 tanks, stored in JNA depots. The Croatians used T-34-85s during Operation 'Flash' in May 1995 in the Slavonia region, and operation 'Thunder' in August 1995 in Krajina. A dozen or so T-34-85s survived the hostilities and were later scrapped. (However, at the end of the 20th century, a few T-34-85s were known to be stored at a military base in the town of Benkovac).

Many tanks of this type also equipped Bosnian Serb units. Some were retrofitted with provisional additional armour for better crew protection. Based on available photographs it seems that the added protection mostly consisted of thick rubber matting (possibly to make the tanks less visible through thermal imaging). The tanks were used mainly in the infantry support role as self-propelled artillery. Information about the use of T-34-85s during the Balkan conflicts is still fragmentary, which results in part from the fact that the tanks were used not only by military units but also local militias.

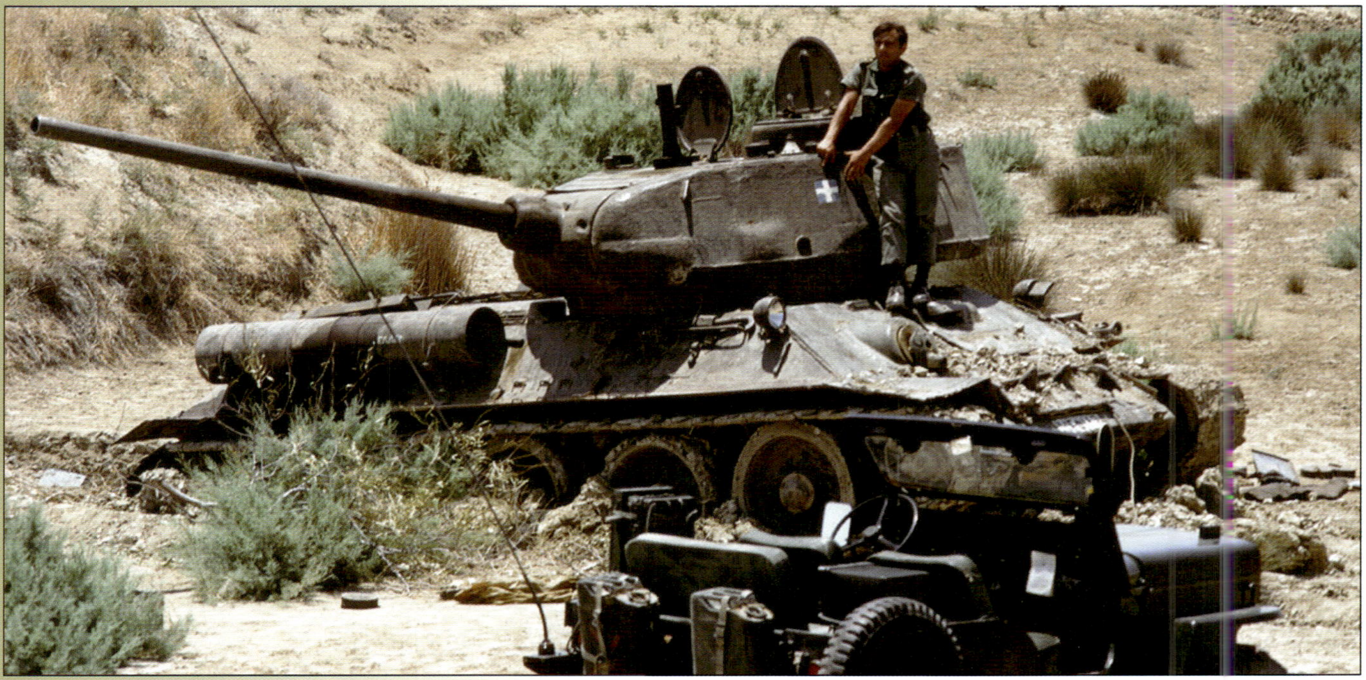

A Turkish soldiers inspects a T-34-85 (Plant No. 183) operated by the Cypriot Greeks in 1974.

Until recently it seemed that the last use of a T-34-85 in Europe took place during anti-government riots in Budapest in October 2006, involving a tank that had been on display at an exhibition commemorating the Hungarian uprising of 1956. However, in 2014, after the outbreak of fighting in eastern Ukraine, the T-34 saw combat again. Museum exhibits and tanks taken from monuments were used by pro-Russian separatists. It is not known, how many tanks were put into operation, but at least two such cases are known. One ex-museum T-34-85 was used in Lugansk and another one, with additional improvised armour, was used by the so-called National Cossack Guard in the town of Antratsit. It should be noted here that the first case of combat use of a T-34-85 tank taken from a monument probably took place in the early 1990s during hostilities in Nagorno-Karabakh. The tank was taken from a monument (or, according to other sources, stolen from a museum) by Armenians and used in combat for about a month. As the original engine was not serviceable, a diesel engine from a Kamaz truck was installed instead.

It is worth mentioning that during 2014-15, attempts to smuggle several T-34s seem to have been prevented. It is hard to determine if these were attempts to reinforce one of the sides of the Russo-Ukrainian conflict, but they show that nearly 80 years after its birth the T-34 is still a desirable weapon.

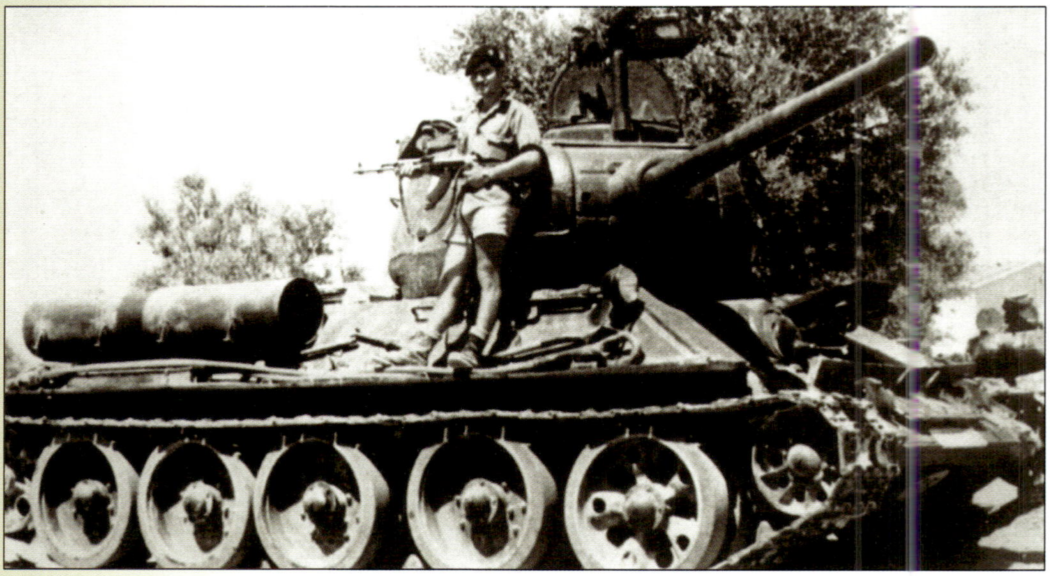

One of T-34-85s operated by the Cypriot Greeks, mid-1970s. The tank was modified to Model 1969 standard, but not all wheels were changed to so-called Starfish wheels. The bridge classification number is visible on the forward lower armour plate.

In the Bay of Pigs

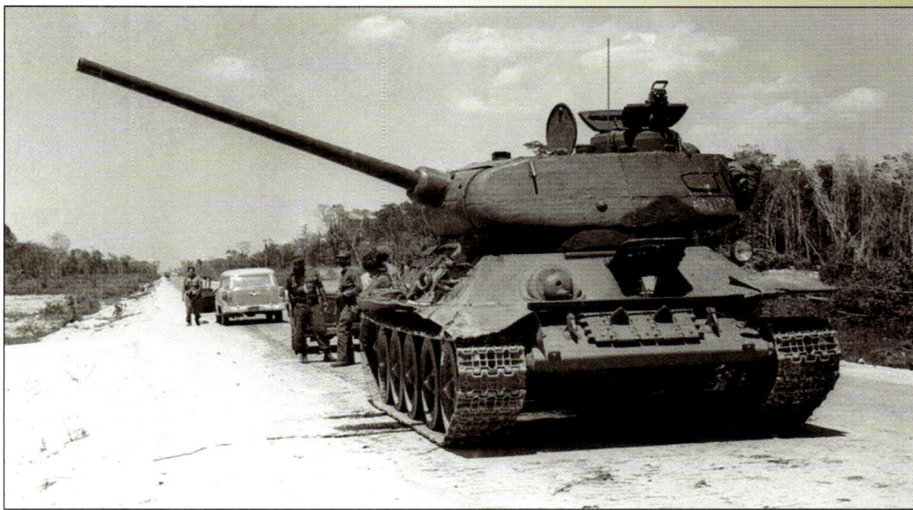

A Cuban T-34-85 (of wartime production – the shape resembles turrets from Plant No. 183, but the trace of joining suggests the 8-part pattern of the Plant No.112 turret) on its way to the Bay of Pigs, April 1961. The tank has no markings. According to legend, this tank was commanded by Fidel Castro.

The only American country to operate T-34-85 tanks was Cuba. The Cubans commenced negotiations with the USSR about the delivery of the tanks in 1960 and the first T-34-85s arrived at the end of that year or beginning of the next. It is estimated that about 500 tanks of that type were delivered to this country from the USSR during 1960–63 (some came from Czechoslovakia). At the beginning of the invasion of US-trained insurgents at the Bay of Pigs on 17 April 1961, the crews of Cuban tanks were undergoing training at a base in Managua. Due to this fact only five T-34-85 tanks were sent to fight back the landing near Playa Giron and Playa Larga. During the first attack on the positions of 'Brigade 2506' the insurgents burned one T-34 with bazookas. During the next day a dozen or so T-34-85s and Su-100 self-propelled guns arrived at the scene. The insurgents had only five M41 Walker Bulldog tanks at their disposal (some sources say that Brigade 2506 was equipped with M4 Sherman tanks and M8 armoured cars, but this is not borne out by most evidence). By 20 April 1961 the Cuban army defeated the enemy forces. On that day one of the T-34-85s reportedly shelled the insurgent supply ship *Houston*. A legend says that 'El Commandante' Fidel Castro himself took part in the action. In total during four days of fighting the Cubans lost five T-34-85s destroyed by the fire of M41 tanks, bazookas and 57 mm recoilless guns. One Walker Bulldog was destroyed by T-34-85 crews (the other ones were destroyed by other Cuban units or abandoned due to lack of ammunition).

Later the Cubans developed astonishing modifications of the T-34-85s, building self-propelled guns and howitzers on their chassis, or fitting 100 mm KS-19 and 130 mm KS-130 anti-aircraft guns or 122 mm D-30 howitzers to the existing hull. Tanks of this type were also placed along the Cuban coast as fixed firing points, defending the island against invasion.

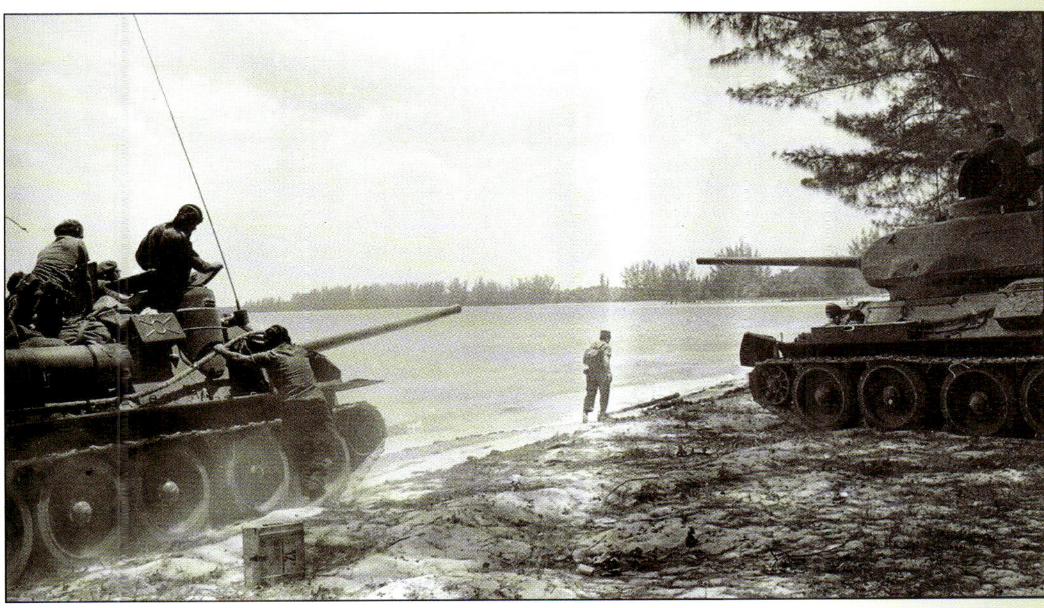

A T-34-85 tank and Su-100 self-propelled gun in the Bay of Pigs area after having defeated the invasion, April 1961. Probably it is a staged propaganda photo taken after the end of the fighting.

PAINT SCHEMES AND MARKINGS

EUROPE

ALBANIA

This is one of the least known European T-34-85 operators. During 1955–56 a total of 138 tanks of this type were received from the USSR. According to some sources, 'eighty-fives' were also delivered to Albania from China, but this is improbable. About 70 tanks were in the Albanian army inventory in the early 21st century.

Based on the few photos available, it can be presumed that the standard T-34-85 paint scheme was olive green. The tanks sported white, three-digit tactical numbers on the turret sides.

A column of T-34-85 tanks (with various turret versions) on a mountain road near the Greek border, 1960s.

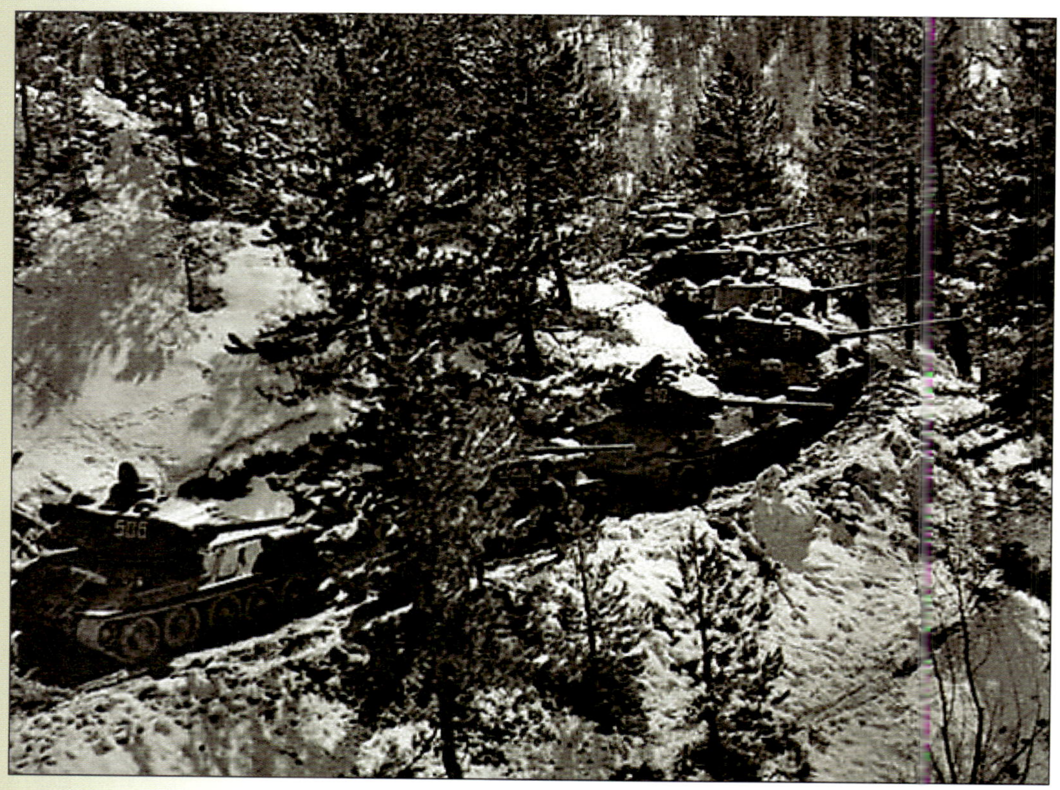

Austria

In 1955 Soviet occupation forces leaving Austria handed over 27 T-34-85 tanks and several (probably ten) T-34T armoured recovery vehicles. The tanks were operated by *Panzertruppenschule* and *Panzerbatallion* 33, remaining in Austrian service until 1964. Later the tanks or their turrets were used as firing points in fortified regions, primarily on the Yugoslavian border.

The Austrian T-34-85s were painted overall in olive green. Initially this was Soviet 4BO paint, but after overhauls was probably replaced with Austrian *Bronzegrün*.

The tanks sported three-digit tactical numbers (for instance 111, 131, 132) painted in solid white or a white outline. They were painted on the turrets (sides and rear) and fenders (front and rear). Combined letter-digit markings were painted on command tanks (for instance I01). Some vehicles also sported unit tactical markings on the fenders (white). During the T-34-85 service the national marking in the form of an inverted white triangle in a red circle was used. The national markings were painted on the forward section of the turret, ahead of the tactical number.

Photographs of Austrian 'eighty-fives' with unit insignia painted on the turret are known from the period of the tank's service in the *Panzerbattalion* 33.

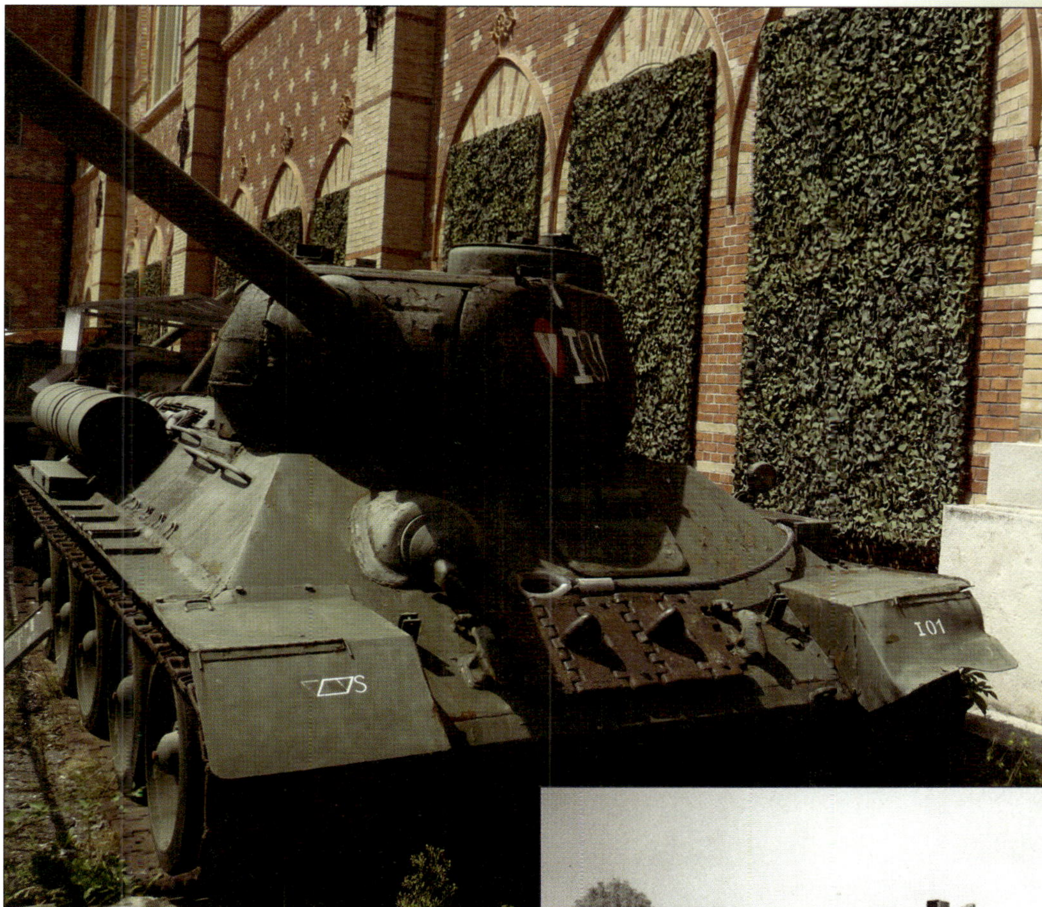

T-34-85 (of Plant No.183 production) preserved at a military museum in Vienna. The tank has the number I01 and marking of headquarters company.

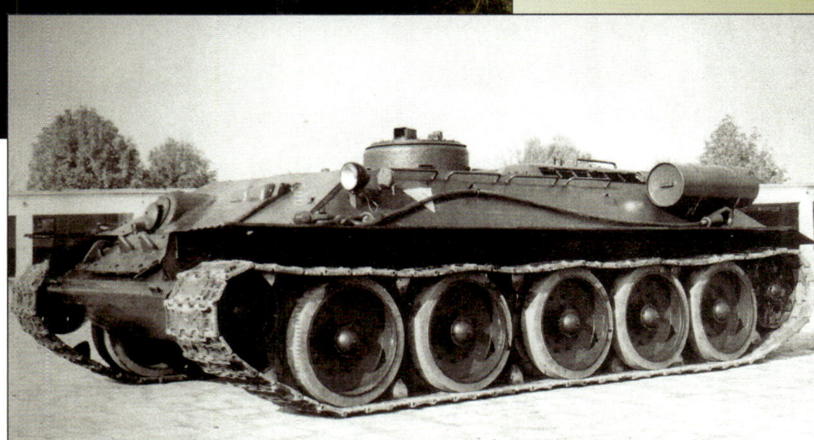

The Austrians operated also T-34T recovery vehicles based on T-34-85 tank.

Right: *Albanian soldiers jump off a T-34-85 tank with tactical number 759. This method of tank marking was characteristic for tanks of the Albanian army.*

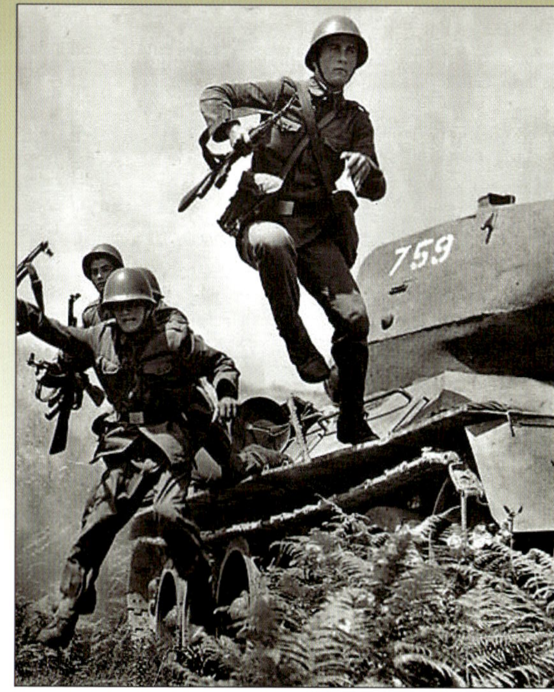

Albania

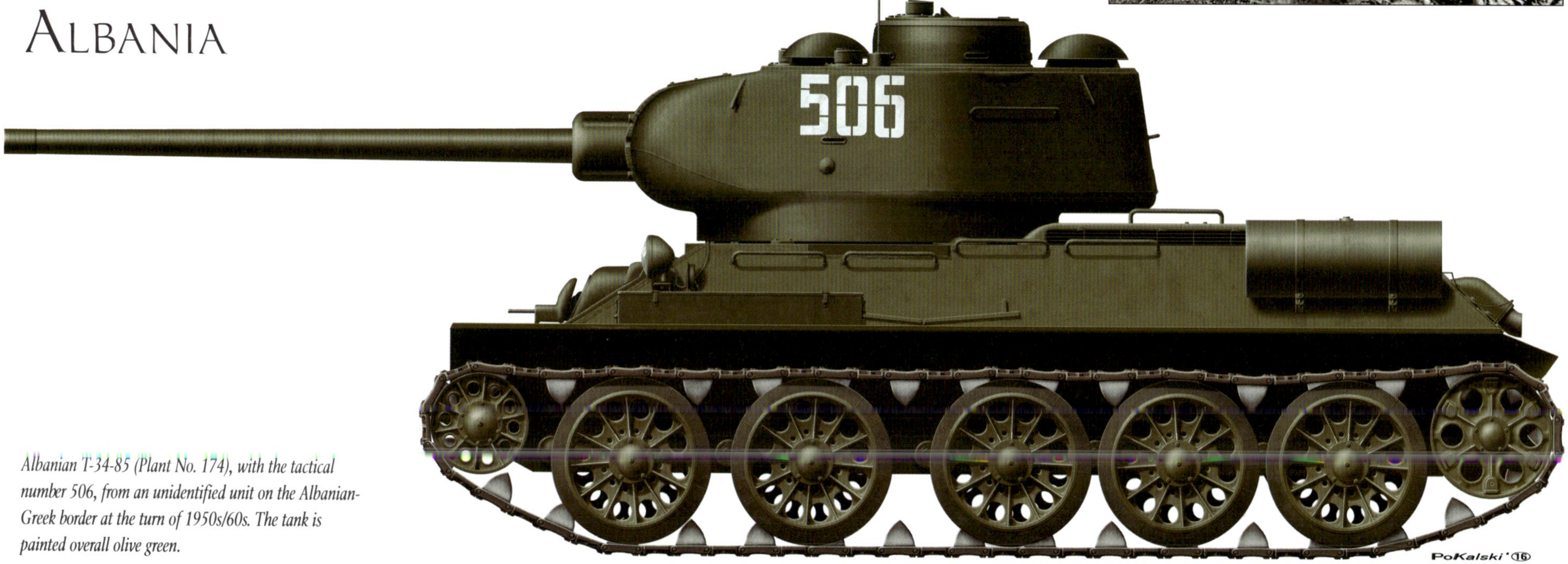

Albanian T-34-85 (Plant No. 174), with the tactical number 506, from an unidentified unit on the Albanian-Greek border at the turn of 1950s/60s. The tank is painted overall olive green.

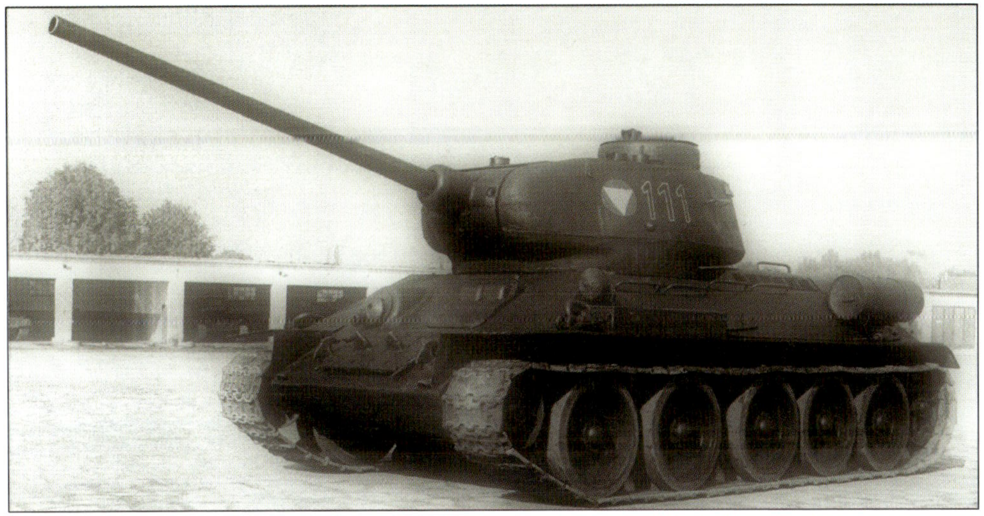

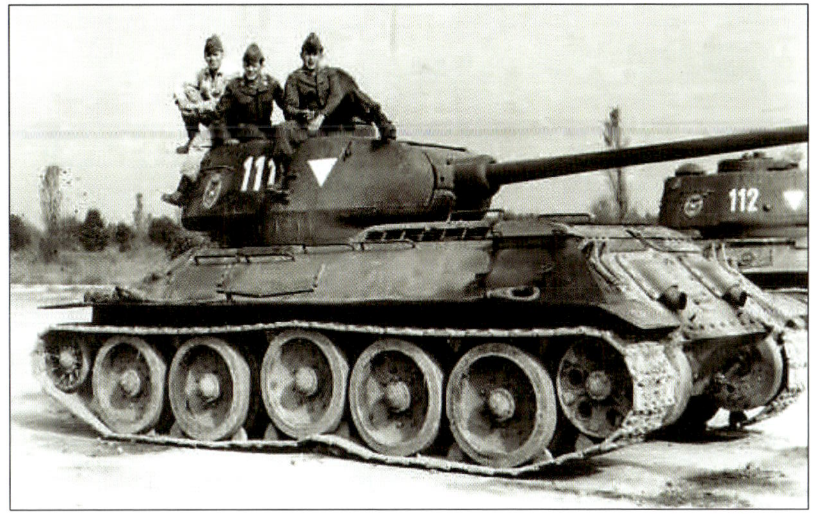

Austrian T-34-85 (of Plant No.183 production) with tactical number 111 and unit emblem painted on the rear part of the turret.

AUSTRIA

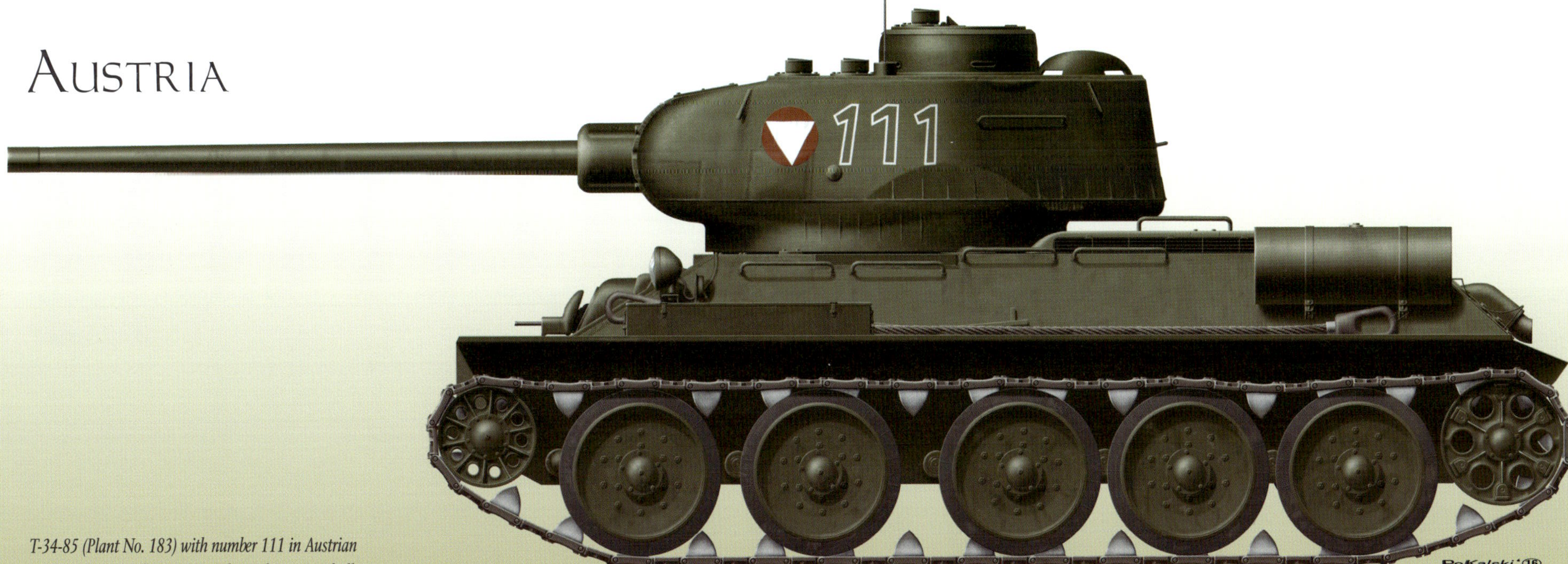

T-34-85 (Plant No. 183) with number 111 in Austrian colours, the turn of 1950s/60s. The tank is painted all-over olive green.

Bulgaria

Bulgaria received 398 T-34-85 tanks from the USSR during 1946–48. They equipped the 1st Armoured Division and two armoured brigades, which were merged into to the 2nd Armoured Brigade in the early 1950s. After further deliveries from the USSR and Czechoslovakia in the mid-1950s the number of Bulgarian T-34-85s increased to almost 1,000.

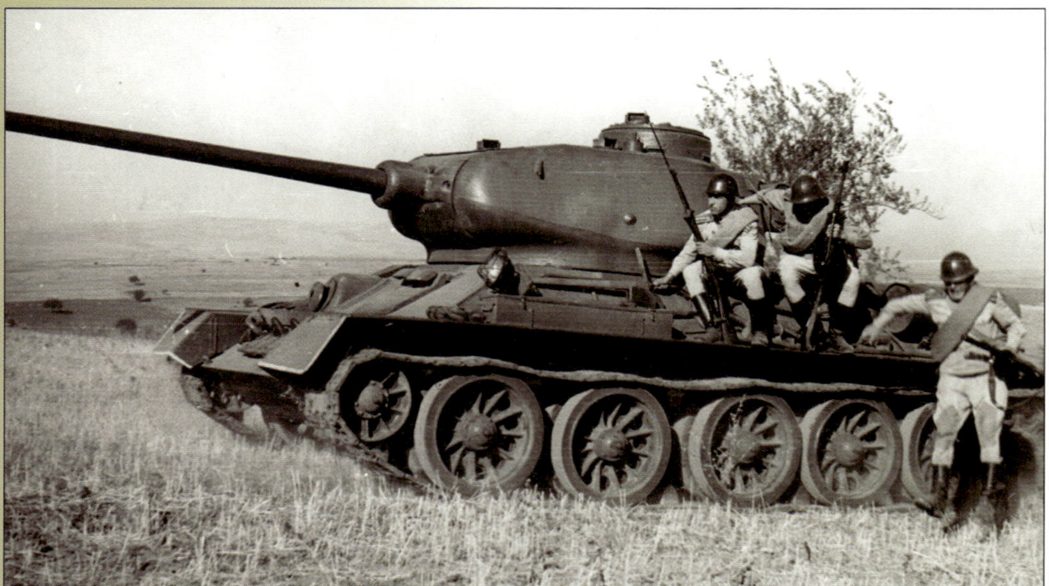

Bulgarian T-34-85 of Czechoslovak production during an exercise with infantry in the 1950s. The tank has no tactical markings, which was a common practice in the early period of service in Bulgarian armoured units. Note fender edges painted white.

Around the end of the 1960s, the Bulgarian tanks underwent modernisation consisting of the installation of brackets for two 200-litre barrels on the rear hull, the addition of a box on the left side of the hull and, primarily, in the addition of a short cupola with an anti-aircraft machine gun mount on the loader's hatch. After the retirement of the T-34-85, the tanks' turrets were used in fortifications on the borders (mainly with Turkey).

The Bulgarian T-34-85s were painted all-over olive green. Initially this was Soviet 4BO paint, then, following overhauls, the tanks were re-finished in Bulgarian paints which had a dark green shade. Tactical numbers were white, usually of three-digit configuration. Red stars were sporadically painted on the turret or fenders. Some tanks had a wide white or yellow stripe painted on the turret. This was probably a marking used during manoeuvres and exercises.

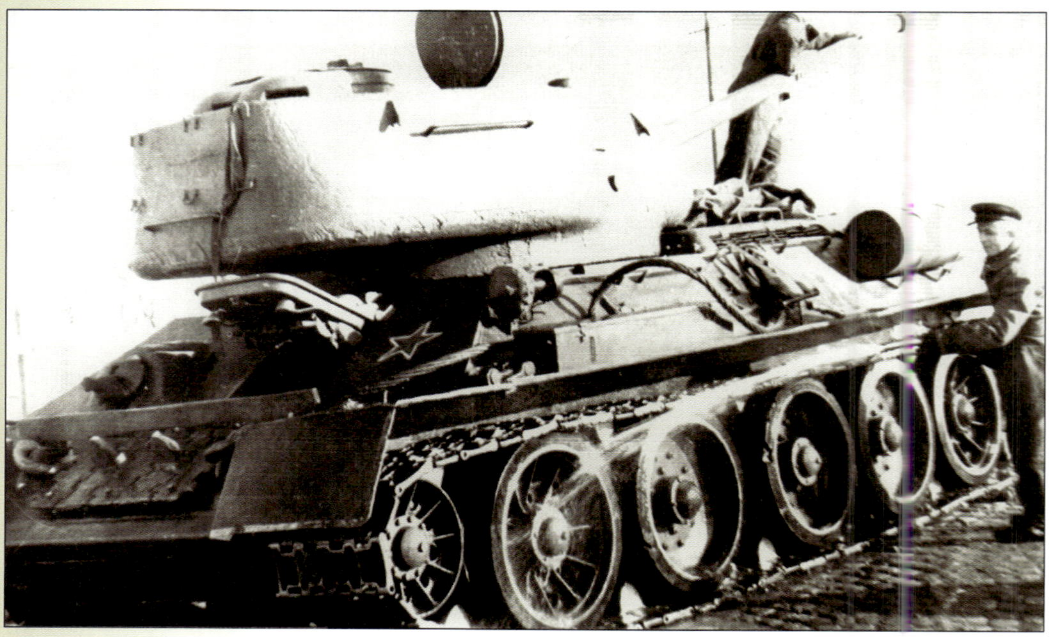

A Bulgarian T-34-85 being washed after an exercise, the turn of 1940s and 1950s. Note the lack of tactical markings and the red star on the forward armour plate.

Cyprus

The tanks that arrived in Cyprus in 1965 were painted overall olive green. During exercises in the late 1960s and early 1970s, some vehicles received improvised camouflage patterns applied with sand-coloured paint or mud. These schemes resembled the camouflage of the Turkish tanks, and tanks sporting these schemes may have played the role of 'enemy' vehicles.

Almost all tanks used by the Greeks during the fighting in Cyprus in the summer of 1974 were olive green. However, a photograph taken near Nicosia airport shows an 'eighty-five' in a two-colour disruptive pattern. According to some sources this provisional camouflage was made with mud. Two-colour camouflages – probably olive green and sand – appeared on the T-34-85s again, probably in the late 1970s and early 1980s, as shown by photographs of the tanks taken on the island.

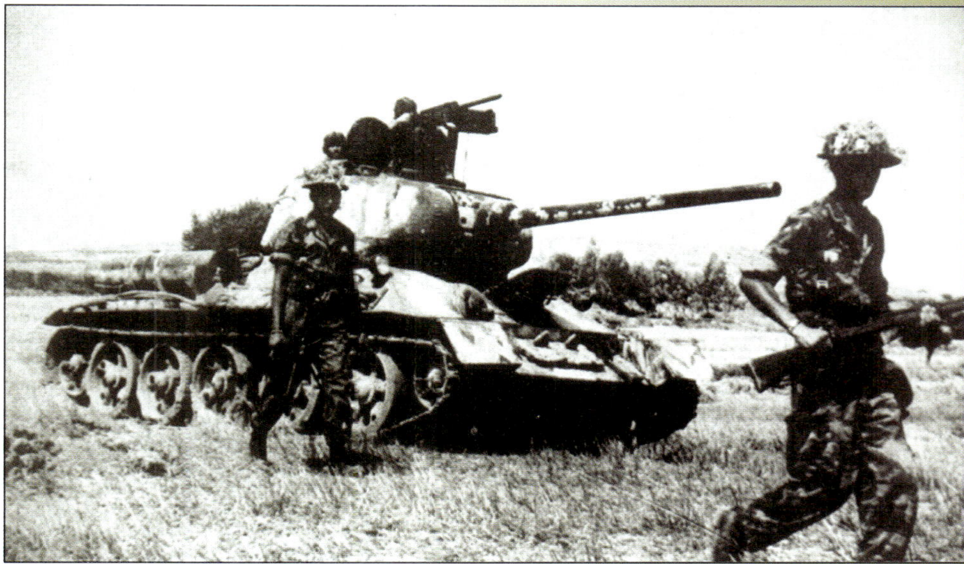

Modified Cypriot T-34-85 Model 1969 during exercises with infantry, probably early 1970s. The tank wears provisional camouflage made with mud.

No tactical numbers were painted on the turrets of Cypriot T-34-85s, the only markings being the insignia of the Greek armed forces – a white cross in a light blue square or shield. An identification number, the same as that of the Greek armed forces, was painted on rear and front hull. This consisted of the Greek armed forces marking and two letters and three digits, e.g. EΦ110. The numbers were all in the 101–132 range. On the lower plate of the hull tub, bridge classification numbers were painted. Some tanks used in the fighting with the Turks in 1974 had propaganda slogans painted on the turrets.

Many 'eighty-fives' were captured by the Turks during the fighting in summer 1974 in Cyprus. However, paint schemes of these tanks are not known.

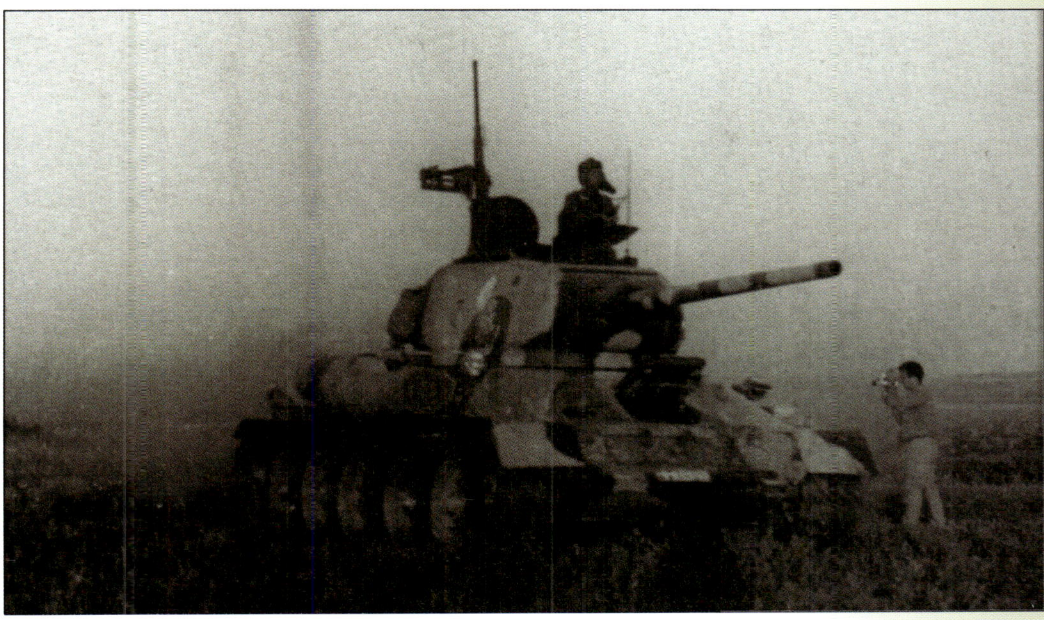

A Cypriot T-34-85 photographed during exercise. It is hard to determine the date of the photograph, but it was probable the turn of 1970s and 1980s, when two-colour camouflages were used.

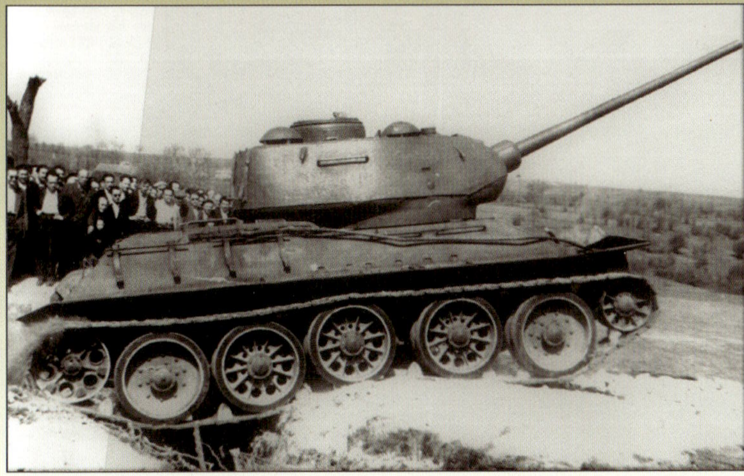

T-34-85 (Plant No. 174, turret with two single ventilators) during a display for civilians, late 1940s.

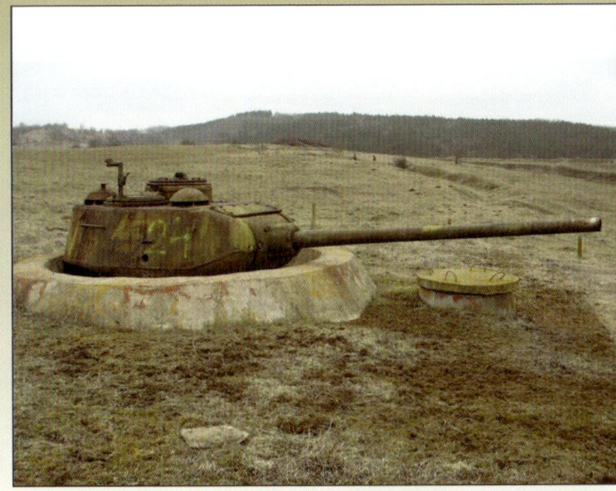

After the withdrawal of T-34-85 tanks from service their turrets were used as firing points in the fortifications on Bulgarian-Turkish border.

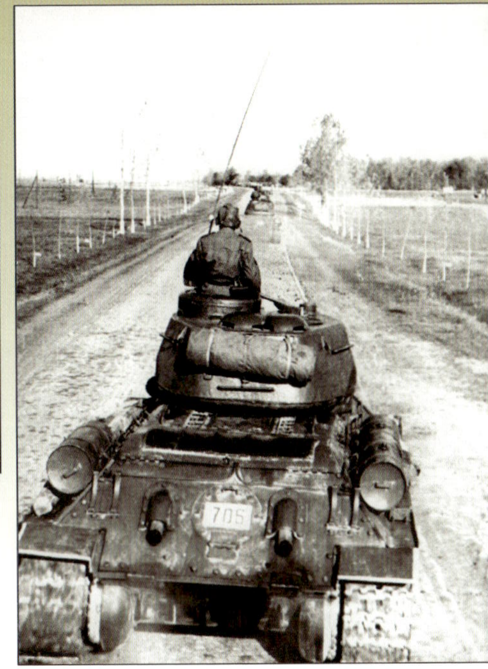

A column of Bulgarian T-34-85 in transit. Note the provisional tactical number 705 on transmission gear compartment cover.

Bulgaria

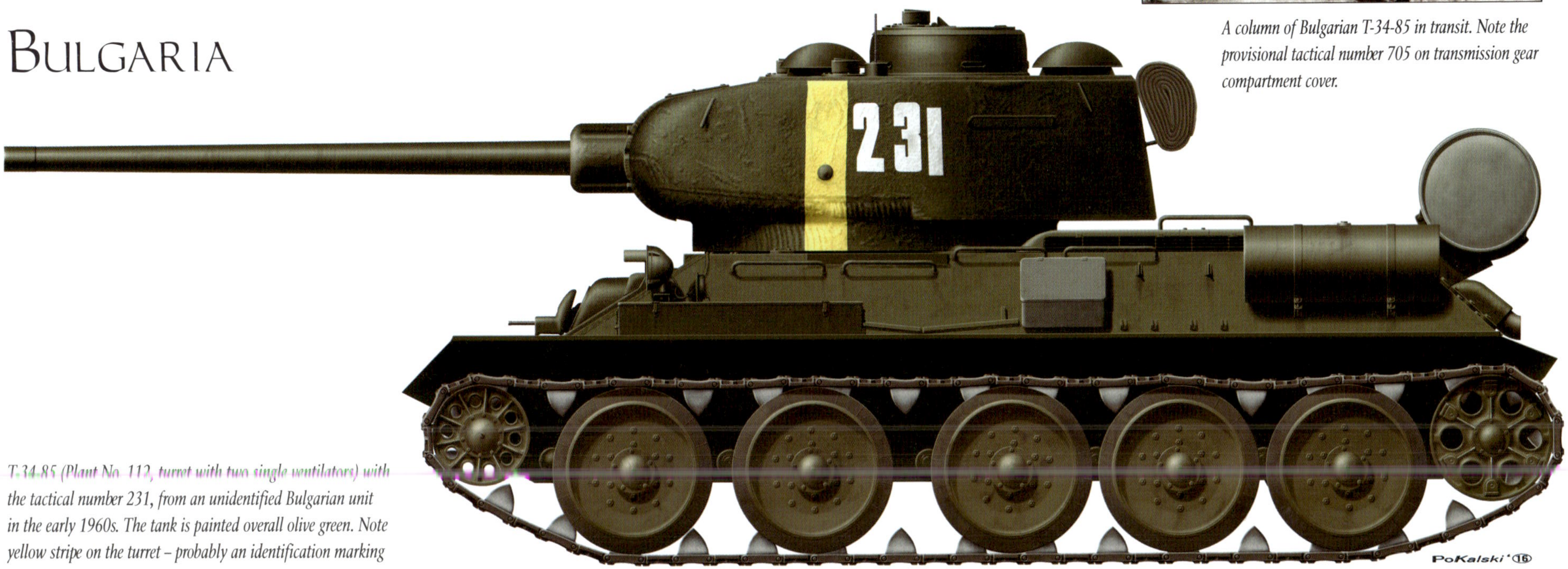

T-34-85 (Plant No. 112, turret with two single ventilators) with the tactical number 231, from an unidentified Bulgarian unit in the early 1960s. The tank is painted overall olive green. Note yellow stripe on the turret – probably an identification marking used during exercises.

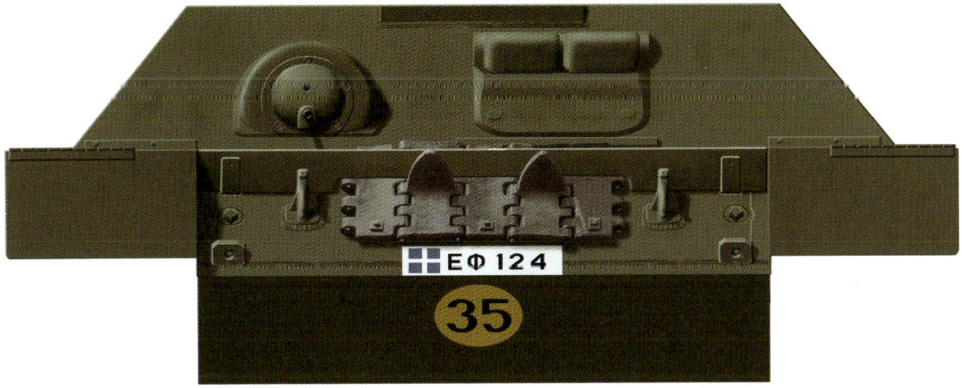

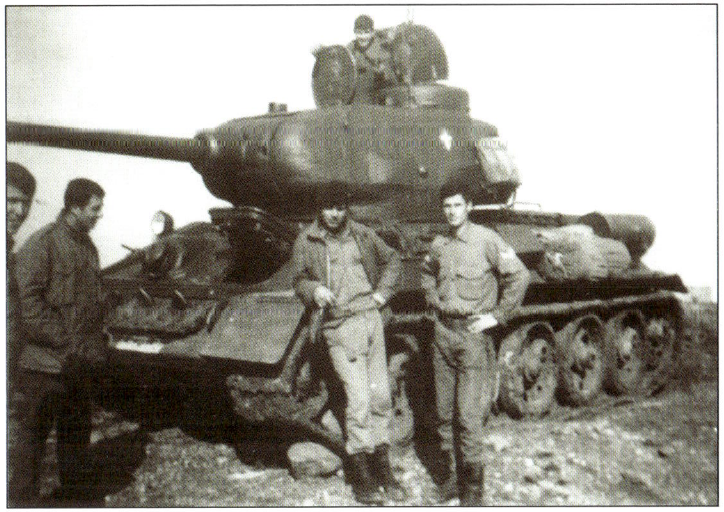

A modified Cypriot T-34-85 (Plant No. 183 turret, IR searchlight, fuel pump stowage box, T-44 wheels) in overall green paint scheme, probably during the period after the hostilities of 1974.

CYPRUS

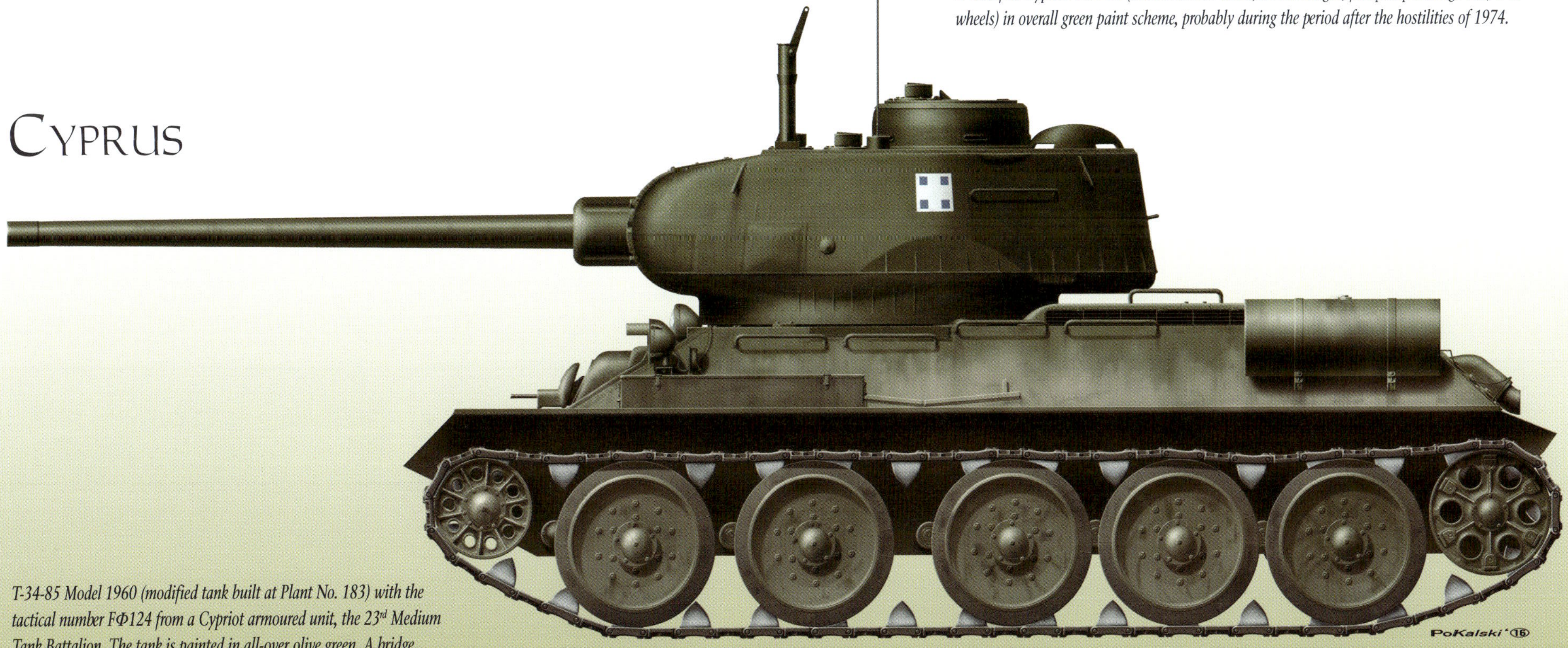

T-34-85 Model 1960 (modified tank built at Plant No. 183) with the tactical number FΦ124 from a Cypriot armoured unit, the 23rd Medium Tank Battalion. The tank is painted in all-over olive green. A bridge classification number is painted on the front armour plate.

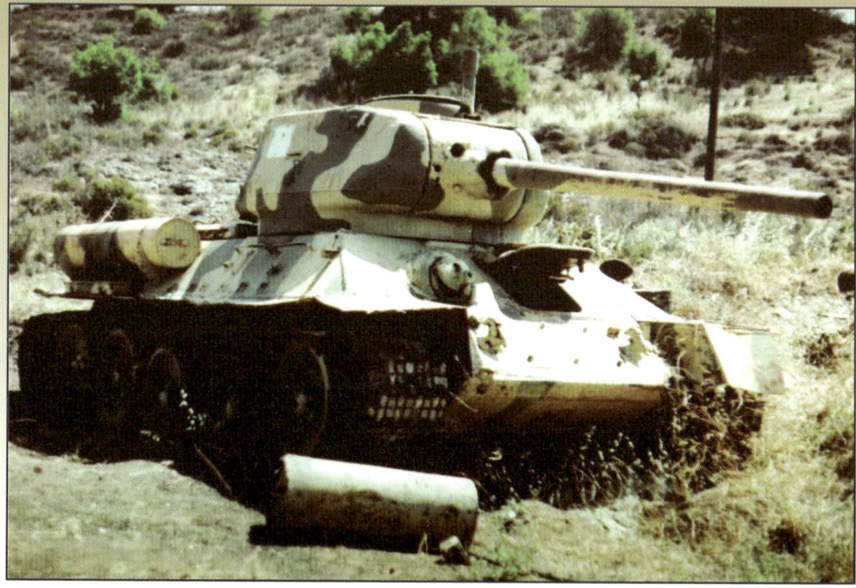

T-34-85 (Plant No.183) in two-colour camouflage, introduced on the turn of 1970s and 1980s. Until now such tanks can be met in Cyprus as monuments or museum exhibits.

Cyprus

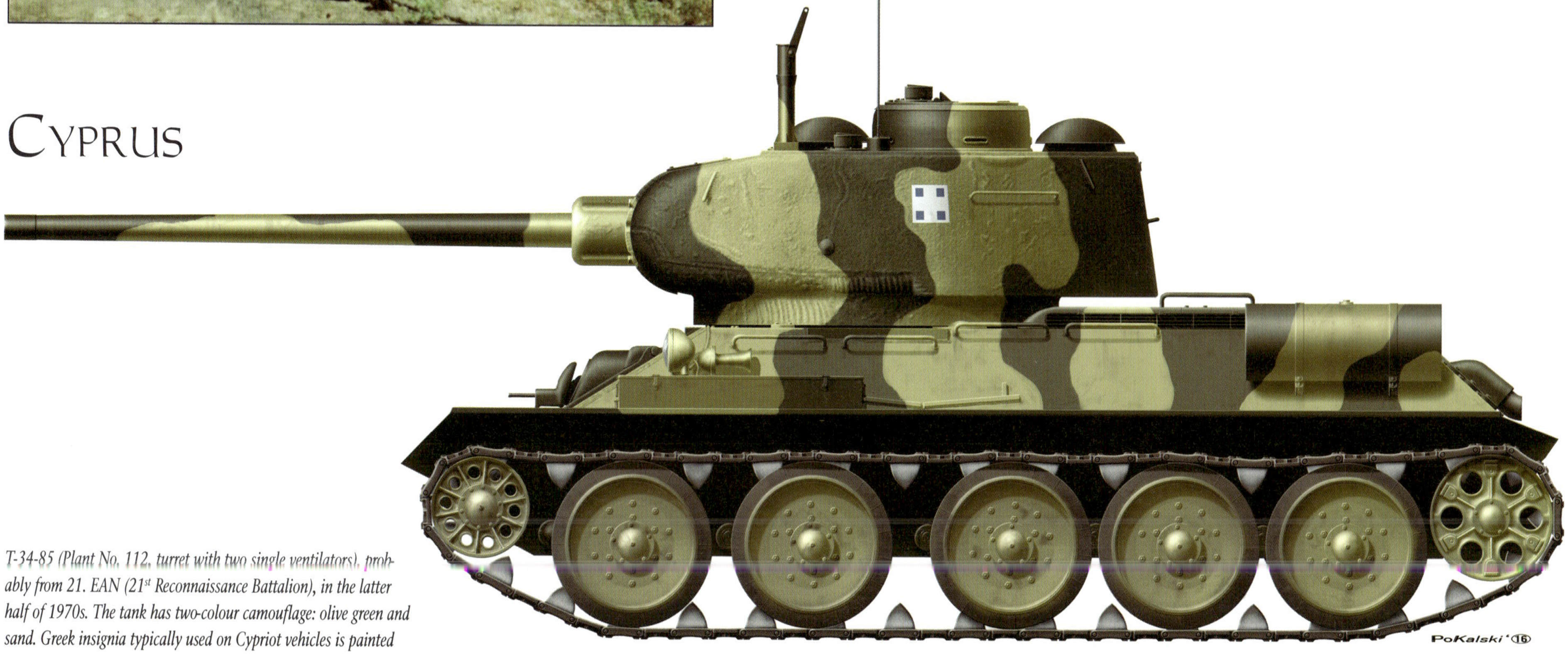

T-34-85 (Plant No. 112, turret with two single ventilators), probably from 21. EAN (21st Reconnaissance Battalion), in the latter half of 1970s. The tank has two-colour camouflage: olive green and sand. Greek insignia typically used on Cypriot vehicles is painted on the turret.

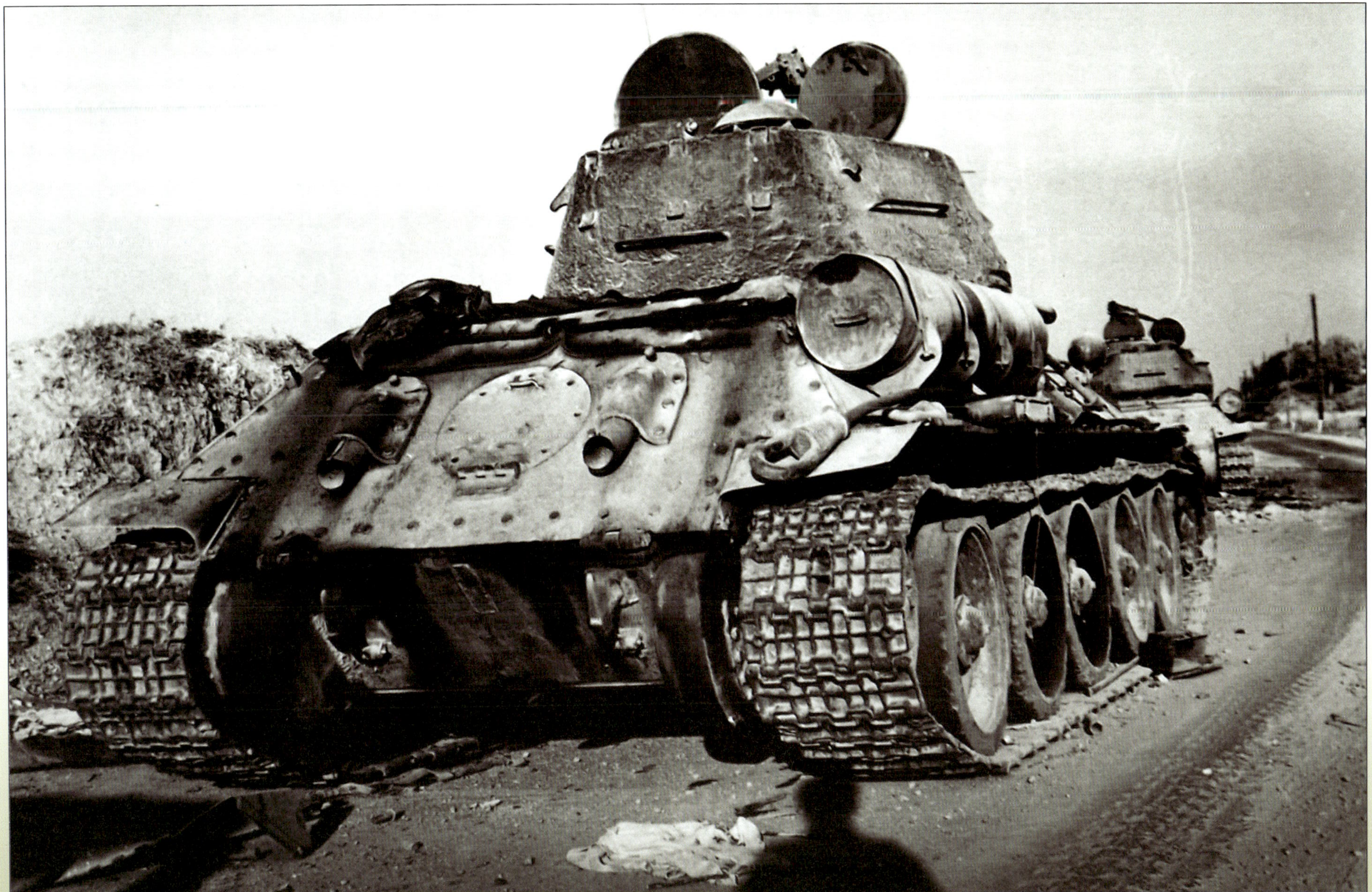

Cypriot T-34-85 tanks destroyed in the fighting with Turkish forces in 1974.

Czechoslovakia

During the first years after the end of the Second World War, T-34-85 tanks were delivered to Czechoslovakia from the USSR. A total of 297 tanks were delivered to Czechoslovak units by 1950. More were licence built in Czechoslovakia. The ČSLA received a total of 1,437 tanks of domestic production (731 made by ČKD and 706 by ZJVS). The year 1956 saw the largest number of T-34-85s in the inventory of the Czechoslovak army, with 1,701 tanks recorded. Over the following years these were gradually replaced by the tanks of T-54/55 family, though as late as 1971, a total of 780 T-34-85s were still in the inventory of ČSLA. In late 1980s these tanks, of which around 90 vehicles remained, were operated only by training units.

Two Czechoslovak T-34-85a (Plant No.112) with markings used immediately after the end of the Second World War. Large 1 and 2 digits seem to be platoon or display markings.

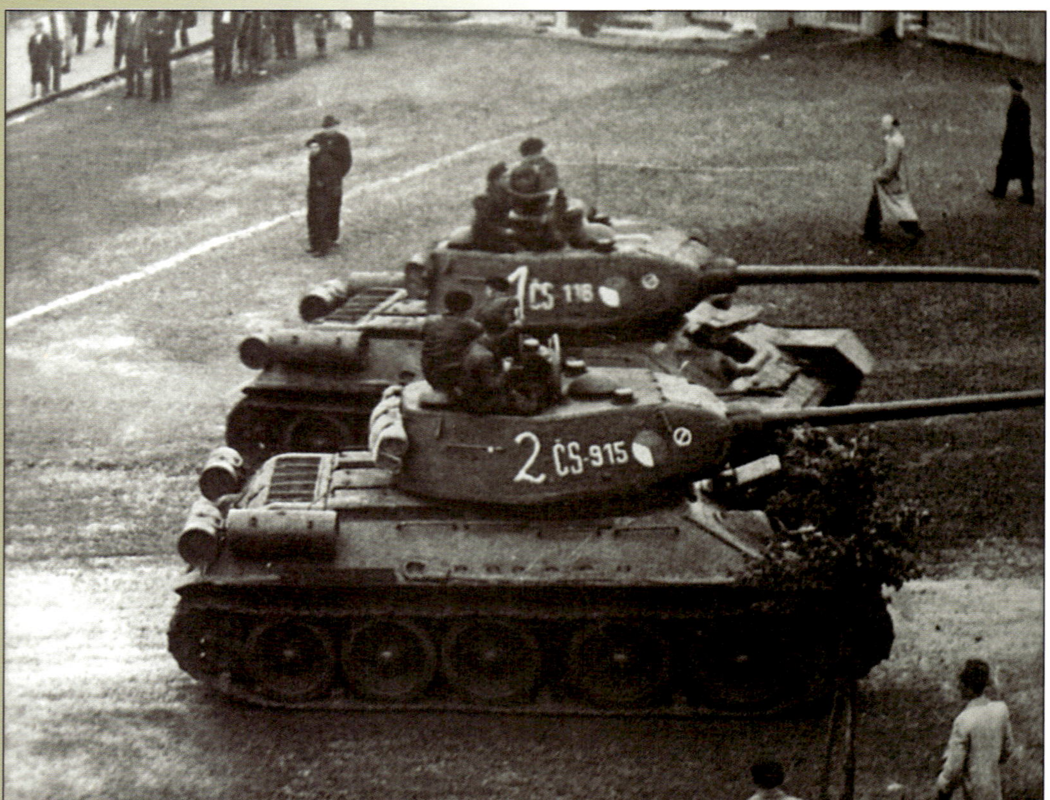

In the initial period after the end of the Second World War, Czechoslovak T-34-85s retained wartime paint schemes. Some tanks were painted all-over olive green (Soviet 4BO paint), while others sported an olive green (4BO) and dark brown (6k) disruptive pattern. Later the tanks were painted all-over khaki of slightly lighter shade than the Soviet paint. In winter, especially during exercises white camouflage patches were applied. According to official documents, on the T-34-85s multi-coloured disruptive patterns, including sand and brown

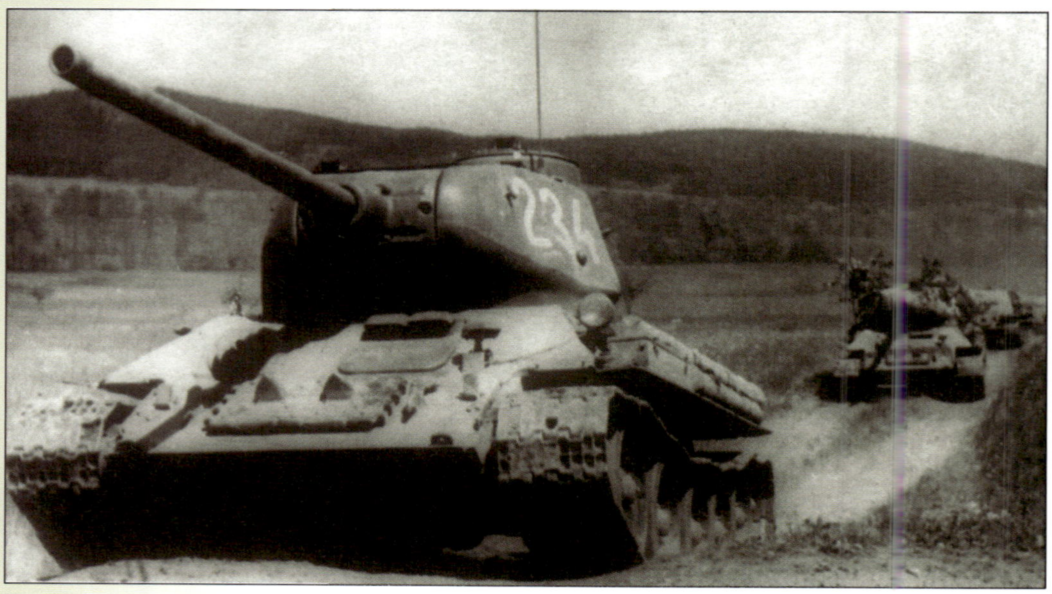

A T-34-85 of Czechoslovak production with number 234 in transit, 1950s. Note light on the front armour plate is visible.

paint were to be applied. The instruction that was initially in force in the ČSLA was a translation of a Soviet document, even mentioning Soviet 6K and 7K paints. In the 1960s new rules of applying multi-coloured camouflages were developed in Czechoslovakia. However, it is hard to find photographs confirming the application of such paint schemes to the T-34-85s in practice.

Just before the end of the Second World War the national insignia (red-white-blue roundels divided radially into thirds, the blue part uppermost) were painted on the T-34-85s of the 1st Independent Czechoslovak Armoured Brigade. This rule was retained in the early post-war period. After the war, tactical markings, consisting of the letters ČS and a number, e.g. ČS-673 and ČS-774 were added. On some tanks the pre-war *utočna vozba* marking of combat vehicles (a white circle with a slanting arrow inside) was applied.

In the 1950s roundels in national colours were not applied on Czechoslovak T-34-85s, but some tanks sported small red stars on their turrets, usually in front of the tactical number. At the end of the 1950s and beginning of the 1960s, new markings appeared. Initially this took the form of a red star with a Czech lion inside. In 1962 the Czech lion in a pentagonal shield, in a thin red outline, became the new national marking for a brief time. On 27 December 1962, an order was issued saying that from February 1963 the national marking on all ČSLA vehicles would be the three-colour roundel. The diameter was 15 cm and the roundel had a 5-mm blue outline. The blue part of the roundel faced forward.

The tactical numbers were usually three-digit, less frequently two-digit. Their standard colour was white and they were placed on the sides of the turrets and sometimes also on the rear. The aforementioned order of December 1962 specified that the number was to be 50 cm long and 25 cm wide. However it seems that these dimensions were not strictly adhered to.

In the 1950s on ČSLA vehicles, including tanks, the identification numbers were applied. In the case of the T-34-85 these were five-digit (e.g. 86197) or six-digit (e.g. 132 136) numbers. White digits were painted on a black rectangular plate mounted at the front and rear of the hull.

During exercises, various markings were used, usually in the form of stripes painted on the turrets. A photograph is known to exist of a Czechoslovak T-34-85 with large letter ‘A’ on the forward hull. Other examples of non-standard markings include names written on the turrets, such as “Janošik”, “Lidice”, “Ležáky”. These may have been applied for parades and displays only.

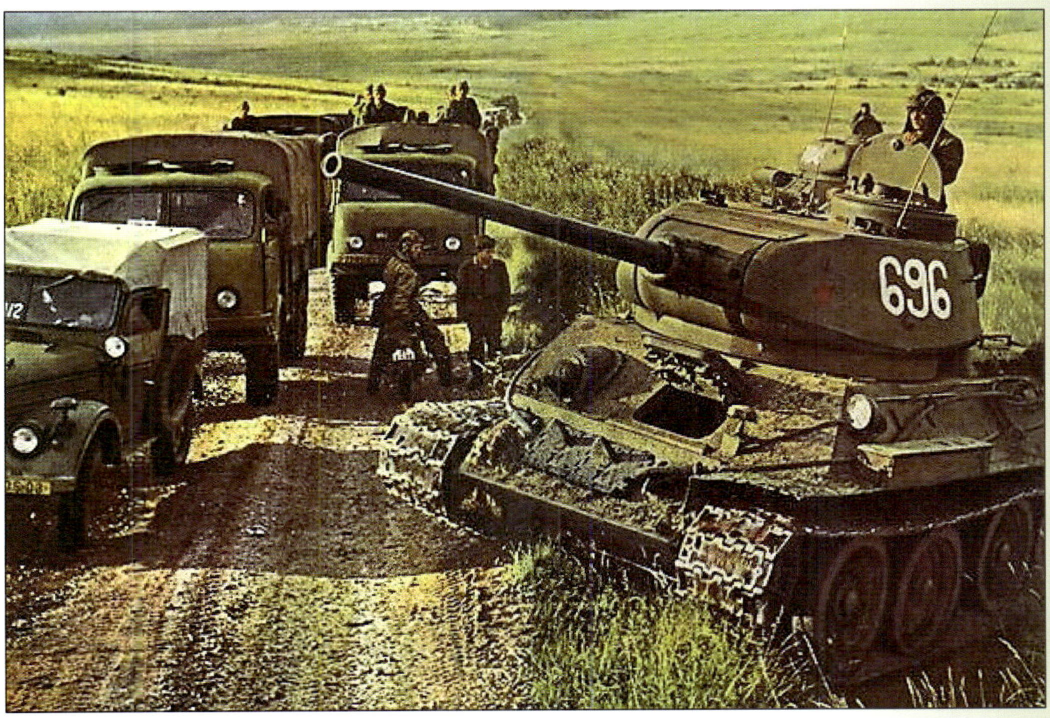

Czechoslovak military vehicles during exercise in the 1950s. A T-34-85 of domestic production with number 696 is visible in the foreground. Note the red star painted on the turret.

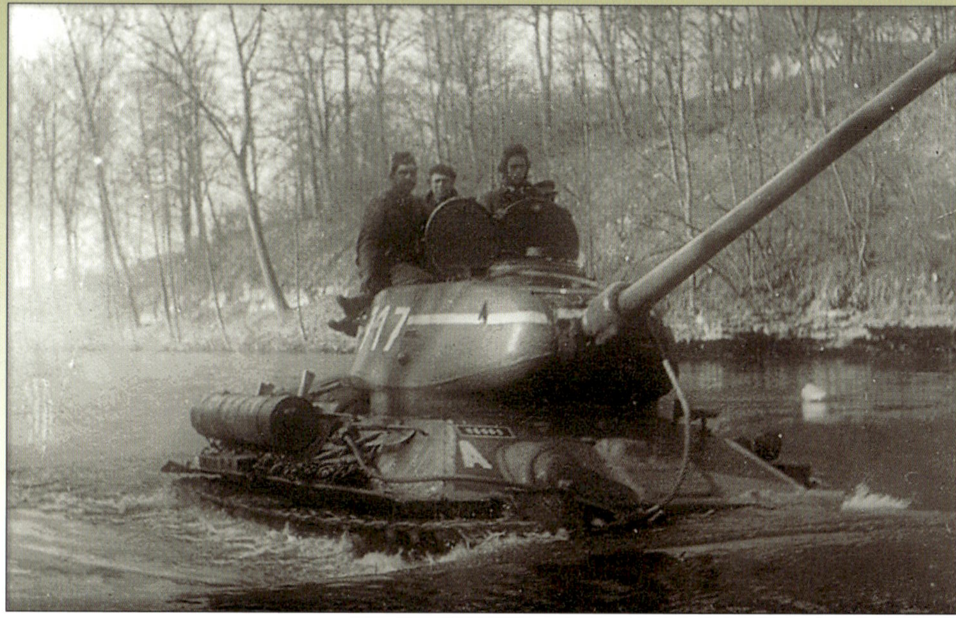

Photographs of a Czechoslovak T-34-85 taken during army maneuvers in the 1950s. The tank number 117 has very interesting markings – a registration plate on the front armour plate, the letter A on the hull and white identification stripe on the turret.

CZECHOSLOVAKIA

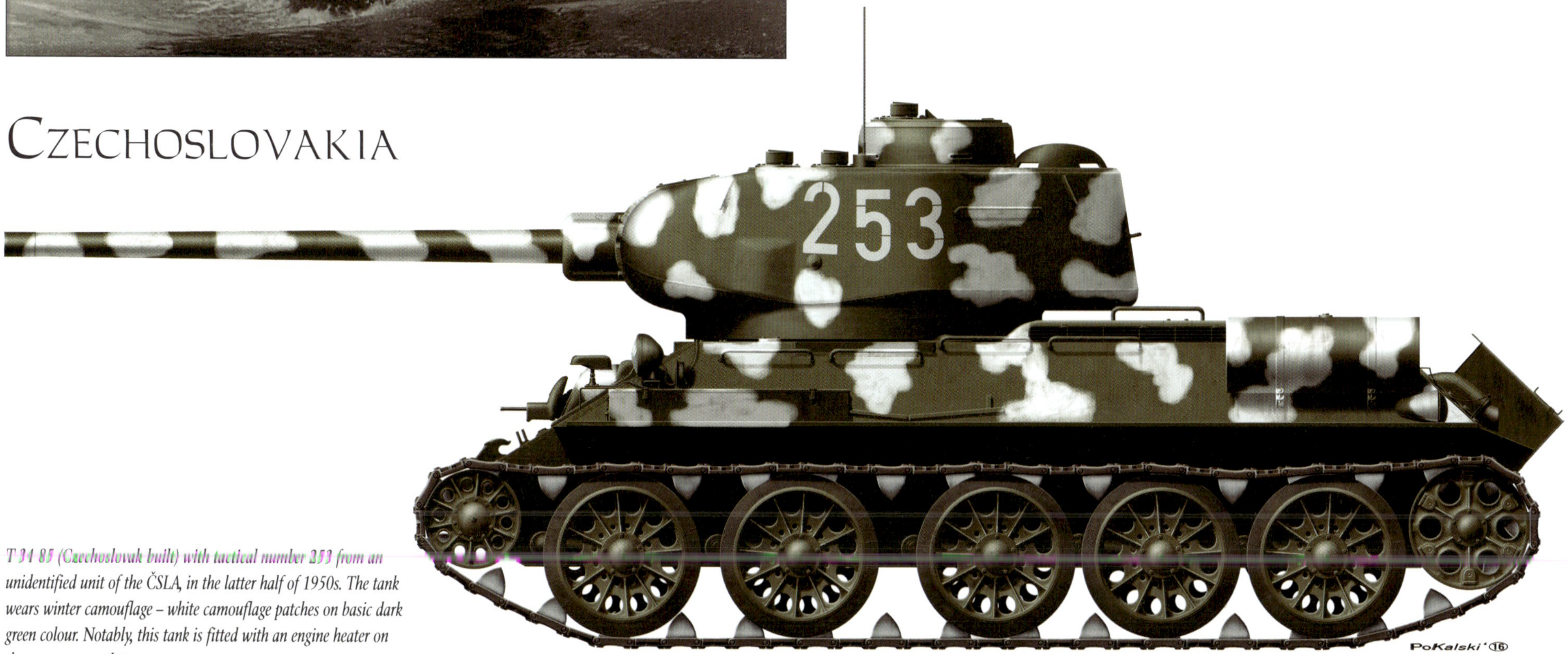

T-34-85 (Czechoslovak built) with tactical number 253 from an unidentified unit of the ČSLA, in the latter half of 1950s. The tank wears winter camouflage – white camouflage patches on basic dark green colour. Notably, this tank is fitted with an engine heater on the rear armour plate.

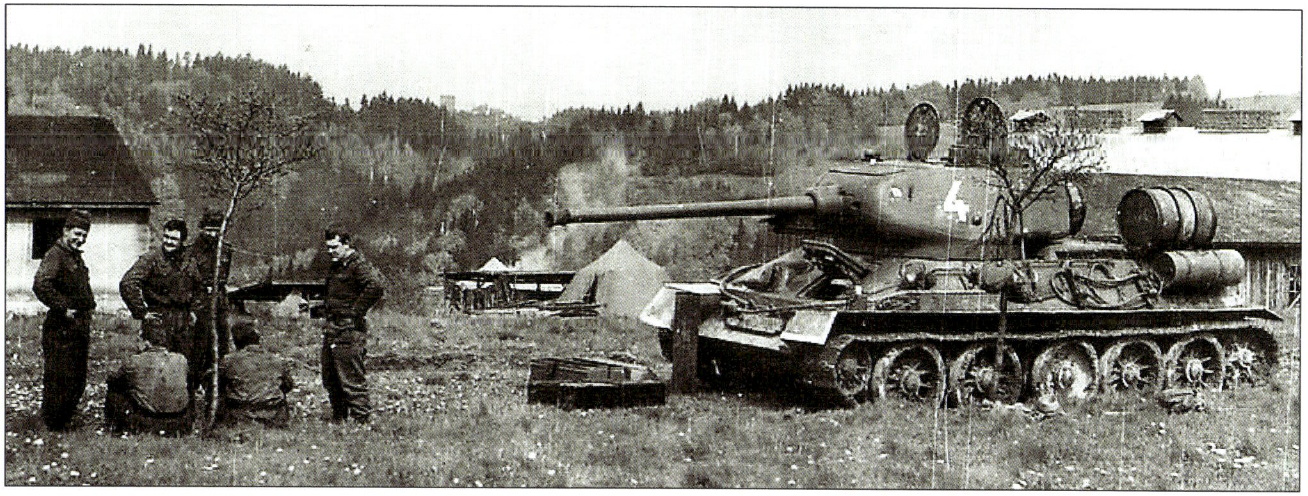

A Czechoslovak T-34-85 with number 4 and three-colour roundel – national insignia introduced on the turn of 1962 and 1963.

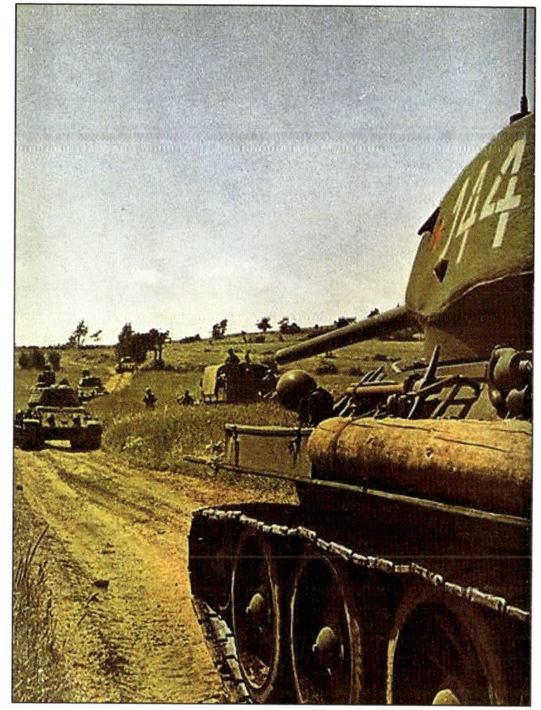

Czechoslovakia

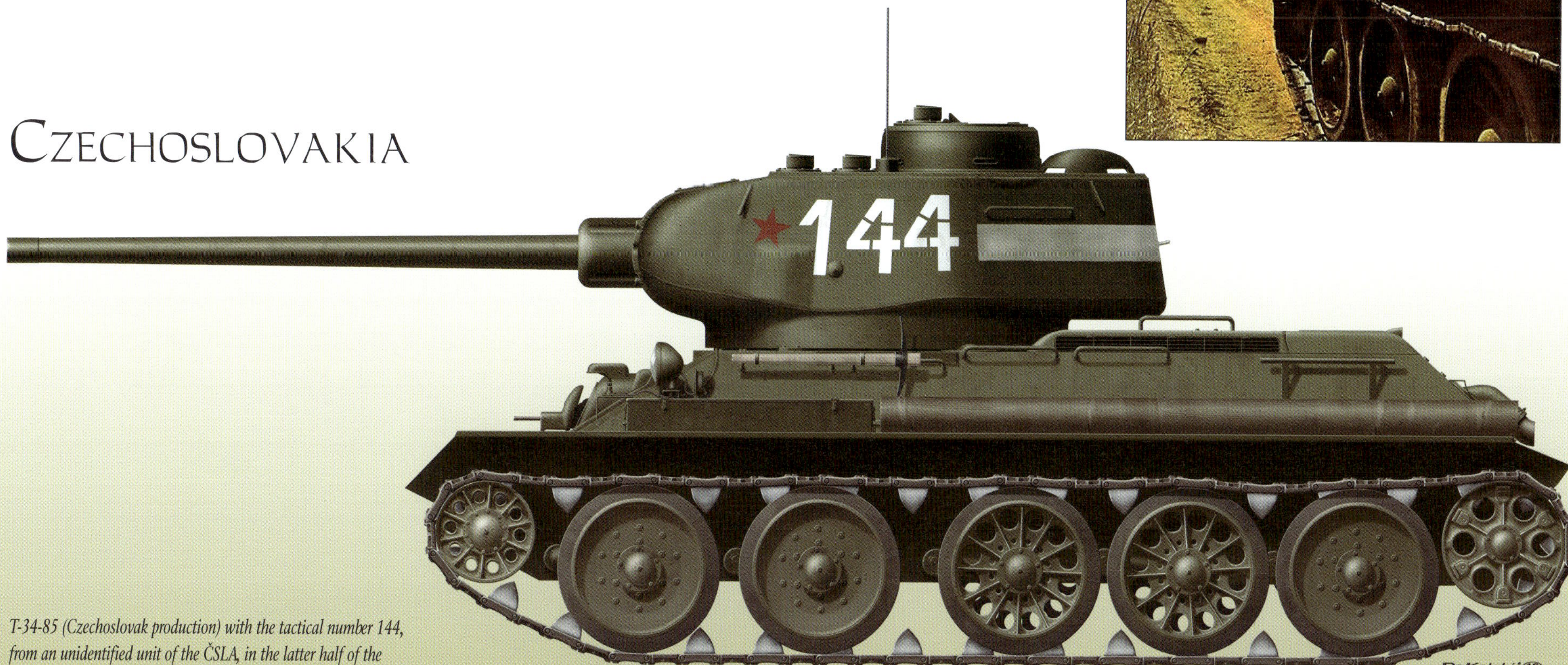

T-34-85 (Czechoslovak production) with the tactical number 144, from an unidentified unit of the ČSLA, in the latter half of the 1950s.

Finland

At the end of the Second World War, the Finns had seven T-34-85 tanks, captured during fighting with the Red Army in the summer of 1944. These vehicles remained in the Finnish Army inventory for the purpose of crew training, and, despite technical problems, they remained in service in this role until the end of the 1950s. The last T-34-85 was written off in September 1962. The T-34-85s operated by the Finns were modified by the installation of fender reinforcements, folding lights and the addition of toolboxes and baskets.

During the post-war period the vehicles received one-colour paint schemes – all surfaces were painted Moss Green. Finnish registration numbers (PS.245-1 through PS.245-7) were retained, painted on the front and rear of the hulls. On the turrets (sides and rear) the national white-blue-white roundels were applied.

Finnish T-34-85 (Plant No. 183), tactical number Ps 245-7 of PsR Parolannummi, summer of 1952. The tank, wearing standard Finnish post-war markings underwent modifications in Finland – new fenders, stowage boxes and equipment.

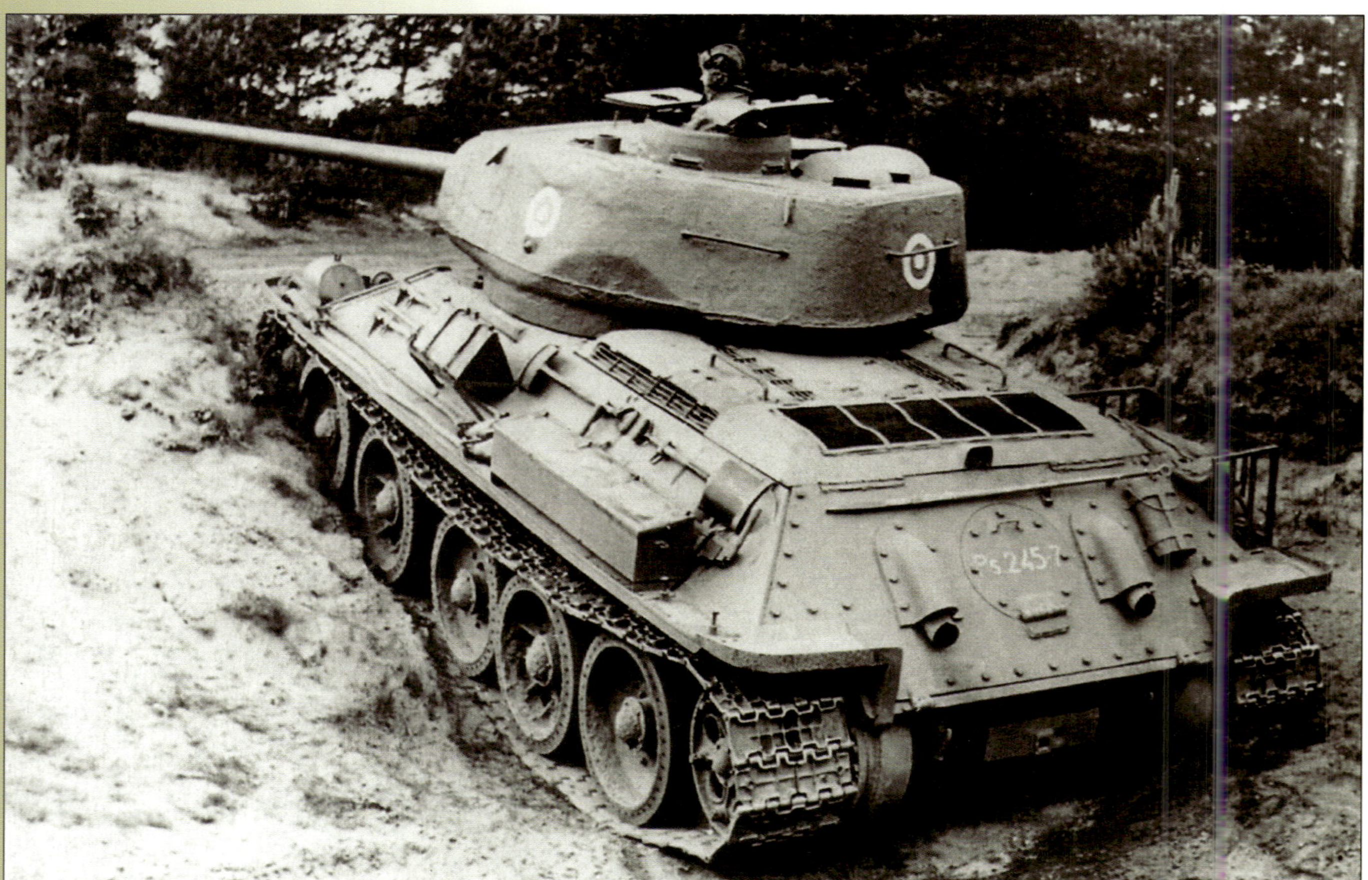

Yugoslavia: Serbia-Croatia-Bosnia and Herzegovina

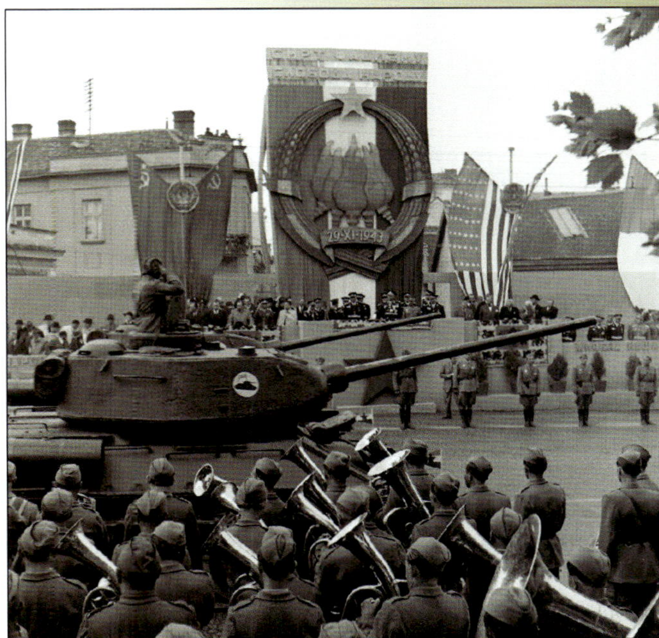

Yugoslav T-34-85s on a parade in the 1950s. In the foreground is a tank of Plant No.174 production, with an interesting emblem on the turret – a silhouette of a tank on white background.

During the Second World War, Yugoslavia received 65 T-34-85 tanks from the USSR, which equipped the 2nd Armoured Brigade. After the end of the war the Soviets delivered 66 more tanks, which equipped the 5th Armoured Brigade, followed by a further 308. Following the deterioration of Yugoslav-Soviet relations, local factories commenced production of spare parts for T-34-85 tanks and V-2-34 engines, to become independent from Soviet supplies. Further deliveries of the tanks from the USSR took place during 1966-68, following the improvement of political relations. A total of 600 modified T-34-85 Model 1960 tanks then arrived in Yugoslavia, receiving the local designation T-34B. Some of the tanks (including those delivered previously) were modified by the Yugoslavs. The most characteristic alteration was the addition of an anti-aircraft machine gun (12.7 mm Browning M2) on the turret and installation of an additional light on the right side of the hull.

The T-34-85 tanks operated by the Yugoslavian army were painted olive green. In the early period after the war this was Soviet 4BO paint. After overhauls and modernisations the tanks were painted with coatings of domestic production, slightly lighter and more green than the Soviet paint. Initially, three-digit white tactical numbers were painted on the turrets. Later new, smaller, four- and five-digit tactical numbers, also white, superseded the three digit numbers.

The T-34-85s operated by the Croatians wore diverse paint schemes. Some were olive green. On others, brown camouflage patches were applied (such paint schemes were used in the early period of fighting, 1991–92). Some tanks sported three- or four-colour camouflage – light green and brown patches on an olive green background. In four-colour schemes, black was added to the above colours. On the turrets and hull fronts, shields in the Croatian white and red chequer

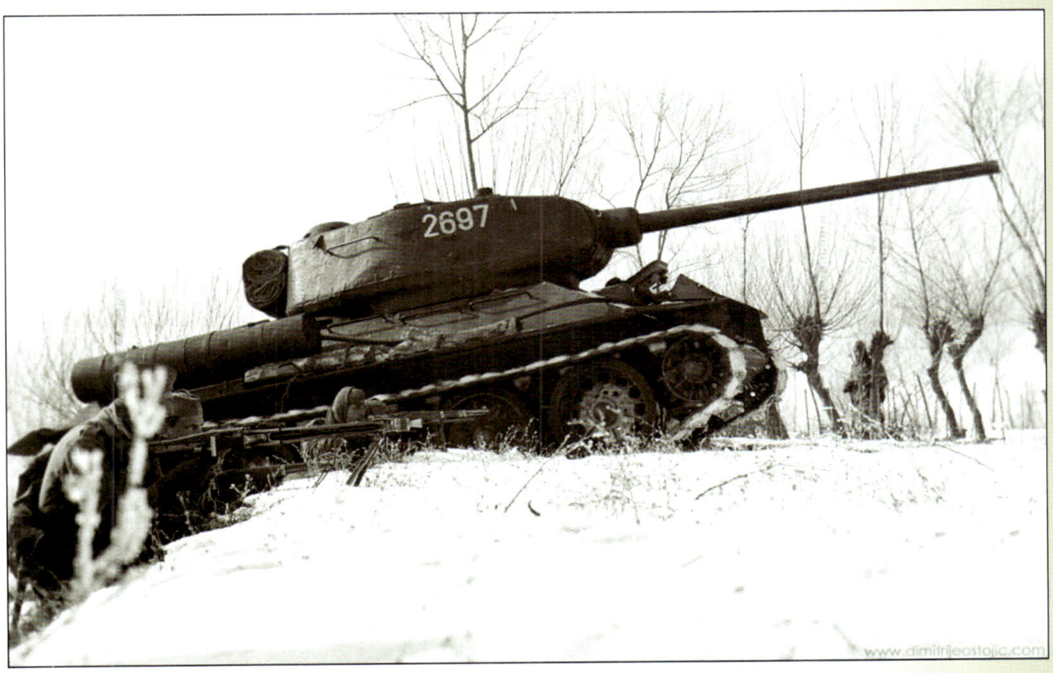

A Yugoslav T-34-85 (Plant No.183) at an exercise in the 1970s. The tactical number 2697 and small red star are well visible.

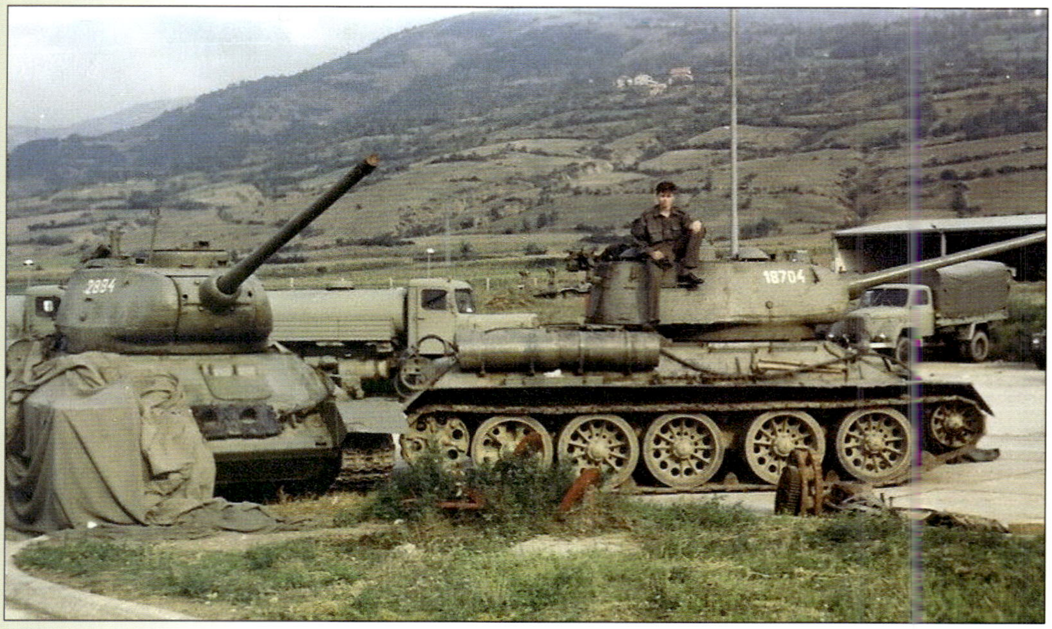

Yugoslav T-34-85s in one of JNA depots. Interestingly, one of the tanks has four-digit number (2884) and the tank next to it – a five-digit number (18704). The photograph shows the shade of the basic green colour , in which Yugoslav army vehicles were painted.

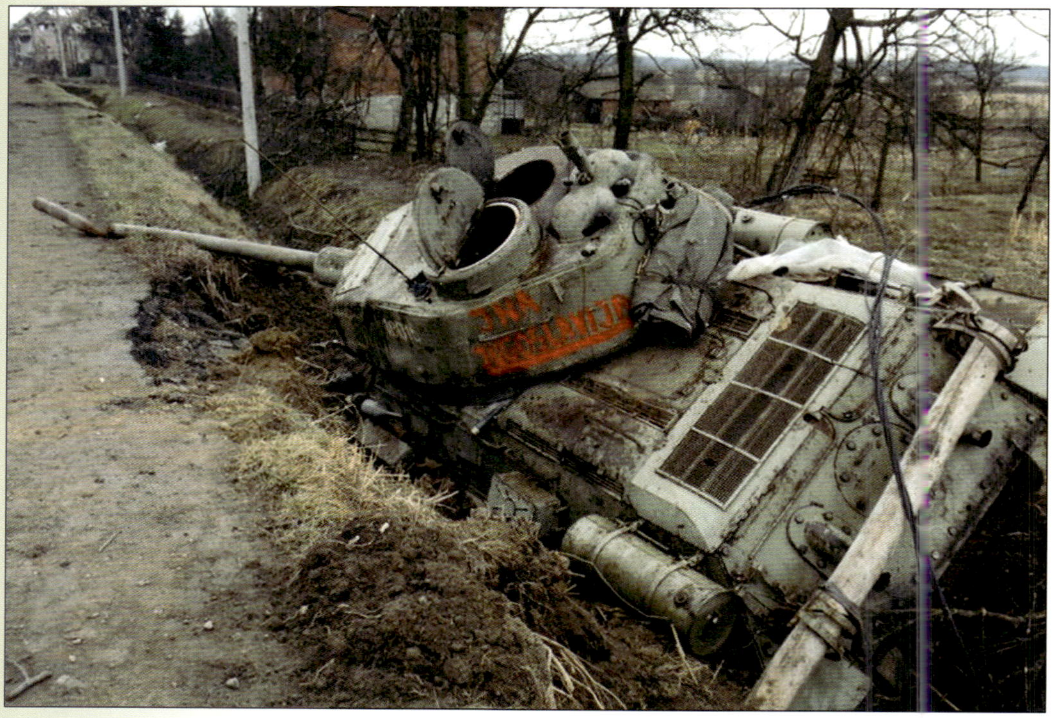

A Serbian T-34-85 (modified tank of Plant No. 183 production) damaged during battle of Stary Grabovec near Vukovar in 1991. Note inscription on the turret – JNA Jugoslavija. *Moreover, the tank has old Yugoslavian tactical number 18018 and a new one – 6 - on the forward part of the turret.*

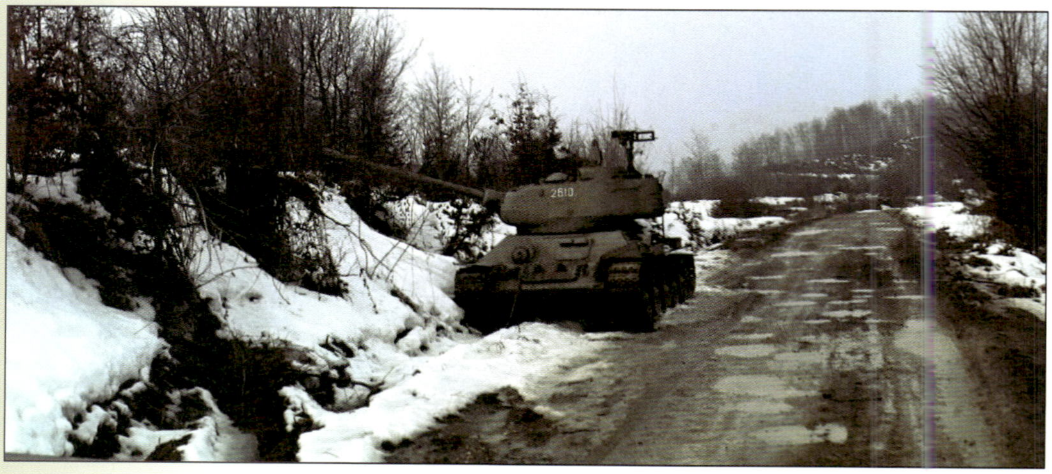

Abandoned Serbian T-34-85, tactical number 2610, Operation Joint Endeavor, February 1996.

pattern were painted. Some tanks had individual names applied, such as “Belaj Bager”, “Demon”, “Mungos”, “Malo Bijelo”, “Pas”, “Sv.Kata”, and “Babo-ZNG”.

Interesting paint schemes, unfortunately poorly documented with photographic evidence, were apparently worn by tanks used during combats in Bosnia and Herzegovina by the Bosnians and Bosnian Serbs. Some received camouflage of brown and/or sand camouflage patches applied on basic olive green. A photograph exists of a tank with the shield insignia and lettering ‘BiH’. Some tanks with additional covers made of thick rubber on the hull and turret had markings (e.g. death’s heads) and names (e.g. Deliye) painted on these temporary covers.

After Macedonia gained independence in the autumn of 1991, four T-34-85 from the JNA inventory, which Serbs did not manage to evacuate, were found in the new state. These vehicles were for a short time on the equipment of the Macedonian army, and then they were withdrawn (probably went to the monuments and to the museum). Unfortunately, it was impossible to get the details of their short service, as well as information about their camouflage and marking.

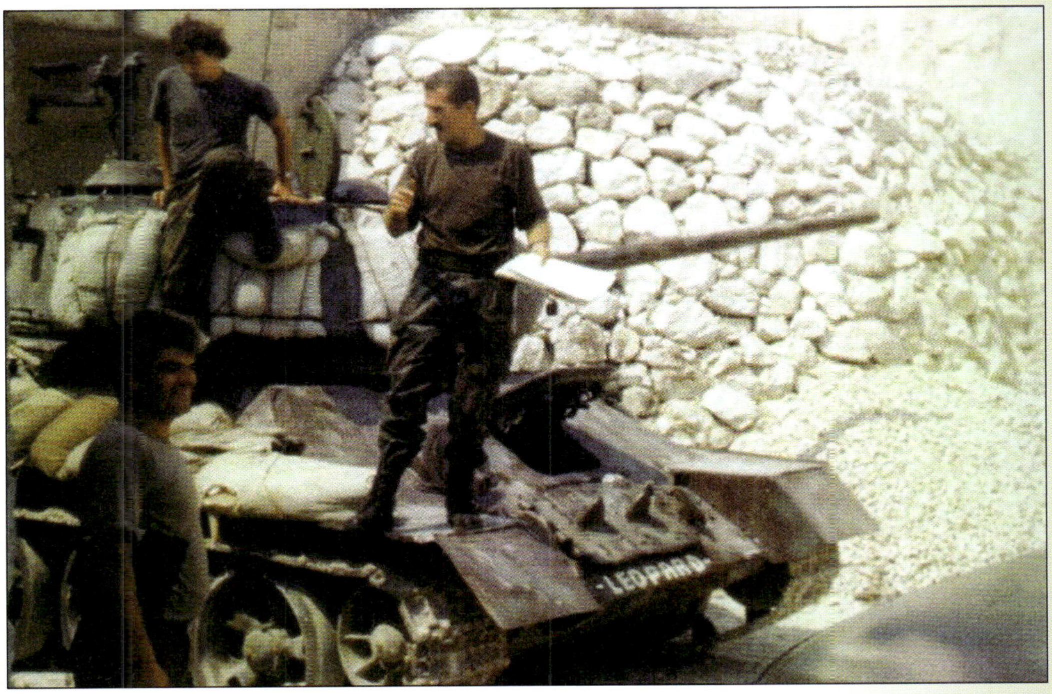

T-34B (modernized T-34-85), named “Leopard”, operated by the Croatians near Dubrovnik in 1991–1992. Note provisional sandbag protections. The tank wears a two-colour camouflage.

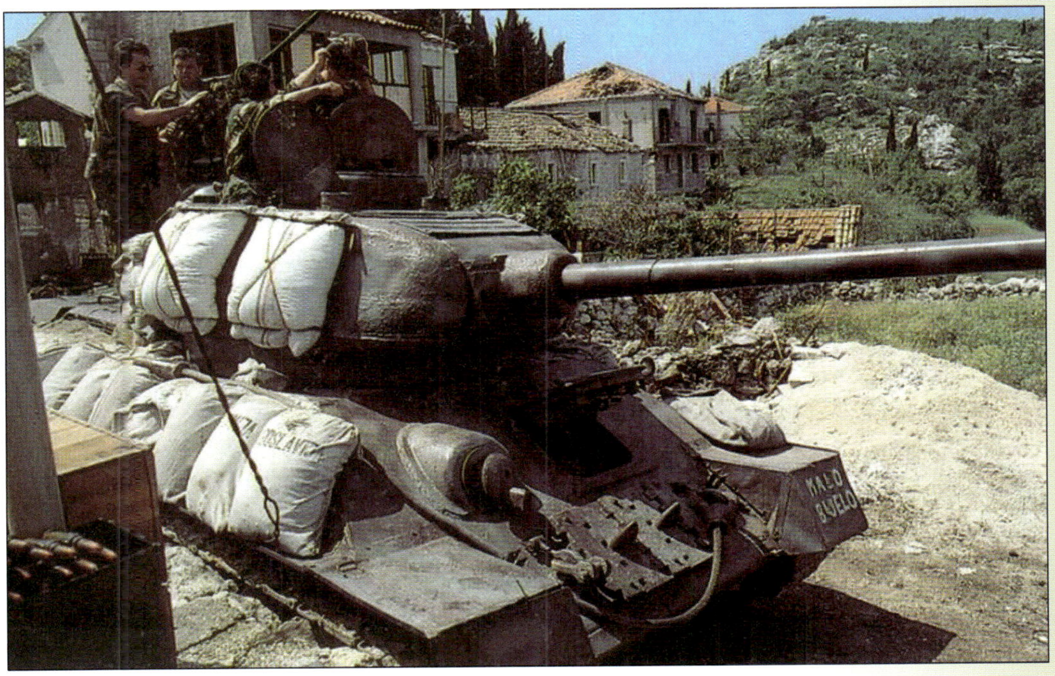

One of the most famous Croatian T-34-85s “Malo Bijelo”, which survived two antitank shell hits in the early period of the hostilities and its crew destroyed several enemy vehicles. The tanks wears two-colour camouflage. In the photo showing the left side of the tank the inscription “Sokol” on the gun barrel is visible.

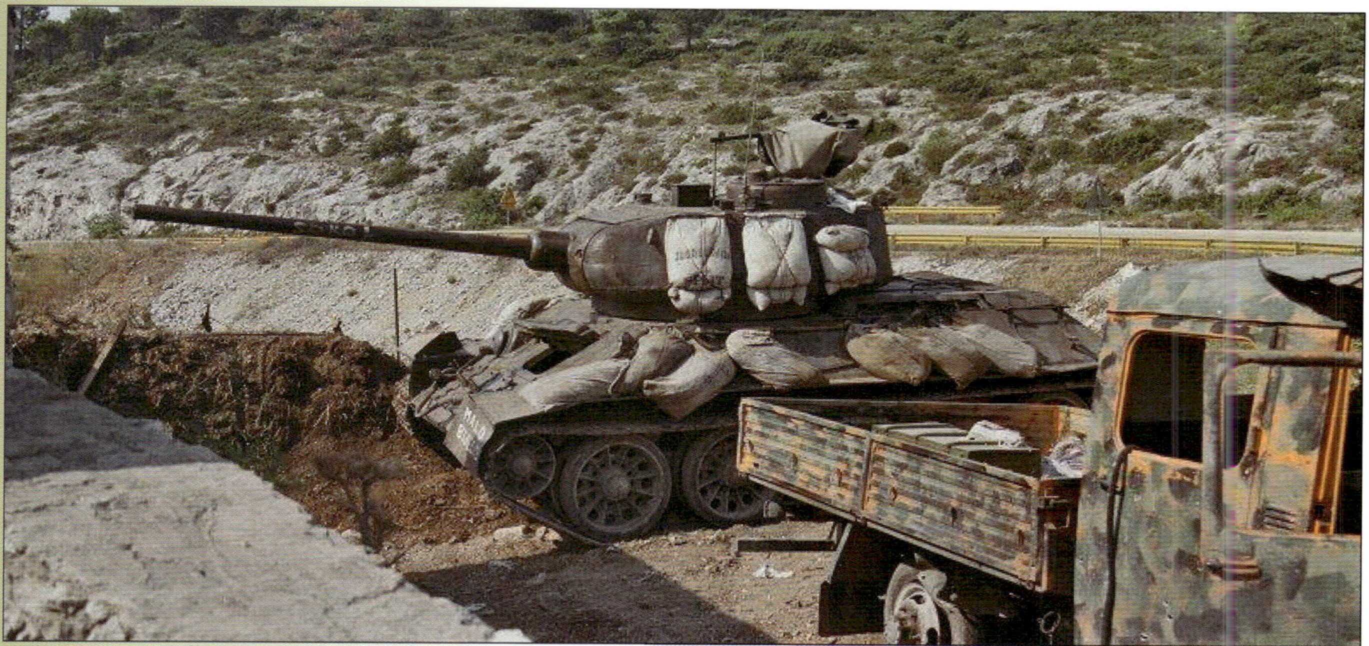

Croatian T-34B (modernized T-34-85) with white and red shield on the front armour plate. The tank wears two-colour camouflage and sandbag protections. According to some authors it was characteristic for the tanks operated by the Croatians near Dubrovnik during 1991–1992.

Croatian T-34-85 tanks at Benkovac military base, late 1990s or early 2000s. The photo is interesting because it shows not only various versions of the tanks, but also various paint schemes.

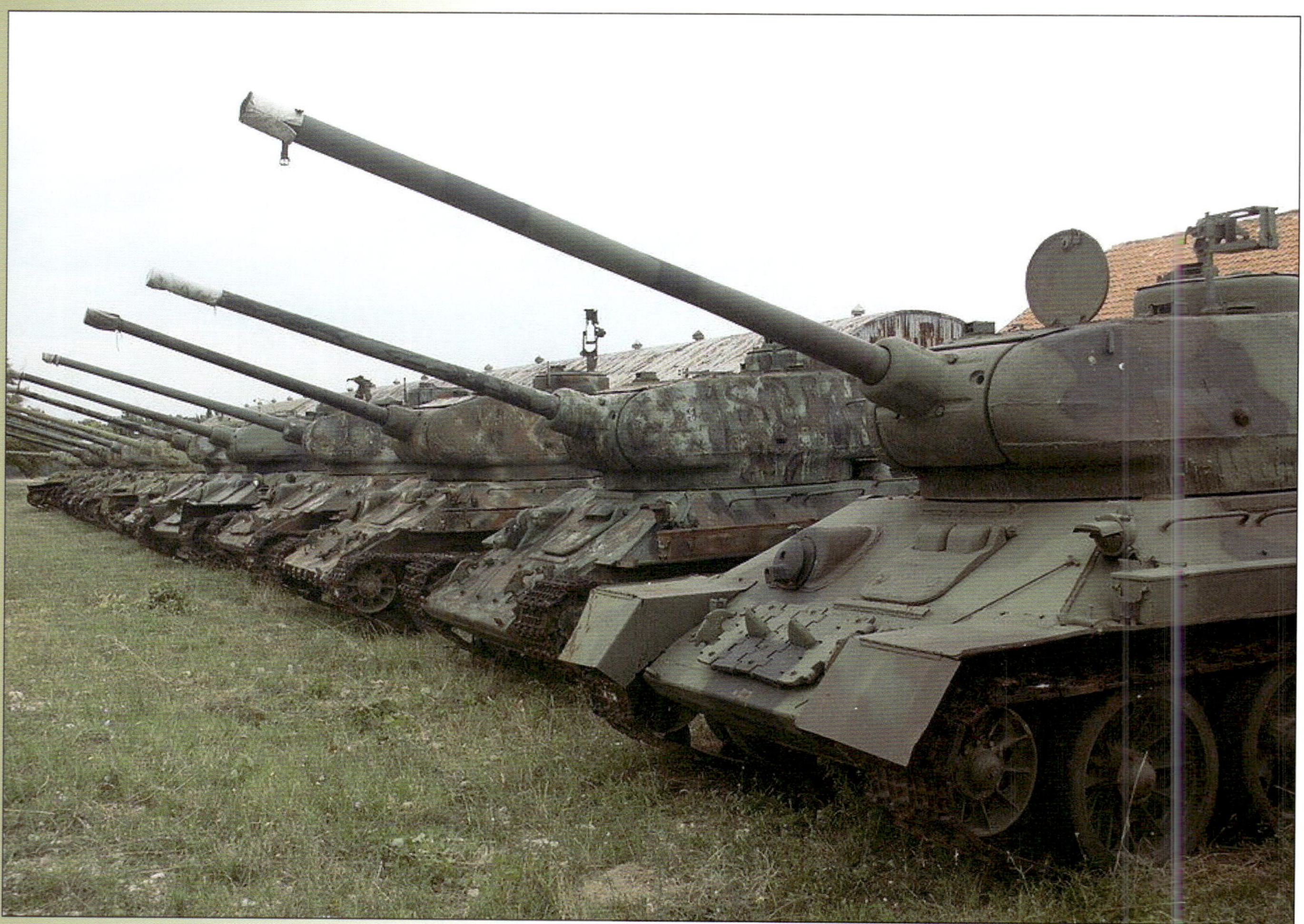

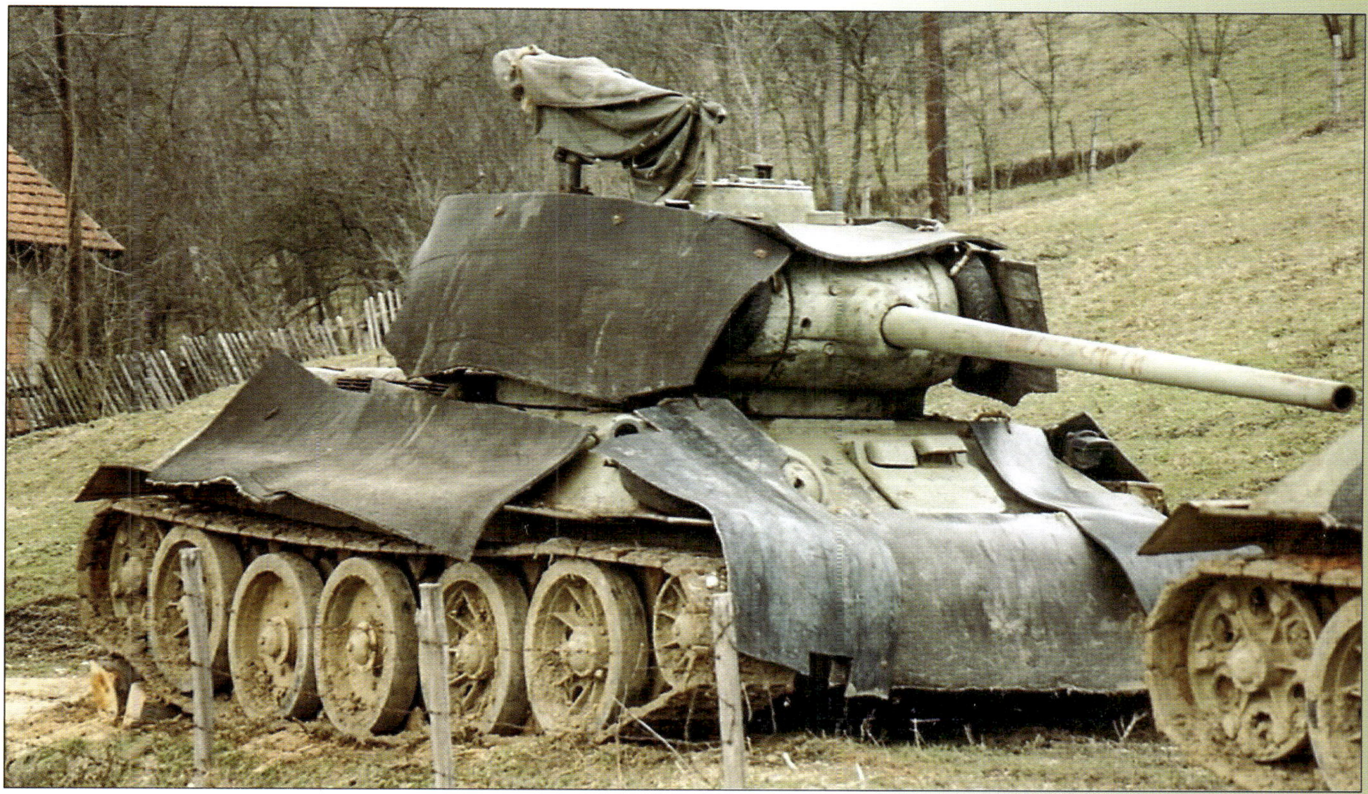

Bosnian (ex-Yugoslavian) T-34-85 with additional covers made of thick rubber, near the town of Doboj, spring of 1996 (so after the end of the hostilities). Such provisional "armour" was frequently carried by tanks operated by Bosnian units.

One of the most interesting photographs of a T-34-85 in Bosnian hands, taken probably in 1993. The tank wears two-colour camouflage (sand splotches on basic green background) and the Bosnian coat of arms with the lettering BIH on the turret. The back of the turret is covered with rubber skirts.

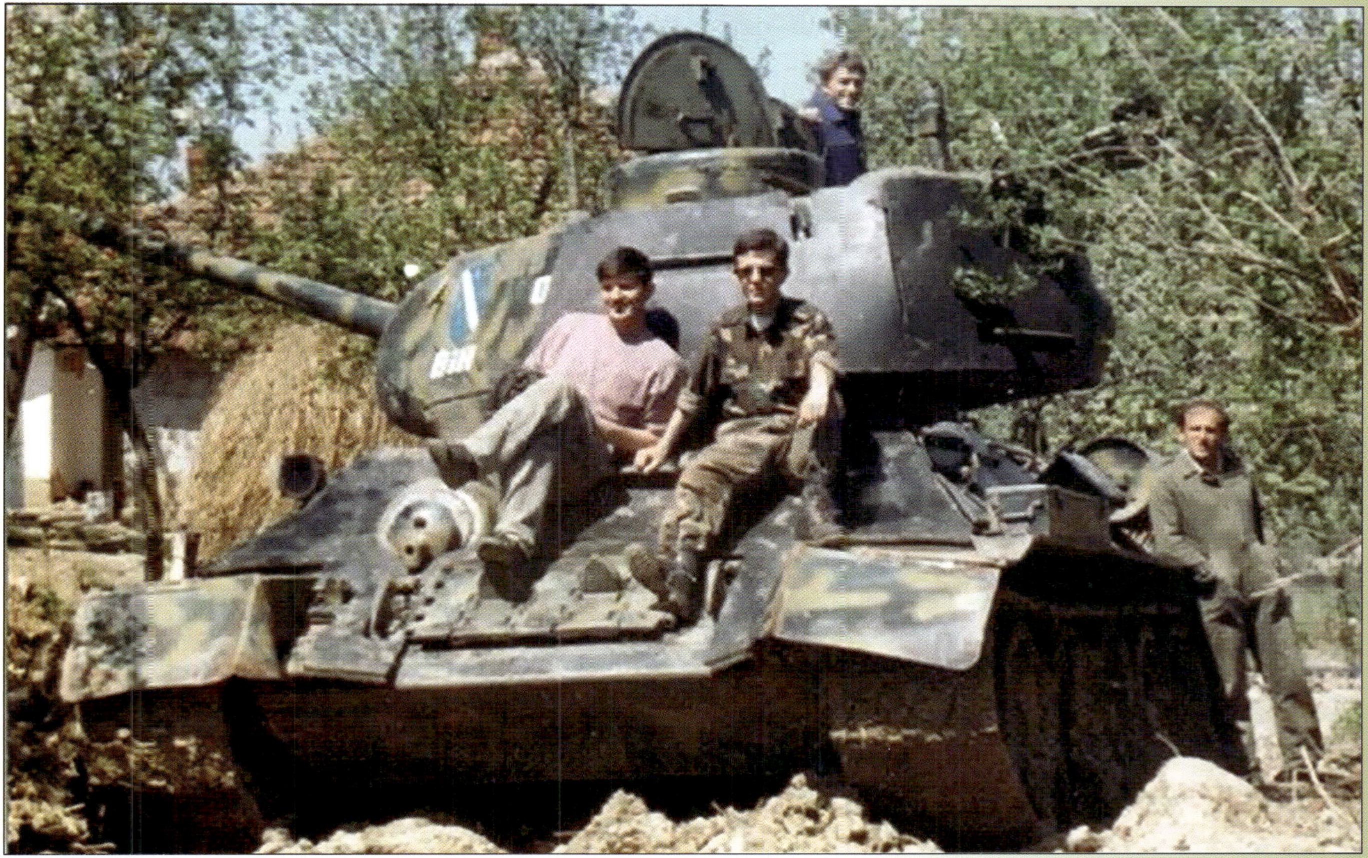

Finland

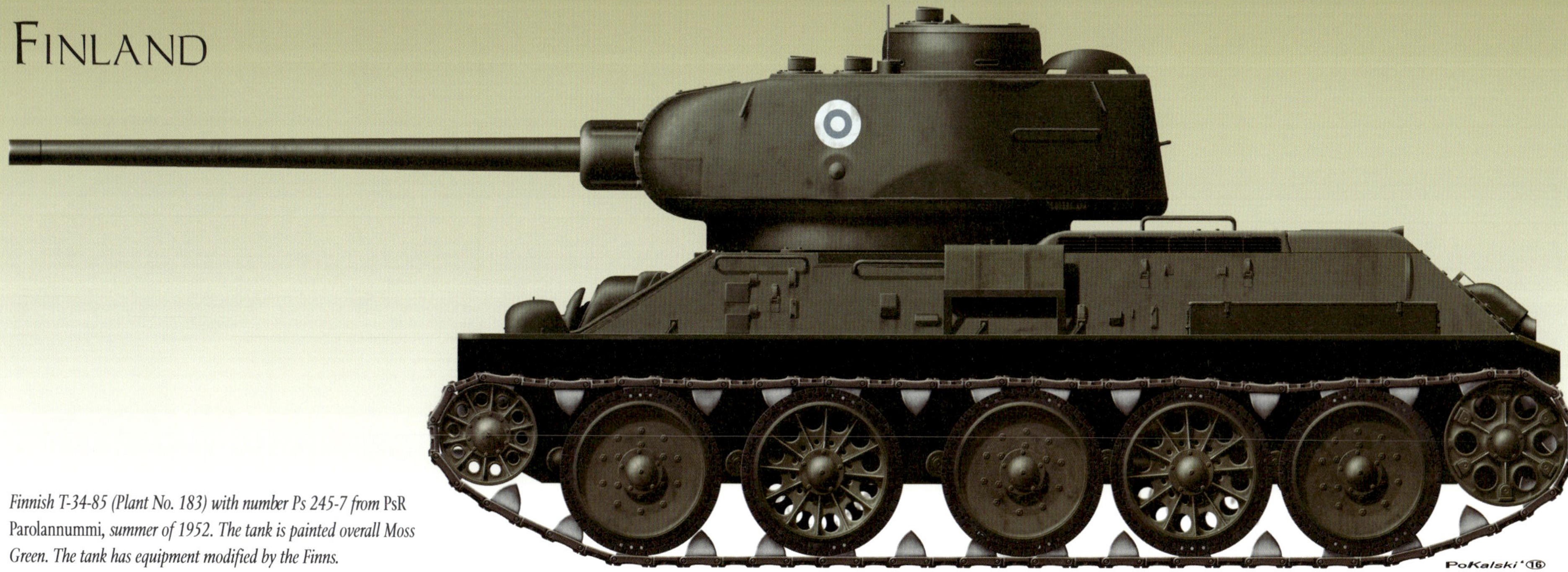

Finnish T-34-85 (Plant No. 183) with number Ps 245-7 from PsR Parolannummi, *summer of 1952. The tank is painted overall Moss Green. The tank has equipment modified by the Finns.*

Croatia

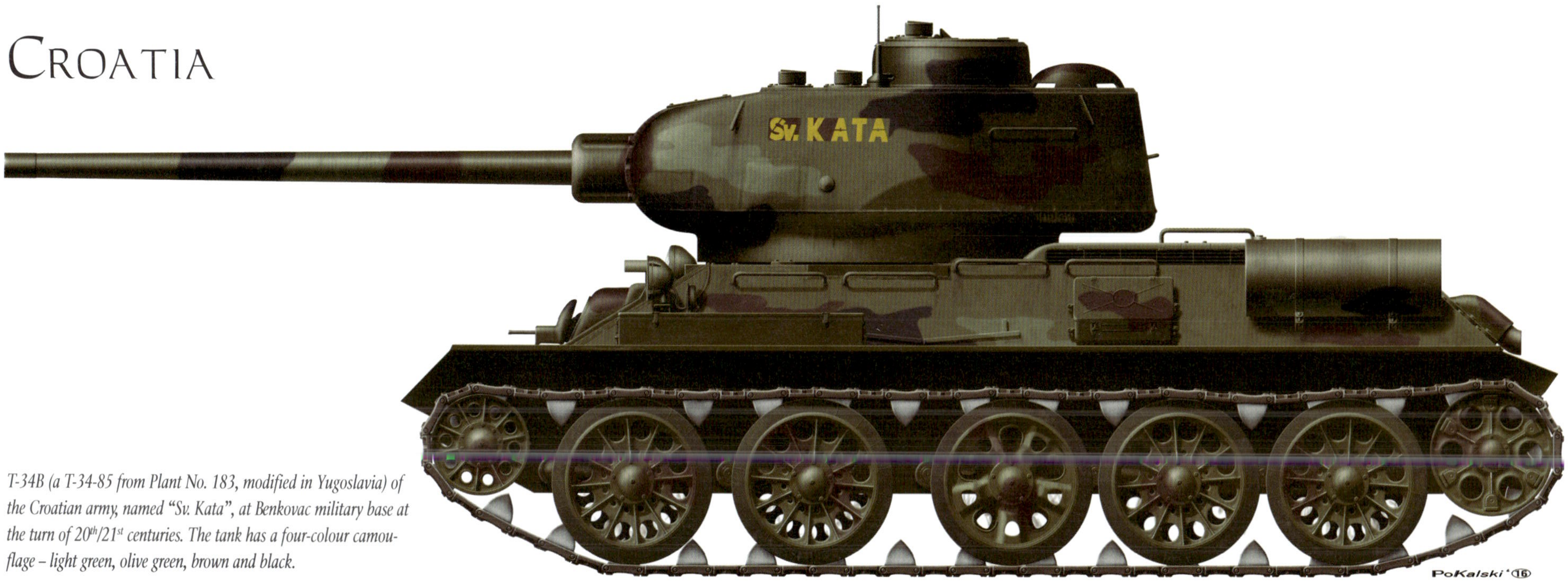

T-34B (a T-34-85 from Plant No. 183, modified in Yugoslavia) of the Croatian army, named "Sv. Kata", at Benkovac military base at the turn of 20th/21st centuries. The tank has a four-colour camouflage – light green, olive green, brown and black.

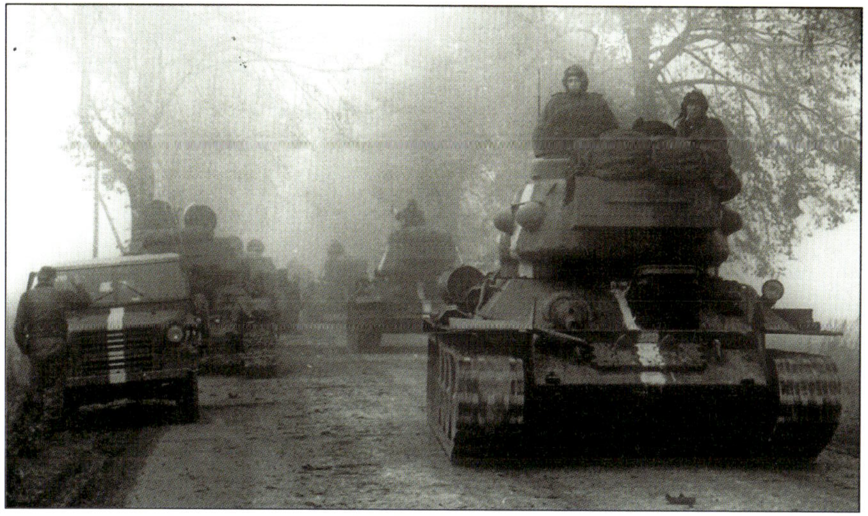

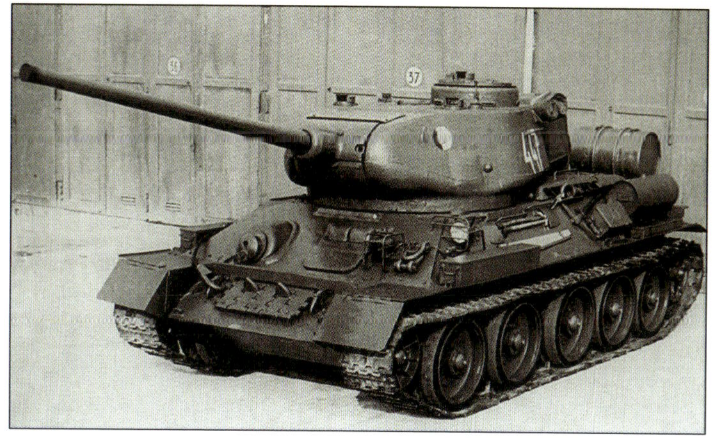

***Left:** A column of East German T-34-85m tanks during Operation "Danube", August-September 1968. Note white stripes – quick identification markings applied to vehicles of the Warsaw Pact forces during invasion of Czechoslovakia.*
***Right:** A model example of modernization of the East German "thirty-four" to T-34-85m standard (tank of Polish production). Analyzing the photos one may see that not all tanks underwent the full modernization. The tank sports complete markings – tactical number and national insignia.*

East Germany

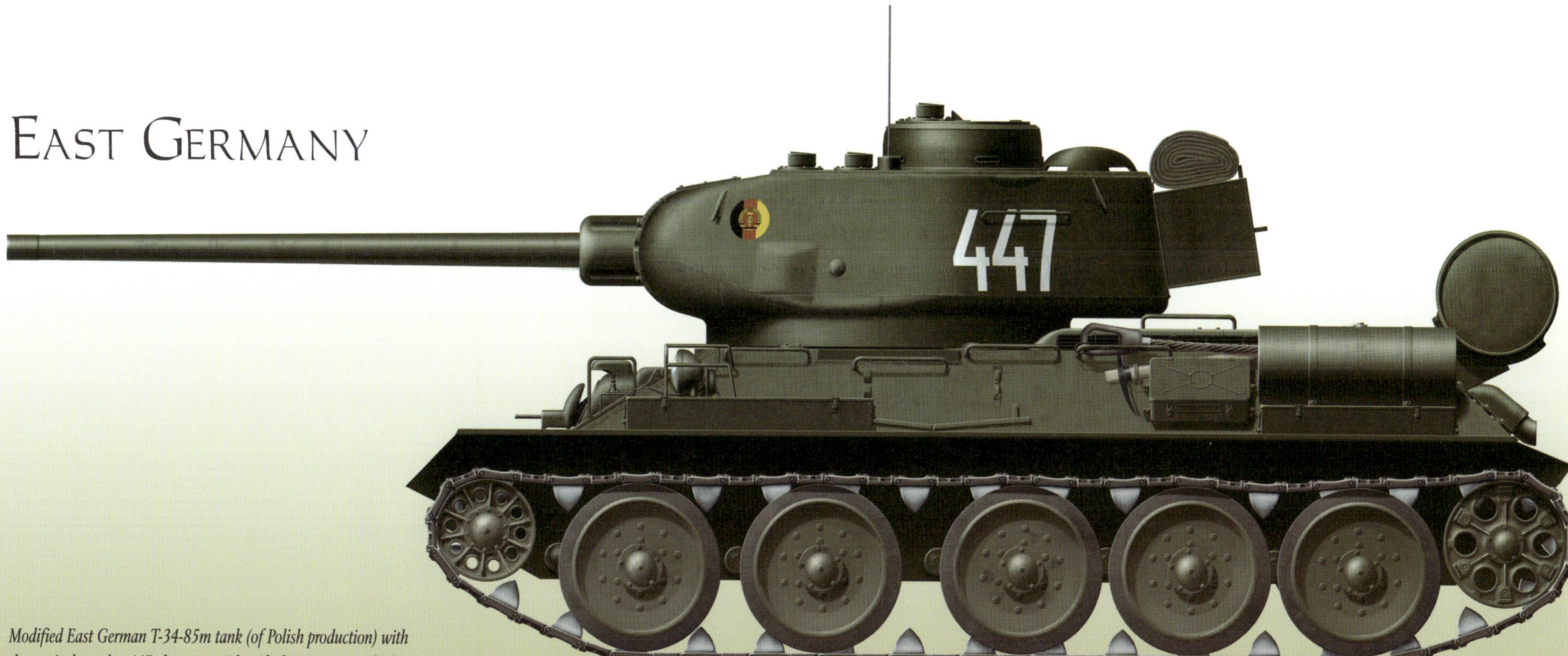

Modified East German T-34-85m tank (of Polish production) with the tactical number 447, from an unidentified NVA unit, in the latter half of the 1960s. The tank is painted all-over olive green.

East Germany

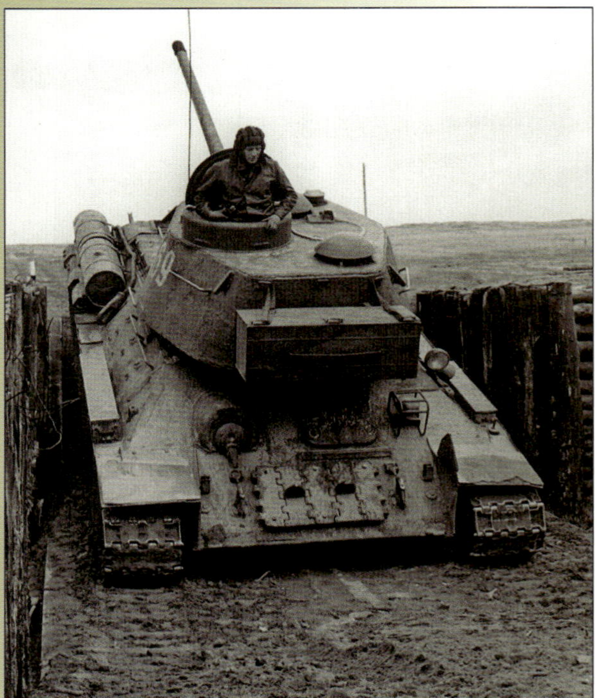

A T-34-85m (Plant No. 112) during drivers' exercises, June 1964. A stowage box on the back of the turret is visible.

In the post-war period T-34-85 tanks equipped East German units. A total of 1,346 tanks of this type were operated by the *Kasernierten Volkspolizei* and then the *Nationale Volksarmee*, including 285 tanks delivered from Poland during 1955–56[1]. East German 'eighty-fives' underwent a number of modernisations. In the late 1950s some received special air heaters, facilitating operation at low temperatures. The air heater was installed on the rear armour plate. These vehicles were designated T-34-85 m.O. (*mit Ofen* – with heater). However, this was not indigenous German design, but an adaptation of a Russian one. Work began on a tank adapted for fording water obstacles, and another that could swim. In the 1960s, a programme of modernisation consisted of the installation of 24-volt electric system, R-113/26 wireless set, more efficient air filters, new boxes for tools (on the hull) and for crew's equipment (on the back of the turret), 200-litre fuel drums on the rear hull and light shrouds. These tanks were designated T-34-85m. About 100 tanks were upgraded to the command version, designated T-34-85m(K), with the addition of a further wireless set.

East German T-34-85s were painted all-over olive green. Initially only tactical numbers (two- and three-digit) were painted on the turrets. At the turn of 1950s and 1960s, three-digit numbers, painted on the middle section of the turret, were introduced with the insignia of the DDR ahead of the number.

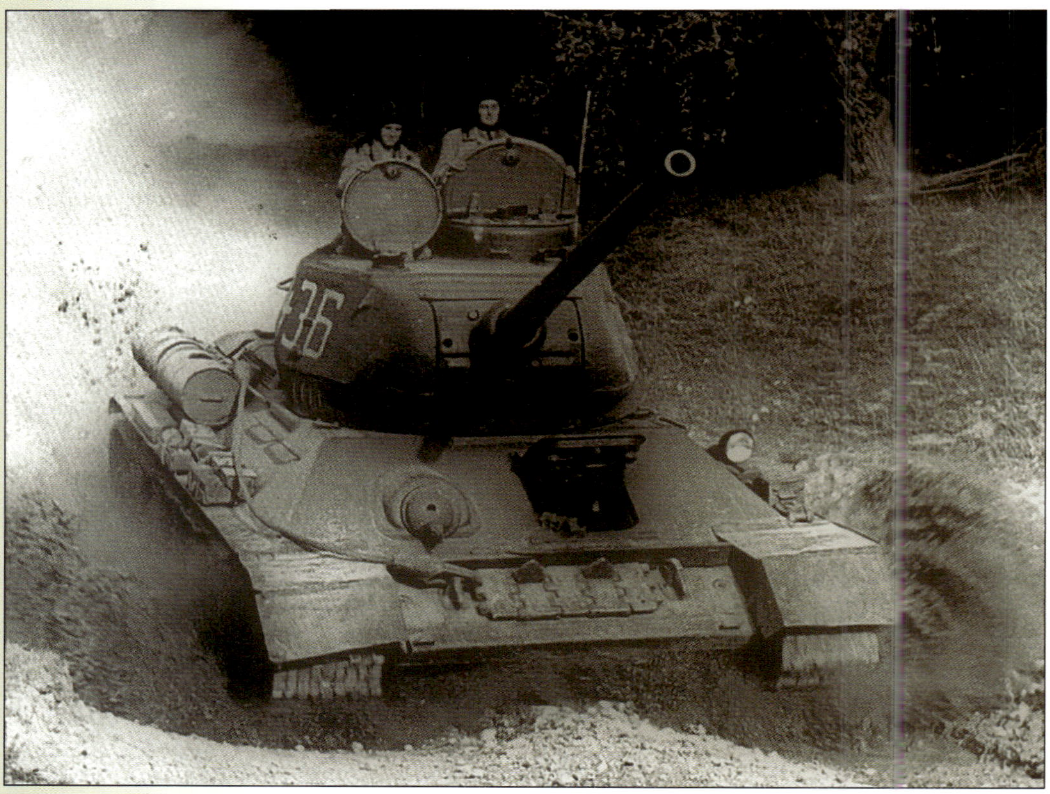

T-34-85 (Plant No.183) of the NVA with tactical number 436 during exercise in late 1960s.

1. The price of a tank delivered from Poland amounted to 214,834 DM.

Poland

After the end of the Second World War paint schemes and markings of Polish T-34-85s did not change – the tanks were painted overall Soviet olive green (4BO). From the early 1950s, Polish dark green (khaki) paint began to be used. In the mid-1960s, regulations for multi-colour disruptive patterns were developed, which consisted of three or four colours. In the case of three-colour patterns, the colours were dark green (khaki), yellow-khaki (dark sand) and black, while the four-colour pattern added light green. Both patterns were intended for the period from spring to autumn (and was thus called summer camouflage). As during the Second World War, a white paint scheme was stipulated for operations in snowy landscape. Casein paints were used and removed following the spring thaw. The extent to which such paint schemes were used is questionable. It seems that only a small number of tanks received such paint schemes. Photos of T-34-85s, probably taken in the late 1960s, show multi-colour camouflages. According to some sources, these were worn by tanks of a training regiment, probably being part of the Warsaw Military District. No photograph showing a T-34-85 in multi-colour winter camouflage complying to the rules developed in the mid-1960s appears to have been published yet. Sometimes all surfaces of the tank were painted white, quite precisely and sometimes the white camouflage was made up only of white patches and streaks. Interestingly, often only the turrets were camouflaged with white and the hulls remained dark green (khaki).

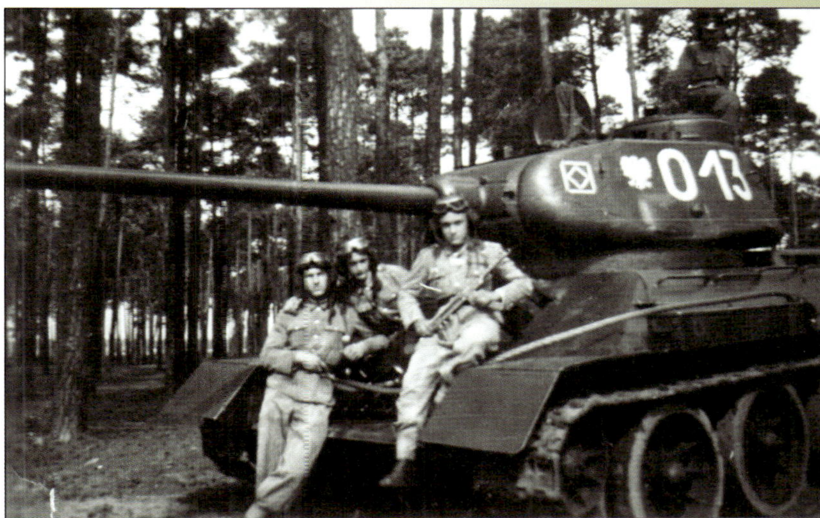

A T-34-85 of Polish production, tactical number 013 in the 1950s. The tactical marking indicates that the tank is assigned to 22nd Medium Tank Regiment. This name was used from 1957, previously the unit was named 22nd Independent Tank Regiment (till 1954) and 22nd Tank and Self-Propelled Gun Regiment (1954-1957).

In the early post-war years, approximately until 1948, wartime tactical markings were used. After that, three- and four-digit numbers were introduced, although in some units, exceptions in the form of single or two-digit numbers could be found. Also the size and shape of the digits were diverse. In the 1950s, large digits, almost to the full height of the turret, prevailed, usually painted on the sides of the turret, but sometimes on the back. Sometimes small numbers were also placed

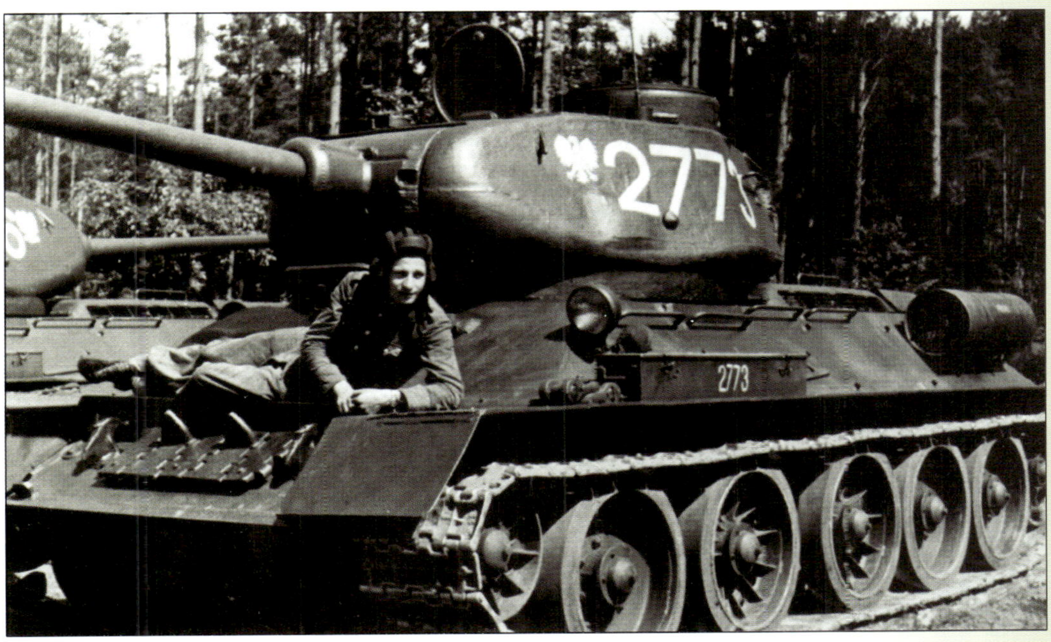

A T-34-85, tactical number 2773 from an unidentified Polish Army unit, 1950s. Note the tactical number repeated on the ramrod box and fuel drums.

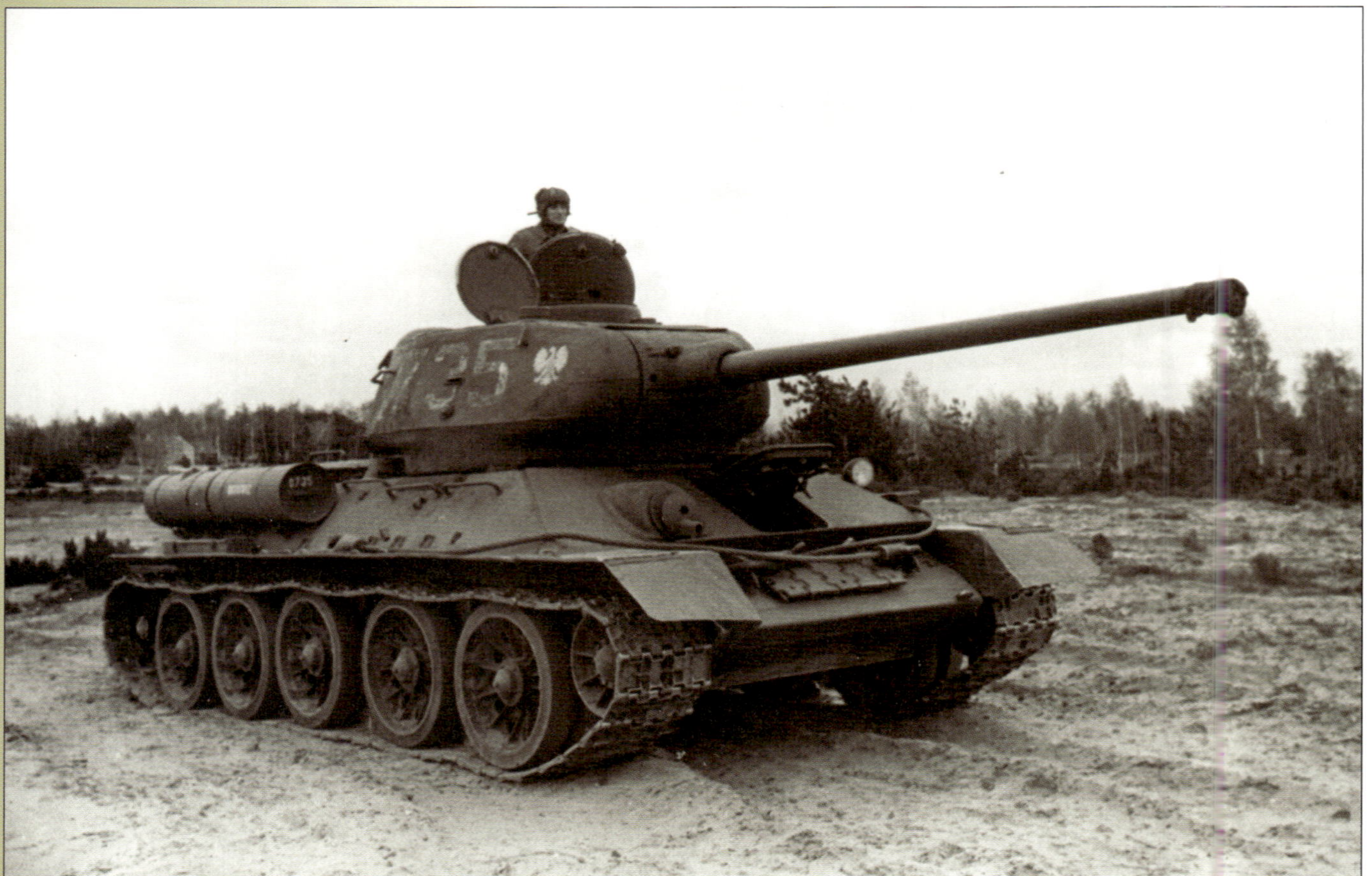

A Polish T-34-85 (Plant No. 183), tactical number 8735 from an unidentified Polish Army unit, 1950s. The number on the turret seems to be purposely soiled (stark contrast with the eagle).

on toolboxes, fuel tanks and even unditching beams. In the 1960s and 1970s, smaller numbers were applied, usually only on the turret sides. Some units (of training regiments, probably of the Warsaw Military District) used very distinctive tactical numbers, painted in the form of a dotted outline. These were usually applied on tanks in multi-colour camouflages.

From the late 1940s to the early 1960s, the white eagle was the national insignia painted on Polish T-34-85s. The shape of the eagle was similar to that of the state coat of arms. Its size was 30–50 cm and it was placed on the sides of the turret (on the forward section, ahead of the tactical

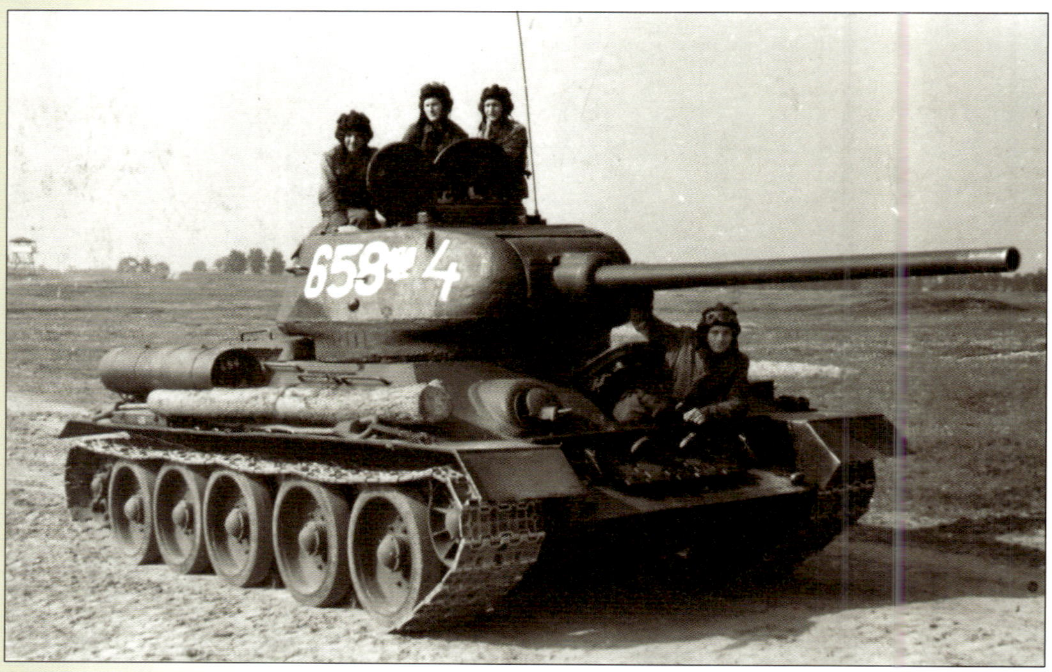

A T-34-85 (Plant No. 183), from an unidentified Polish Army unit, 1950s. The tanks has interesting markings – tactical number 658 and number 4 ahead of the eagle. It could be a marking of a subunit or used during exercise.

number. The tanks belonging to Coastal Defence Unit had an eagle merged with an anchor painted on the turrets. In the 1960s the insignia was changed – the eagle was replaced by a white and red rhombus.

Tactical markings were sporadically applied to the Polish T-34-85s, apparently most often taking the form of geometric figures (rectangles, rhombuses, circles), though this is very poorly documented. Some of the T-34-85 tanks which were seen on the streets of Poznań in June 1956, and previously in exercises at Wędrzyn and Biedrusko training areas, bore these markings. The tactical symbols were usually located on the turrets and often also on front hull armour plates. However, it cannot be ruled out that some of the tactical markings were applied only during training exercises and manoeuvres. On the tanks participating in the exercises, other markings, indicating assignment to individual units, were also applied. Photographs of Polish T-34-85s with large digits or identification stripes painted on the turrets and/or hulls for the duration of exercises are known.

The anchor was a particular tactical marking, painted on the front armour plates of tanks assigned to Coastal Defence Unit.

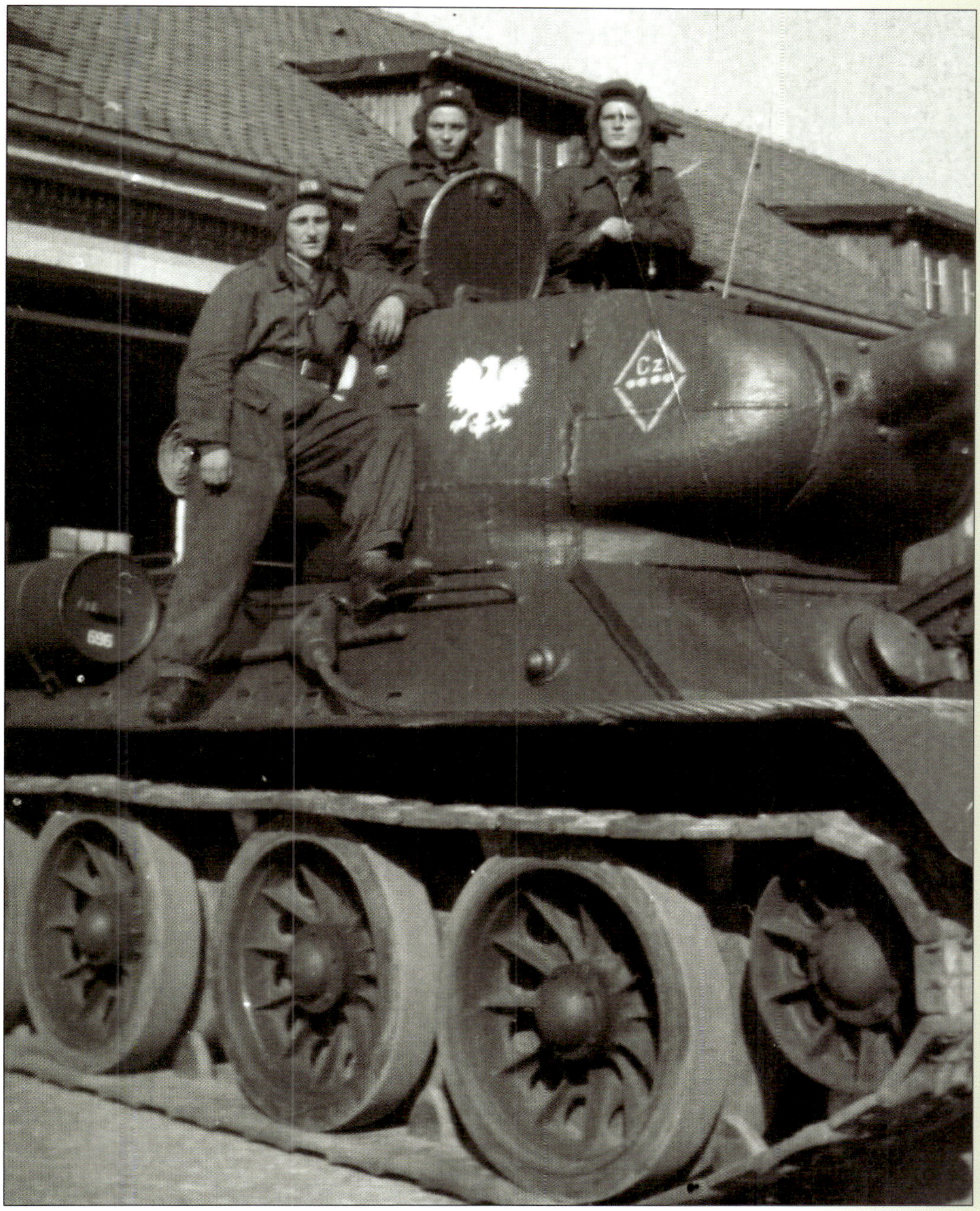

A Polish T-34-85 (Plant No. 174, with etalon-type turret) with tactical number 696 and very interesting tactical marking.

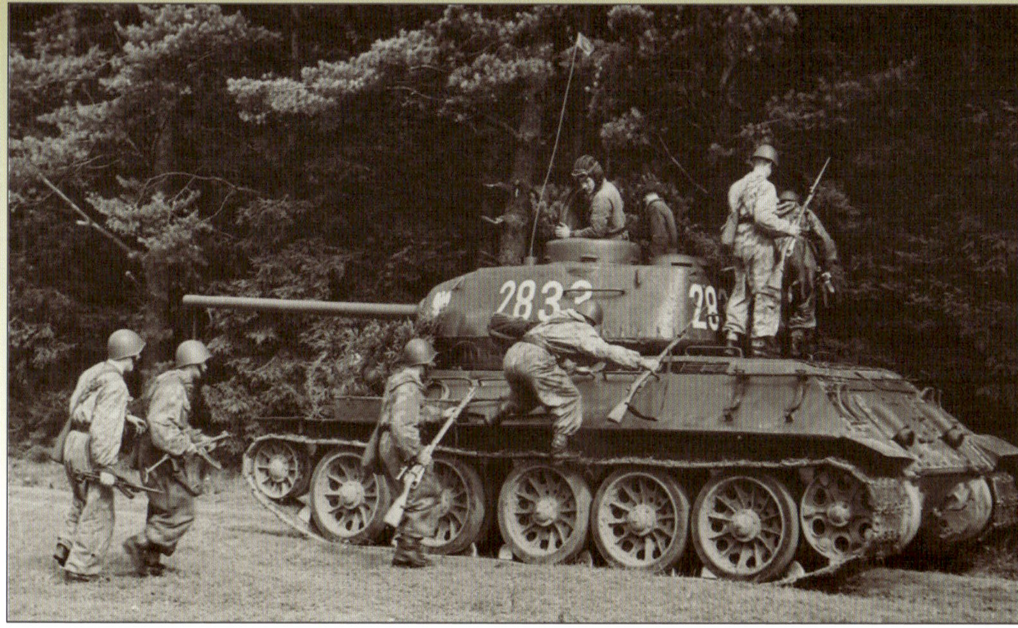

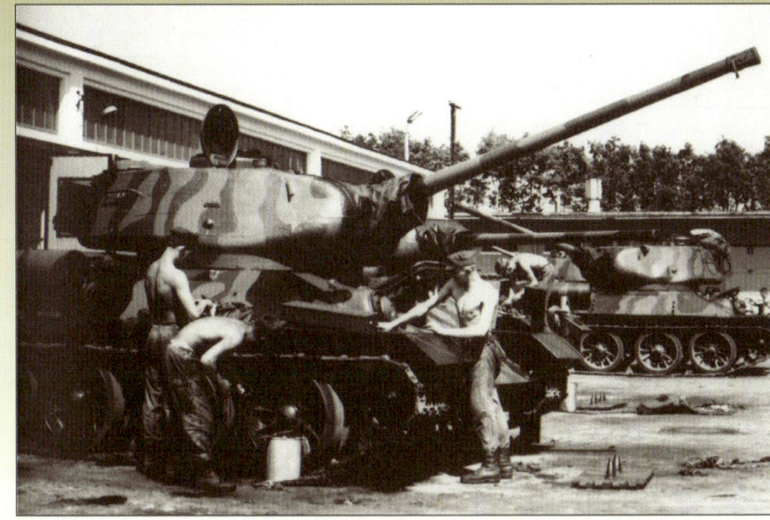

A very interesting photo, taken probably in the 1960s, showing a T-34-85M2 (of Polish production) in three-colour camouflage, compliant to the spring scheme of multi-colour camouflage developed in the 1960s.

POLAND

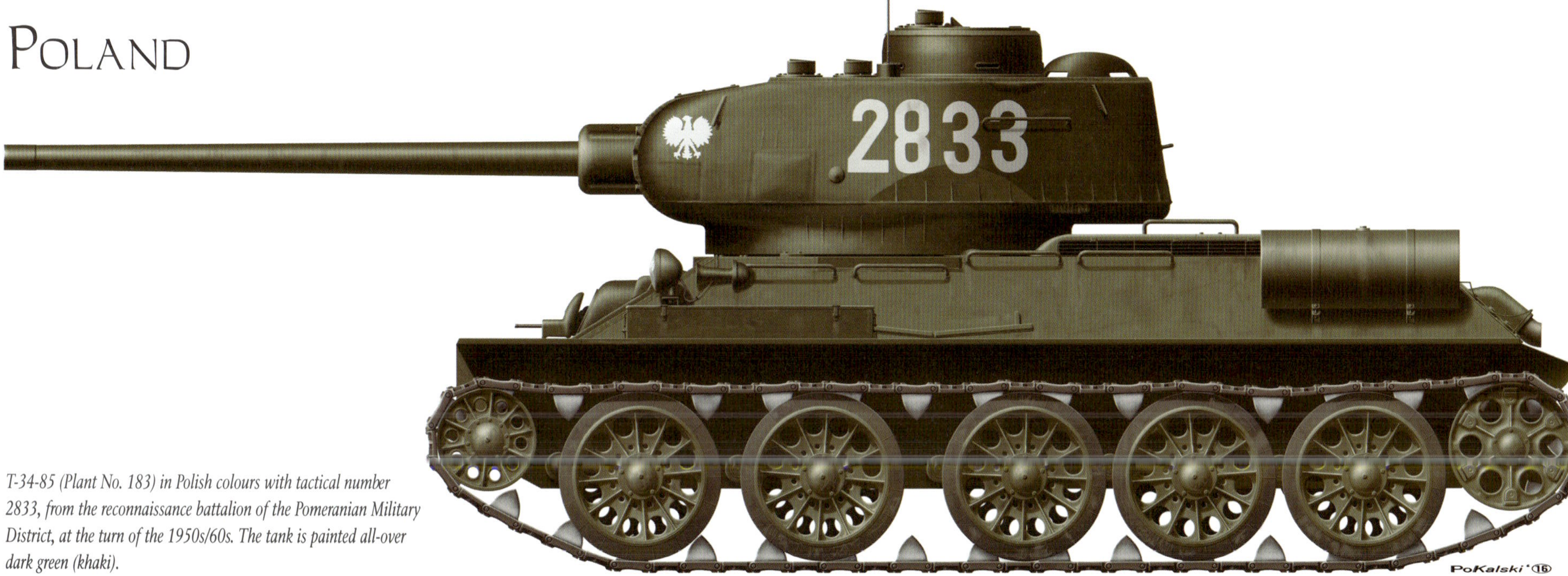

T-34-85 (Plant No. 183) in Polish colours with tactical number 2833, from the reconnaissance battalion of the Pomeranian Military District, at the turn of the 1950s/60s. The tank is painted all-over dark green (khaki).

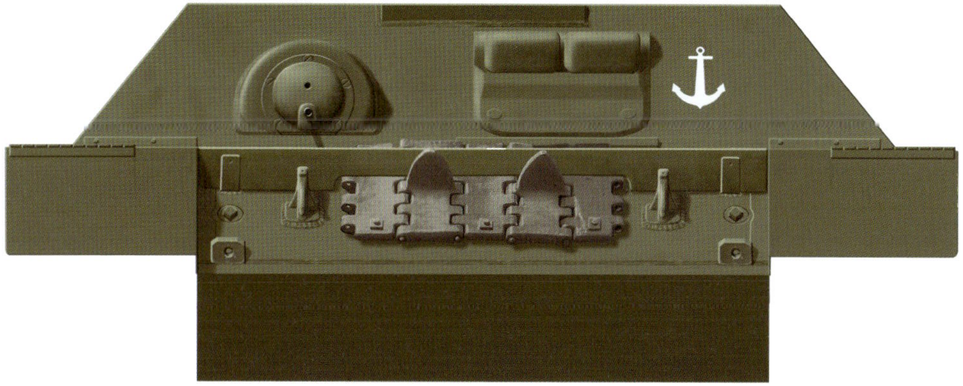

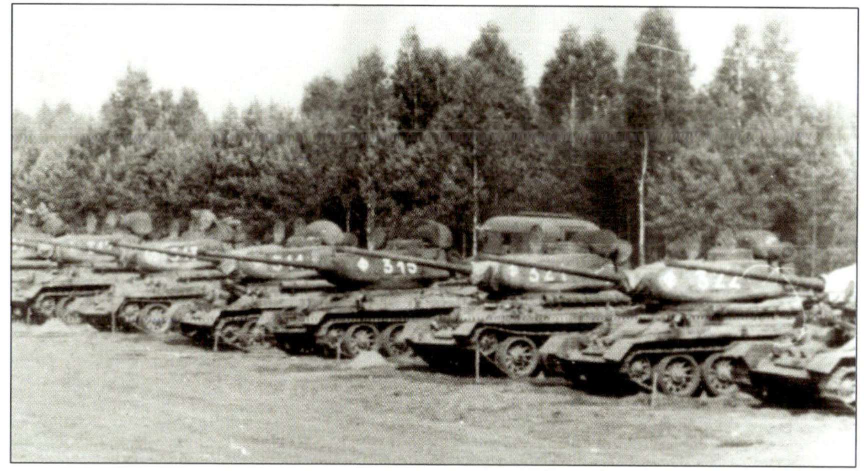

Modernized Polish T-34-85M2 tanks from an unidentified Polish People's Army unit, 1970s. The tanks wear a national insignia in form of white and red rhombus. The tanks in the photograph have three-digit tactical numbers. On some tanks they must have been painted quite recently, because rectangles blanking out previous numbers are visible.

Poland

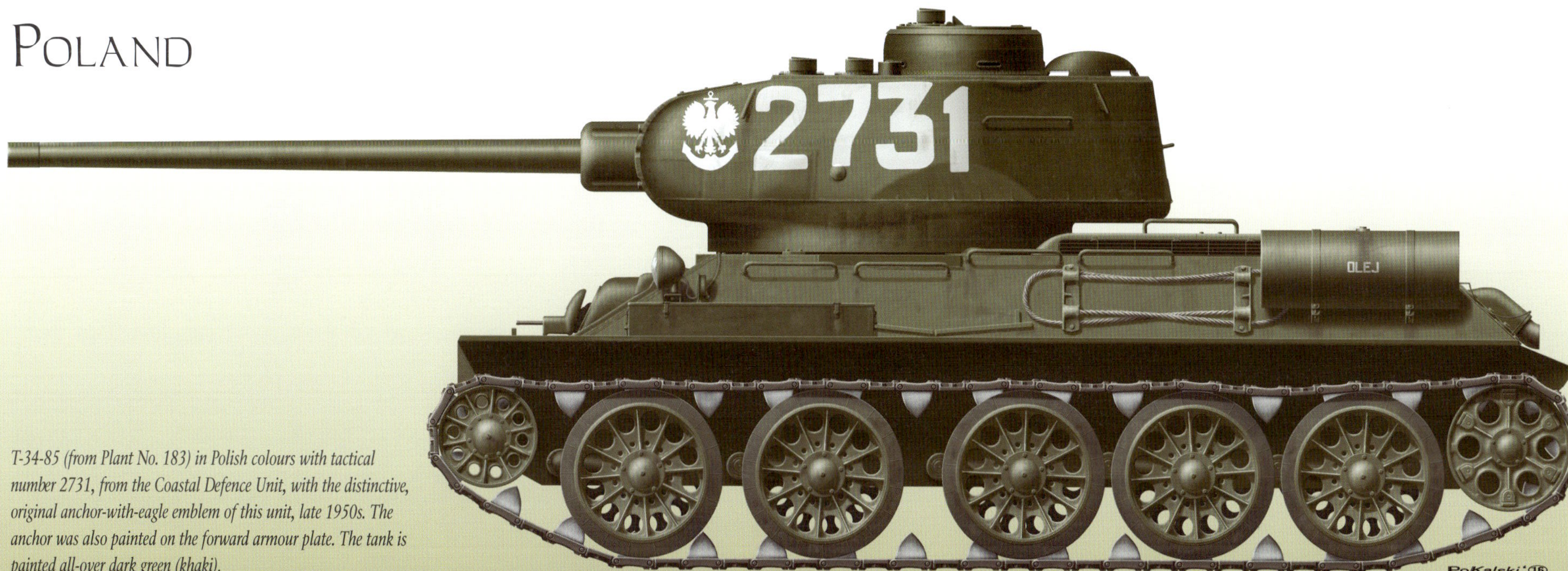

T-34-85 (from Plant No. 183) in Polish colours with tactical number 2731, from the Coastal Defence Unit, with the distinctive, original anchor-with-eagle emblem of this unit, late 1950s. The anchor was also painted on the forward armour plate. The tank is painted all-over dark green (khaki).

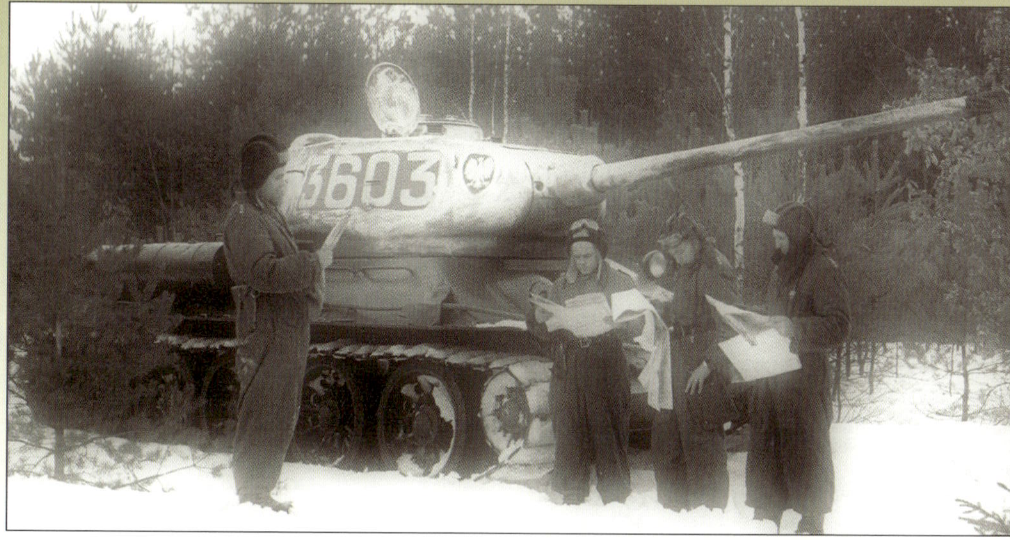

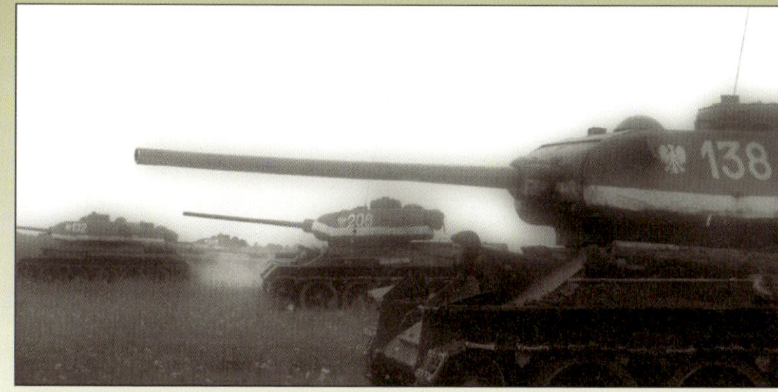

T-34-85 tanks (produced by various plants) of the Polish Army during exercises in the 1950s. White stripes are quick identification markings used during maneuvers.

POLAND

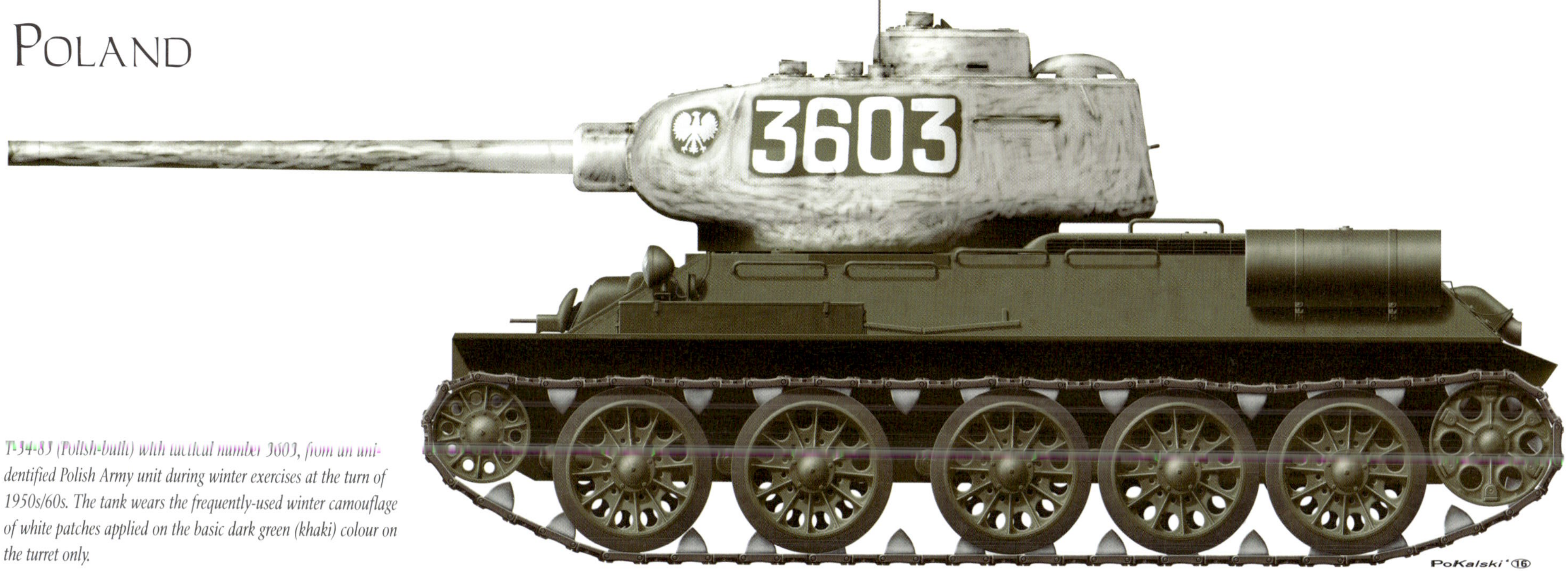

T-34-85 (Polish-built) with tactical number 3603, from an unidentified Polish Army unit during winter exercises at the turn of 1950s/60s. The tank wears the frequently-used winter camouflage of white patches applied on the basic dark green (khaki) colour on the turret only.

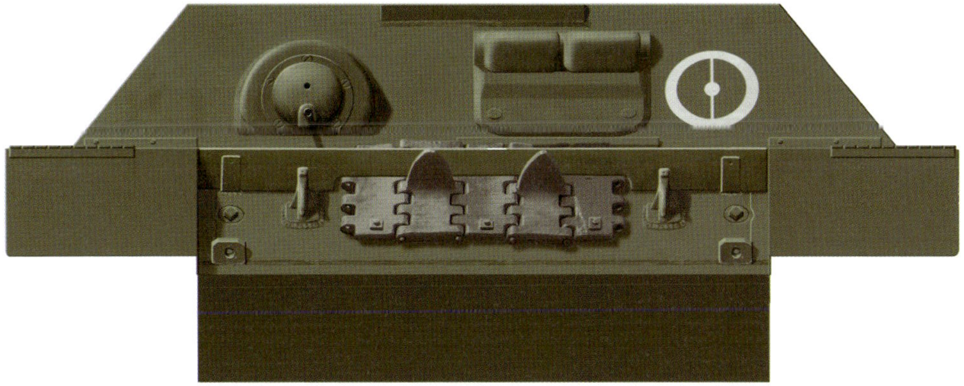

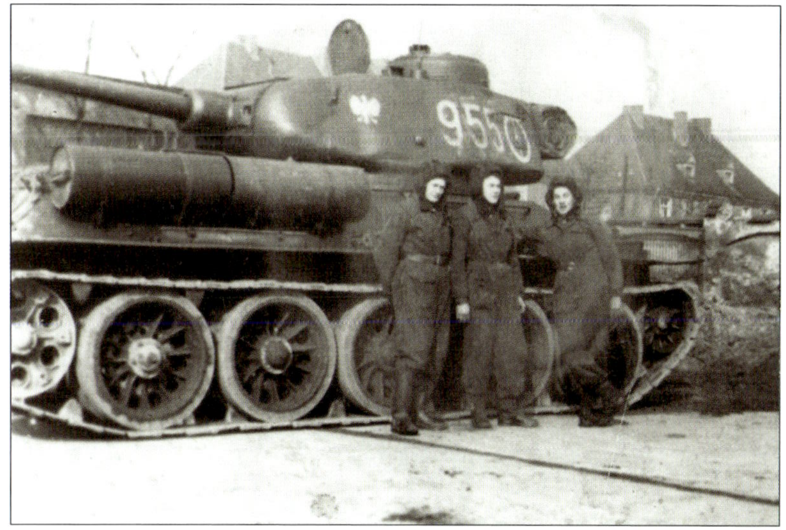

A Polish T-34-85 (Polish production), with tactical number 955 and tactical marking on the back of the turret. Such markings were worn by some tanks used in June 1956 to suppress the uprising in Poznań.

Poland

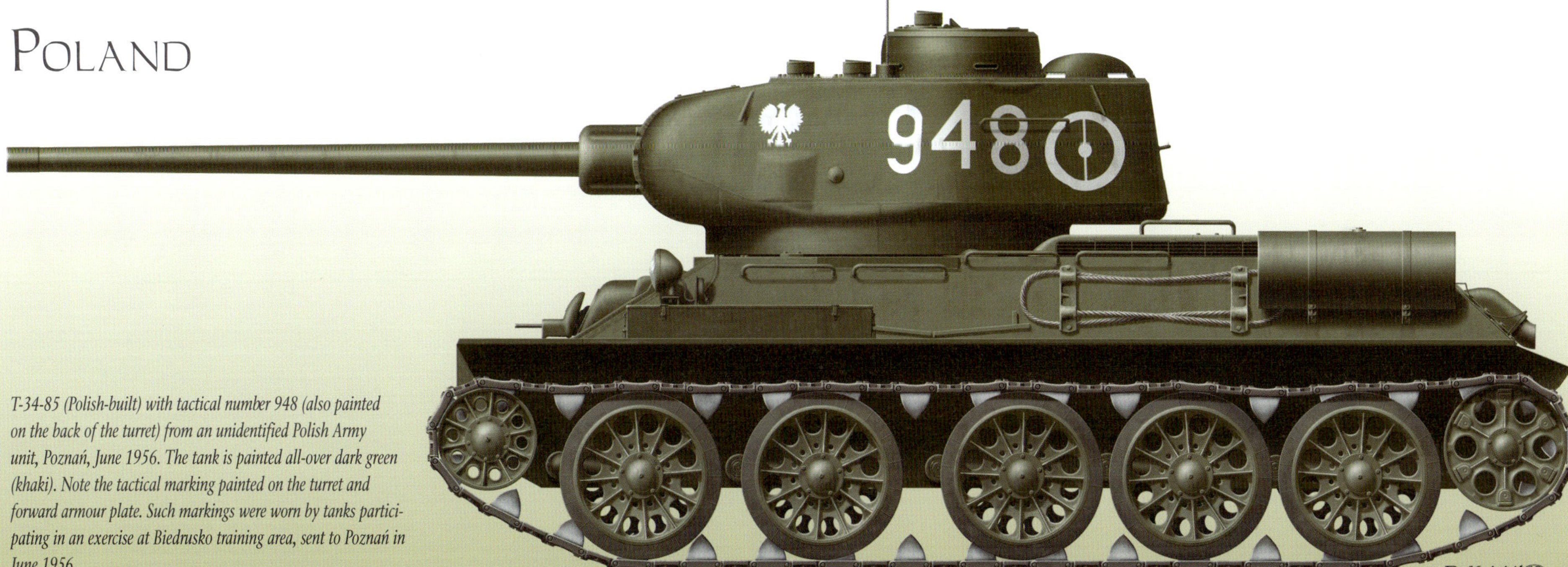

T-34-85 (Polish-built) with tactical number 948 (also painted on the back of the turret) from an unidentified Polish Army unit, Poznań, June 1956. The tank is painted all-over dark green (khaki). Note the tactical marking painted on the turret and forward armour plate. Such markings were worn by tanks participating in an exercise at Biedrusko training area, sent to Poznań in June 1956.

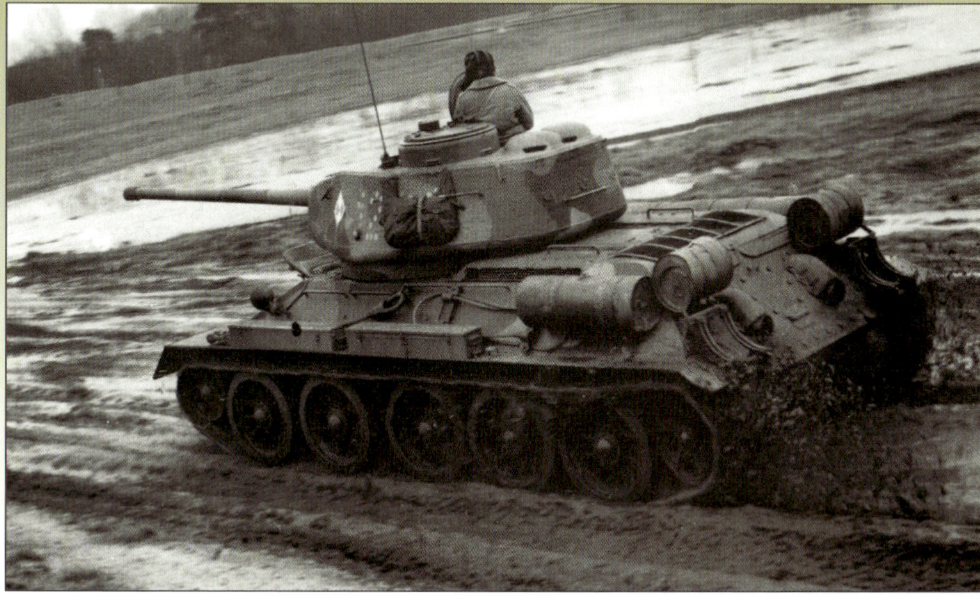

A modernized Polish T-34-85M in multi-colour camouflage scheme (summer camouflage), unidentified training unit, probably of the Warsaw Military District, late 1960s or early 1970s. Note the tactical number painted with dotted line.

Poland

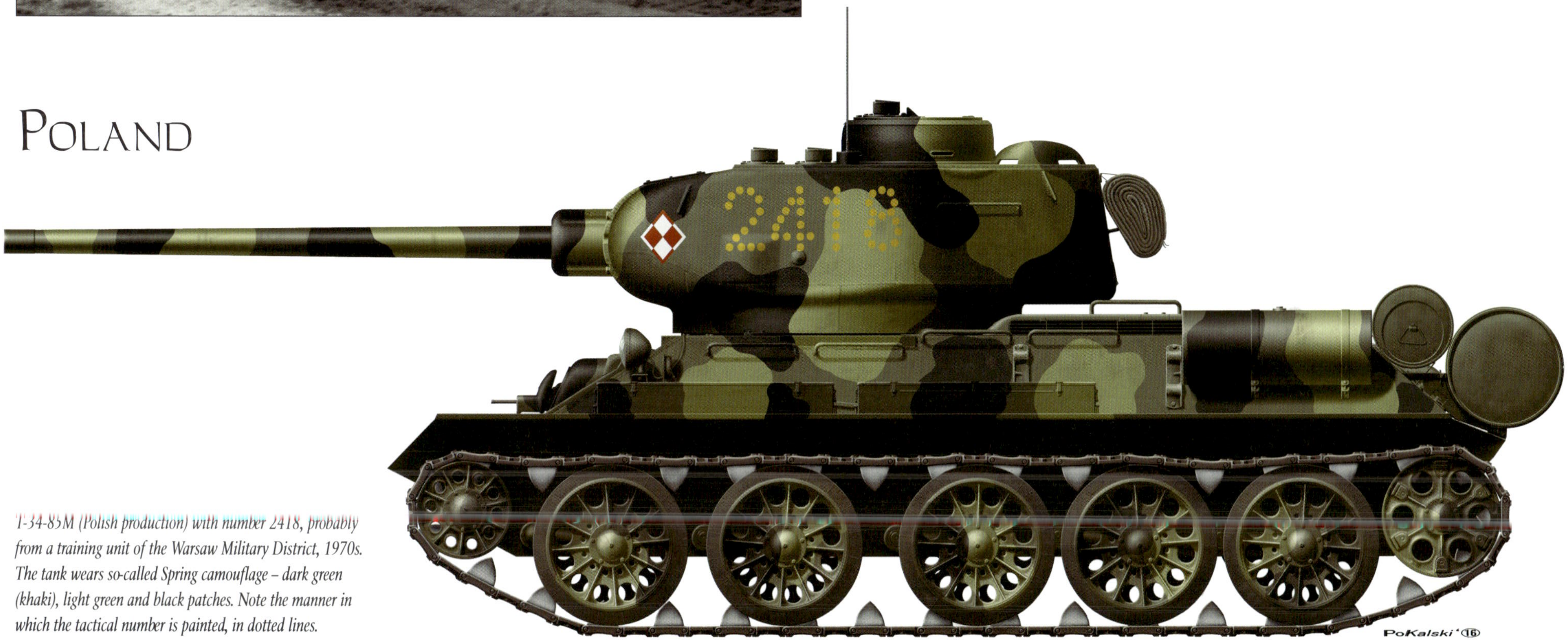

T-34-85M (Polish production) with number 2418, probably from a training unit of the Warsaw Military District, 1970s. The tank wears so-called Spring camouflage – dark green (khaki), light green and black patches. Note the manner in which the tactical number is painted, in dotted lines.

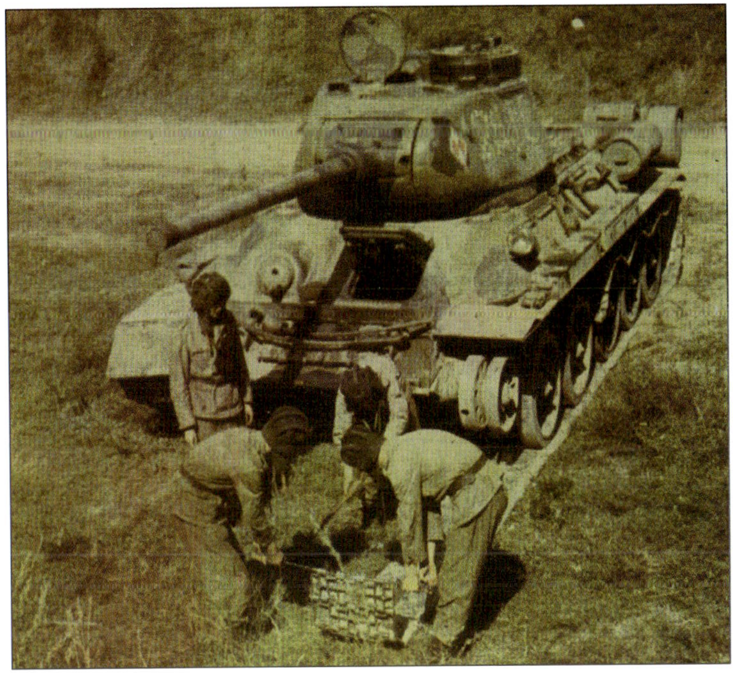

A modernized Polish T-34-85M in multi-colour camouflage, 1970s.

Poland

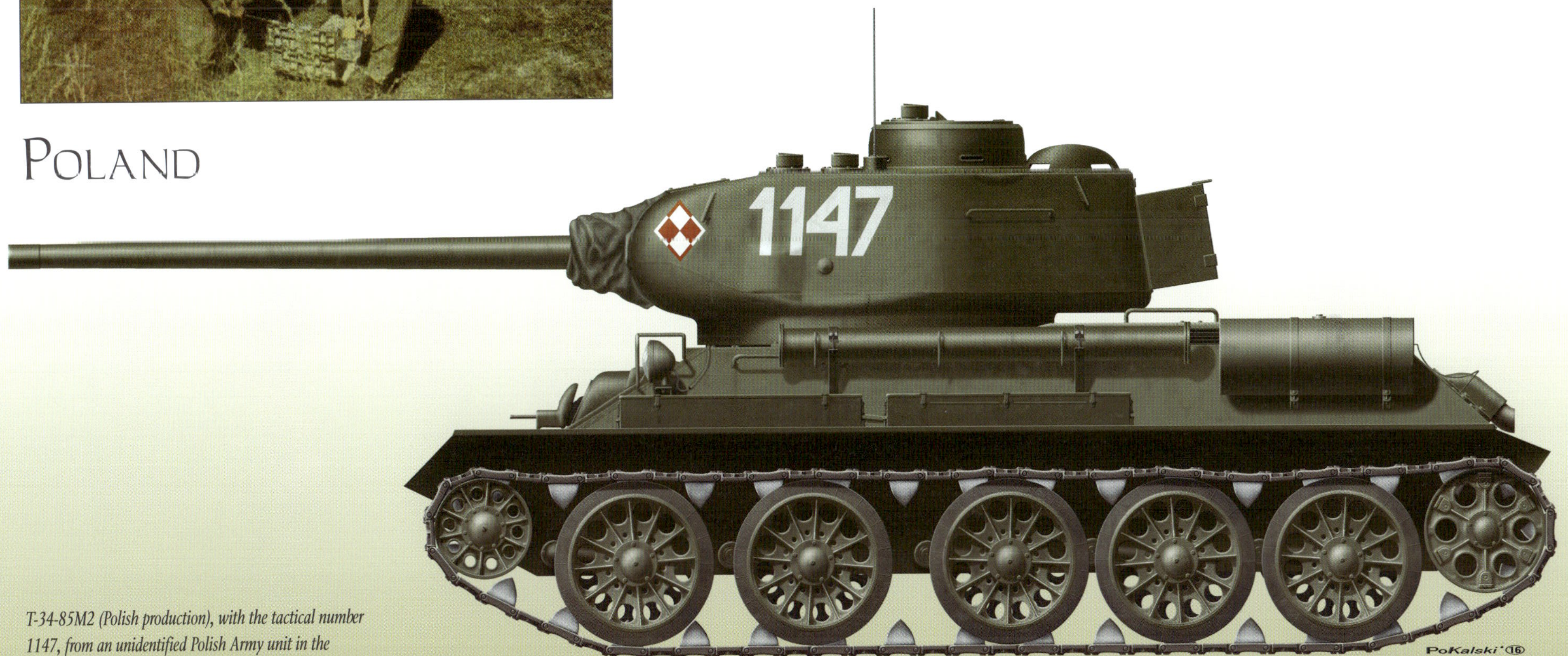

T-34-85M2 (Polish production), with the tactical number 1147, from an unidentified Polish Army unit in the 1970s, The tank is painted overall dark green (khaki).

Romania

During 1952–54 the Romanian army received 250 T-34-85 tanks, delivered from Czechoslovakia. Romania also received around 60 tanks from the USSR. Some Romanian 'eighty-fives' were probably modernised at the turn of the 1960s and 1970s by the installation of locally made water obstacle crossing systems. Some tanks were also retrofitted with additional boxes mounted on the fenders.

Initially the Romanian T-34-85s were painted all-over olive green (probably Soviet 4BO paint). Following overhauls the tanks were painted with Romanian khaki paint. Tactical numbers were usually three-digit. In the 1950s a national marking of a red star in a white circle was painted on some tanks. Later the insignia took the form of a red star with a Romanian roundel inside. In the early 1990s Romanian blue-yellow-red roundels were seen on the T-34-85s remaining in service.

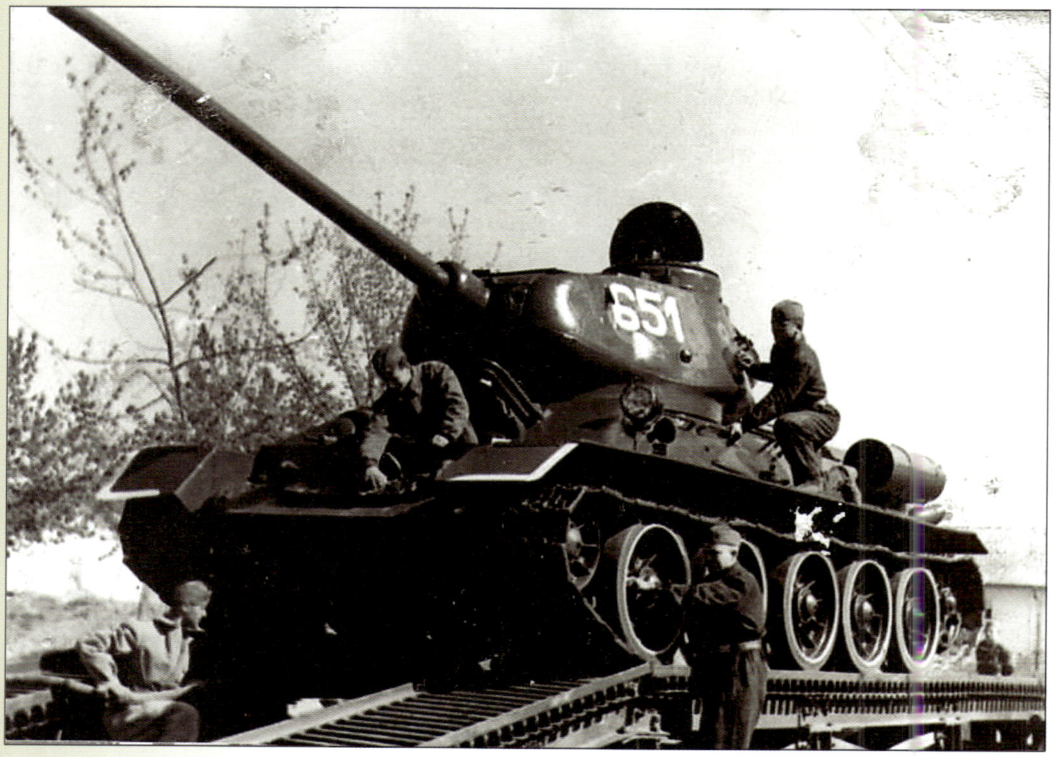

A Romanian T-34-85 (Czechoslovak production) being cleaned after exercise in the 1950s. The tank has the tactical number 651 and national insignia painted aft of the tactical number. The edges of the fenders are painted white.

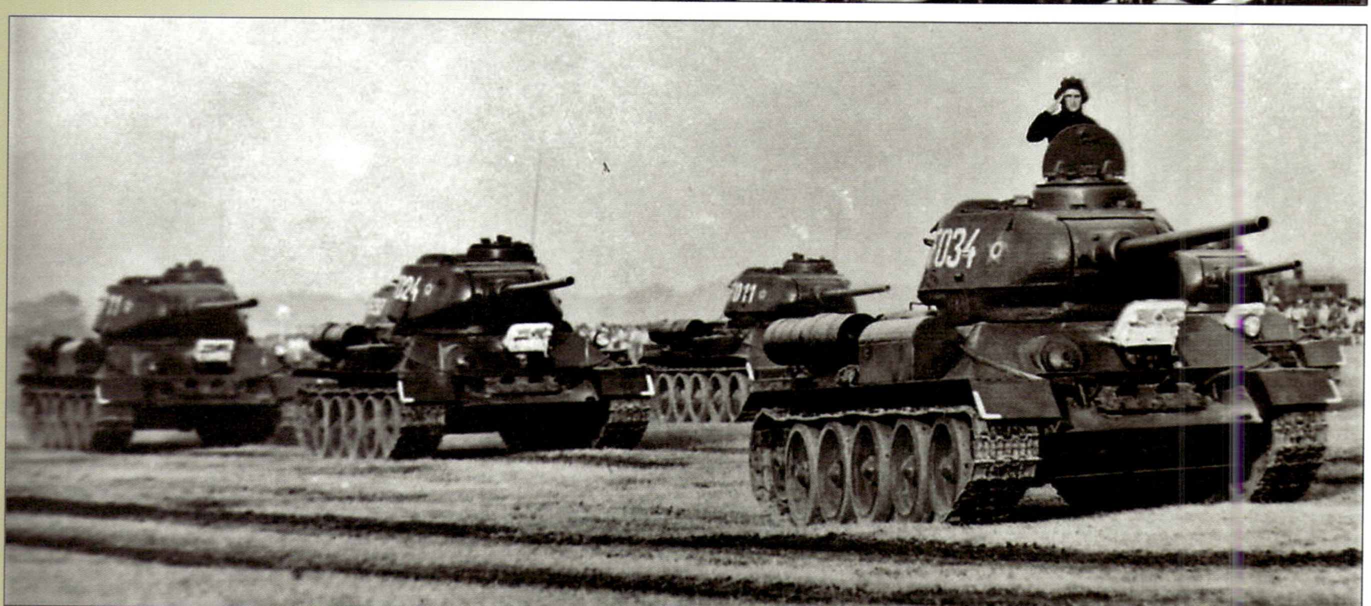

Formation of Romanian T-34-85 tanks, which underwent modernization probably in the 1960s. The tank with number T034 and national insignia ahead of it is visible in the foreground. Fender edges are painted white. Note large toolbox on the fender with lid resembling a coffer. The third tank in the column has a similar toolbox, while two other tanks in the picture have toolboxes with flat lids.

Ukraine

Tanks used by pro-Russian separatists during the fighting in Ukraine in 2014 had diverse paint schemes, mainly those they wore when in the museums or on the monuments they were taken from. However, sometimes additional elements, such as tactical numbers or slogans were applied. An example is the T-34-85 used by the National Cossack Guard in the area of the towns of Antratsit and Perevalsk. The number 135 and inscription "For Antratsit" were painted on its turret.

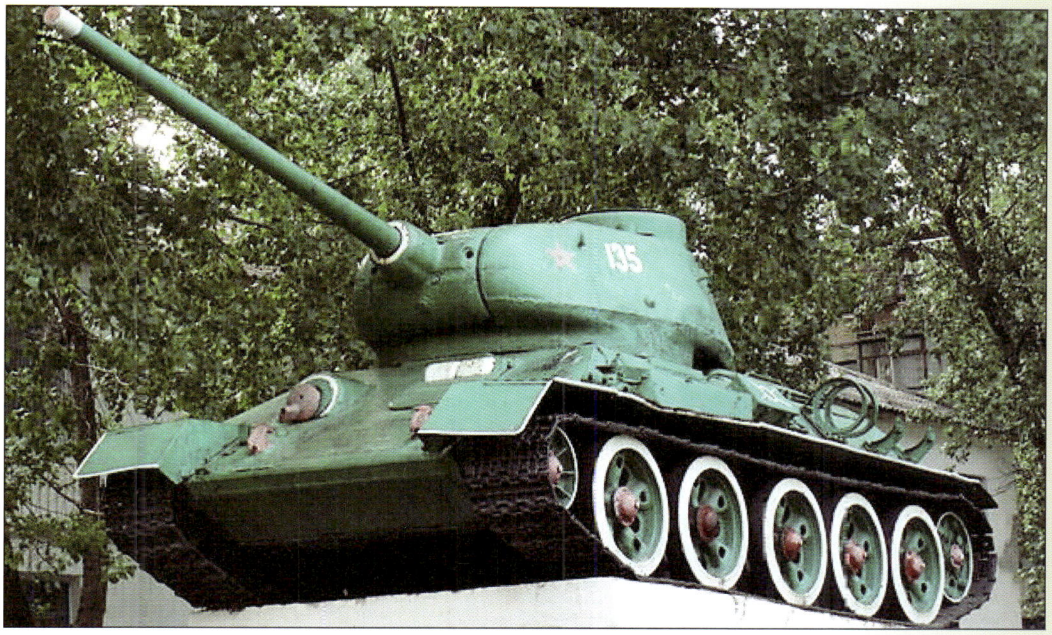

A T-34-85 Model 1969 tank (Plant No. 183 production) on a monument in the town of Antratsit.

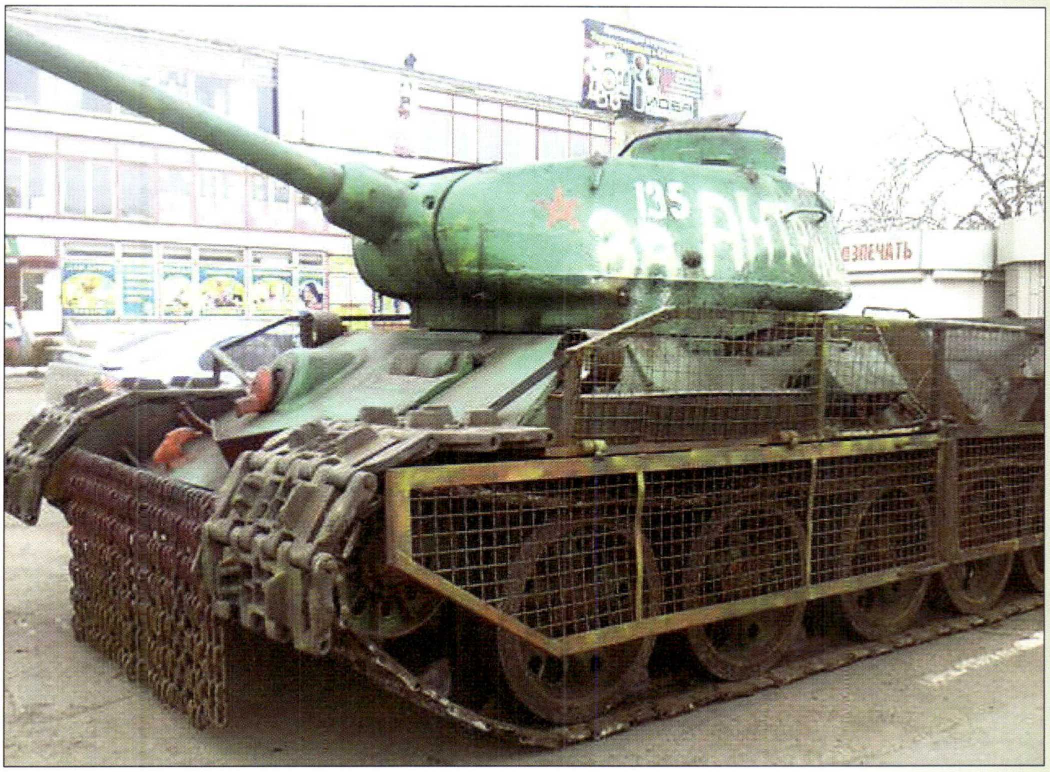

In 2014 the same vehicle saw combat in pro-Russian separatist units after having been taken out from the monument and rearmament.

Hungary

Tanks used by the Hungarian National Army were painted all-over olive green (Soviet 4BO paint). Three-digit tactical numbers were typically applied on both sides of the turret. Many tanks had the national insignia – a red star in a green-white-red circle – painted on the front of the turret. Some tanks had a wide vertical white or yellow stripe painted between the national insignia and tactical number (probably to distinguish them from the tanks used by insurgents).

In the autumn of 1956, some tanks were captured by Hungarian insurgents. Emblems referring to the pre-war Hungarian coat of arms were usually painted on the turrets and sometimes also on the hulls and fenders. On some tanks only the red star in the HNA marking was painted over. Patriotic slogans were spontaneously painted on some tanks.

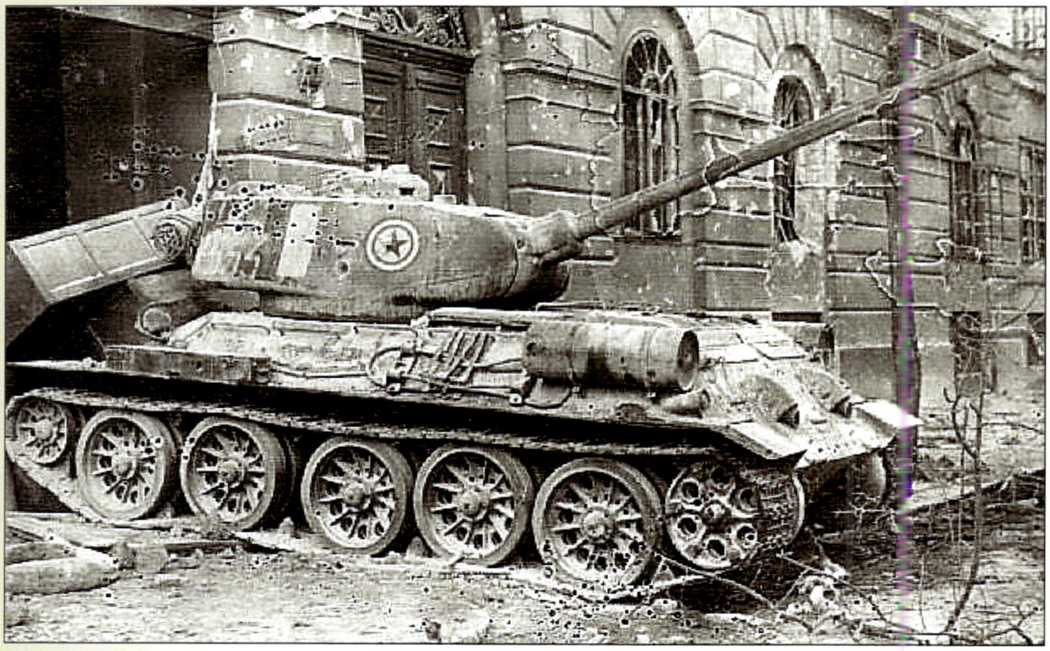

A Hungarian T-34-85 (Plant No.183), tactical number 353, of the government forces, Budapest, autumn of 1956. Note the Hungarian national insignia and white or yellow identification strip. According to some sources it was the tank used by the commander of Hungarian revolutionary forces, General Pal Maleter (1917–1958), although it seems improbable.

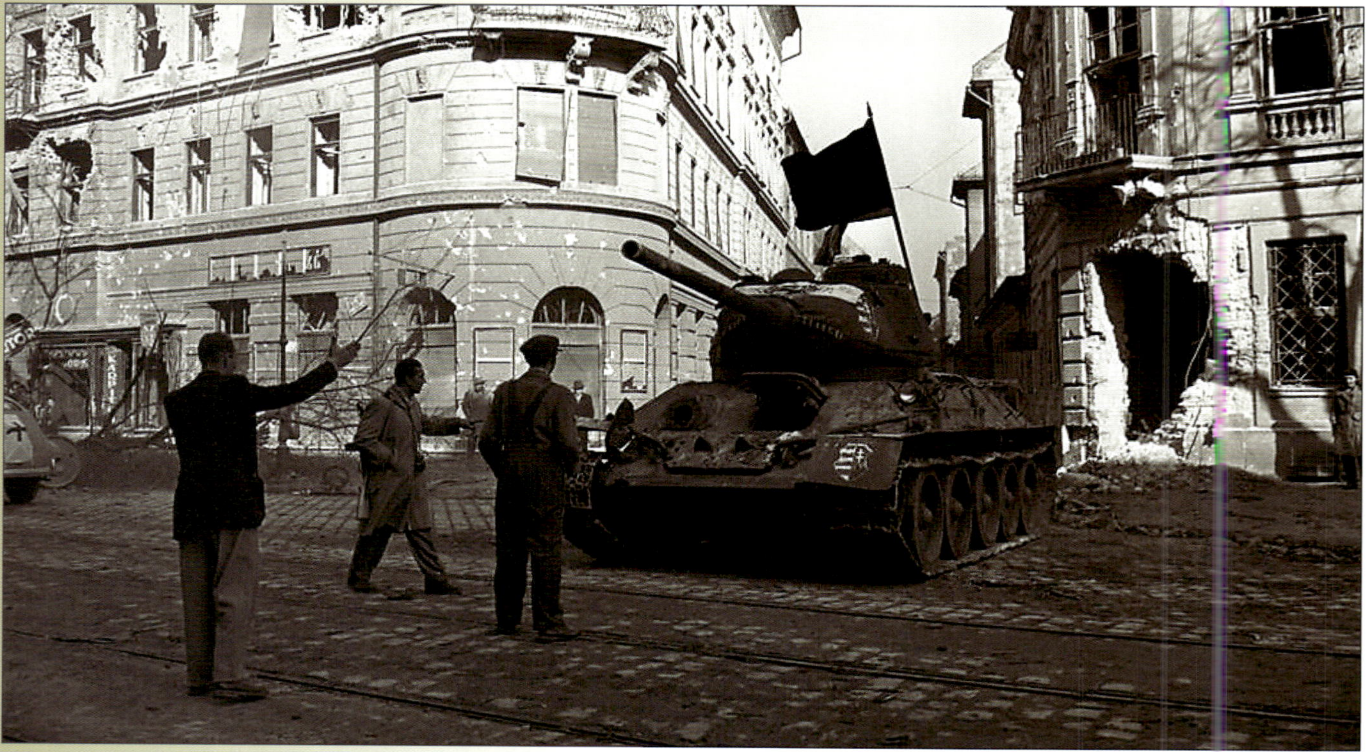

A captured T-34-85 (Plant No. 112 with two single ventilators) in the hands of Hungarian insurgents and with applied new markings. Budapest, autumn of 1956.

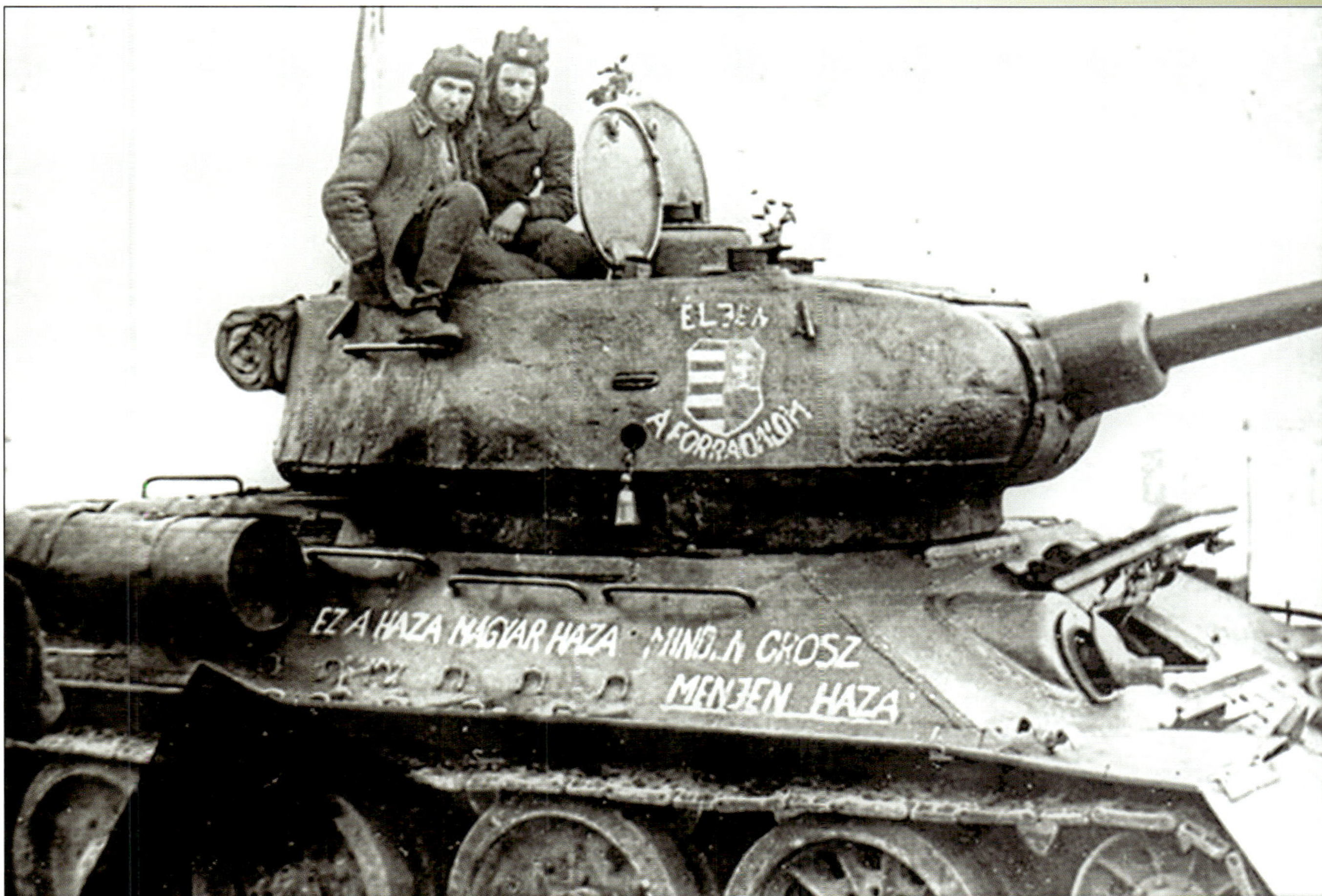

A Hungarian T-34-85 (Plant No.183) with insurrectionist markings and patriotic slogans. Budapest, autumn of 1956.

Two Hungarian T-34-85s (both of Plant No.183 production) blocking a bridge in Budapest autumn of 1956. The photograph is interesting because the tank on the right has a pre-insurgency insignia of the Hungarian army with a red star. The tank on the left has the red star painted over.

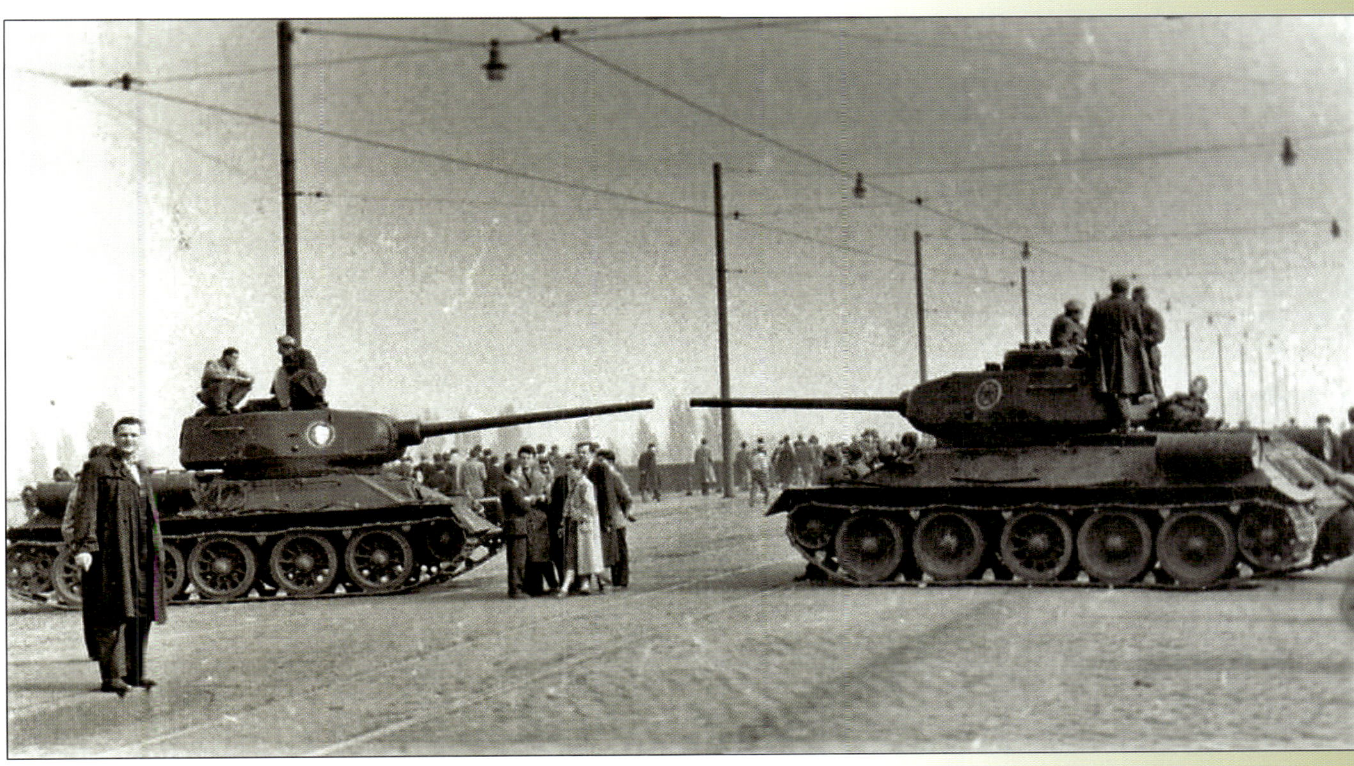

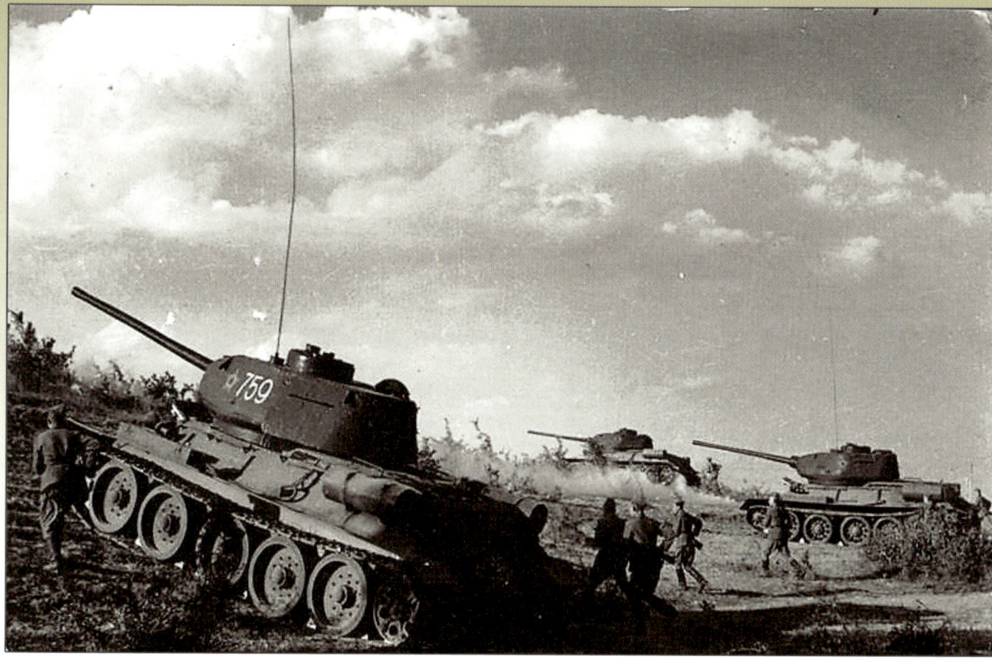

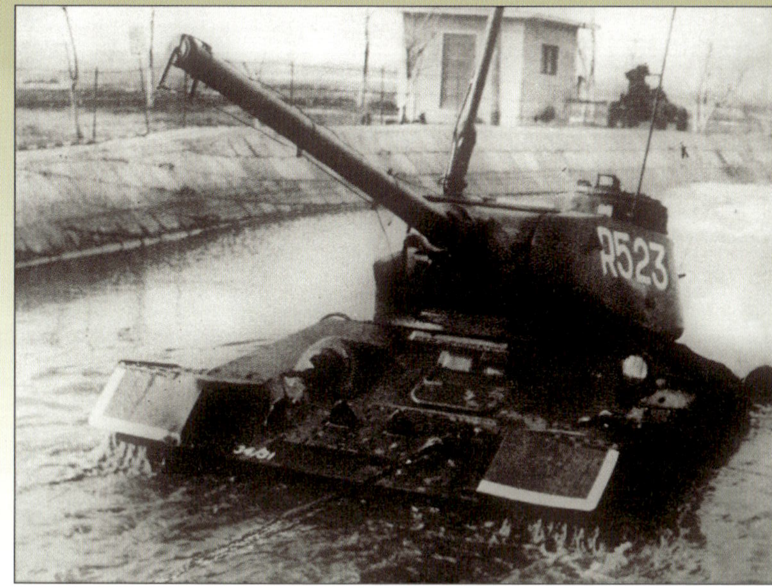

A Romanian T-34-85 (Czechoslovak production) with tactical number R523 crossing a water obstacle. Note the number 34/31 on the front armour plate and white fender edges.

Romania

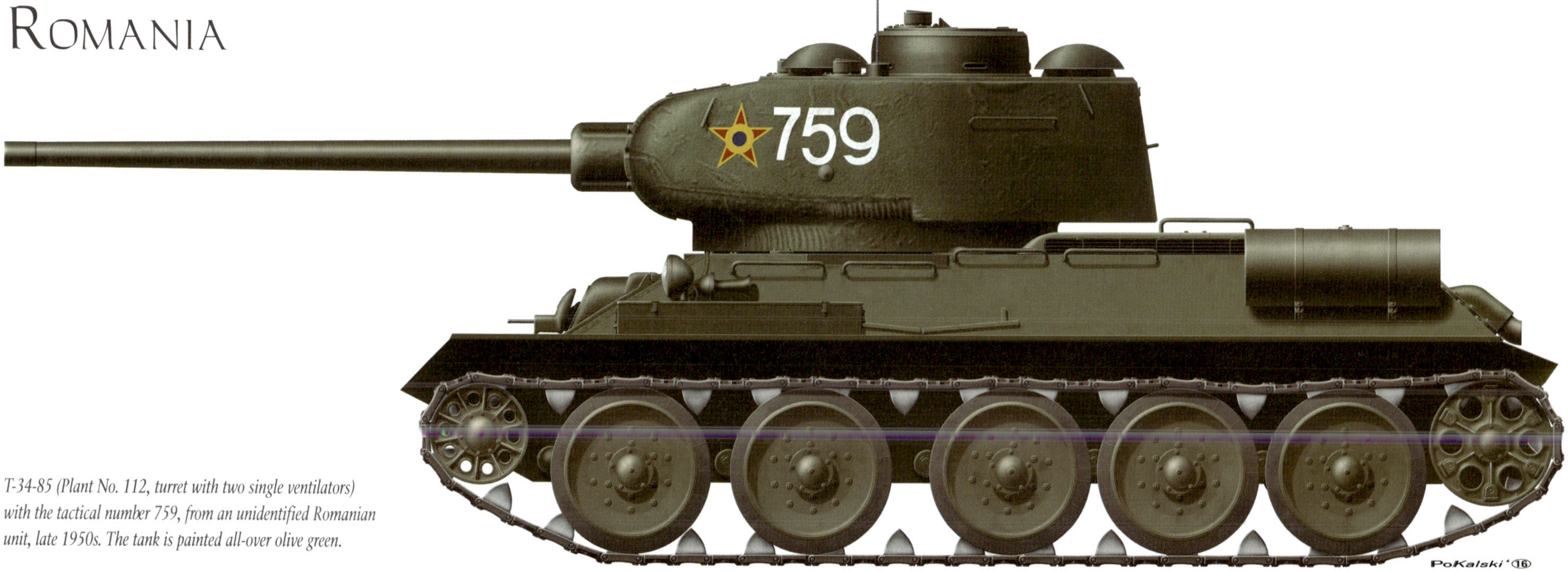

T-34-85 (Plant No. 112, turret with two single ventilators) with the tactical number 759, from an unidentified Romanian unit, late 1950s. The tank is painted all-over olive green.

Ukraine

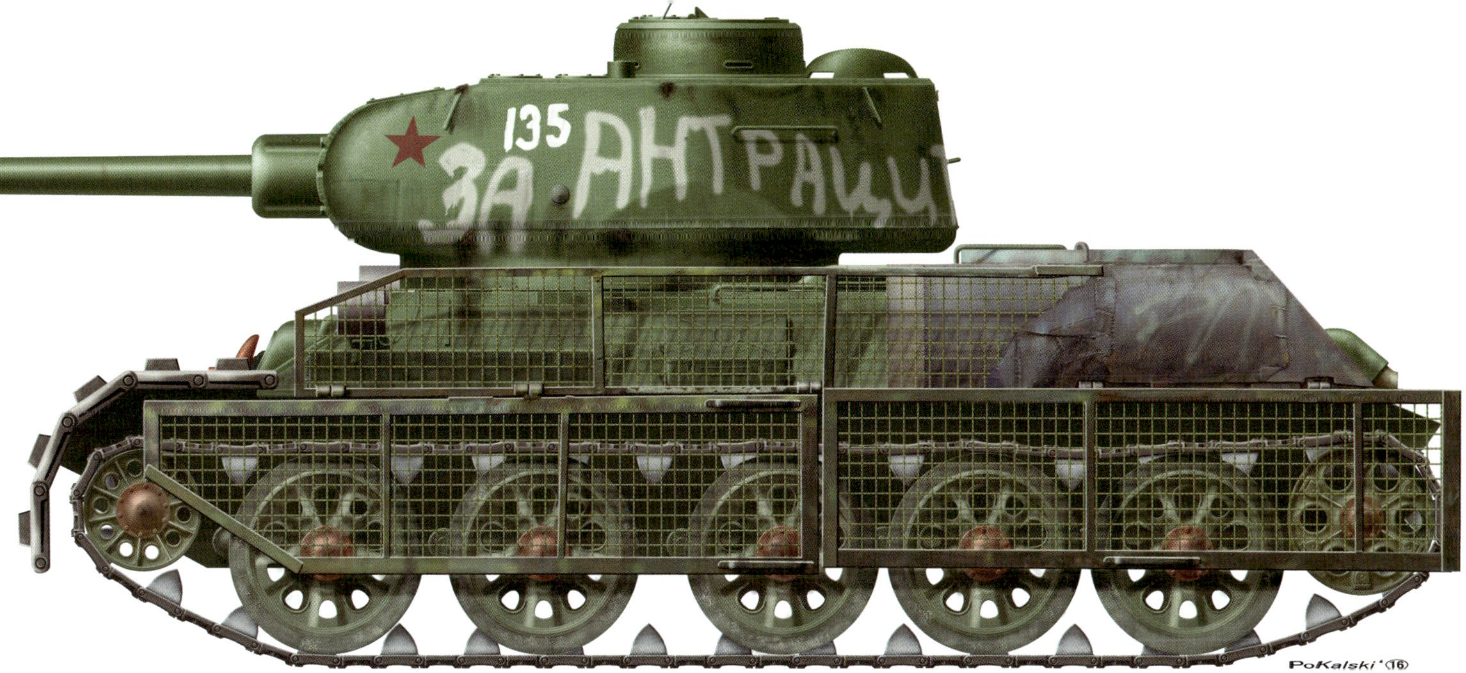

T-34-85 Model 1969 (modernised tank from Plant No. 183) used by pro-Russian separatists in Donbas in 2014. The tank had been taken off a monument and had its armour reinforced, before being used in combat for a period near the town of Antratsit – hence the inscription "For Antratsit" on the turret. Subsequently the tank was again placed on the monument. A truly extraordinary career!

Hungary

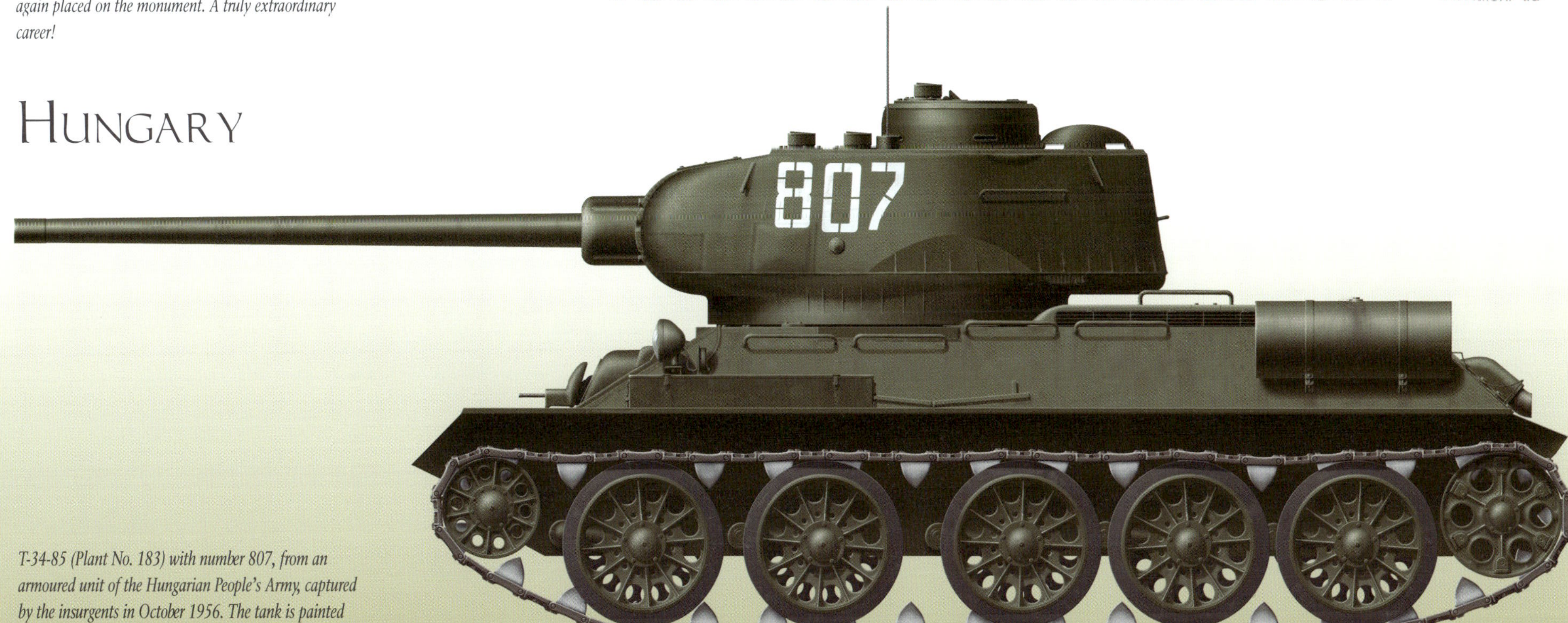

T-34-85 (Plant No. 183) with number 807, from an armoured unit of the Hungarian People's Army, captured by the insurgents in October 1956. The tank is painted overall olive green.

USSR

After the end of the Second World War the Red Army operated about 18,000 T-34-85 tanks. Initially the vehicles retained their wartime paint schemes and markings, but later (in the second half of the 1940s) the paint schemes began to be unified, with all surfaces painted olive green (4BO).

In the case of post-war T-34-85s, geometric tactical markings, widely used by the Soviets during the Second World War, were rarely applied. Tactical numbers were usually two- or three-digit. Sometimes red stars appeared on the tanks – usually on the turrets and sometimes on the fenders.

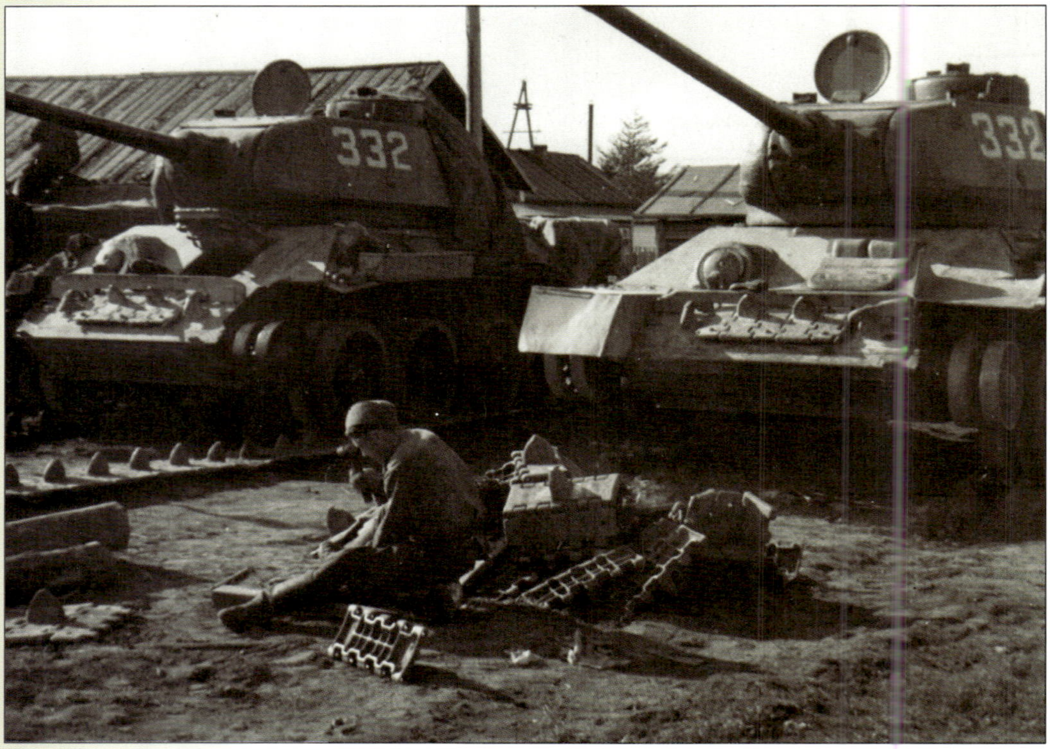

Two Soviet T-34-85 tanks from an unidentified unit based in East Germany, photographed in the 1950s. Interesting is the fact that both tanks have the same tactical number!

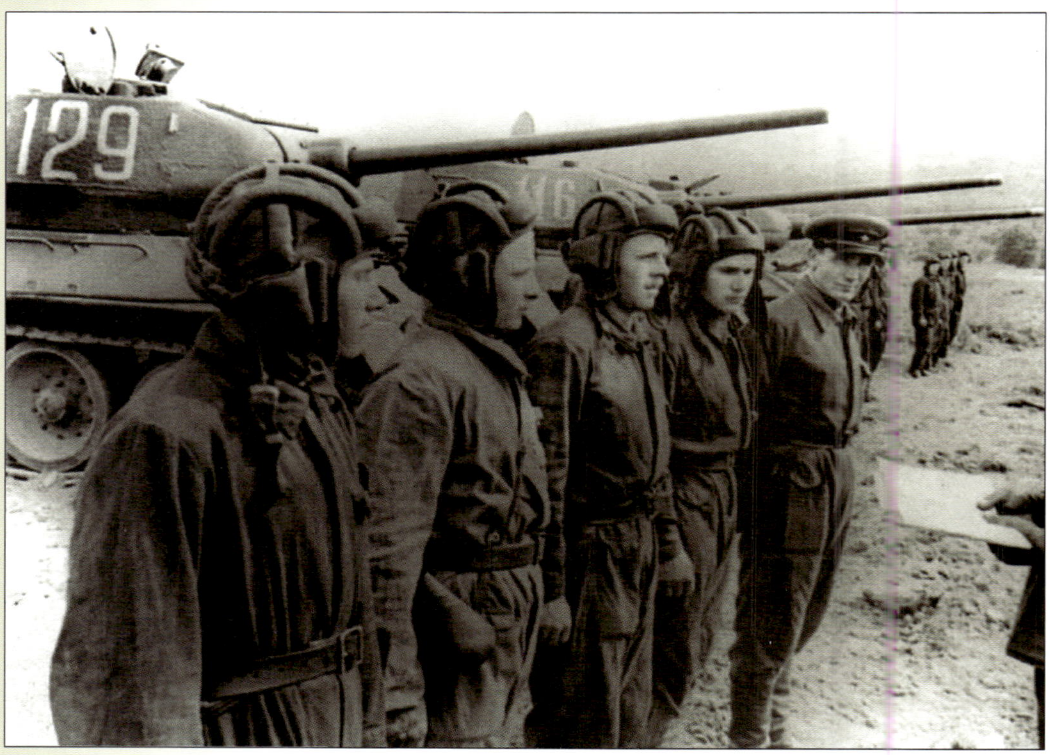

Inspection of crews of Soviet T-34-85s in one of Far East-based units, late 1940s. These are tanks of various versions, but of wartime production. Note different shape of tactical number digits.

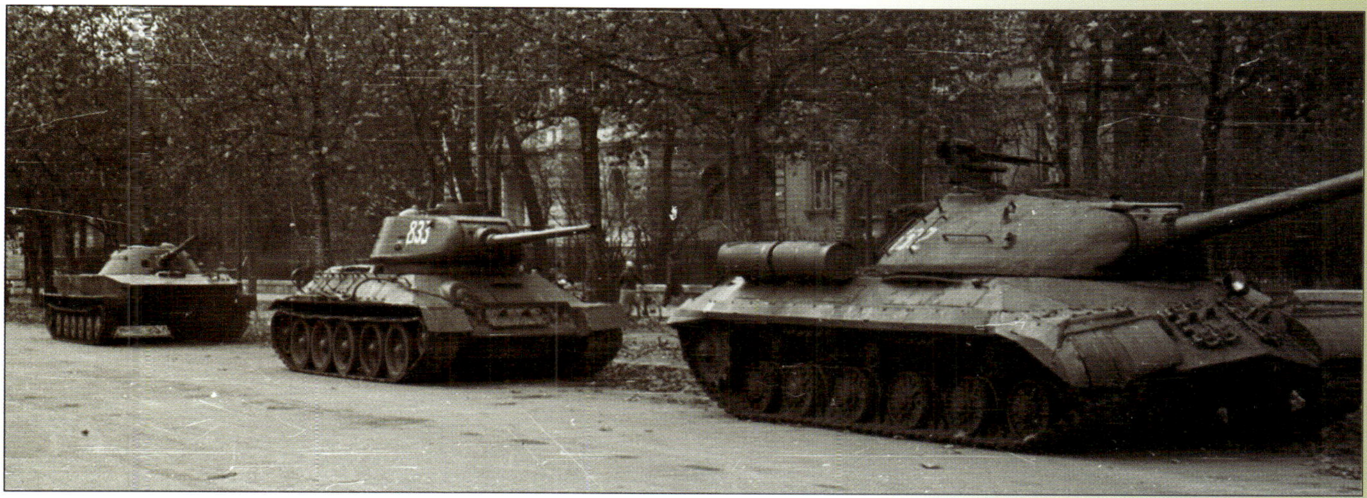

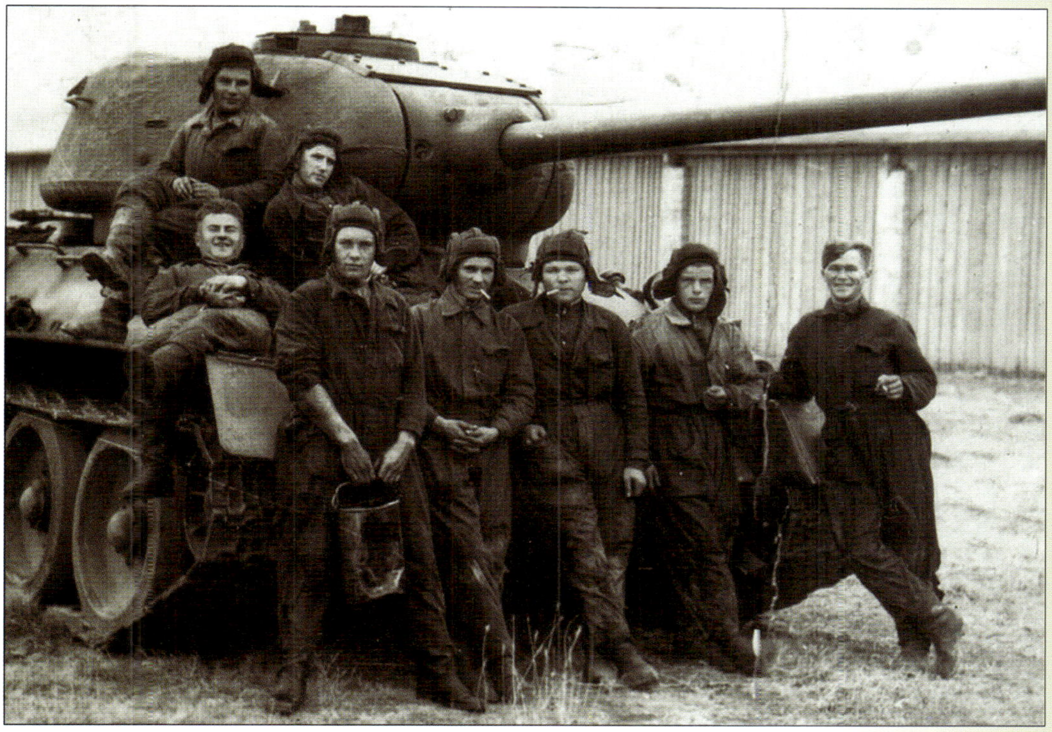

Soviet tank on a Budapest street, October 1956. Surprising is not only the lineup of various types of tanks – PT-76, T-34-85 and IS-3, but also the fact that the "thirty-four", tactical number 833 is a tank of early wartime production with D-5T gun.

Soviet tank soldiers pose next to a T-34-85 (probably of unit, late 1940s/early 1950s.

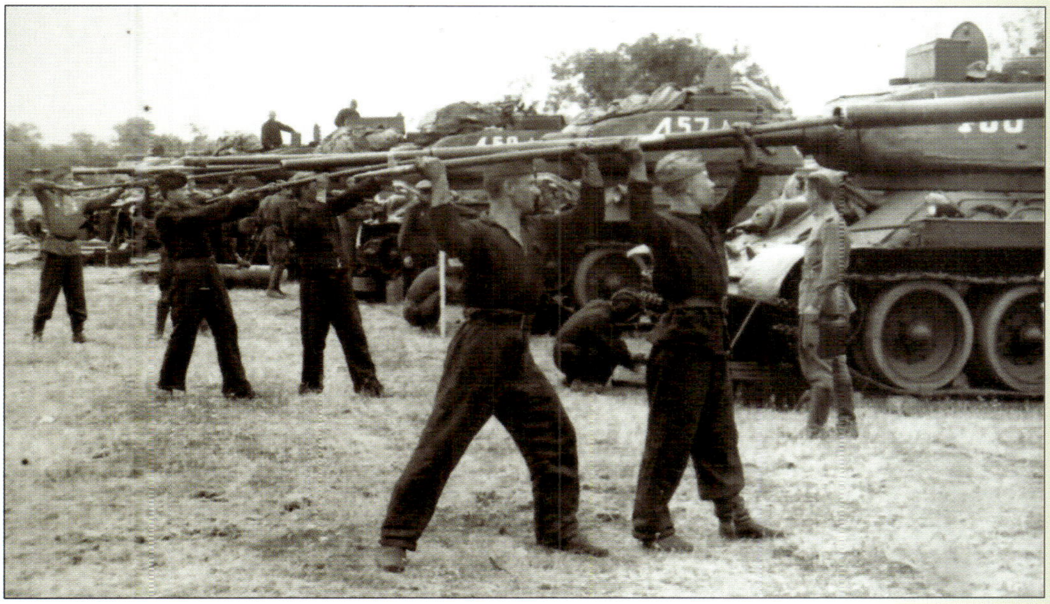

Maintenance work on Soviet T-34-85 tanks from an unidentified unit based in East Germany. Apart from the tactical numbers the tanks have also red stars painted on the turrets.

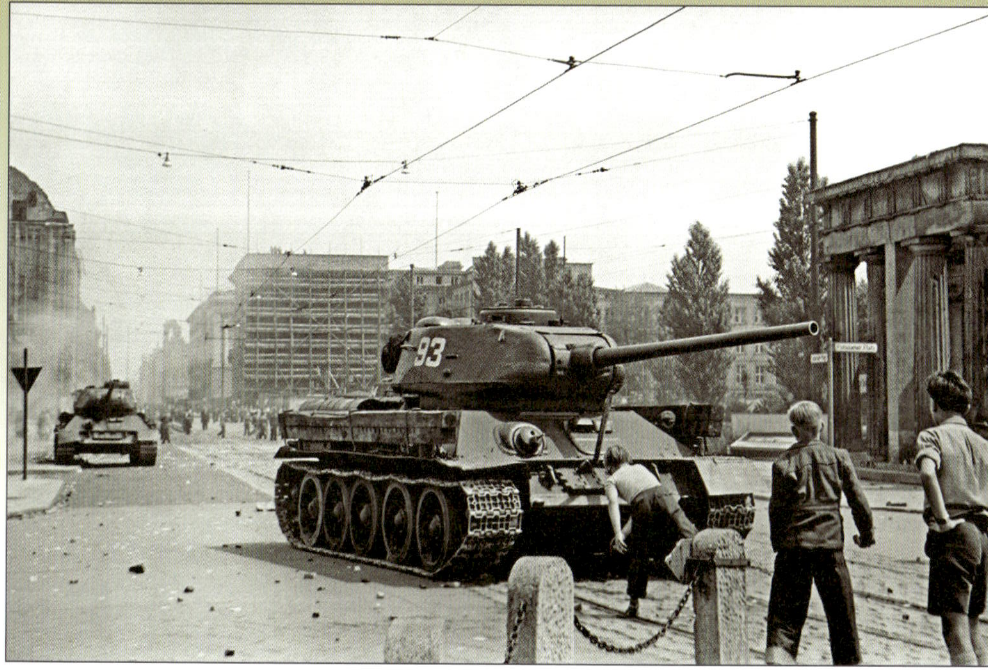

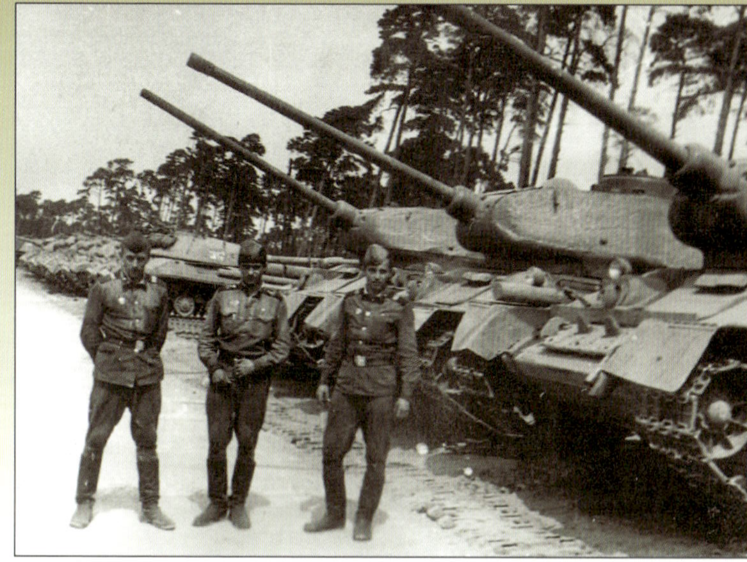

T-34-85 and IS-3 tanks from the 41st Independent Armoured Regiment, based at Forst Zinna (East Germany, near Polish border). It was the training unit of Soviet Army Group in Germany. The T-34-85s have no tactical markings.

USSR

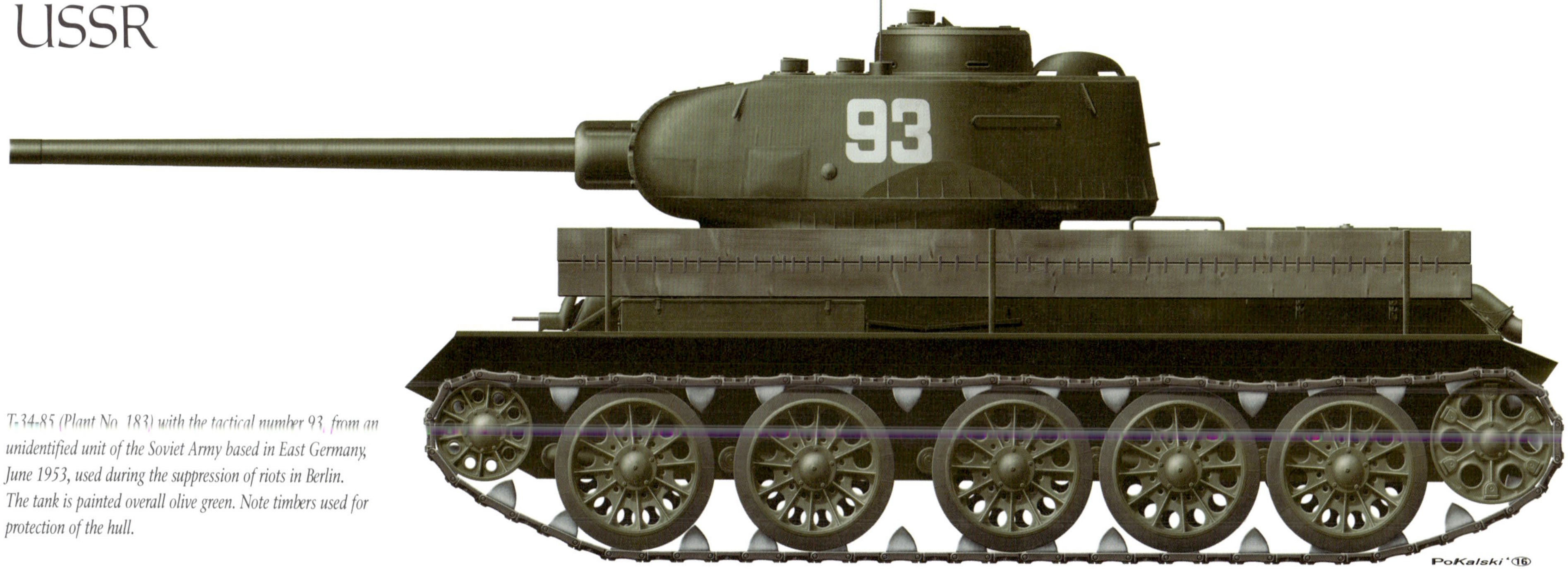

T-34-85 (Plant No. 183) with the tactical number 93, from an unidentified unit of the Soviet Army based in East Germany, June 1953, used during the suppression of riots in Berlin. The tank is painted overall olive green. Note timbers used for protection of the hull.

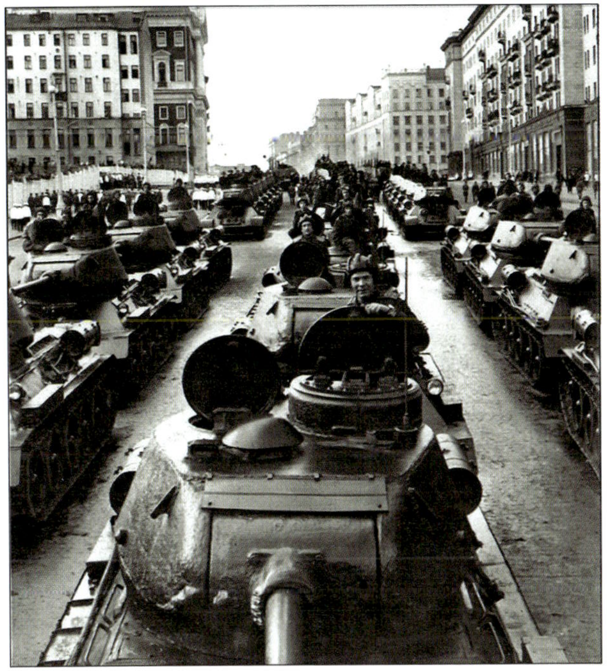

Left: *A column of T-34-85s (mostly of Plant No. 112 production with two single ventilators on the turrets) ready for a parade in Moscow, 1945 or 1946.*

A modified Soviet T-34-85 model 1960, tactical number 338 during winter maneuvers, probably early 1960s.

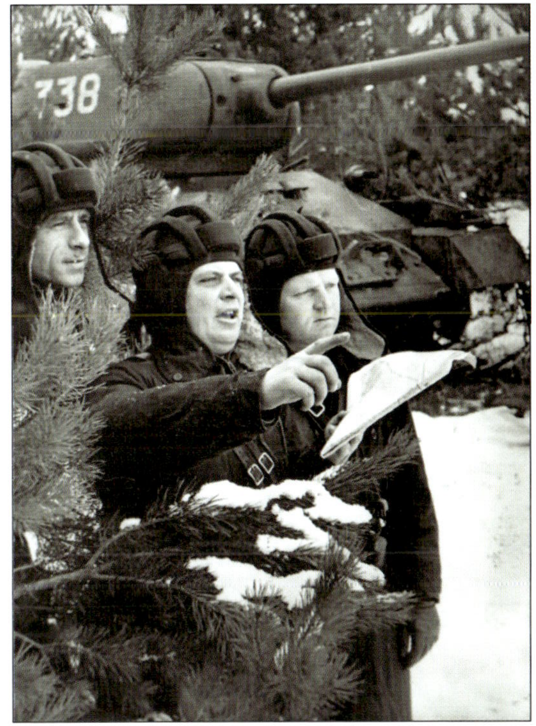

USSR

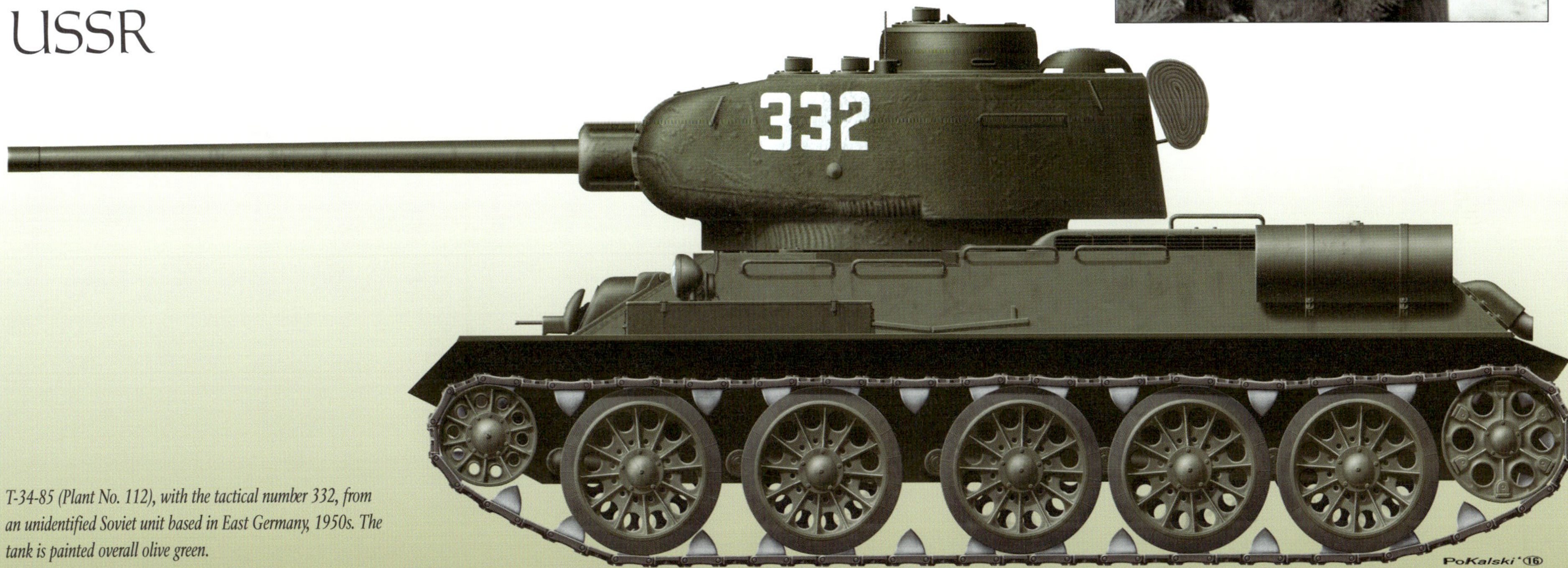

T-34-85 (Plant No. 112), with the tactical number 332, from an unidentified Soviet unit based in East Germany, 1950s. The tank is painted overall olive green.

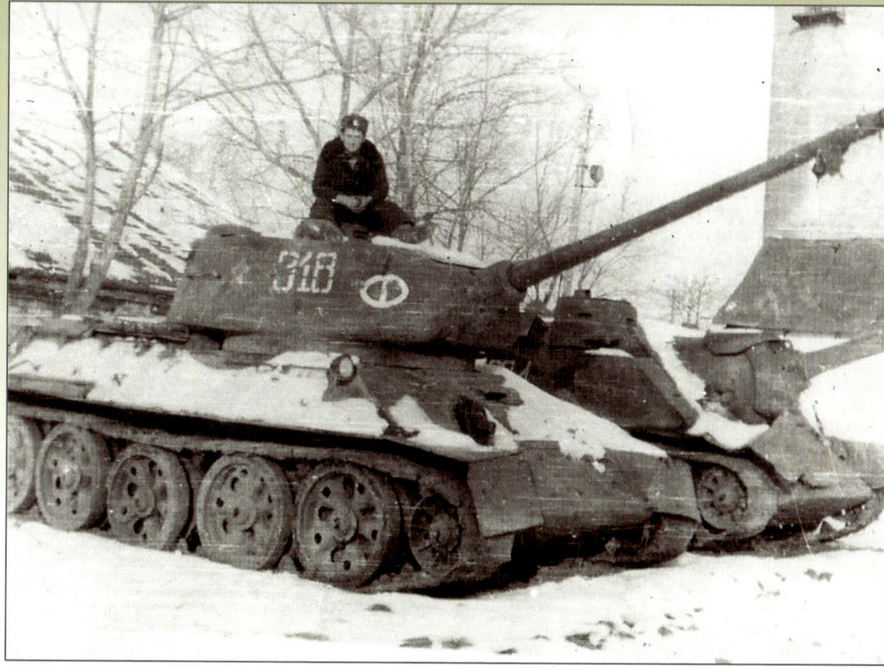

A T-34-85 (Plant No. 174) during military exercise in the Crimea, 1950s. The tank with tactical number 101 sports also an emblem in form of anchor with a red star, which may indicate that the tanks is assigned to a marine unit.

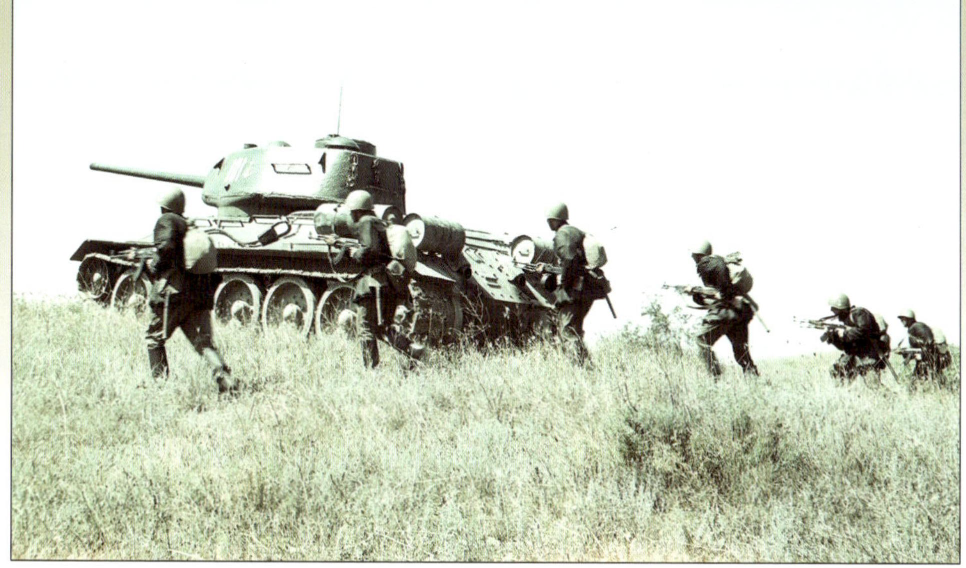

USSR

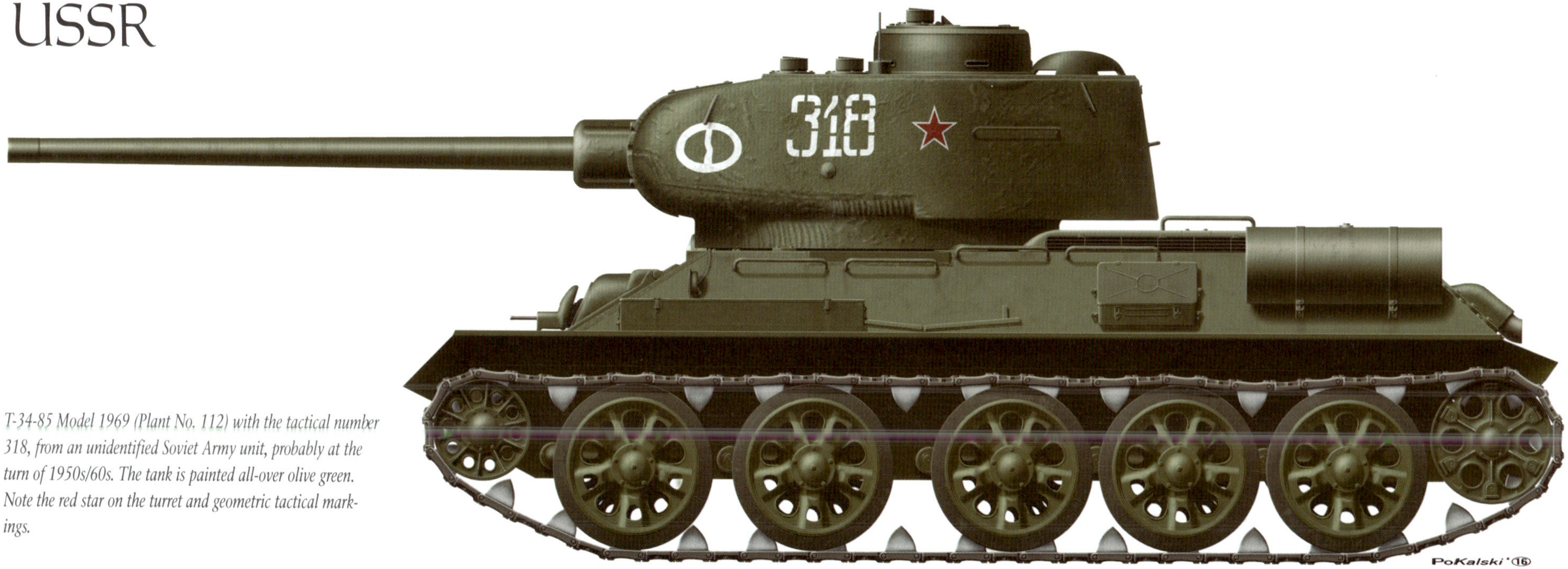

T-34-85 Model 1969 (Plant No. 112) with the tactical number 318, from an unidentified Soviet Army unit, probably at the turn of 1950s/60s. The tank is painted all-over olive green. Note the red star on the turret and geometric tactical markings.

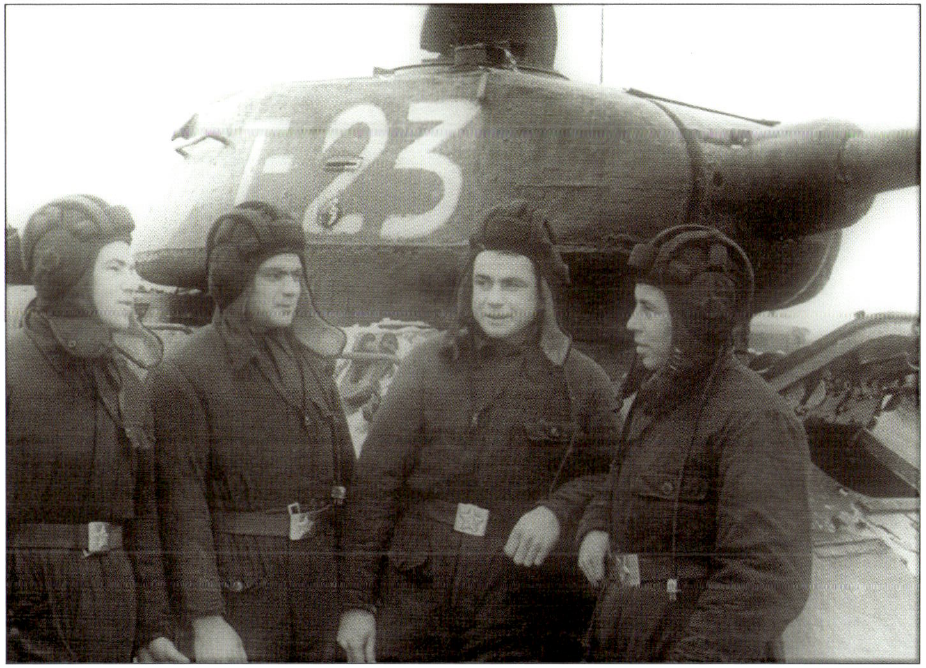

USSR

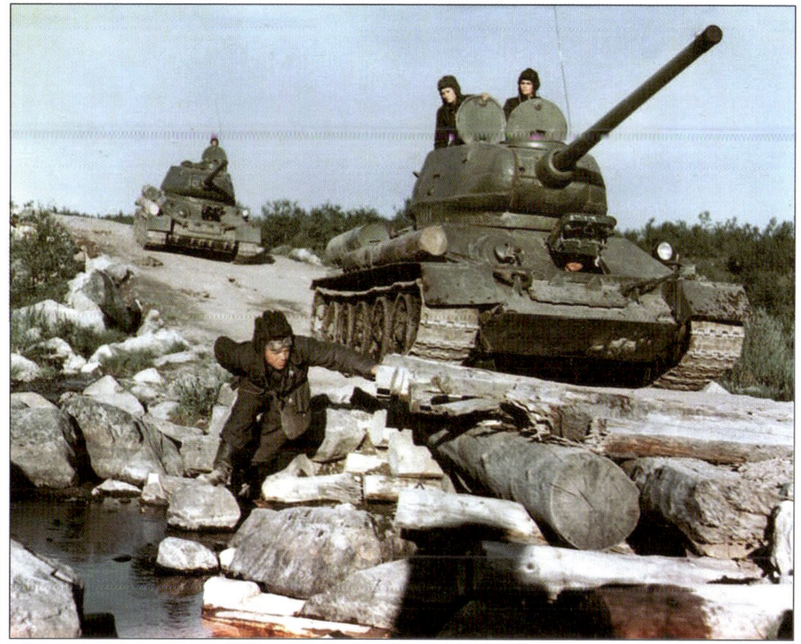

T-34-85 tanks from an unidentified training unit, 1950s. The tanks have no tactical markings and are painted overall olive green (4BO paint).

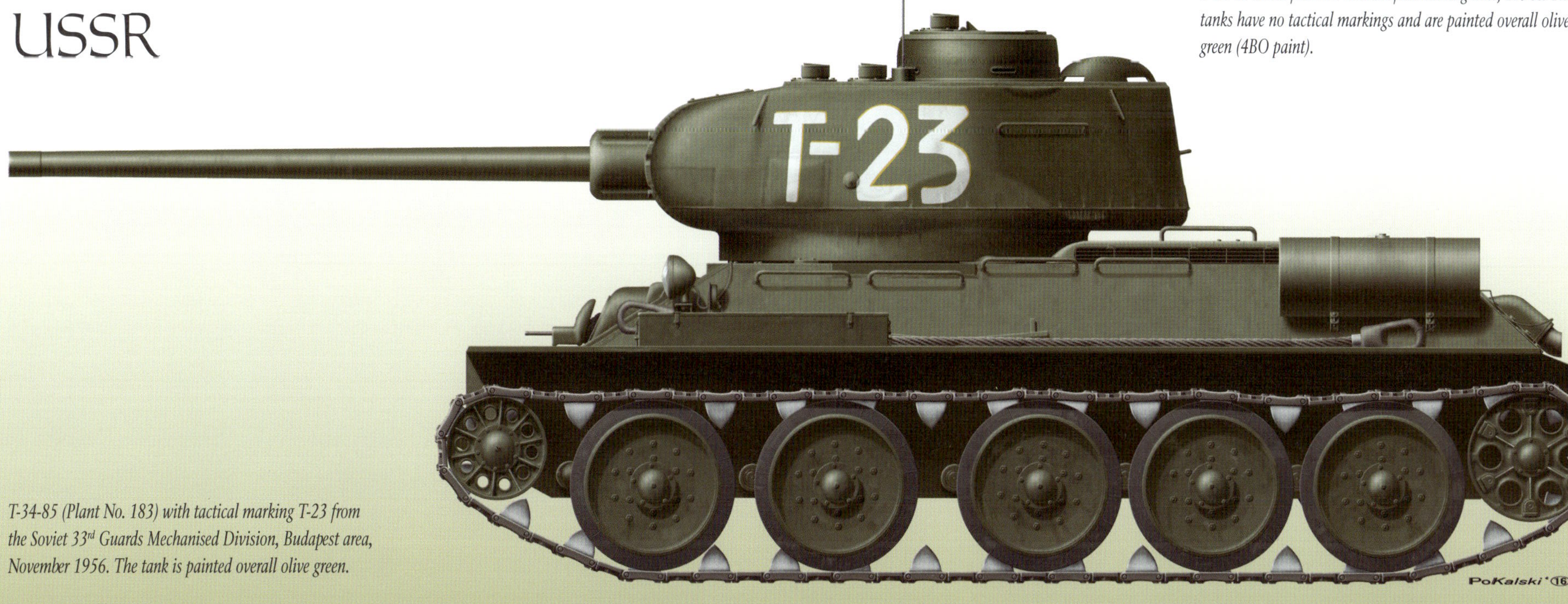

T-34-85 (Plant No. 183) with tactical marking T-23 from the Soviet 33rd Guards Mechanised Division, Budapest area, November 1956. The tank is painted overall olive green.

Asia

Afghanistan

During 1955-57 the Royal Afghan Army received 25 T-34-85 tanks from the USSR. In 1978, when the communists took over, the Soviets sold 150 T-34-85 tanks to Afghanistan. They remained in the inventory until 1987.

The tanks were painted olive green. Three-digit tactical numbers were placed on the sides of the turrets. The national insignia was often painted ahead of the number – initially of the royal army, then of the 'democratic' forces.

Wreck of an Afghan T-34-85 (of Plant 112 production), photographed in the early 21st century. Note the road wheels (Starfish, from T-44) lying next to the wreck – they apparently differ from the wheels of the T-54/55 tank family.

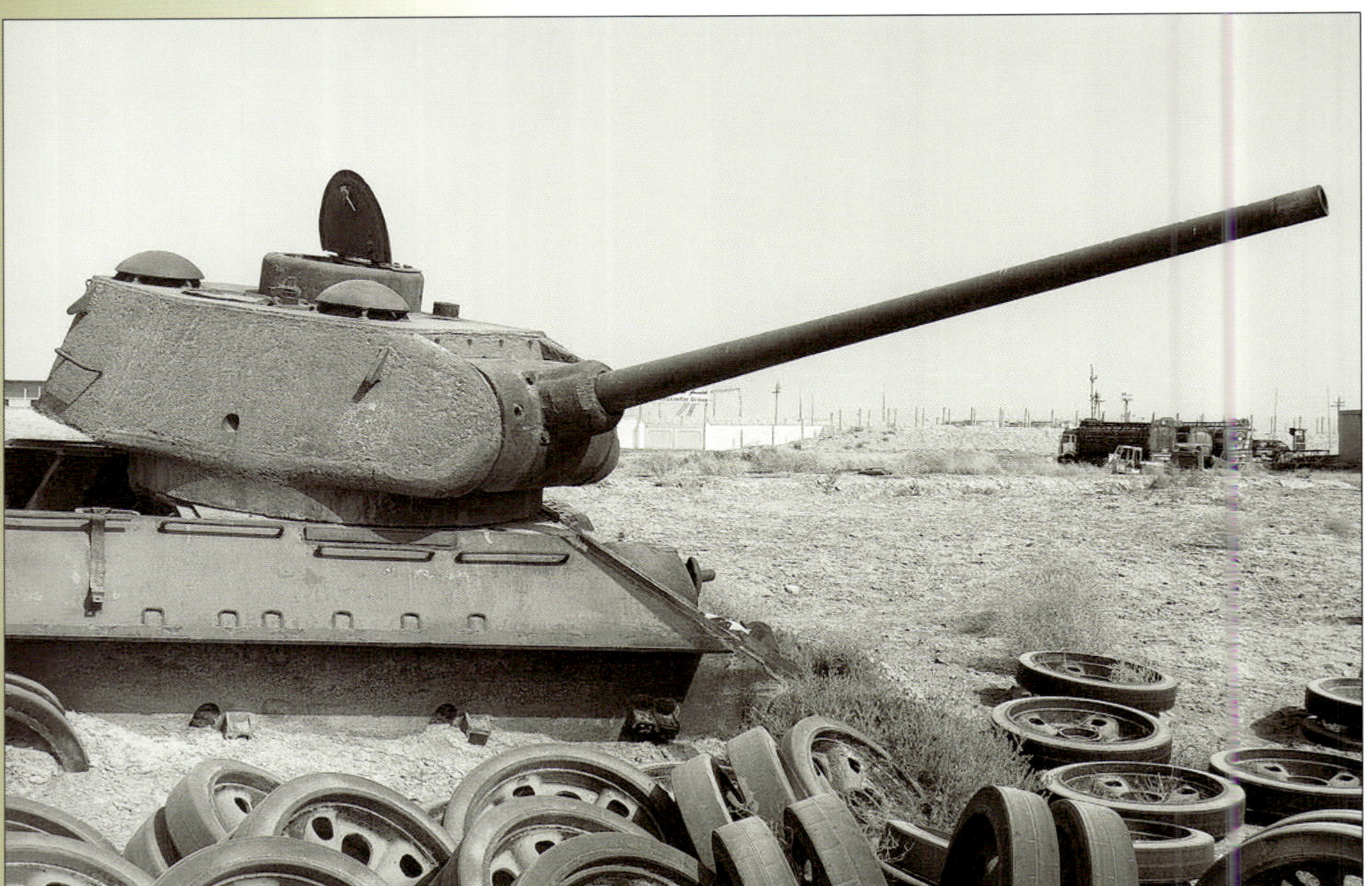

China

At the end of the 1940s and beginning of the 1950s, 1,837 T-34-85 tanks were delivered from the USSR to China (some Chinese sources give the number 1,964, but this also includes tanks armed with 76 mm guns). According to Western sources, vehicles in the inventory of People's Liberation Army were designated Type 58, but this is not confirmed by Chinese sources. Sometimes-stated designations of modified tanks, such as Type-58-I or Type-58-II, were also not used. However, there is no doubt that the tanks underwent some modifications, consisting of the addition of a cupola with 12.7 mm DshK anti-aircraft machine gun mount on the loader's hatch, reinforcement of hinges on the rear hull plate and installation of some components of the Type 59 tank (gunsight, lights and probably road wheels). The Chinese built many interesting vehicles based on the T-34-85. An example of a vehicle that entered series production was an anti-aircraft tank armed with two 37 mm Type 63 cannon. They were operated not only by the Chinese People's Liberation Army, but also the Vietnamese. One of the most interesting modifications was the tank equipped with 12 TPO-50M flamethrowers, mounted in pods on the sides of the turret.

In the early period the Chinese T-34-85s were painted all-over olive green with Soviet 4BO paint. White, three-digit tactical numbers were painted on the turrets. Some vehicles had the national insignia – Chinese red star – painted ahead of the tactical number. The tanks used by the Chinese "volunteers" in Korea sported only tactical numbers.

It is unclear whether or not Chinese tanks ever sported multi-colour paint schemes when in service. Admittedly photographs of such vehicles are known, but these generally depict tanks at shows or in displays of the equipment at schools or military units. Such paint schemes were probably not used during operational service. It is hard to determine when such paint schemes appeared, but it was probably in the late 20th century.

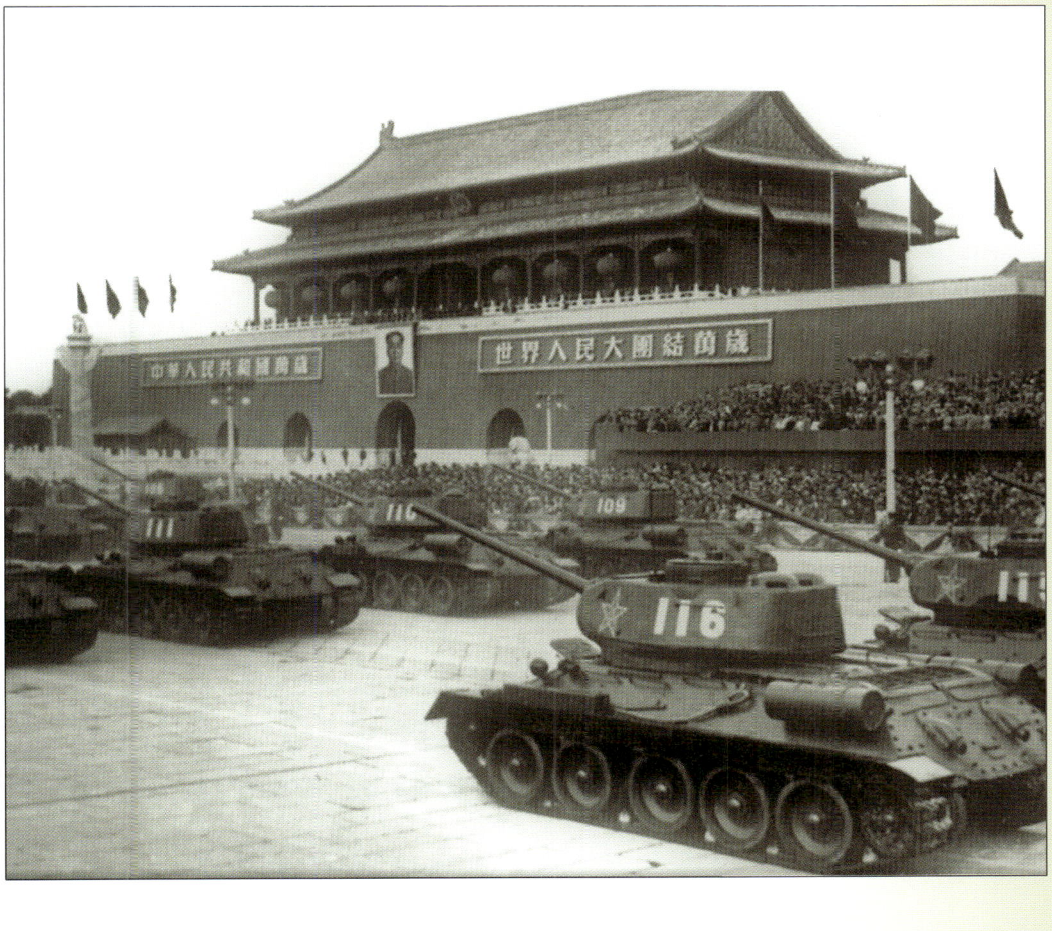

Chinese T-34-85s during a parade at Tienanmen Square in Beijing, early 1950s. Tanks in single colour (olive green) paint scheme with standard markings.

Crews of Chinese T-34-85 prior to a parade in Beijing, early 1950s. The Chinese received tanks made by various Soviet production plants, which is apparent in this photograph. The tanks in the first row were produced by Plant No.112 (left) and No.174 (right). Interesting is the fact that the crews are four-man.

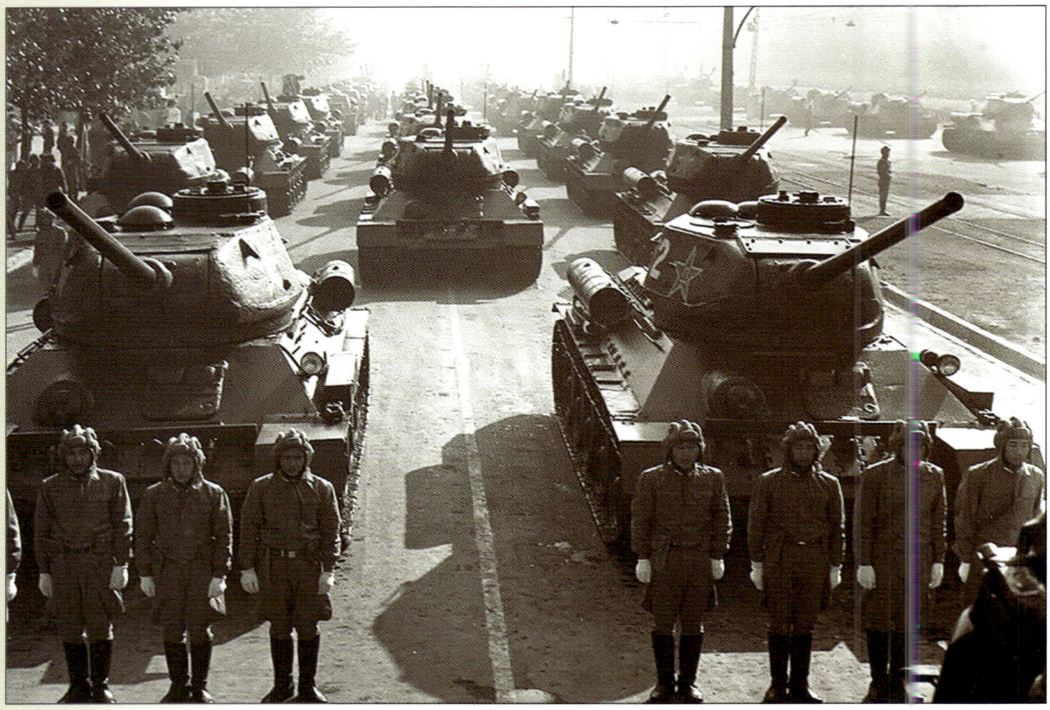

A "volunteer" crew of a Chinese T-34-85 (Plant No.183) with number 215, who distinguished themselves during the Korean War. According to some sources in 1953 they destroyed several enemy vehicles and strongpoints. Unfortunately this information is hard to verify.

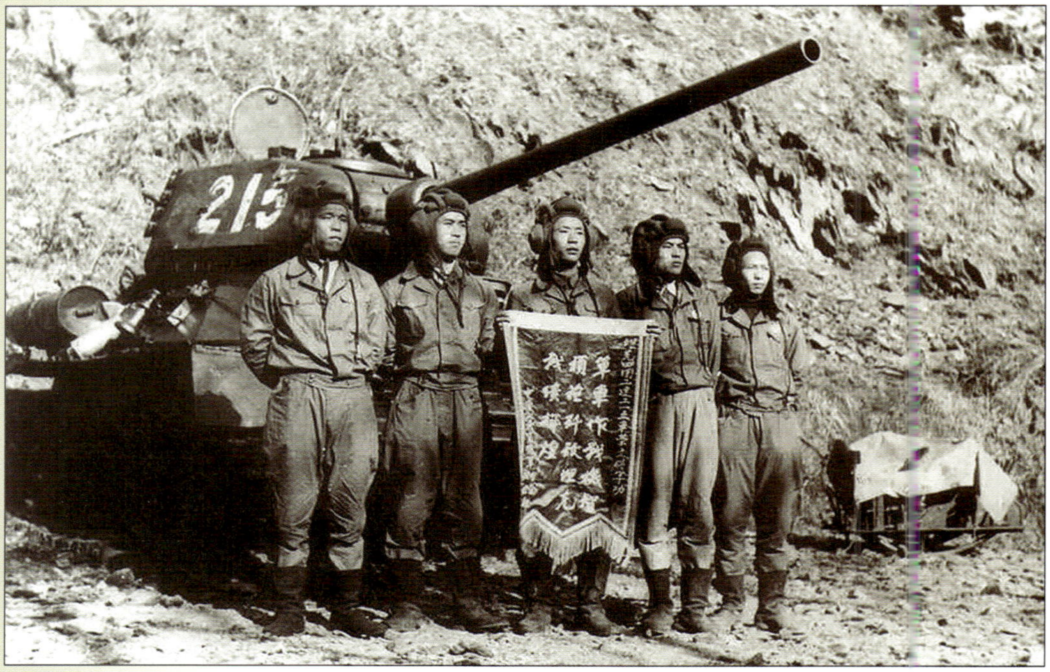

A Chinese T-34-85 (Plant No.183) photographed during exercise, probably in the 1950s. Note very untypical marking on the turret.

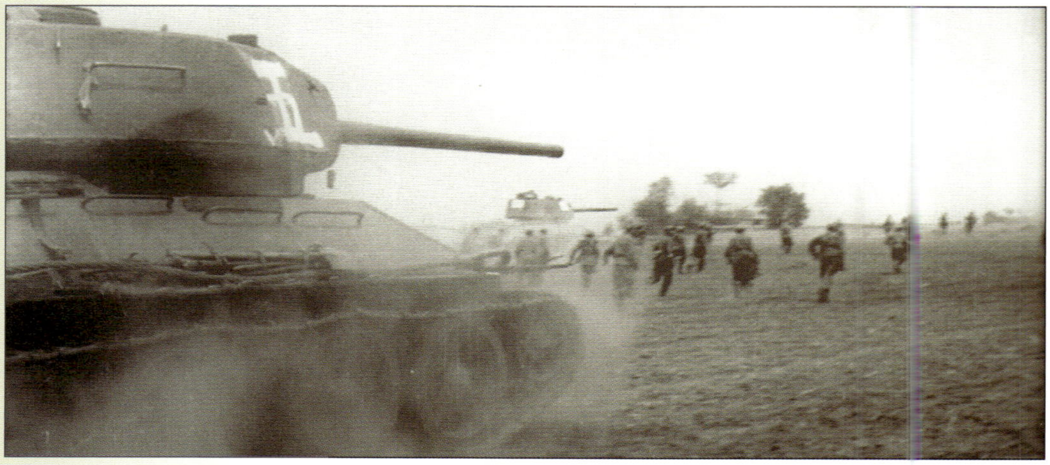

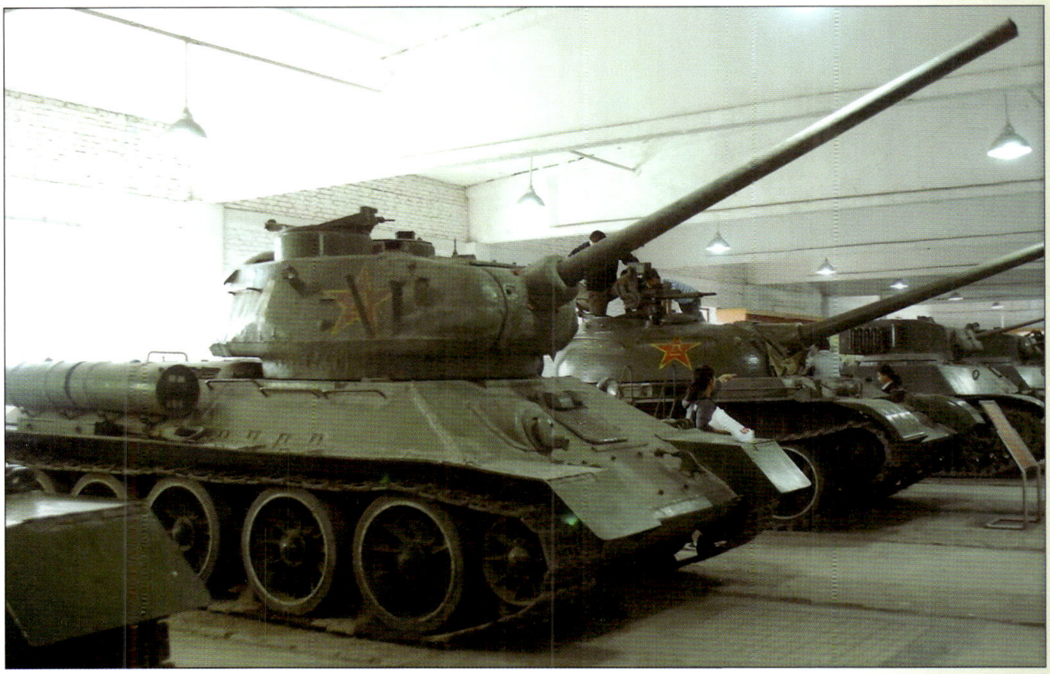

A modified Chinese T-34-85 (Plant No.183) at Chinese military museum in Beijing. A cupola over the loader's hatch is visible.

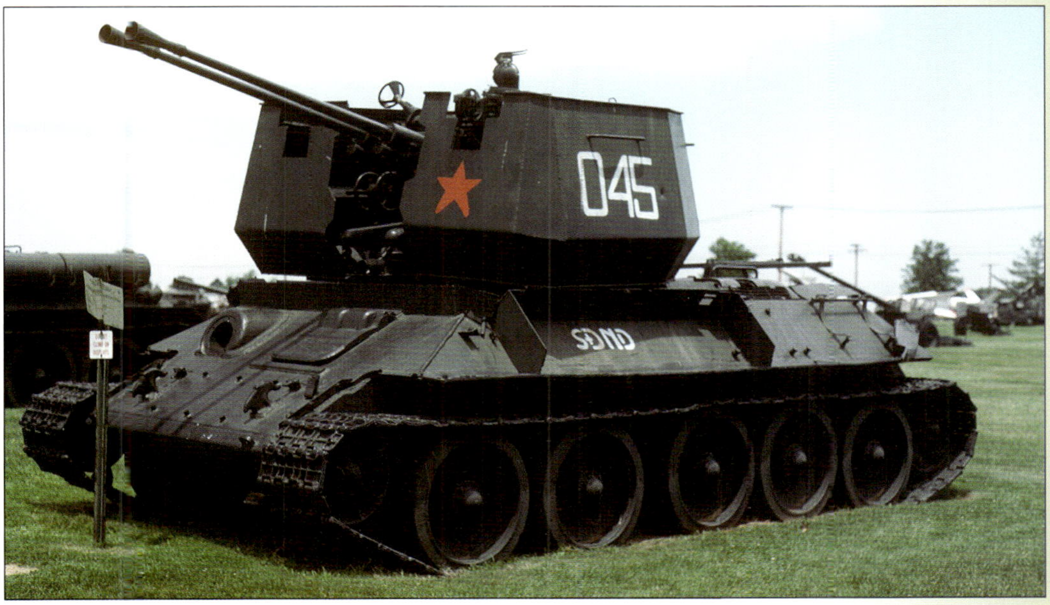

Anti-aircraft tank developed on the basis of T-34-85. It was armed with two 37 mm Type 63 cannons. These vehicles were operated not only in the PRC, but also in North Vietnam. Photographed is the vehicle preserved at Aberdeen museum, USA.

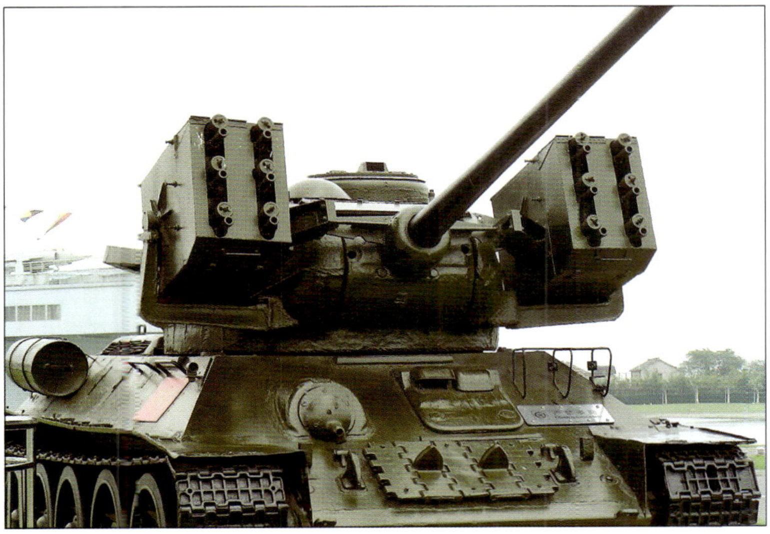

Among the Chinese modifications of the T-34-85 this one seems to be the most weird. Pods with 12 TPO-50M heavy flamethrowers were mounted on both sides of the turret.

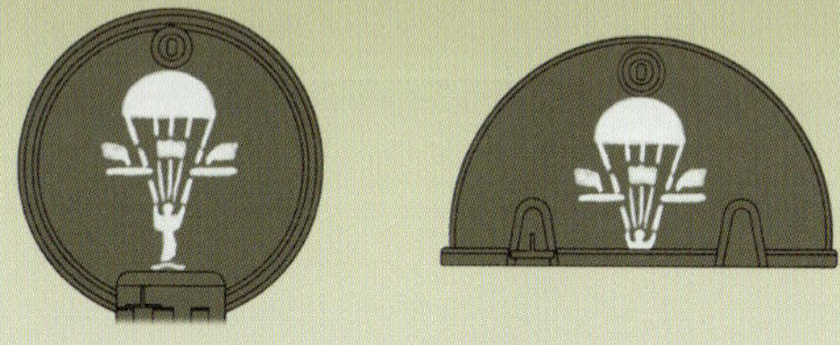

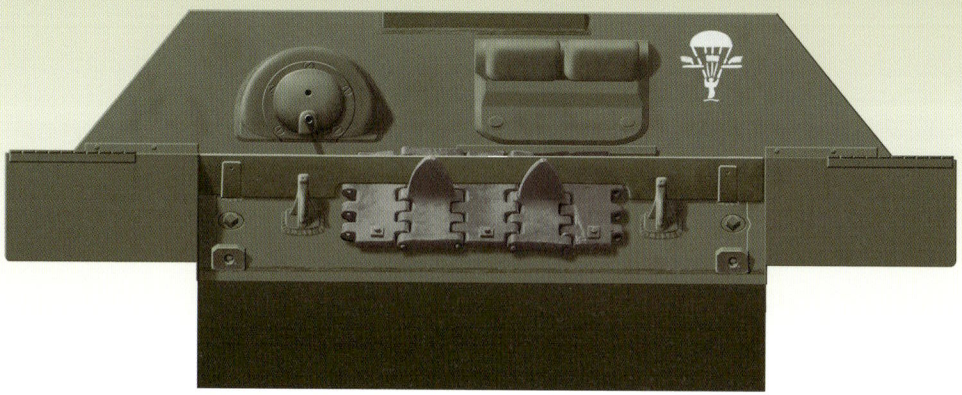

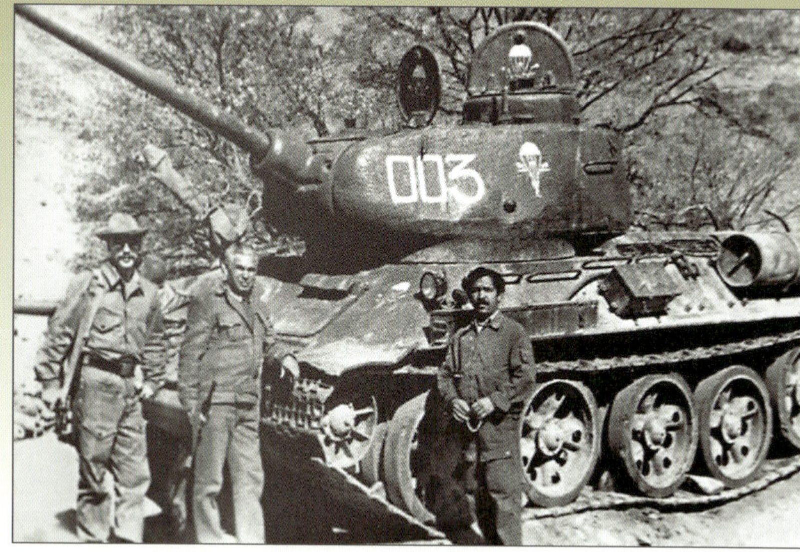

Afghanistan

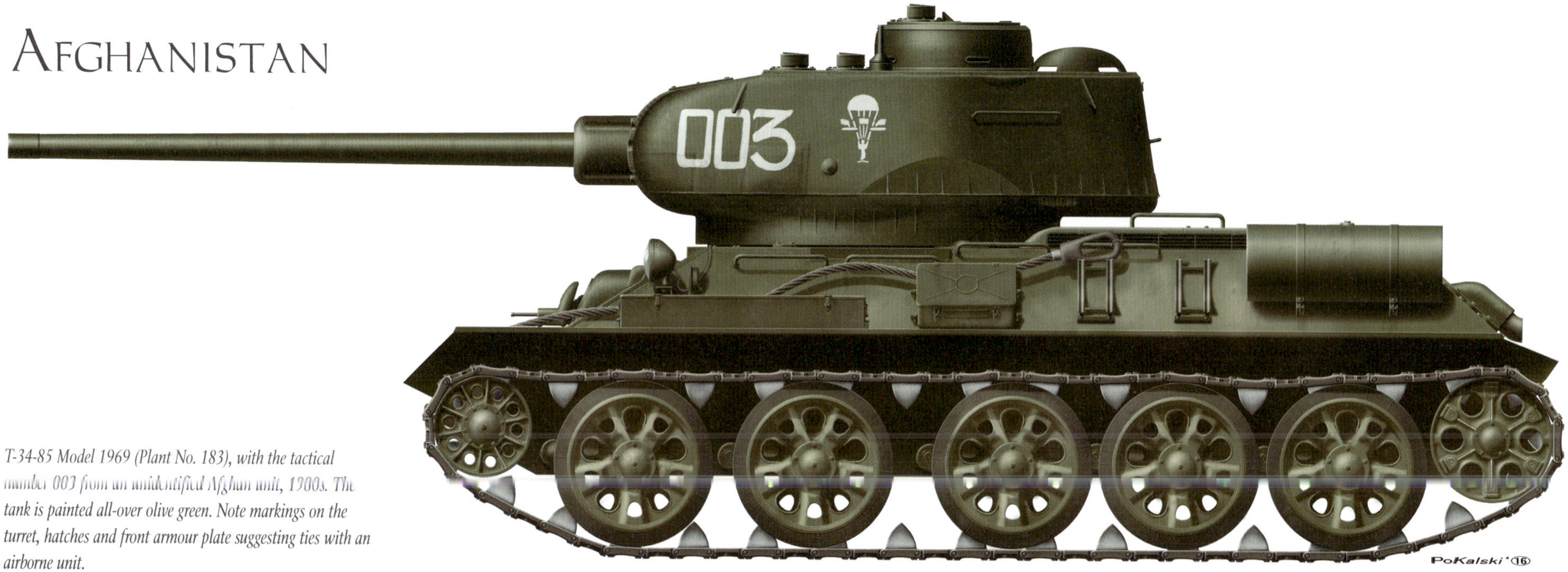

T-34-85 Model 1969 (Plant No. 183), with the tactical number 003 from an unidentified Afghan unit, 1980s. The tank is painted all-over olive green. Note markings on the turret, hatches and front armour plate suggesting ties with an airborne unit.

China

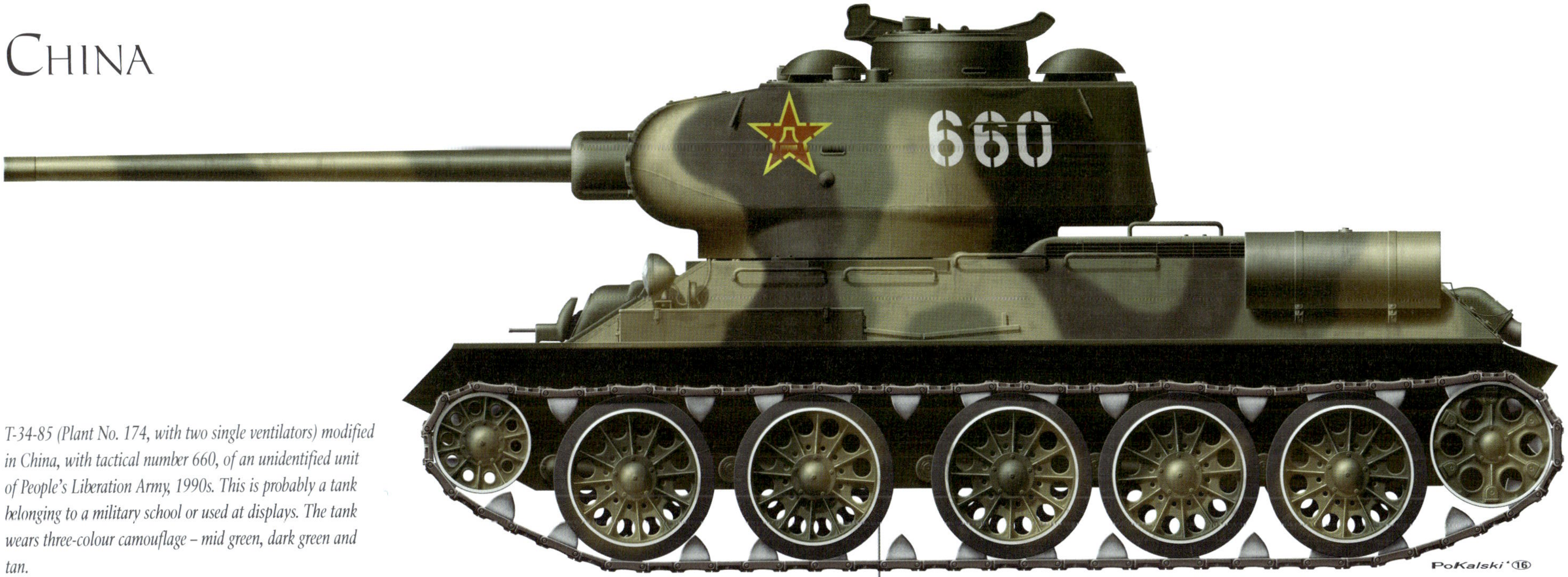

T-34-85 (Plant No. 174, with two single ventilators) modified in China, with tactical number 660, of an unidentified unit of People's Liberation Army, 1990s. This is probably a tank belonging to a military school or used at displays. The tank wears three-colour camouflage – mid green, dark green and tan.

China

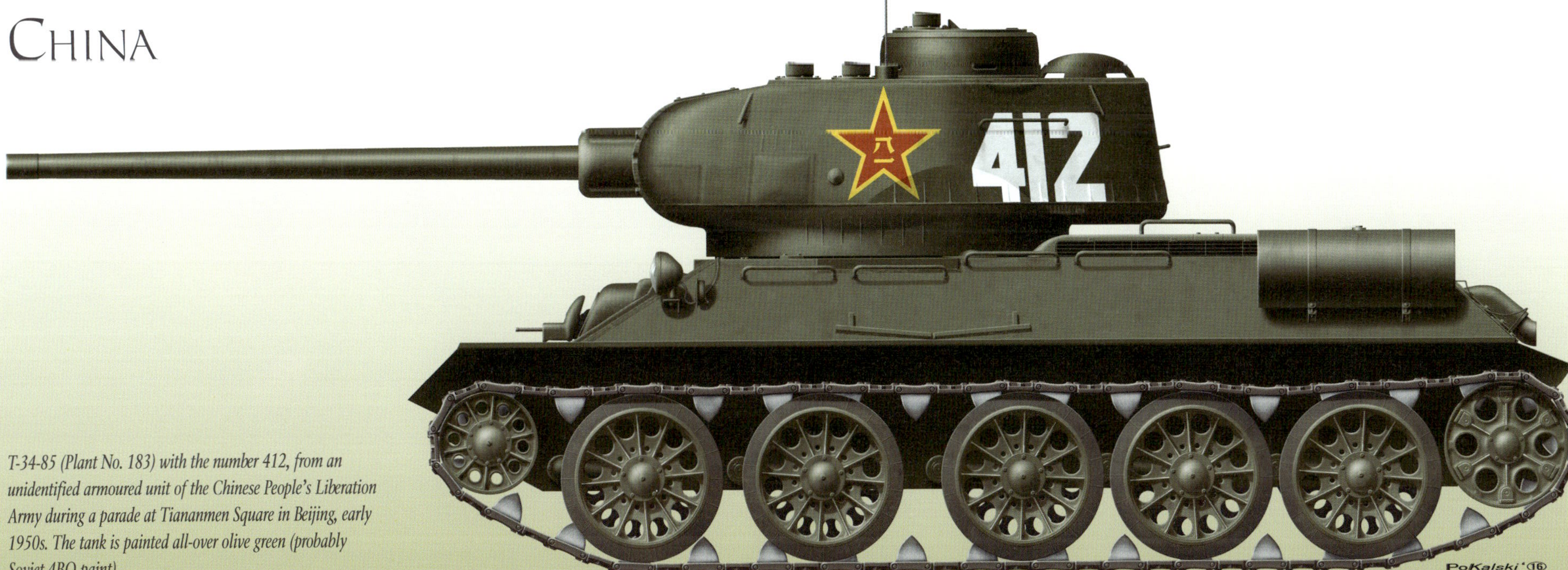

T-34-85 (Plant No. 183) with the number 412, from an unidentified armoured unit of the Chinese People's Liberation Army during a parade at Tiananmen Square in Beijing, early 1950s. The tank is painted all-over olive green (probably Soviet 4BO paint).

North Korea

T-34-85 tanks were delivered to the North Korean army from the USSR and PRC. Their exact number has never been specified, a reasonable estimate indicating about 500. The tanks were painted olive green and had white three-digit tactical numbers painted on the turrets.

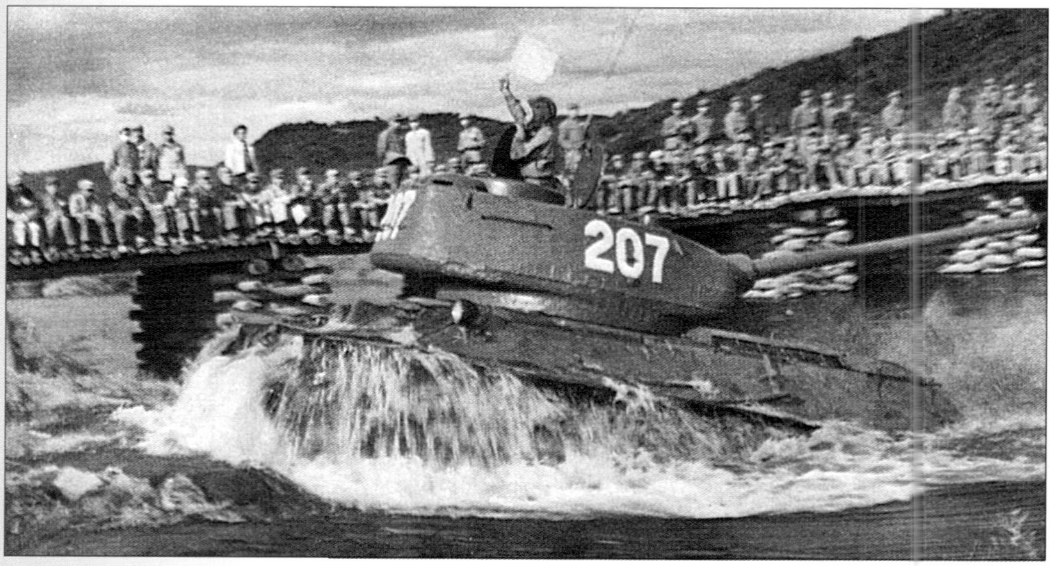

North Korean T-34-85 (Plant No.183), number 207 demonstrating water obstacle crossing.

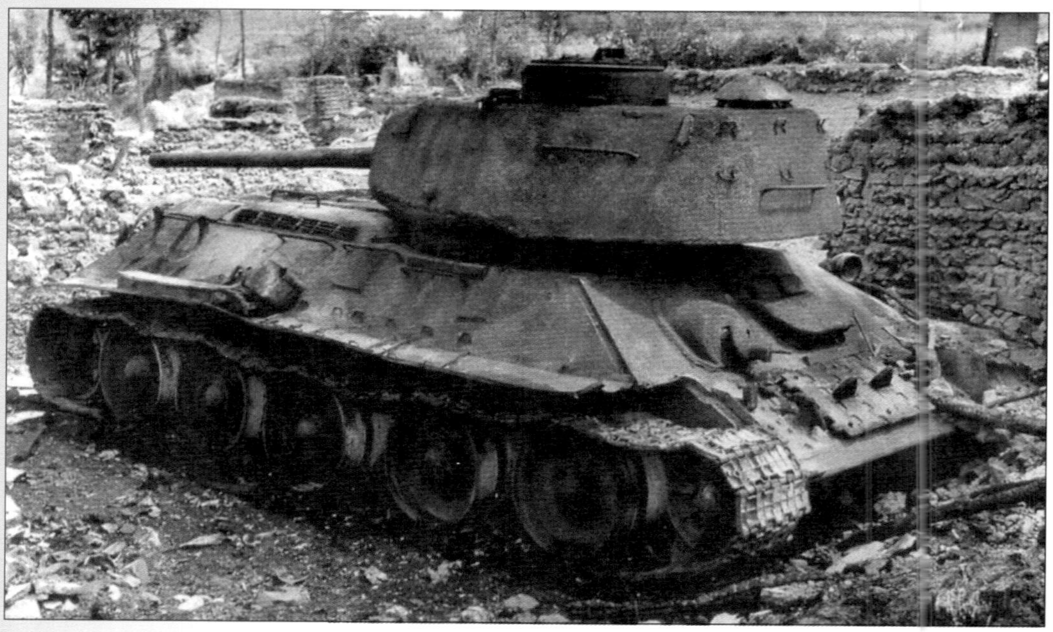

A burnt-out wreck of T-34-85 (Plant No.112 with two single ventilators) from the 16th Armoured Brigade near Yongsan, October 1950.

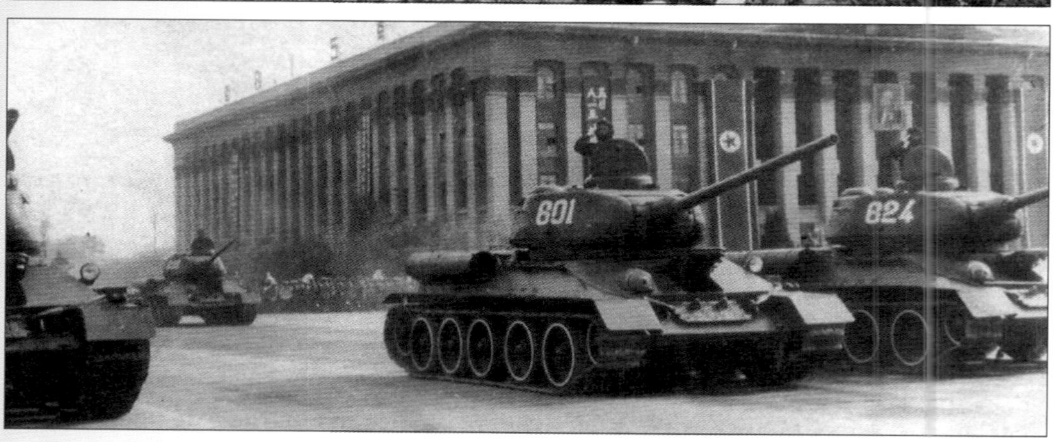

T-34-85 tanks at a parade in Pyongyang on the occasion of the North Korean national holiday, probably in the 1960s. The tanks wear sso-called parade paint scheme, with white wheel trim. Similar schemes were also used by the USSR and some other Eastern Bloc nations.

VIETNAM

Tanks operated by North Vietnamese units were painted olive green, which quickly faded in the monsoon climate. Three-digit tactical numbers (usually yellow or white) were painted on the turrets. On many vehicles, five-pointed stars within dashed-outline circles were painted ahead of the number, both elements in yellow. According to some sources the background of the Vietnamese insignia was red and according to others, red and blue. Photographs confirm both versions were used. It seems that initially the background was red and later red and blue. Interestingly, analysis of the photographs suggests that in the case of the two-colour background, there were versions with the background colours in the order red-blue, and some blue-red.

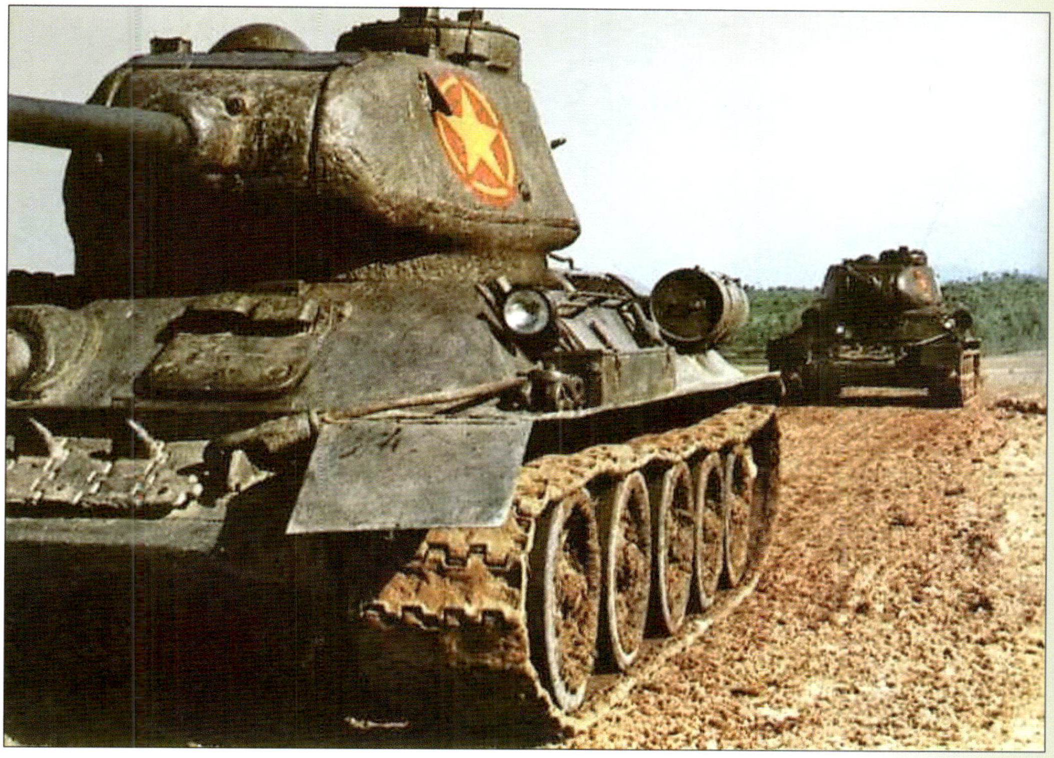

A T-34-85 (Plant No. 112, with two single ventilators) from an unidentified North Vietnamese unit. The tank has the national insignia in the most frequent form, with red background.

T-34-85 tanks of North Vietnamese Army during a night exercise, early 1970s. Visible in the foreground is a tank with tactical number 158, modernized to Model 1969 standard. Note the characteristic method of painting of the tactical number, with a gap in the middle.

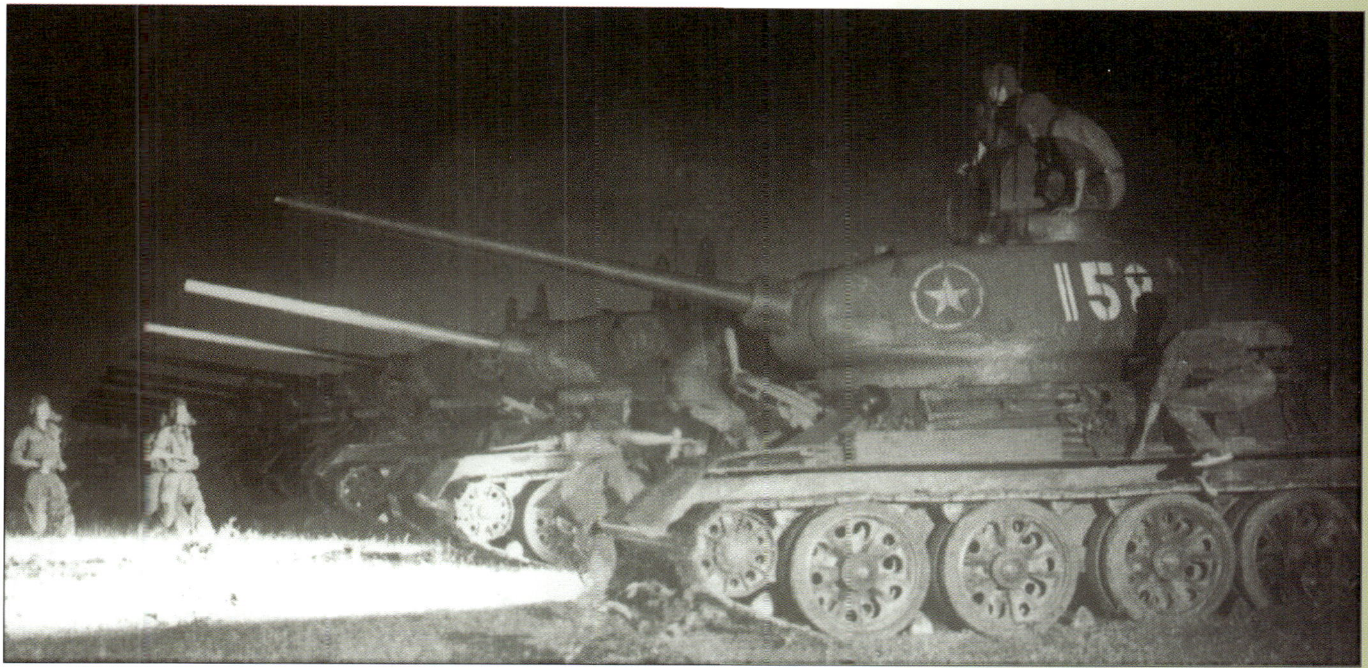

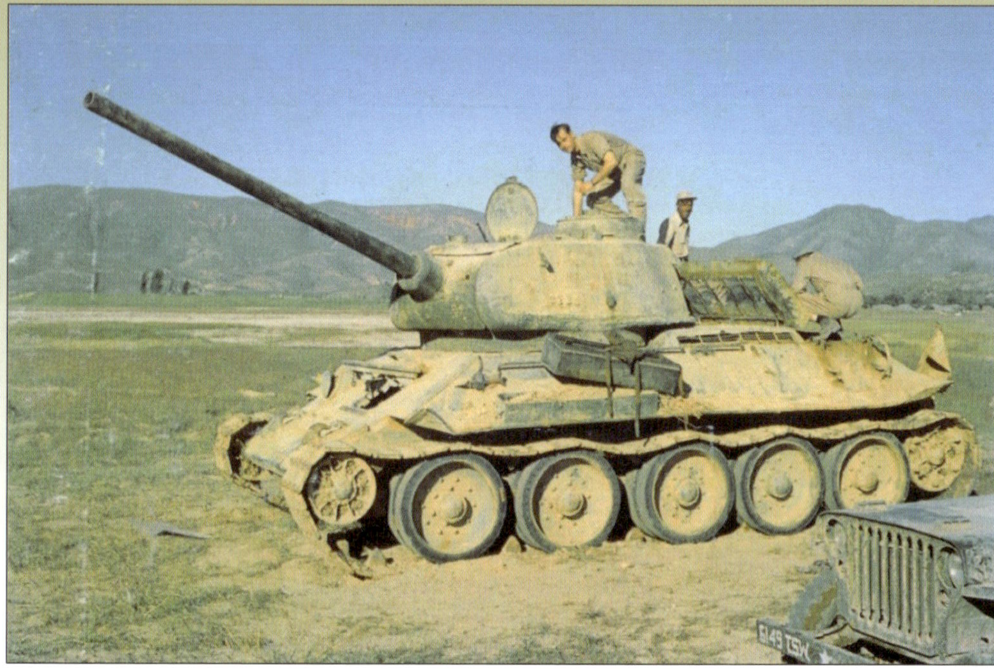

American soldiers inspect a destroyed North Korean T-34-85 (Plant No.112). The tanks is covered with dust, but it seems to have no tactical number.

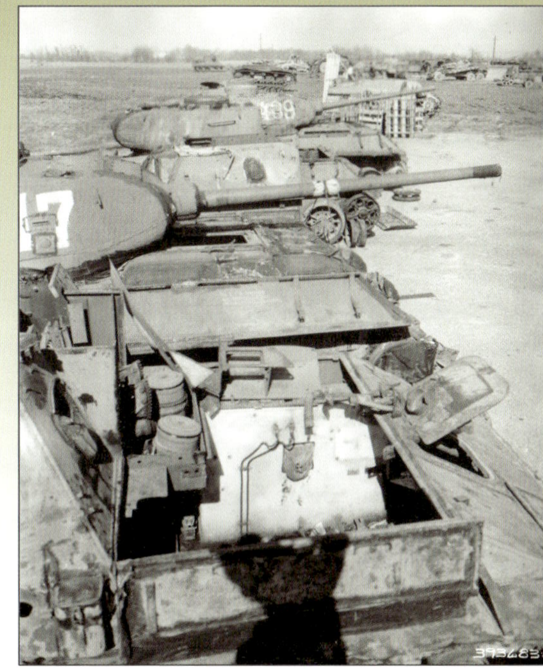

Destroyed North Korean T-34-85 tanks, produced by various plants. The shape of digits of the tactical numbers is also diverse.

North Korea

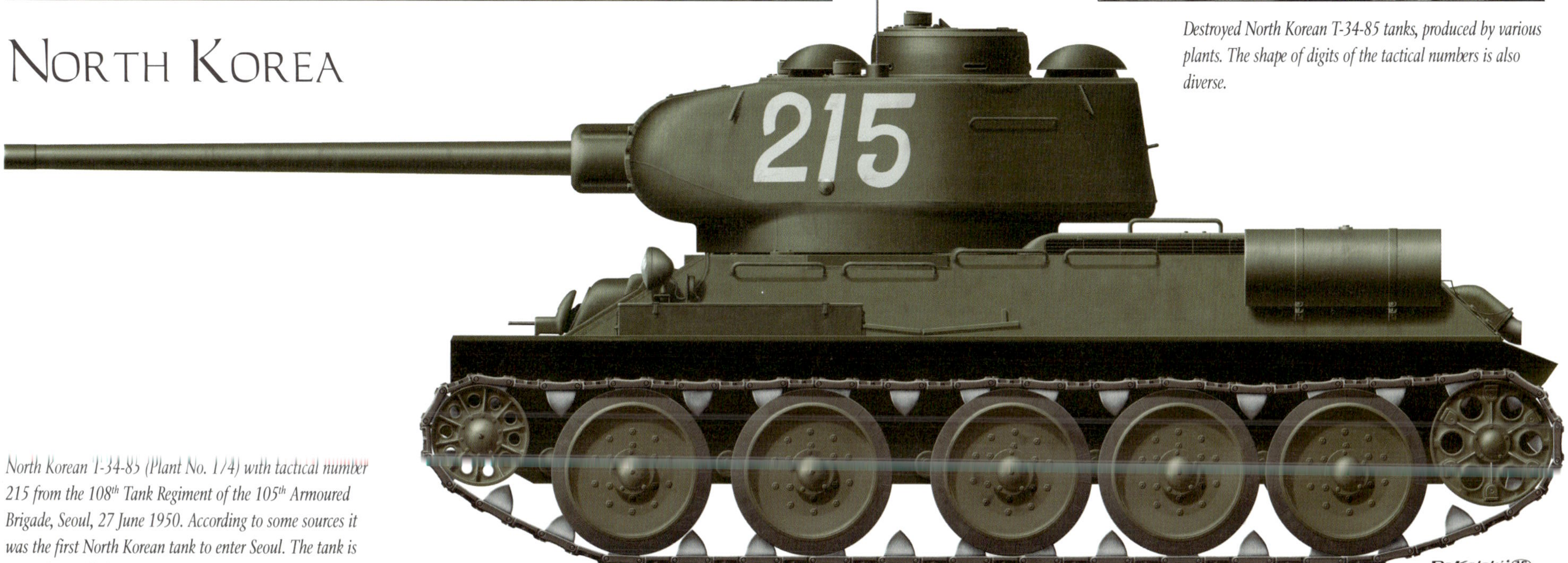

North Korean T-34-85 (Plant No. 174) with tactical number 215 from the 108th Tank Regiment of the 105th Armoured Brigade, Seoul, 27 June 1950. According to some sources it was the first North Korean tank to enter Seoul. The tank is painted overall olive green.

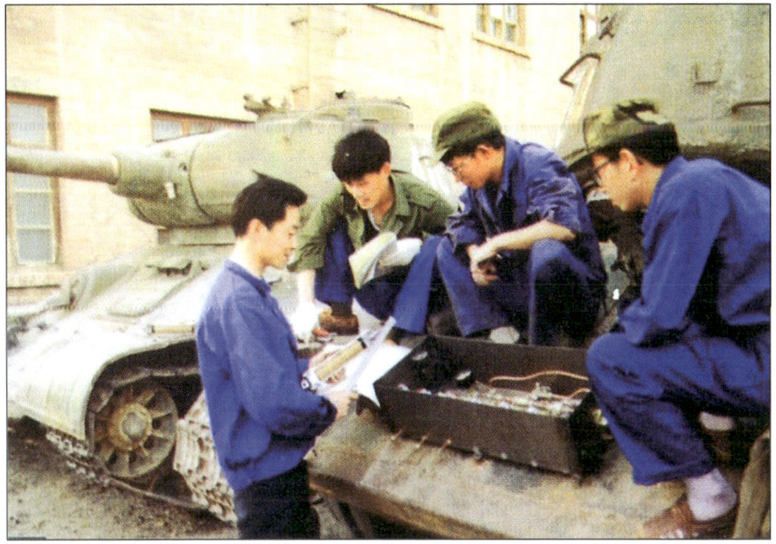

A very mysterious photograph, showing Vietnamese mechanics at a T-34-85 tank. The tank in the background is a vehicle modernized in China. It is difficult to find information confirming that PRC sold such tanks to Vietnam. There is also no information that the Vietnamese captured such tanks during the border conflict with China.

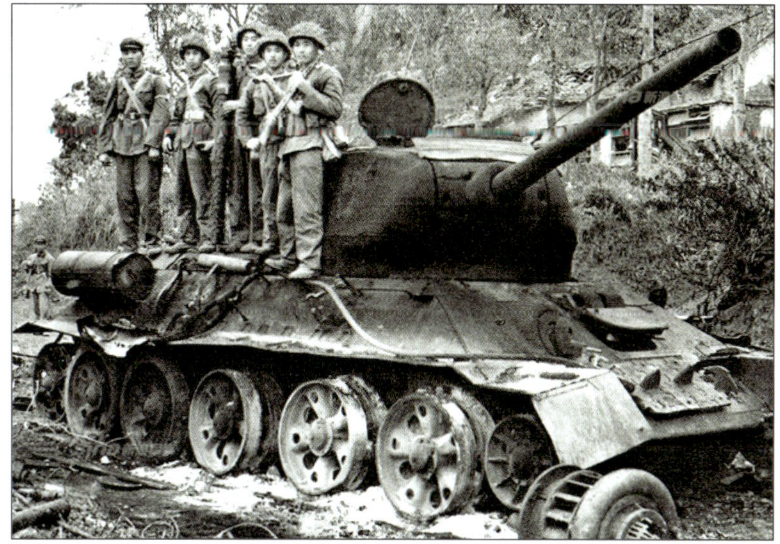

Chinese soldiers posing on a burnt-out wreck of a Vietnamese T-34-85 Model 1969 tank near Lang Son in 1979.

Vietnam

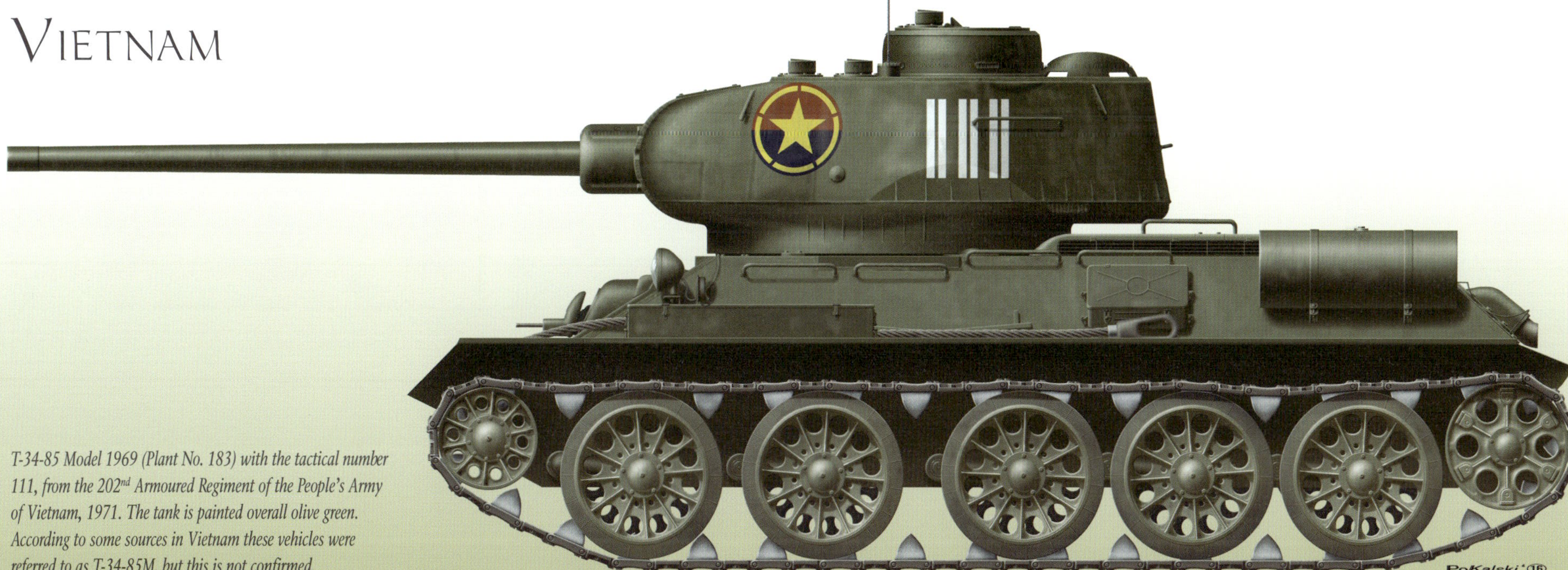

T-34-85 Model 1969 (Plant No. 183) with the tactical number 111, from the 202nd Armoured Regiment of the People's Army of Vietnam, 1971. The tank is painted overall olive green. According to some sources in Vietnam these vehicles were referred to as T-34-85M, but this is not confirmed.

Middle East

In the post-war period the T-34-85s entered service in armoured units of numerous Arab countries. The tanks sported diverse paint schemes – some remained in their original olive green livery, others received desert camouflage, both in single and multi-colour schemes.

Egypt

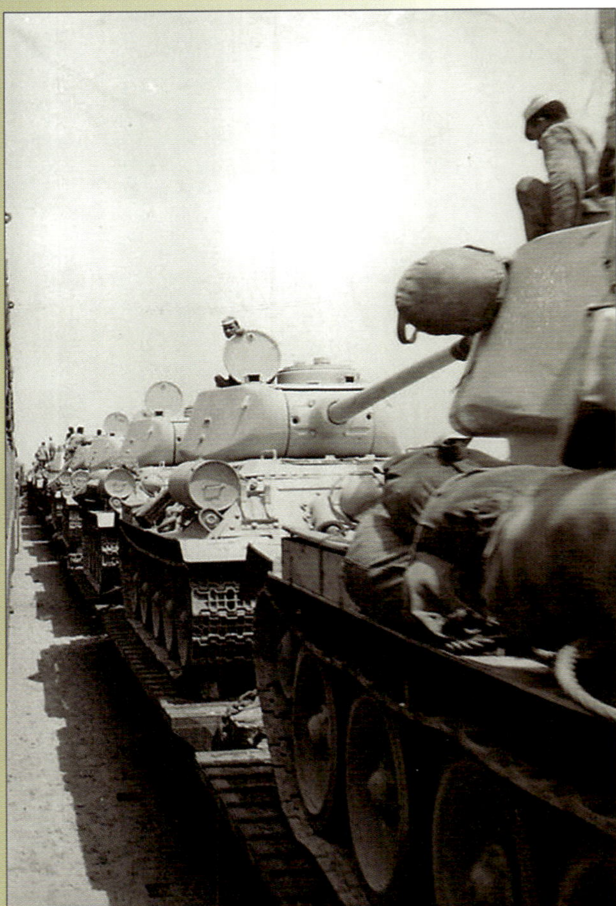

Egyptian T-34-85s (Czechoslovak production) on railway wagons, autumn of 1956.

The Egyptian army was the largest Middle Eastern T-34-85 operator. A total of about 500 tanks were delivered from the USSR and Czechoslovakia (at least 290 of which were delivered during 1955-57). The Egyptian tanks had some distinctive features, making them easily recognisable: the forward section of the fender was slightly upturned, the exhaust pipes were extended and a tool holder was installed on the turret. Some Egyptian tanks had a 12.7 mm DShK anti-aircraft machine gun mount installed on the turret. In the 1970s a modification of T-34-85 was developed by Egyptian No.5 Works, consisting in retrofitting more modern equipment and wheel skirts. This proposal did not enter series implementation.

Paint schemes and markings of Egyptian T-34-85 tanks have been the subject of controversy and disputes between authors focussing on this subject. It seems that during the conflicts in 1956 and 1967 the basic paint scheme consisted of applying sand colour paint on all surfaces. Information about multi-colour (two-tone) paint schemes has not been confirmed by photographic material, although it cannot be ruled out that such paint schemes were worn by T-34-85s. For example, multi-colour camouflage was certainly worn by T-34-122 howitzers used by the Egyptians during the Yom Kippur war.

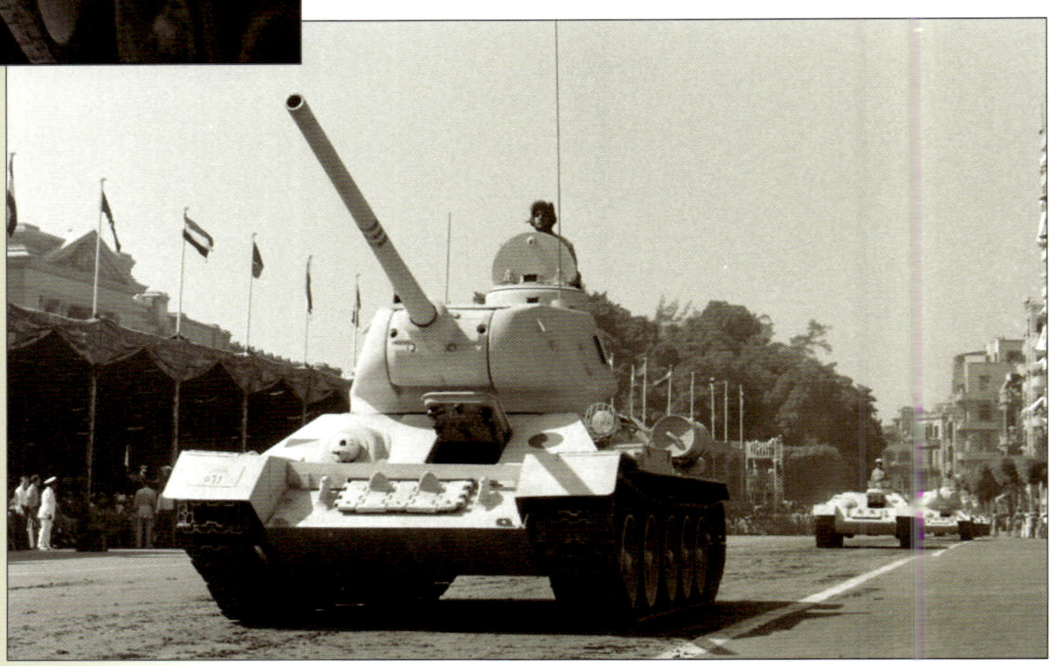

A T-34-85 (Czechoslovak production) during a parade in Cairo, summer of 1956. The tank wears an overall sand paint scheme.

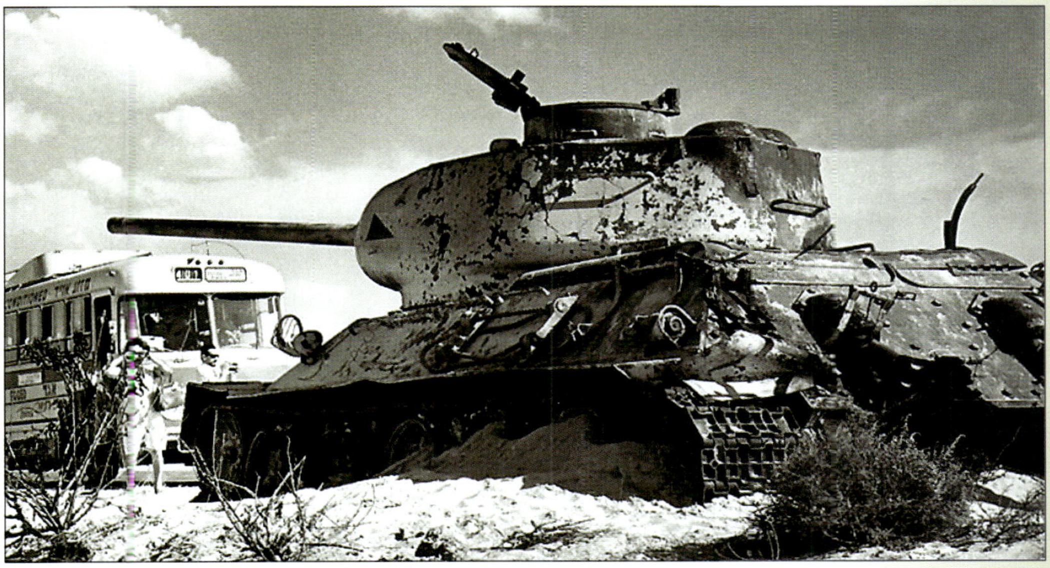

A wreck of Egyptian T-34-85 (Czechoslovak production) destroyed during the Six Day War in June 1967. Note the tactical marking on the turret – two-colour rectangle.

Regarding tactical markings, the Egyptian armoured forces symbol was a green-red or blue-violet rectangle, the colours divided by a diagonal line. During the conflicts in 1956 and 1967 green and red triangles were painted on turrets and forward hulls (usually at the left of the front armour plate) of the Egyptian T-34-85s. However, the identification of these markings is difficult. This is also the case with gun barrel markings, said to consist of wide green (and perhaps also blue) stripes applied in the middle or at the end of the barrel. It can be speculated that the location of the stripe denoted the sub-unit. In photos taken during a parade in Cairo (before the outbreak of the Suez crisis) thin, black stripes (one, two or three) are visible on T-34-85 gun barrels, though again, the purpose of this marking is hard to confirm. Egyptian units used geometric symbols as tactical markings – circles, squares and rhombuses located on the front armour plate, to the left of driver's hatch. Registration plates were placed on the fenders at the front and rear. These contained the inscription "army" in Arabic and a four-digit number. In the late 1960s and early 1970s, three-digit tactical numbers began to be applied to Egyptian T-34-85s on the forward section of the turret, and sometimes also on fenders. According to some sources, some vehicles also had Egyptian flags painted on the turrets. A few photographs confirm that this was the case, but not when the markings were applied as the dates the photographs were taken are unknown.

In the photos from the aforementioned parade in Cairo in 1956, interesting emblems are visible on the turrets of T-34-85s: a rhinoceros, a warthog, an elephant, and pyramids. According to some sources, these were parade markings, but this is not certain as such emblems can also be seen in photos of Egyptian vehicles in combat conditions.

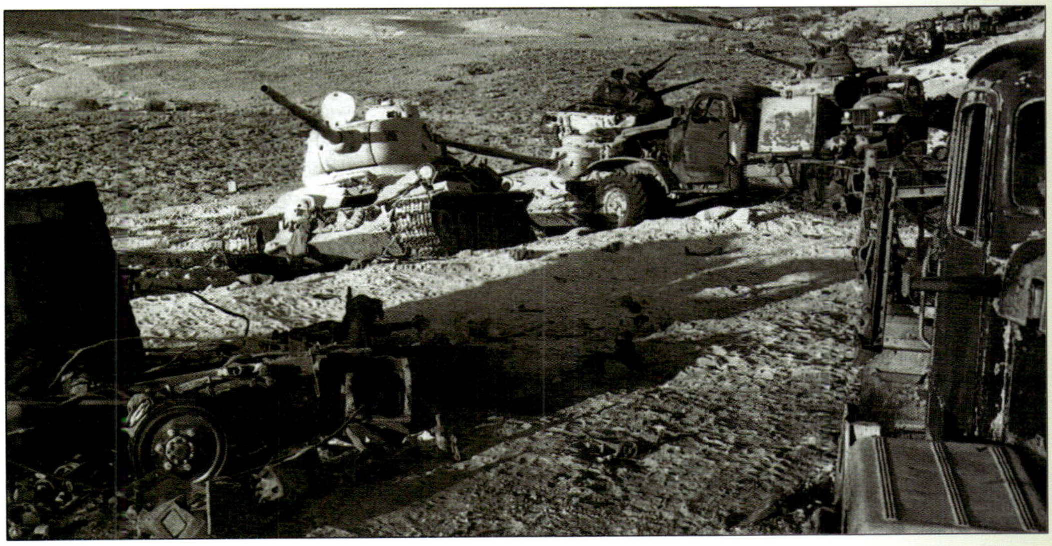

A column of Egyptian military vehicles destroyed during the Six Day War in June 1967. The T-34-85 has a tactical marking in form of rectangle on the turret.

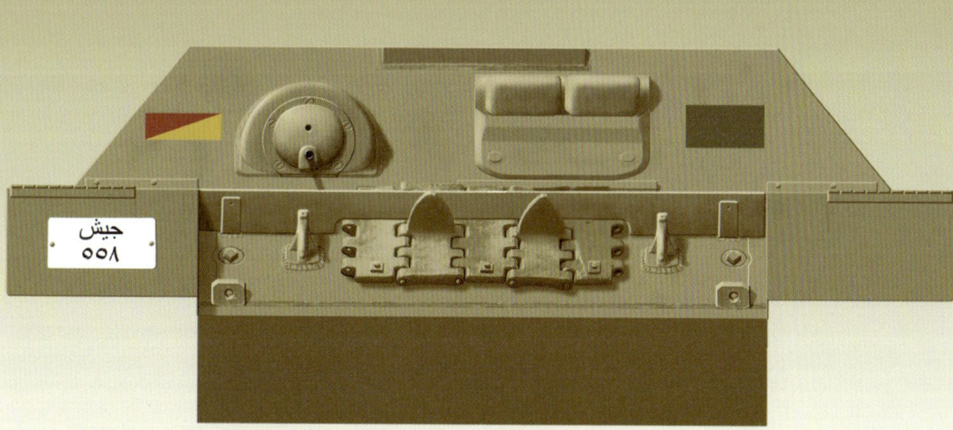

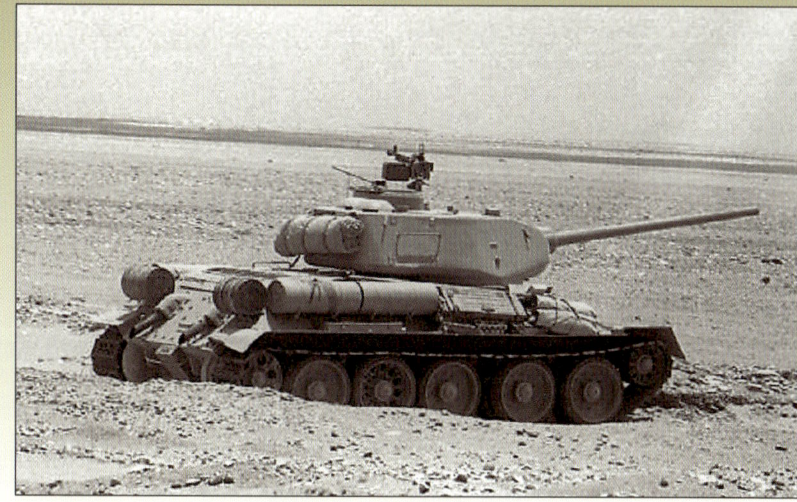

An Egyptian T-34-85 (Czechoslovak production), photographed in the desert, probably late 1960s/early 1970s. The tank has no tactical markings. Of interest are local modifications: DShK machine gun on the turret, raised forward part of the fender, additional boxes, including one in the lower part of the hull and long exhaust pipes.

Egypt

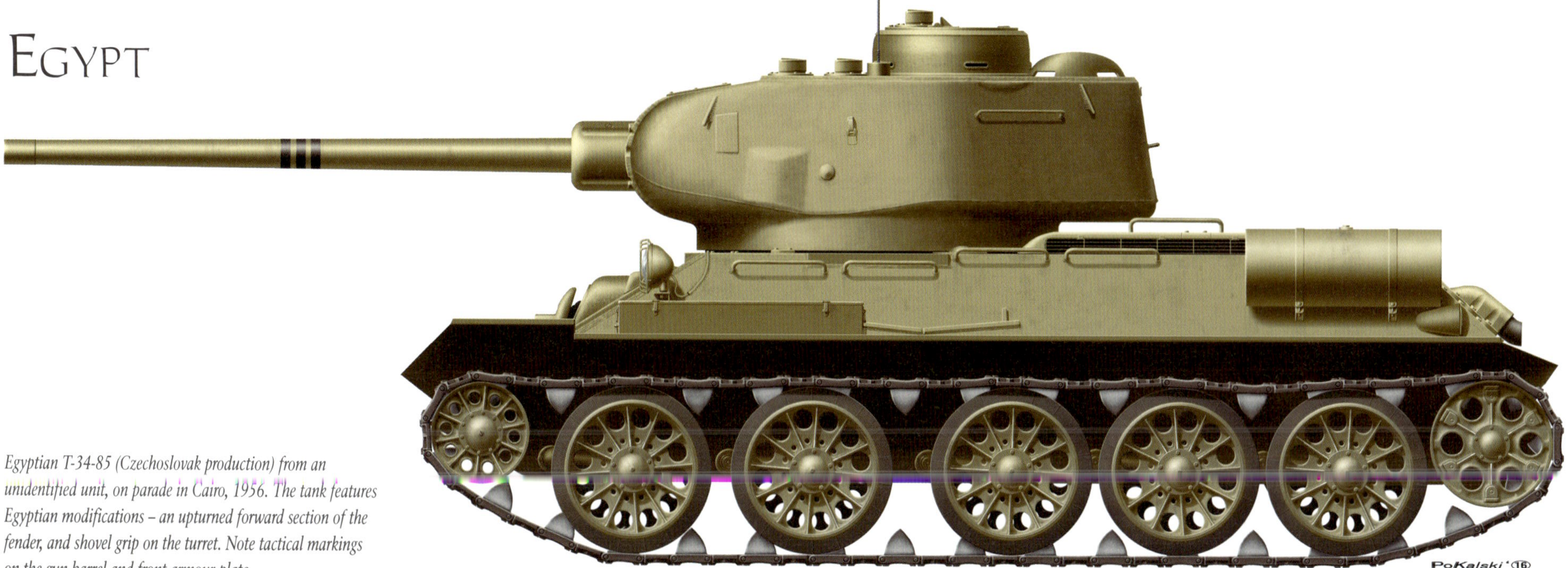

Egyptian T-34-85 (Czechoslovak production) from an unidentified unit, on parade in Cairo, 1956. The tank features Egyptian modifications – an upturned forward section of the fender, and shovel grip on the turret. Note tactical markings on the gun barrel and front armour plate.

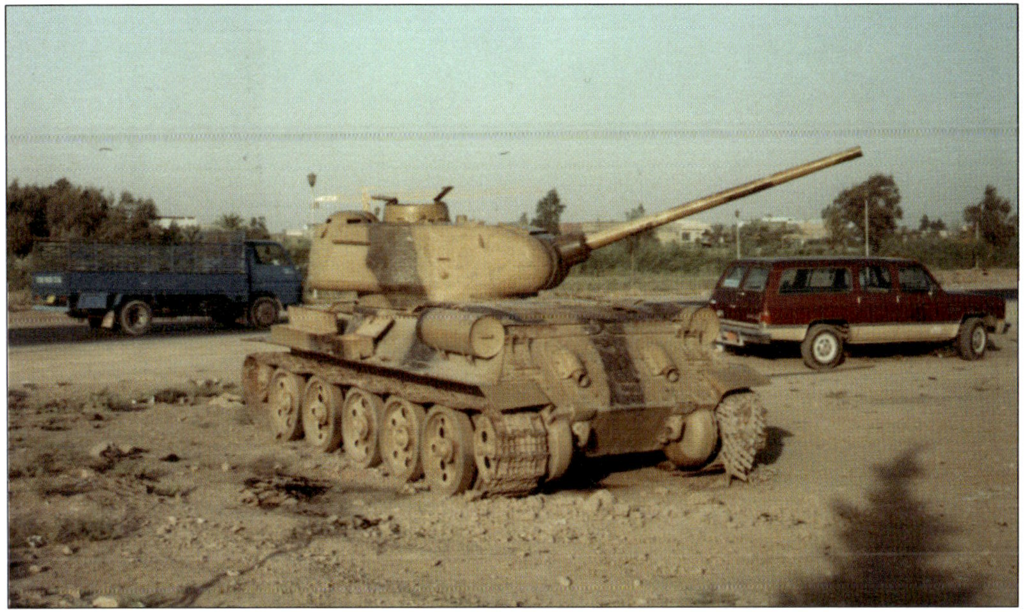

A T-34-85 Model 1969 (wartime Plant No. 174 production with "etalon" type turret) photographed on the outskirts of Baghdad in 1982. At that time the Iraqi army had the "thirty-fours" in their inventory, but it is not certain that the tank in the photograph was operated by a combat unit.

Iraq

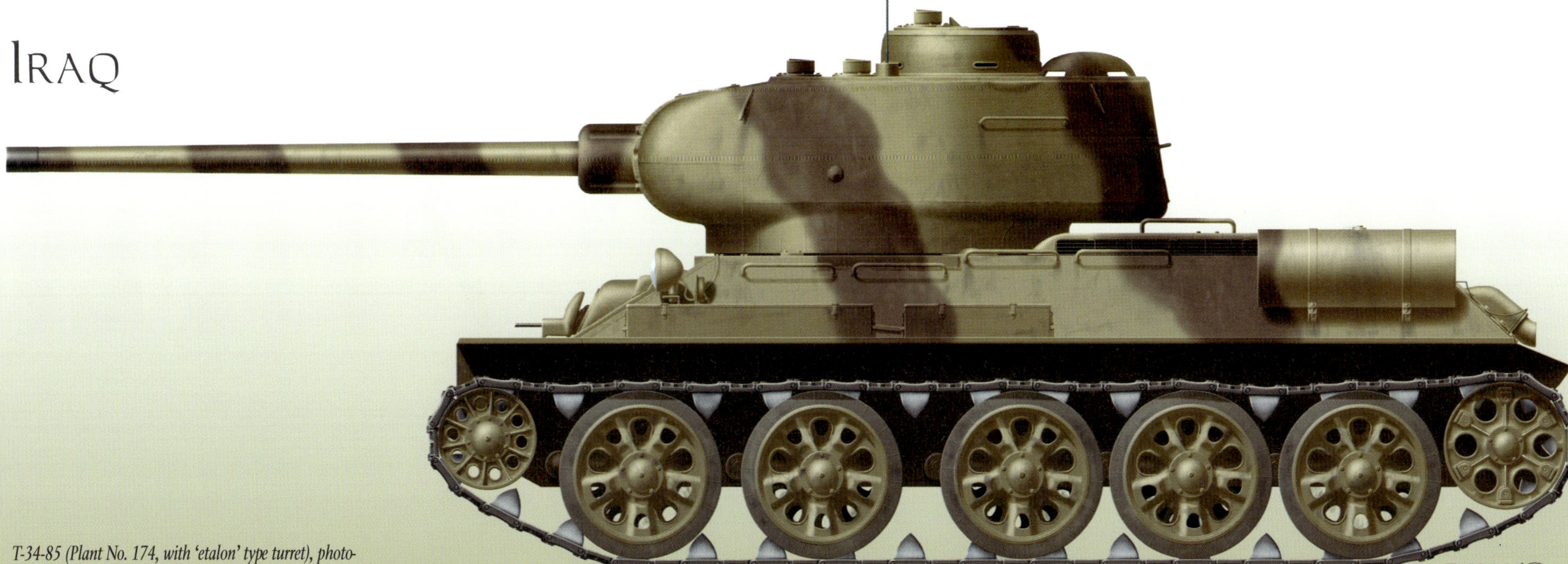

T-34-85 (Plant No. 174, with 'etalon' type turret), photographed on the outskirts of Baghdad in 1982.

Iraq

The Iraqi army operated several hundred T-34-85 tanks, delivered during the 1960s and 1970s. According to some sources, they saw use even during the early period of the Iraq-Iran war, but this cannot be confirmed.

It is very difficult to find information about paint schemes and markings of Iraqi T-34-85 tanks. They were probably covered with an all-over sand colour paint scheme. Multi-colour schemes cannot be ruled out, but the only known photo depicting a T-34-85 in two-tone sand-and-tan camouflage, taken in 1982 on the outskirts of Baghdad, shows a tank acting as monument or children's playground apparatus, and the scheme it wears is not necessarily authentic.

Tanks of the combat units sported three – or four-digit tactical numbers painted on the turrets (forward section). According to some authors, Iraqi flags were painted on the turrets of some tanks, but this information has not been confirmed by photographic evidence.

Israel

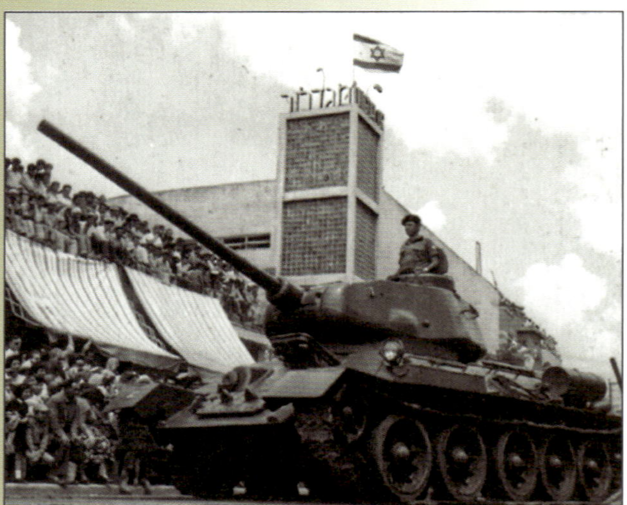

During fighting with Egypt and Syria, the Israeli army captured at least a few T-34-85s. These tanks entered Zahal's inventory, but were not used in combat. The tanks were painted green and sand, and had no markings except for the bridge classification sign – a white number 33 in a dark blue circle with red outline on the right fender.

***Left:** A T-34-85 (Czechoslovak production) displayed at a parade on the occasion of the 9th anniversary of Israel's independence. On this occasion several tanks of this type were displayed. They were probably repainted in Israel. Bridge classification symbol – white number 33 on dark blue circle with red outline is painted on the right fender.*

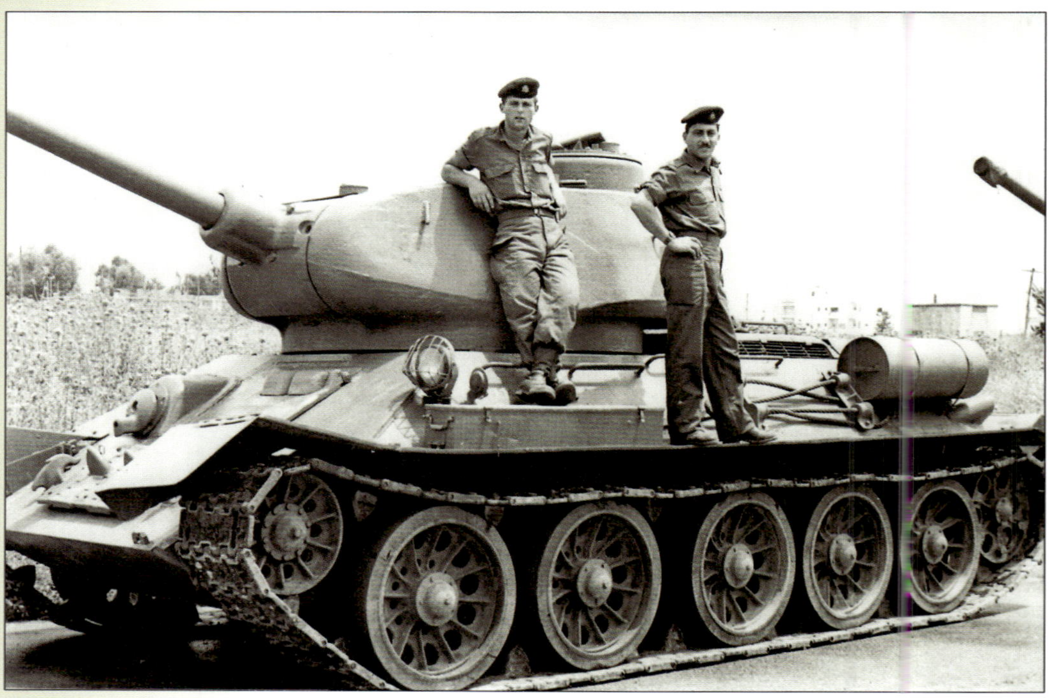

Israeli soldiers posing with a captured T-34-85 (Czechoslovak production). It is an Egyptian tank captured in 1956. Interestingly, the forward section of the fender is upturned, but it is not a raised fender, featured by many Egyptian "eighty-fives".

Yemen

Based on the evidence of a few photos, it can be stated that T-34-85 tanks used during fighting in Yemen in 2015 wore diverse paint schemes. However, usually the tanks had three-colour camouflages: green and tan camouflage patches sprayed onto a basic sand colour. Some tanks probably remained in overall sand livery. No tactical numbers are visible in available photographs.

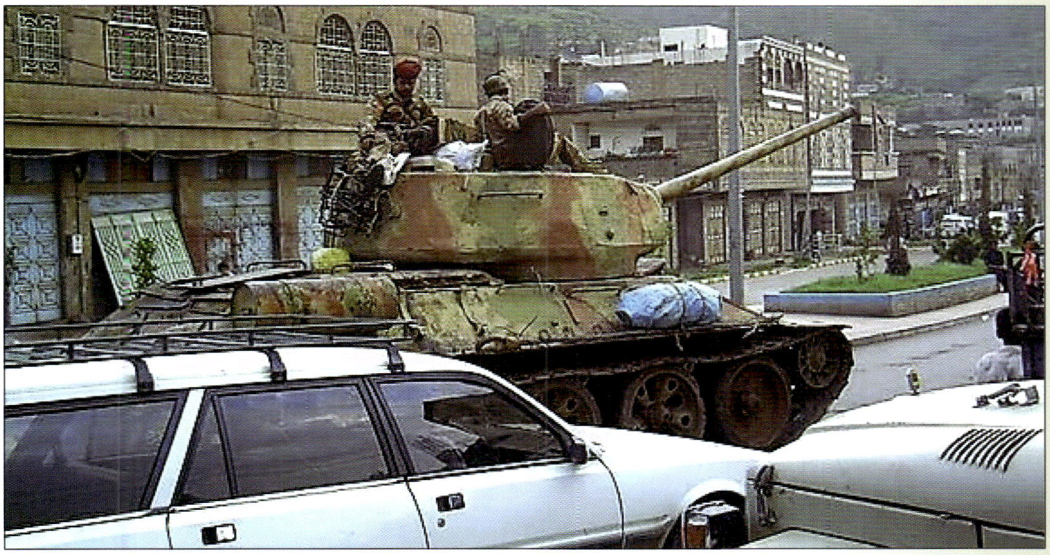

A modified T-34-85 (Plant No. 183) in the street of Yemeni capital Sana in 2015. The tank wears a three-colour camouflage, worn also by Su-100 self-propelled guns.

Lebanon

During the hostilities in Lebanon in the 1970s and 1980s, T-34-85 tanks were operated by units of the pro-Syrian militia and Palestine Liberation Organisation (the tanks had reportedly been delivered from Hungary, but this has not been confirmed). The paint schemes of these vehicles were diverse and seemingly arbitrary, and therefore it is hard to generalise. However, it seems that many vehicles wore a two-colour camouflage, with sand brown patches over a basic olive green colour. The shade of this colour and size of the patches were diverse. Patriotic slogans or even photographs of local heroes were often placed on the tanks.

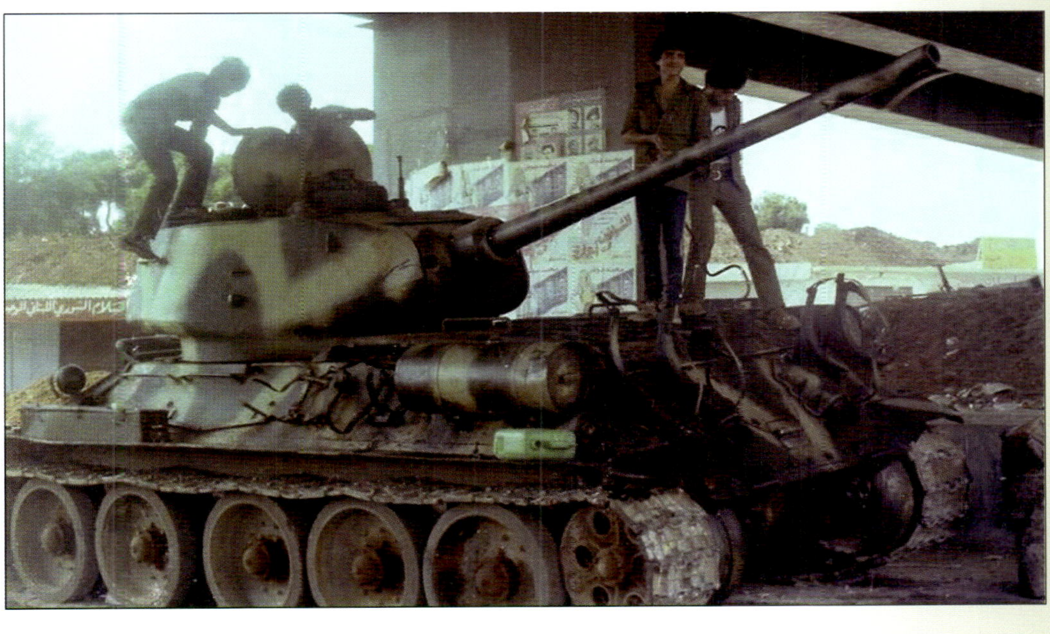

T-34-85 of Czechoslovak production, operated in early 1980s by pro-Syrian militia units during fighting in Beirut. The tanks wears two-colour camouflage – sand splotches applied on basic olive green.

Yemen

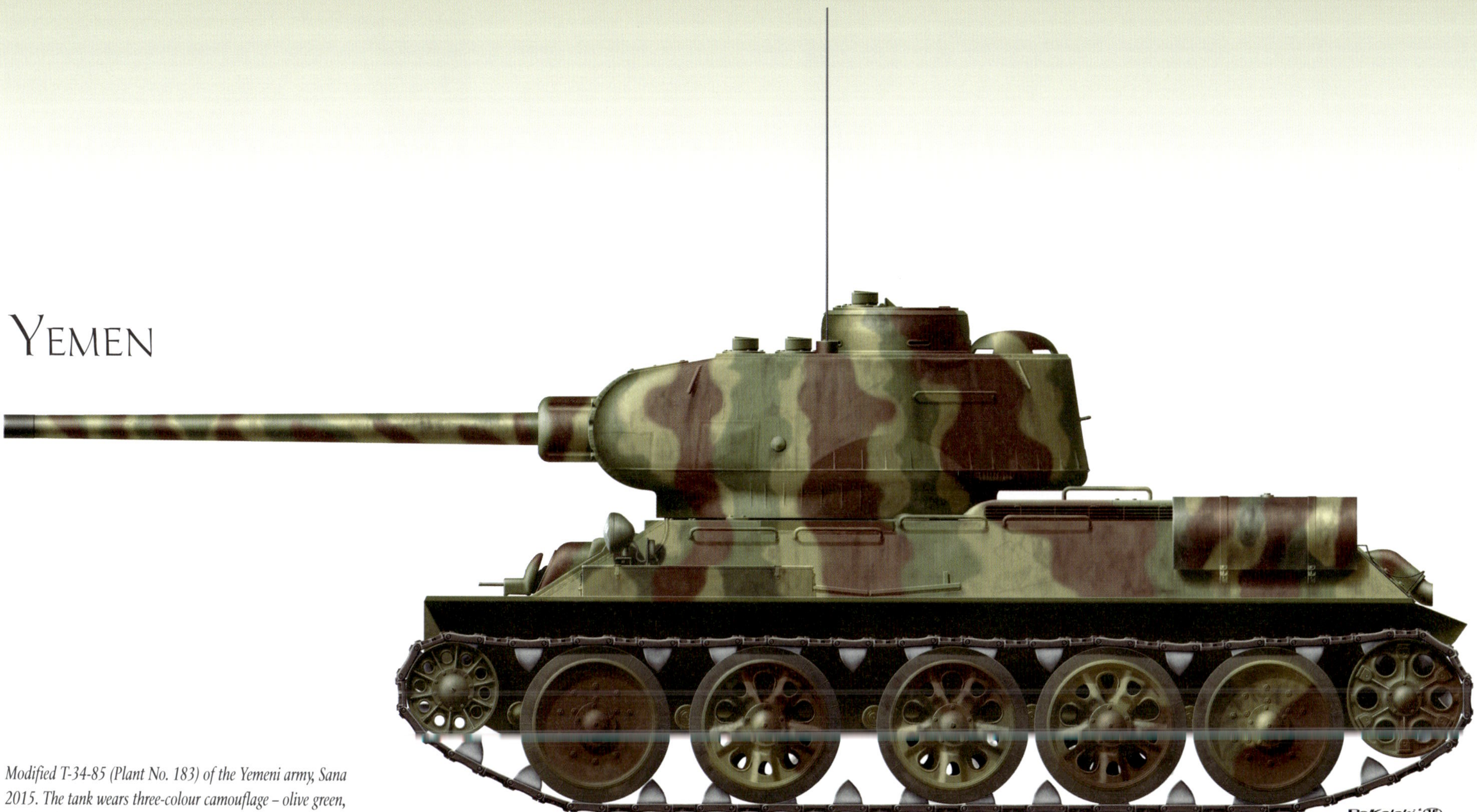

Modified T-34-85 (Plant No. 183) of the Yemeni army, Sana 2015. The tank wears three-colour camouflage – olive green, sand and tan.

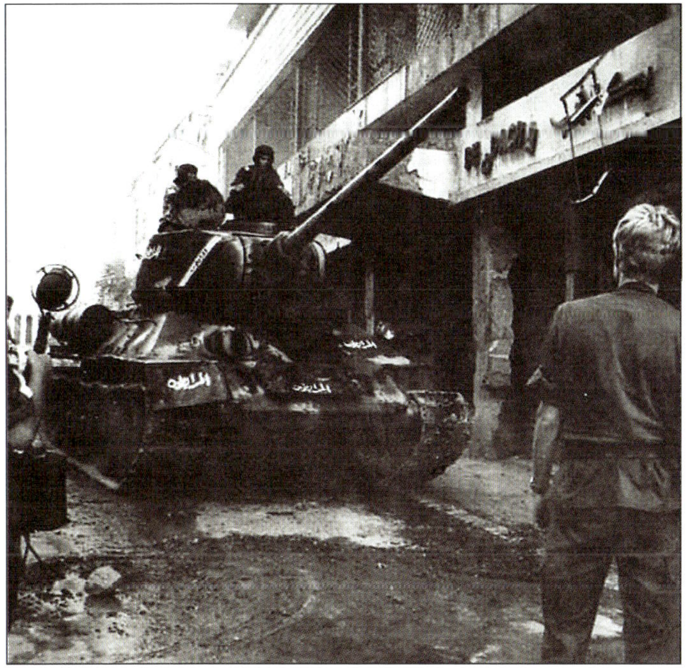

LEBANON

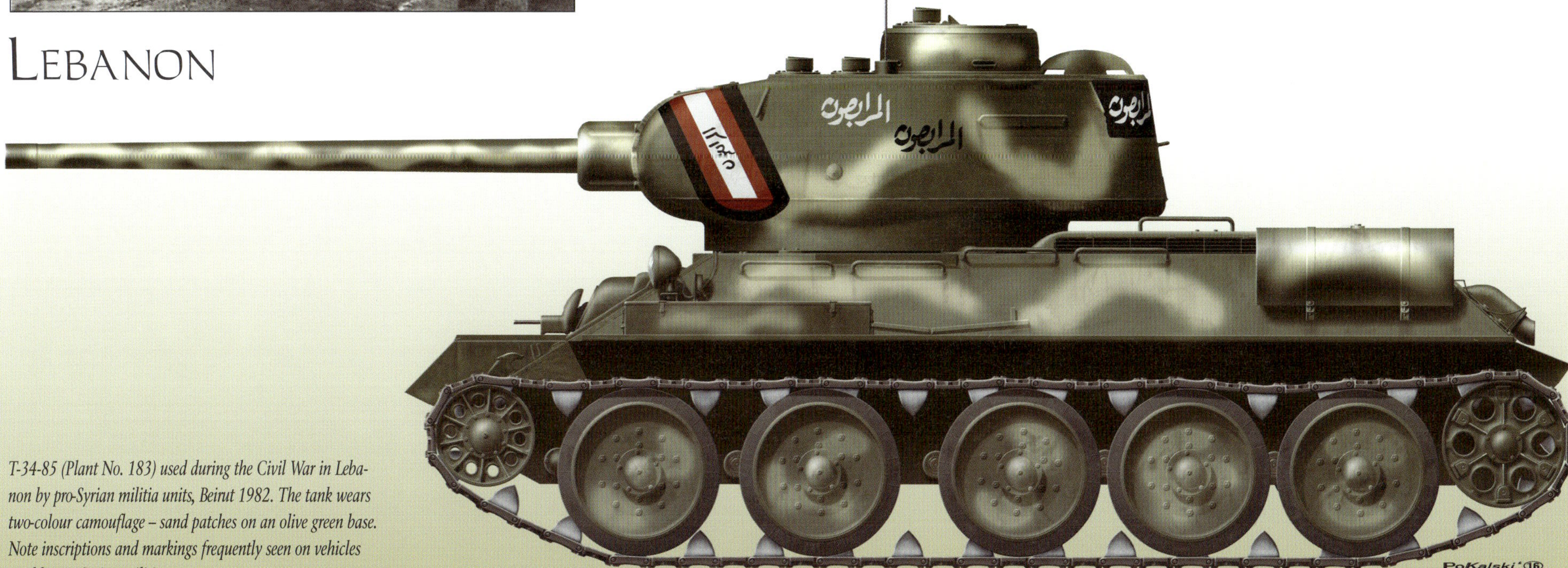

T-34-85 (Plant No. 183) used during the Civil War in Lebanon by pro-Syrian militia units, Beirut 1982. The tank wears two-colour camouflage – sand patches on an olive green base. Note inscriptions and markings frequently seen on vehicles used by pro-Syrian militia.

Syria

T-34-85 tanks were delivered to Syria from the USSR and Czechoslovakia. In total at least 220 'eighty-fives' were delivered to this country. The Syrians made minor modifications, of which the most distinctive was the installation of a 12.7 mm DShK anti-aircraft machine gun mounted on the commander's hatch.

Initially the tanks were painted dark green. However, photographs taken in 1961, during the crisis caused by the breakup of the Egyptian-Syrian union, show tanks participating in a parade wearing disruptive camouflage. It seems that this consisted of tan patches applied over a basic green colour. A few colour photographs, although of poor quality, seem to confirm the multi-colour camouflages. Moreover, photographs of Syrian tanks captured by Israel in 1973 show that some T-34-85s sported three-colour camouflages, with sand and tan patches applied on the basic green colour. Some sources say that the third colour was not tan, but grey. Indeed, in some pictures the camouflage patches appear to be grey.

As far as tactical markings were concerned, distinctive inscriptions could be seen painted on the turrets of some tanks, honouring Syrian heroes of the 1948 war with Israel. They were used from the early 1960s to the early 1970s. At that time, white tactical numbers, usually of three digits, appeared. In the 1960s a small, white (five-digit) serial number and inscription "Army" were painted on the front armour plate. In that decade the Syrians also used geometric tactical markings – circles and triangles. They were usually painted on the turrets, but also on the front fenders. During the Six Day War, white circles were painted on the turret roofs of the Syrian tanks as quick recognition markings for friendly aircraft.

A Syrian T-34-85 (Czechoslovak production) during a parade in Damascus in 1961. The tank wears a typical dark green paint scheme and markings. The name of an Arab hero of the war with Israel was painted on the turret. Registration plate is fitted to the front armour plate and the tactical marking is painted on the fender.

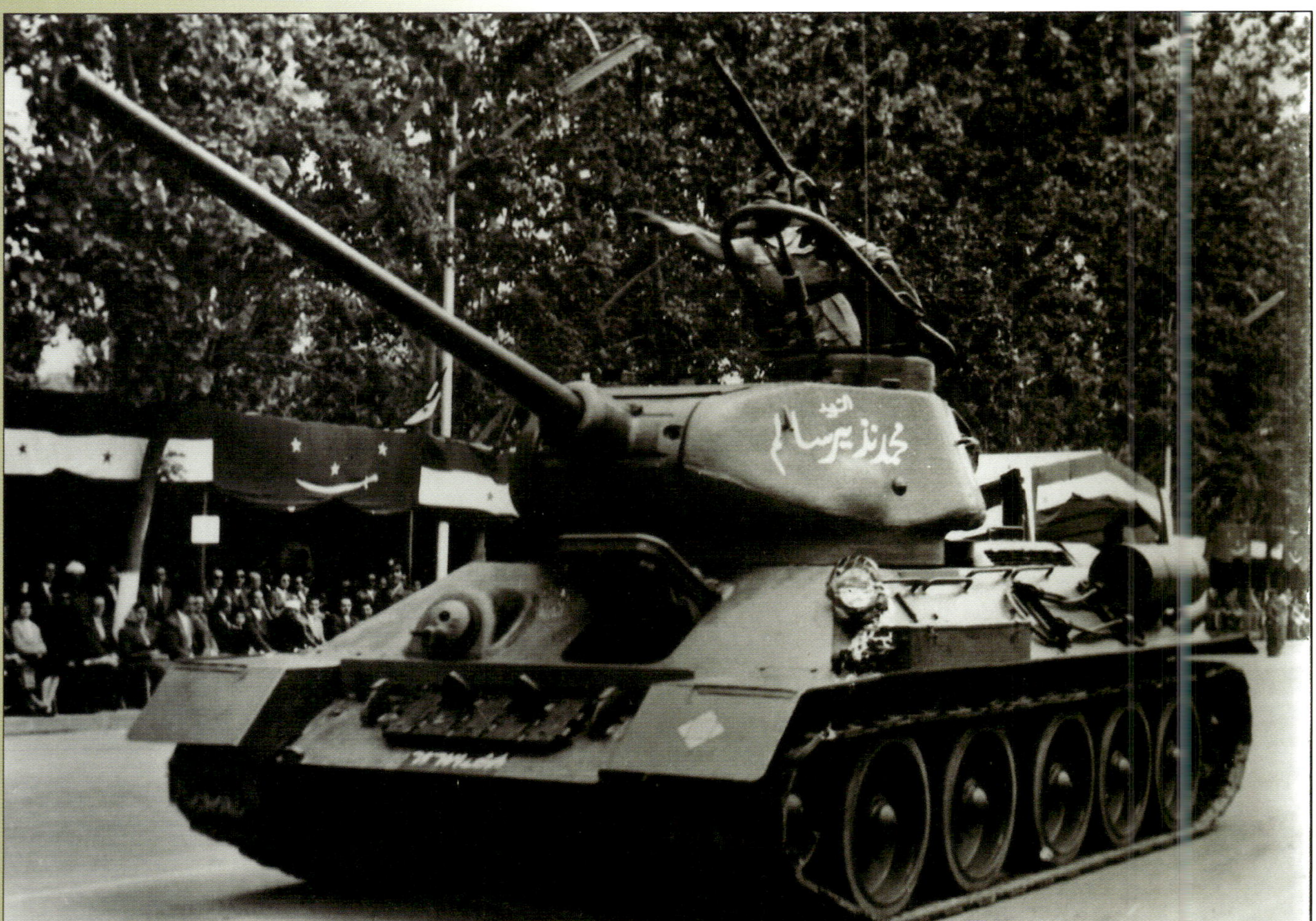

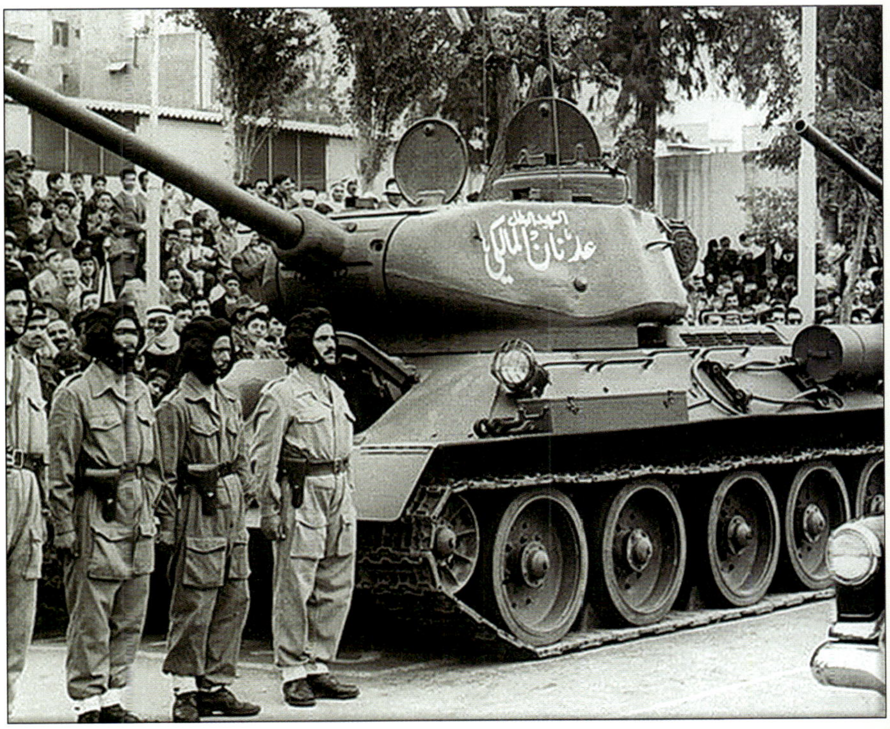

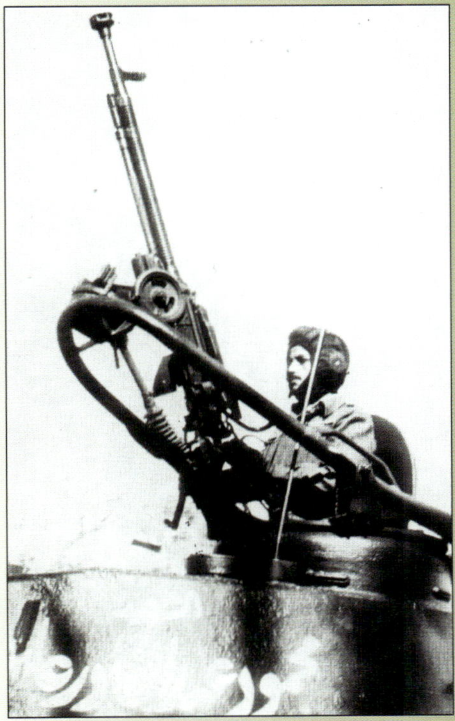

Above, left: *A Syrian T-34-85 (Czechoslovak production) photographed during a military parade in Damascus. According to some sources this photograph was taken in April 1957, which means that the deliveries of these tanks to Syria took place earlier than some sources say (early 1960s).*

Above: *Commander of a T-34-85 tank photographed during Egyptian-Syrian crisis in 1961. The photograph is of poor quality, but the tank might have worn two-colour camouflage.*

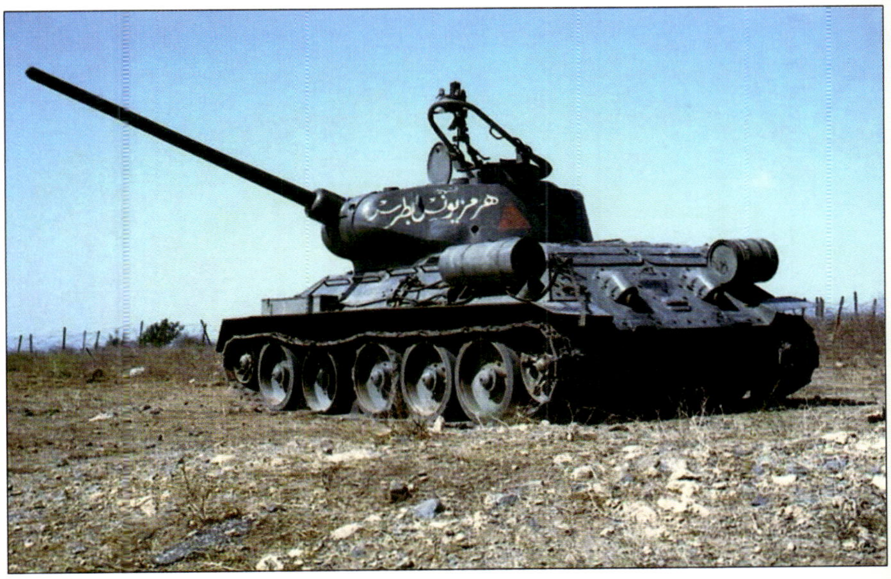

Middle: *Wreck of a Syrian T-34-85 (Czechoslovak production) burnt during the Six Day War in June 1967. The markings suggest that the tank was assigned to the 44th Armoured Brigade.*

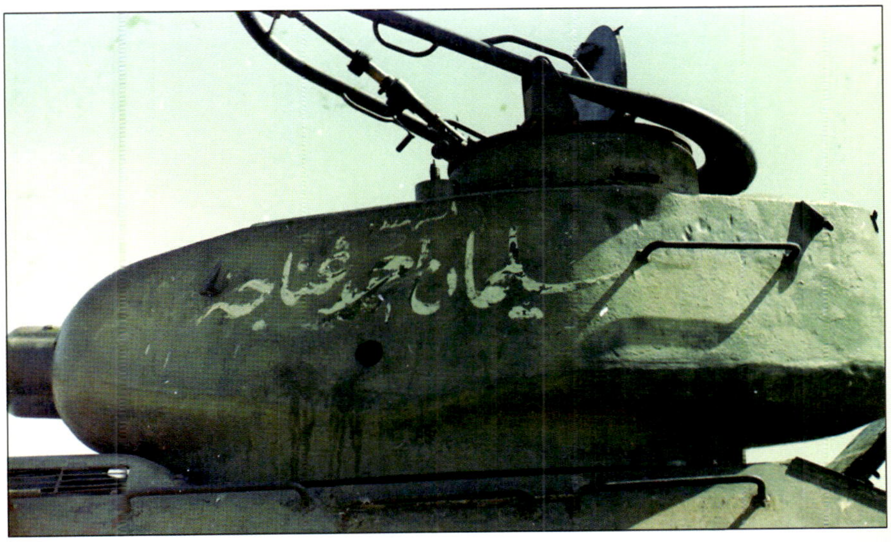

Turret of a destroyed Syrian T-34-85 with lettering (name of a hero of the war with Israel).

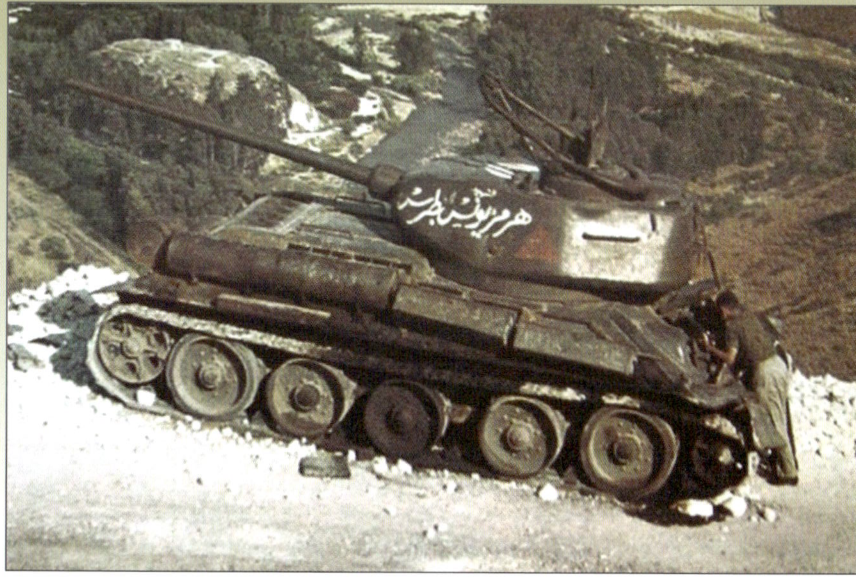

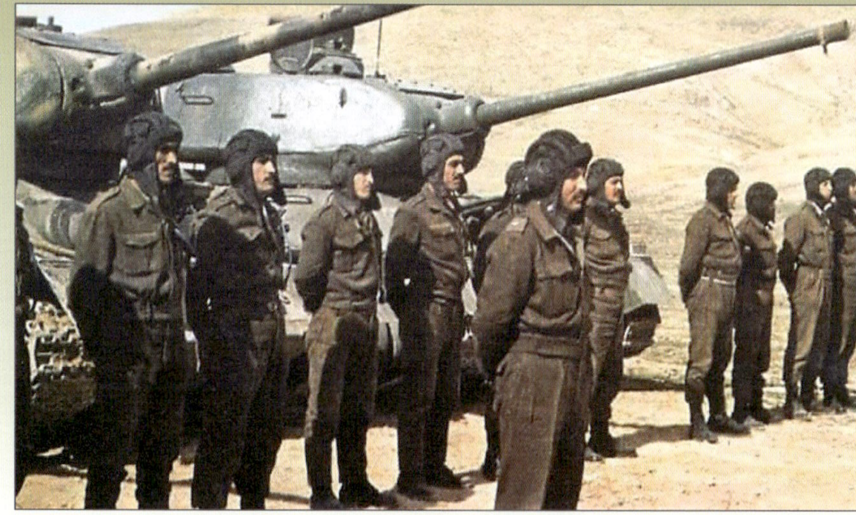

Crews of Syrian T-34-85s in front of their tanks. One of the tanks wears a camouflage pattern similar to that of Syrian T-55 and T-62 tanks in the 1970s.

Syria

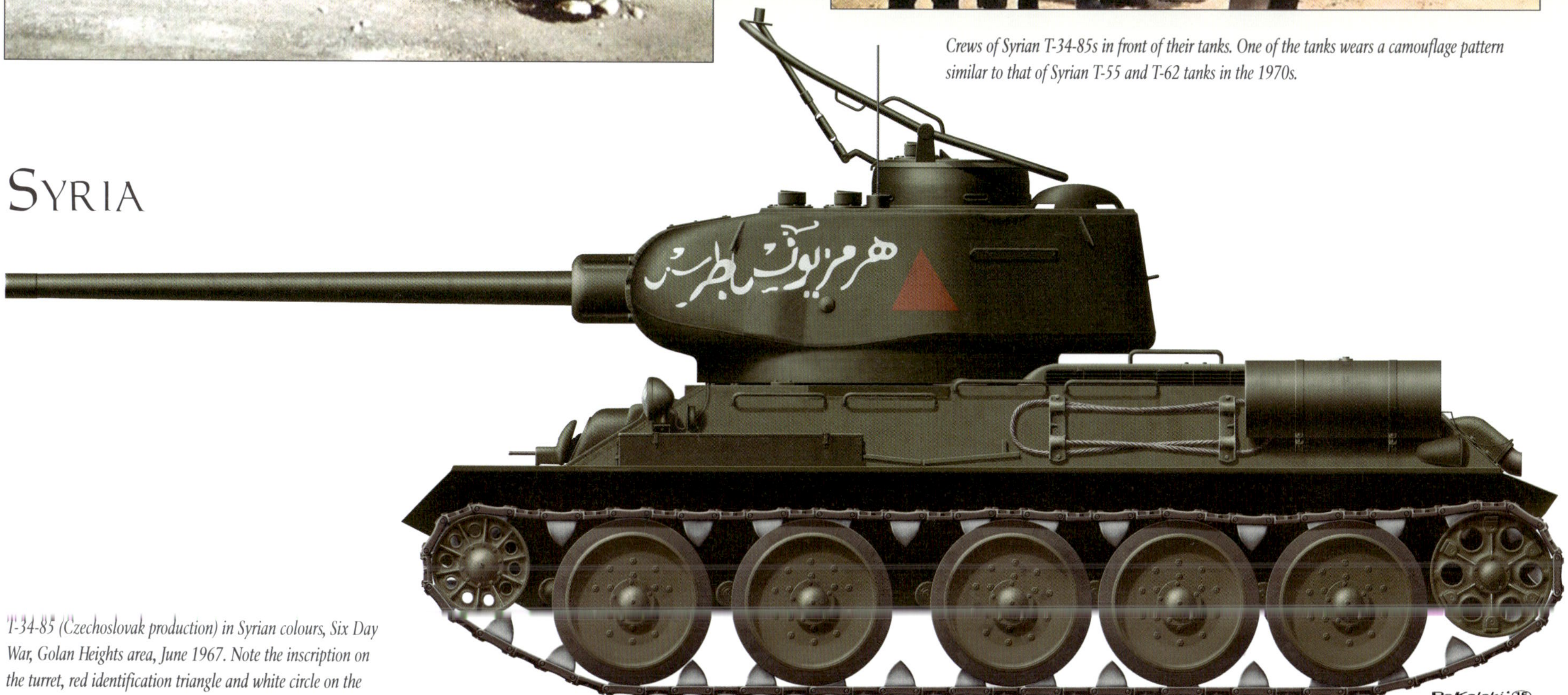

T-34-85 (Czechoslovak production) in Syrian colours, Six Day War, Golan Heights area, June 1967. Note the inscription on the turret, red identification triangle and white circle on the roof of the turret – an aerial identification marking.

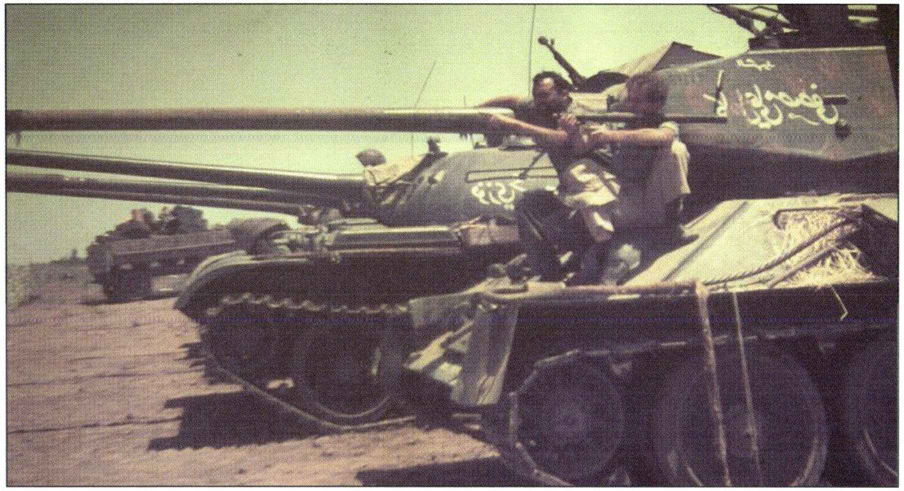

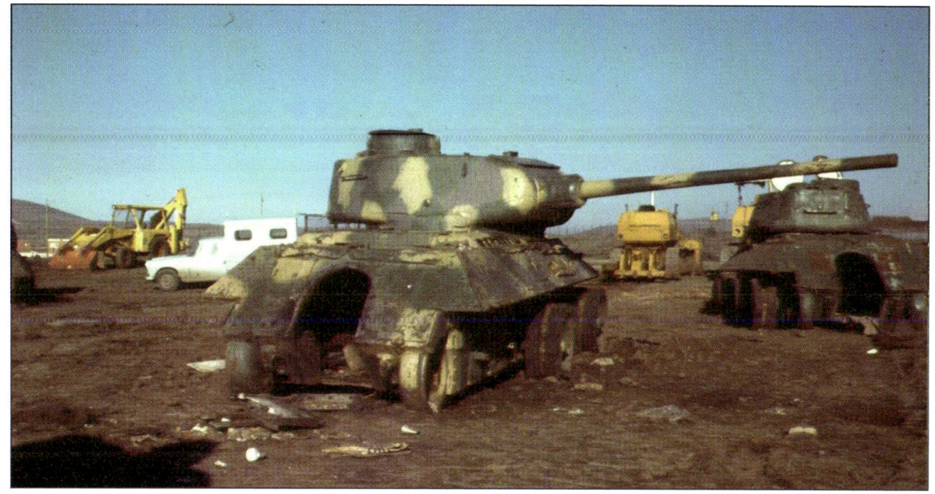

Another proof that Syrian multi-colour camouflage schemes existed. The photograph shows stocks of materiel captured by Israel in 1973. T-34-85 tanks were converted to shelters of fixed firing points.

Syria

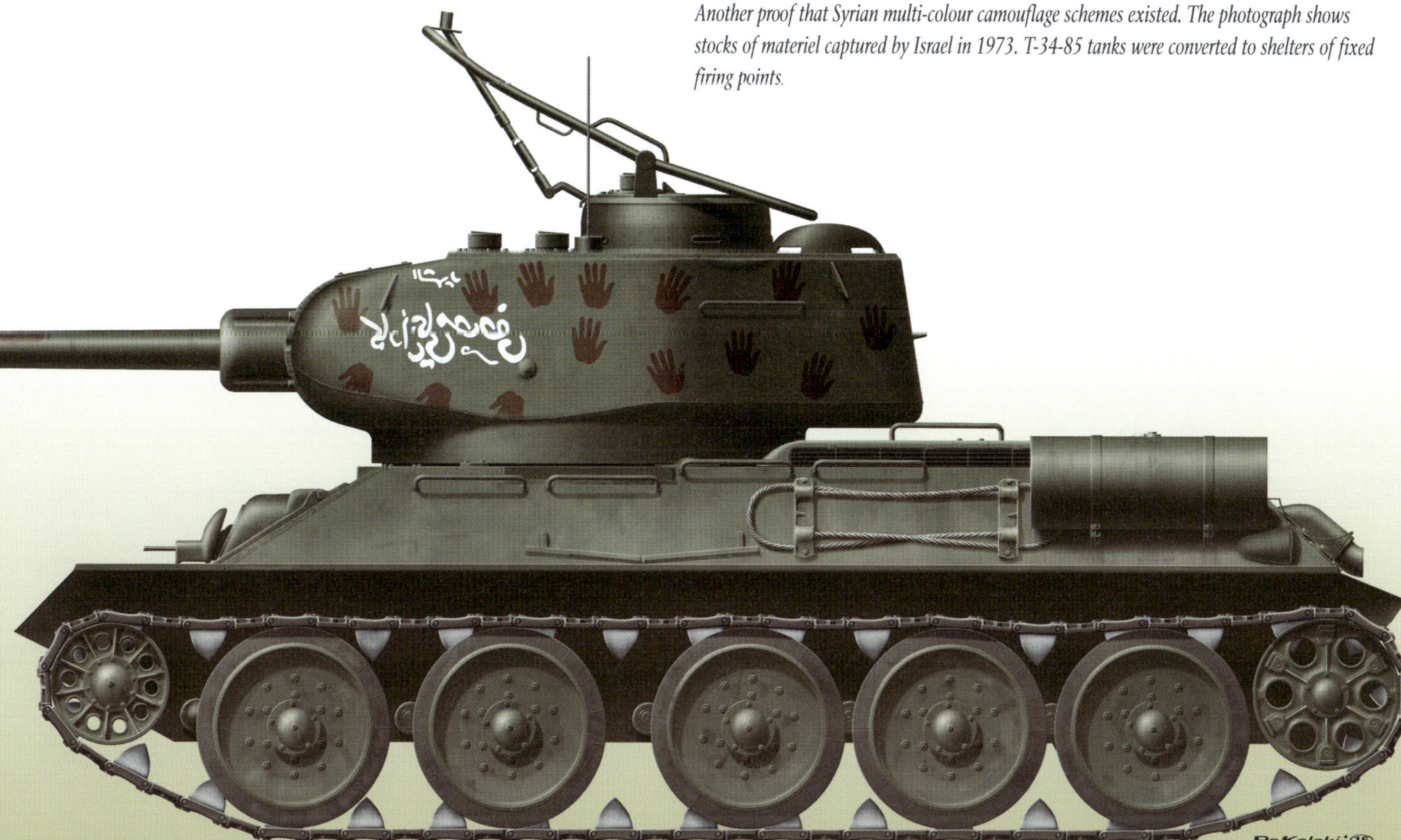

T-34-85 (Czechoslovak production) in Syrian colours, of an unidentified unit, probably at the turn of 1960s/70s. The tank wears an atypical camouflage scheme – brown patches in form of hand prints applied on a dark green background on the turret.

Africa

T-34-85 tanks also proved to be attractive export goods in Africa. They found their way to many countries: Algeria, Angola, Congo, Guinea, Equatorial Guinea, Guinea-Bissau, Ethiopia, Libya, Mali, Mozambique, Somalia, Sudan, Togo and Zimbabwe. Interestingly, in addition to exports from the USSR, numerous other countries exported or re-exported tanks to African nations, including China, Czechoslovakia and East Germany. However, this matter is poorly documented and photographs are rare, and therefore only a selection of paint schemes used in African countries as documented by photographic evidence can be described below.

Angola

The number of T-34-85 tanks operated by Angolan army (FAPLA) units is not known exactly. This uncertainty results from the fact that they had been delivered by the USSR and Czechoslovakia, while Cuba also granted tanks in "fraternal support". It can be estimated that in the 1970s between 125 and 200 T-34-85 tanks were delivered to Angola.

Most tanks wore an overall olive green paint scheme. Analysing photographs of tanks captured by the South Africans and wrecks of tanks destroyed during the hostilities suggests that some may have had camouflage consisting of brown patches on a basic olive green background. As far as tactical markings are concerned, some tanks had none, some had white tactical numbers (usually three-digit), and other tanks had white tactical letter-numeric designations, e.g. 9F1, O-321.

T-34-85 Model 1969 tanks captured by the South Africans during Operation "Protea" in 1981.

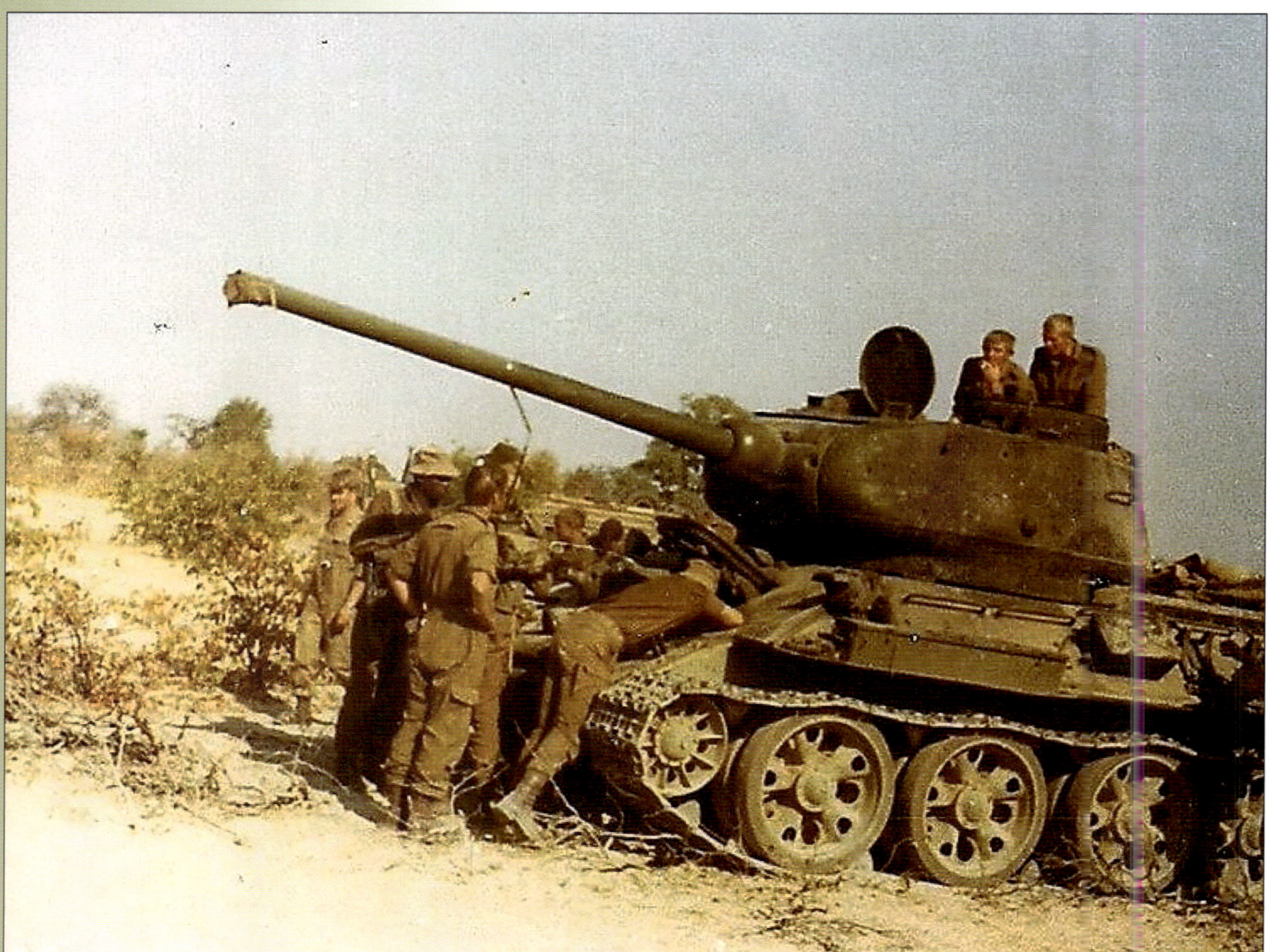

Ethiopia

At the beginning of the 1980s, more than 100 T-34-85 tanks had been delivered to Ethiopia by two countries, the USSR and East Germany. Most tanks featured modifications characteristic of the T-34-85 Model 1960 and Model 1969. Ethiopian T-34-85s took part in the fighting with Somali units in Ogaden province, where their opponents were often other T-34-85s. Several Ethiopian tanks of this type were captured by the insurgents of the Western Somali Liberation Front. Based on the few photos available, it seems that the main colour of Ethiopian 'eighty-fives' was olive green. Tactical markings do not appear to have been used.

Mozambique

About 40 T-34-85s were delivered to Mozambique during 1977–78 from the USSR, Czechoslovakia and East Germany. The tanks were painted olive green, as they had been delivered. There is no information about tactical markings.

Somalia

The first Somali T-34-85s were olive green with white, three-digit tactical markings (e.g. 122, 212). It cannot be ruled out that some tanks had four-digit numbers. However, the size and shape of the digits were not standardised. As far as national insignia are concerned, there were two types: the first was a black and red square divided in half, with dark circle and a white star inside. The other type was much simpler – a red and black square divided diagonally. On some tanks, white stars in a white-outlined circle were also painted (usually on the forward armour plate). This was probably a marking used only during military parades. Tanks used in the late 1970s had registration plates on the front and rear hull, with the Arabic inscription "Army" and a four-digit number. The quality of available photographs does not allow individual numbers to be established, unfortunately.

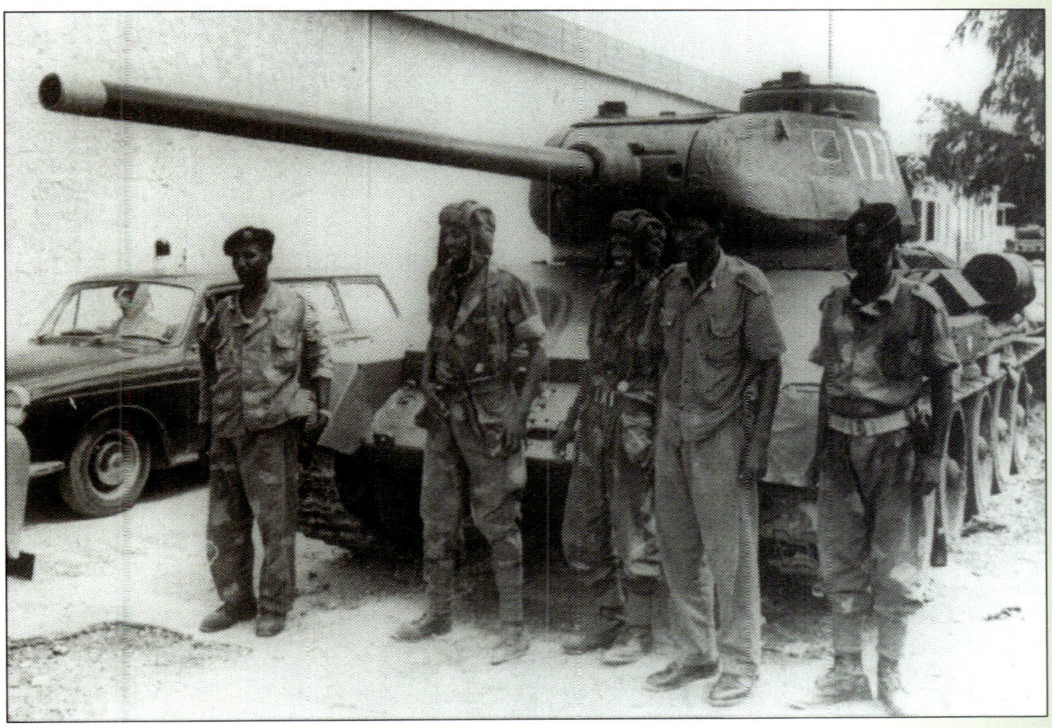

The crew of a Somali T-34-85 Model 1969 pose in front of their tank. The photograph was taken in 1978, during the conflict with Ethiopia. Note bright painted muzzle of the gun, early version of the national insignia (black and red square) and tactical number 122.

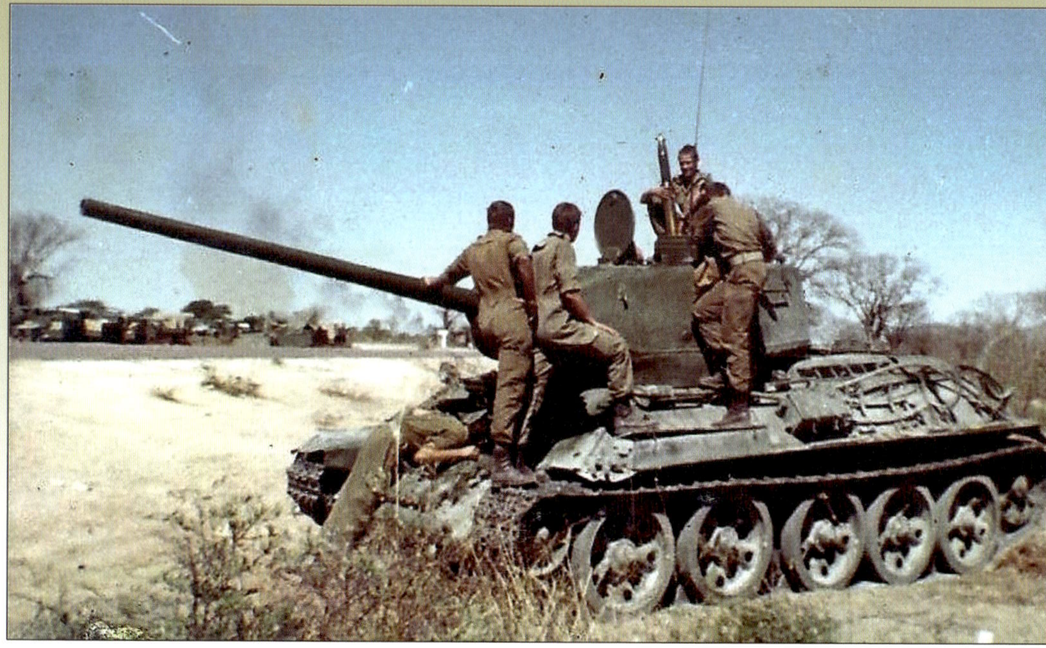

T-34-85 Model 1969 tanks captured by the South Africans during Operation "Protea" in 1981.

Angola

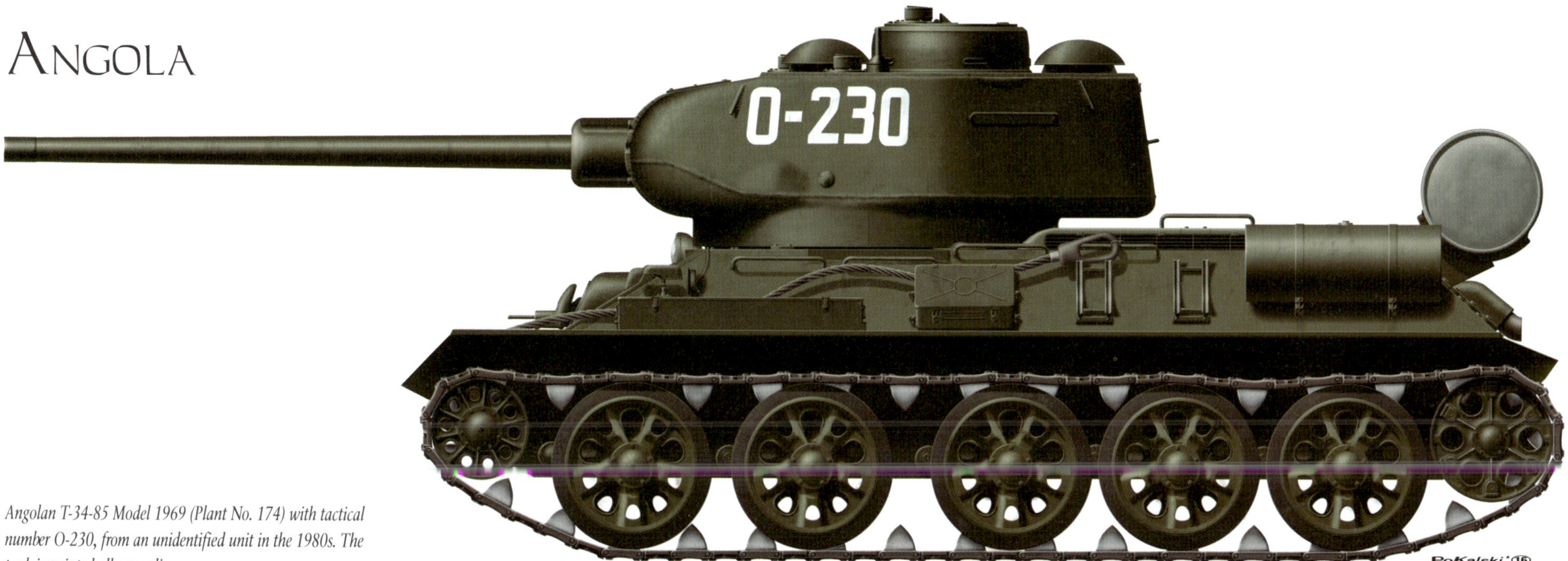

Angolan T-34-85 Model 1969 (Plant No. 174) with tactical number O-230, from an unidentified unit in the 1980s. The tank is painted all-over olive green.

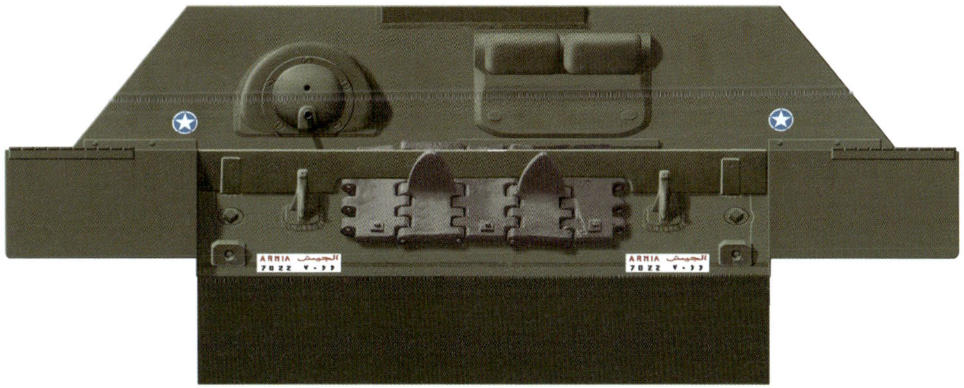

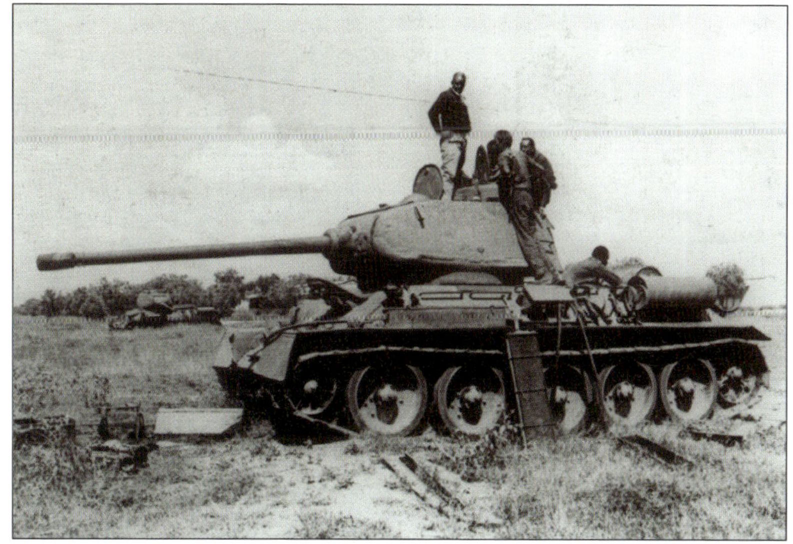

During the Somali-Ethiopian war in Ogaden province in 1978 both sides of the conflict operated T-34-85 tanks. The photograph shows an Ethiopian tank captured by the Somalis. It is a tank produced by Plant No.112 (with two single ventilators), modernized to Model 1969 standard. The wheels remained unchanged.

Somalia

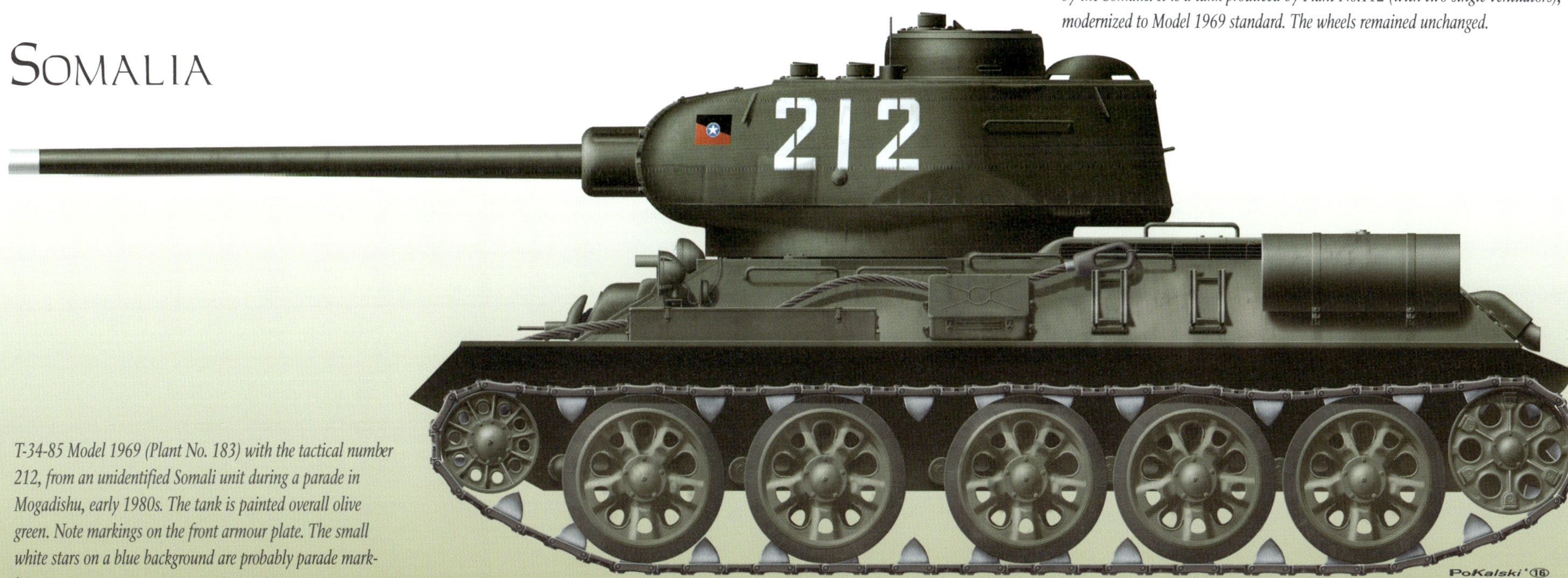

T-34-85 Model 1969 (Plant No. 183) with the tactical number 212, from an unidentified Somali unit during a parade in Mogadishu, early 1980s. The tank is painted overall olive green. Note markings on the front armour plate. The small white stars on a blue background are probably parade markings.

Zimbabwe

The units of the guerrilla organisation called the Zimbabwe People's Revolutionary Army (ZIPRA), which was the armed force of the Zimbabwe African People's Union, operated around 10 T-34-85 Model 1960 tanks. There is no information where the tanks were delivered to Zimbabwe from, and what their subsequent fate was, other than one such tank preserved at a military museum in Gweru.

The tanks probably had two-colour paint schemes of olive green with brown camouflage patches. The shade of the brown paint appears to have varied greatly, though it should be remembered that in the African climate, paints tend to fade very quickly.

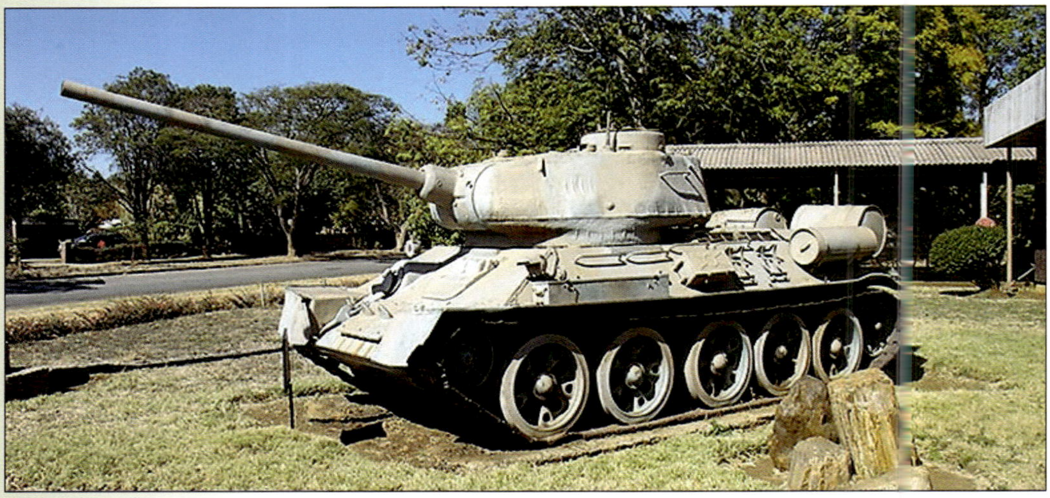

A T-34-85 Model 1969 tank (Plant No. 183 production) preserved at Gweru military museum. The tank has two-colour paint scheme, although it is difficult to make conclusions about tanks operated in Zimbabwe judging by the museum exhibit.

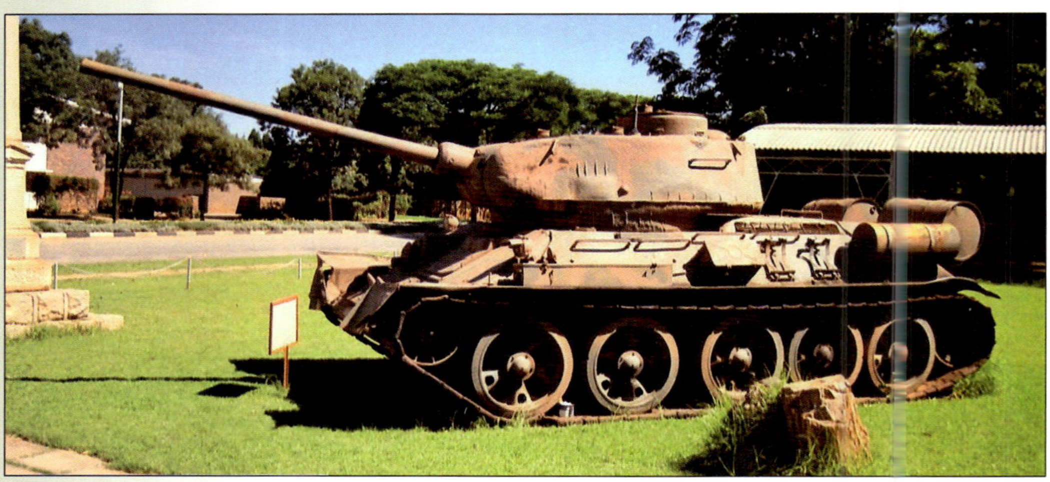

America

Cuba

The first T-34-85 tanks delivered to Cuba, and used to repel the invasion in the Bay of Pigs, were painted olive green. At that time the tanks had probably no tactical numbers.

Later the tanks were probably painted dark green. White, three-digit tactical numbers were applied on the turrets. Some tanks had a small star painted near the tactical number. Small, white stars were also sporadically painted on front fenders.

MODERNIZATIONS
CZECHOSLOVAK T-34-85

T-34-85 tanks of Czechoslovak production preserved at Lešany, Králíky, Rokycany and Smržovka museums. These tanks, although very similar to each other, differ in some details.

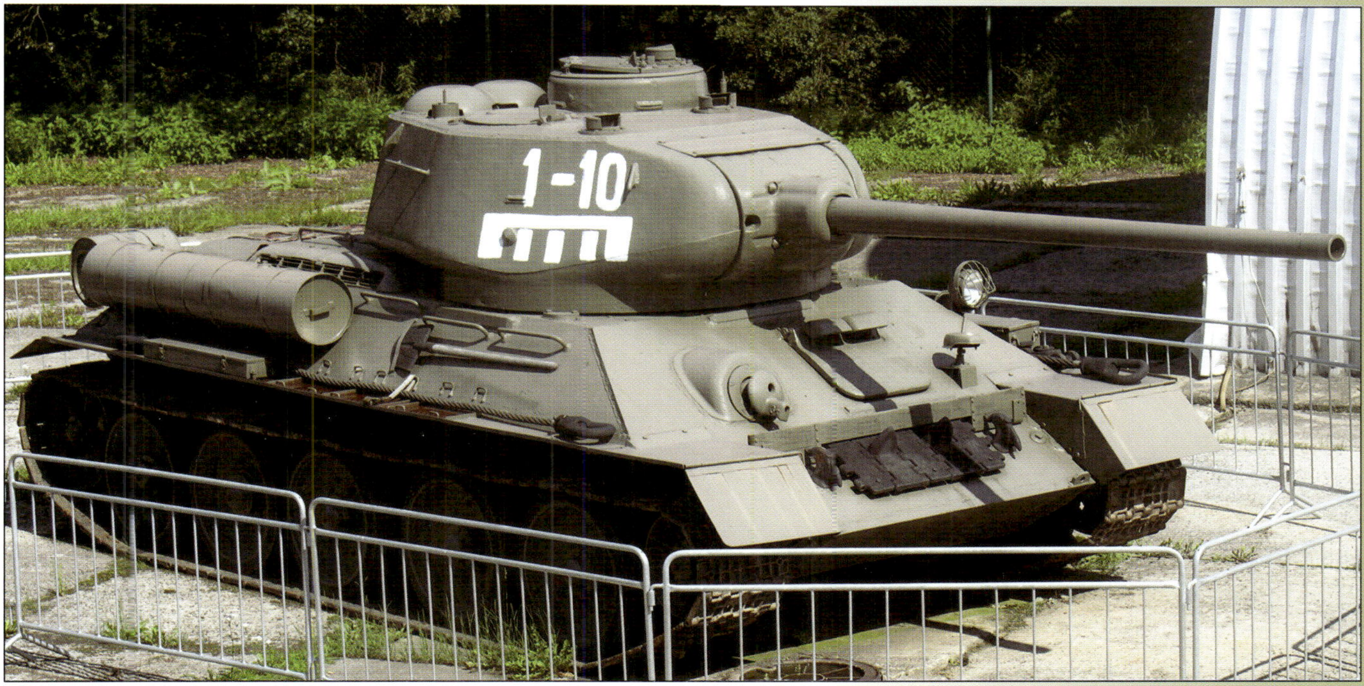

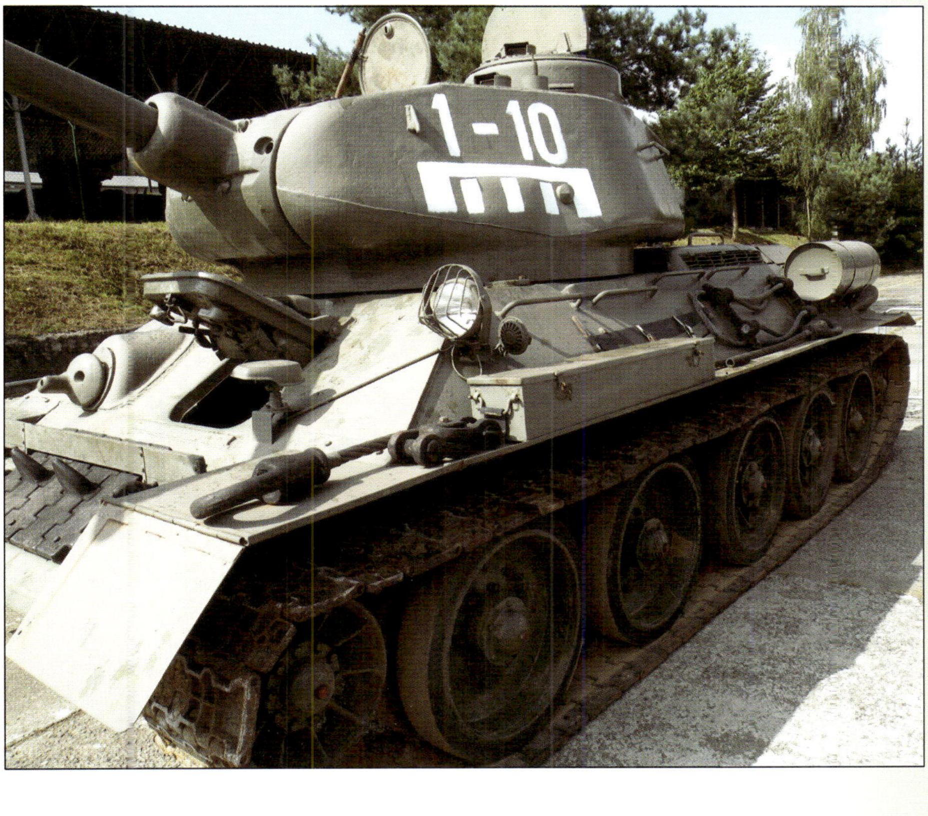

A Czechoslovak T-34-85 preserved at Lešany museum. The tank has the equipment of early 1950s.

A Czechoslovak T-34-85 displayed at Cihelna show in Králíky. The tank has equipment modernized in the 1960s.

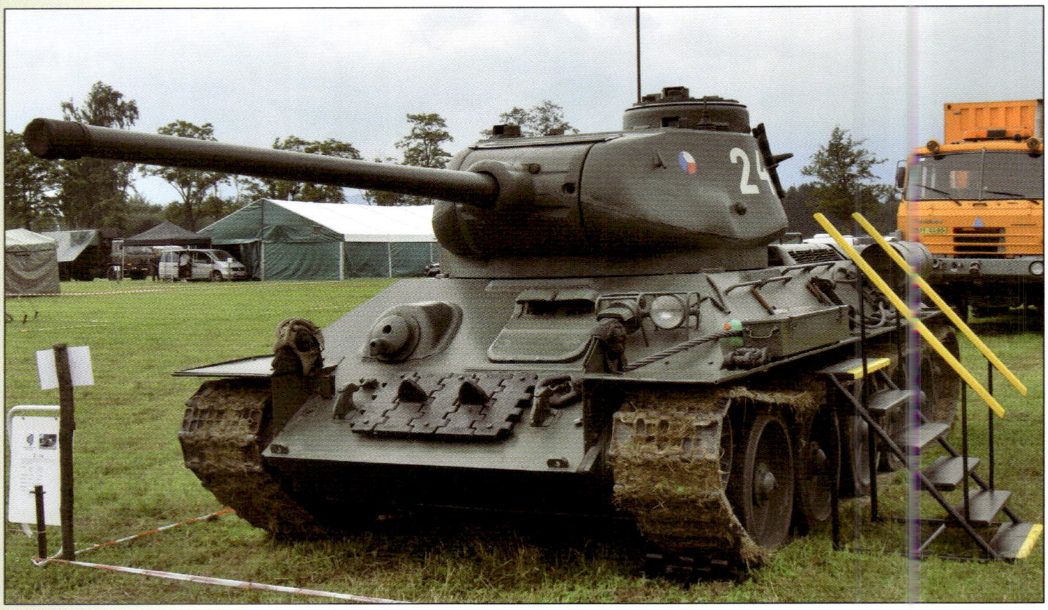

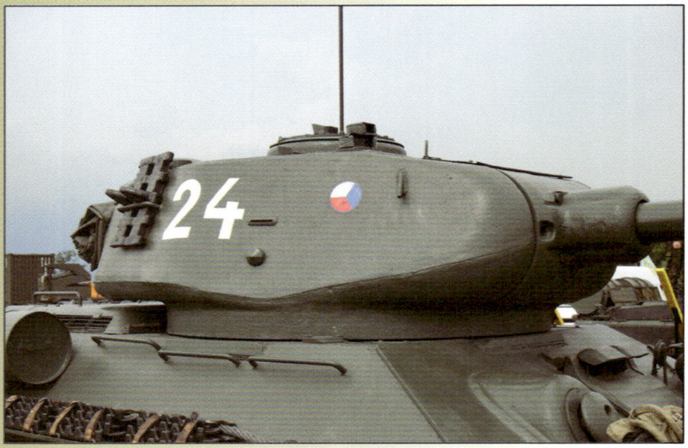

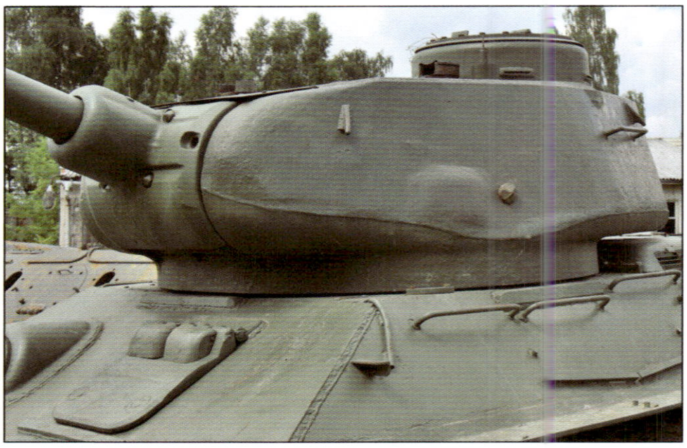

Details of the turret of Czechoslovak production. Note the quality of the casts and additional antenna mount on the turret roof.

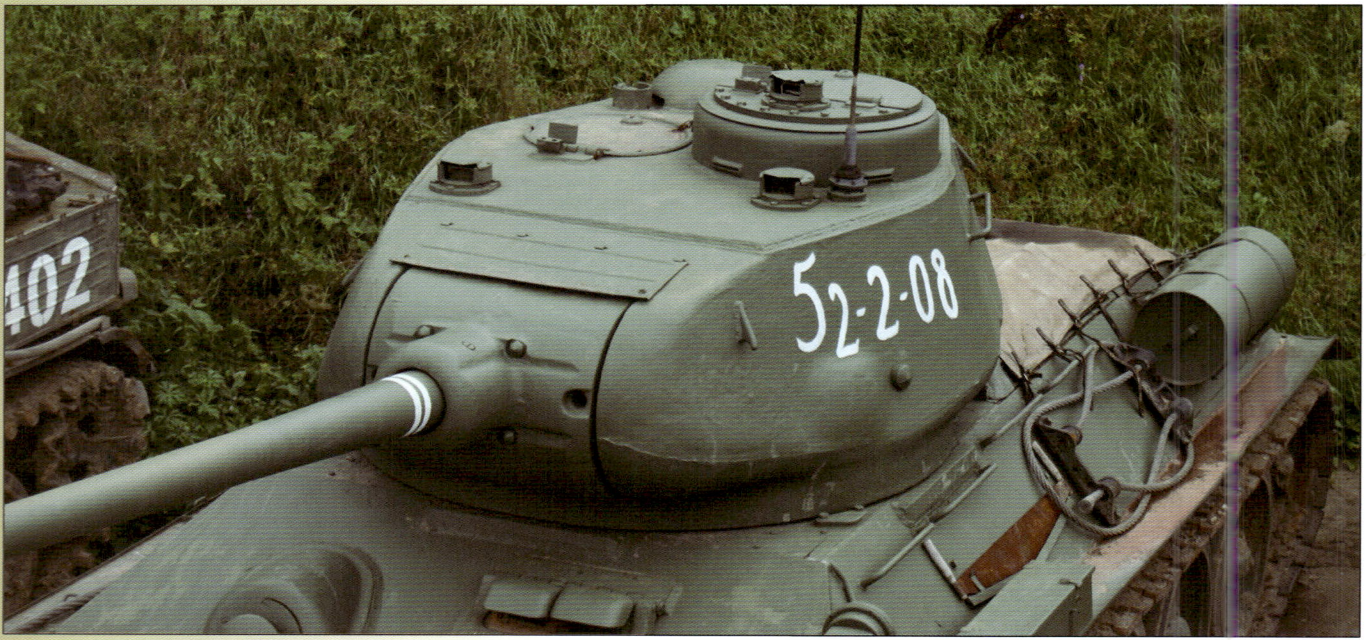

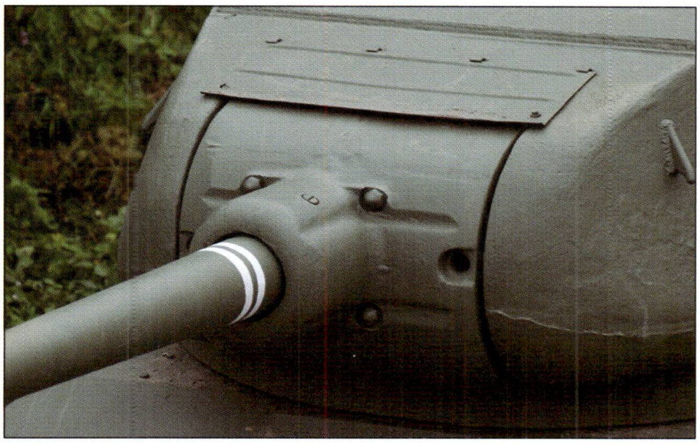

Gun yoke of a Czechoslovak T-34-85.

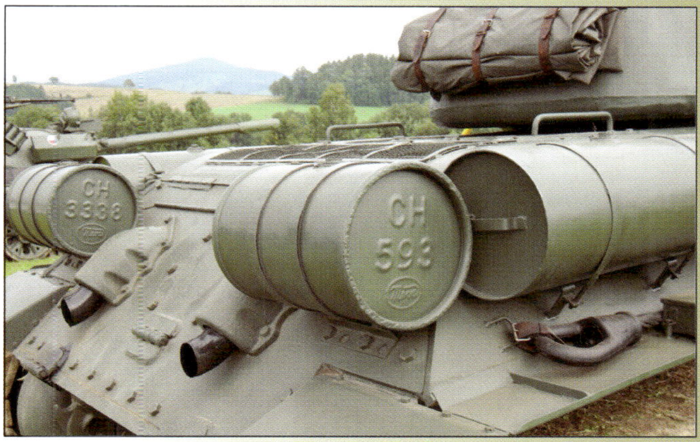

Rear section of the hull of a Czechoslovak T-34-85 with external fuel tanks. Note wide hinges on the rear armoured plate (6-segment, not 5-segment as the Soviet ones).

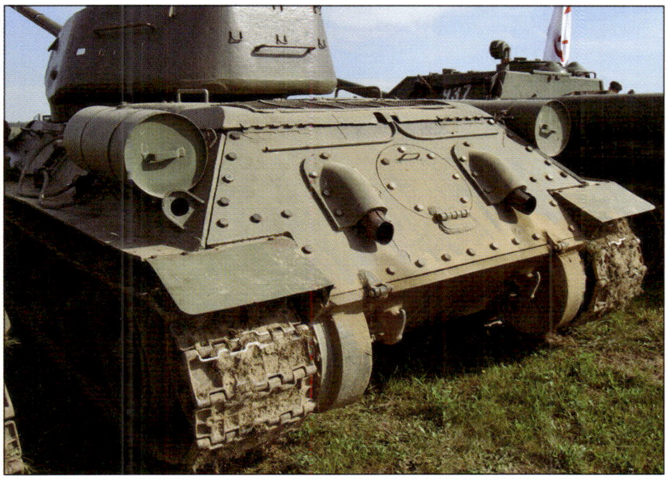

Rear section of the hull of another T-34-85 of Czechoslovak production with narrow hinges.

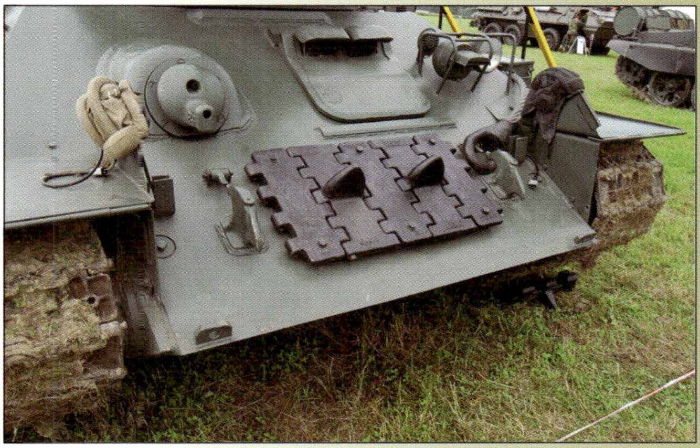

Forward section of the hull of a T-34-85 of Czechoslovak production.

Below, left: *Lights with shroud.*

The signaling device for communication between the desant and crew characteristic for tanks of Czechoslovak production.

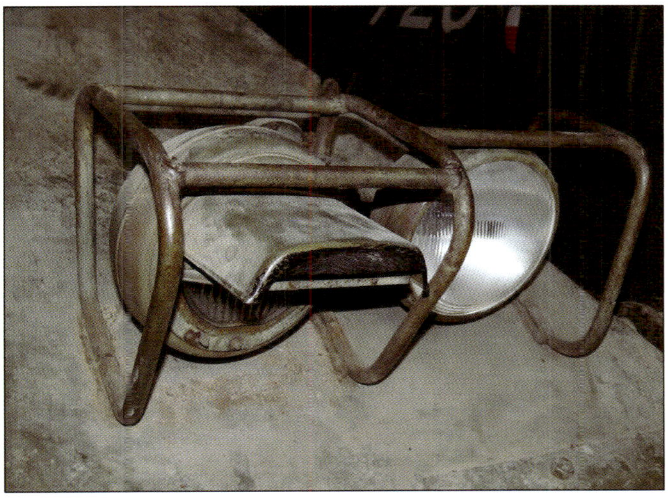

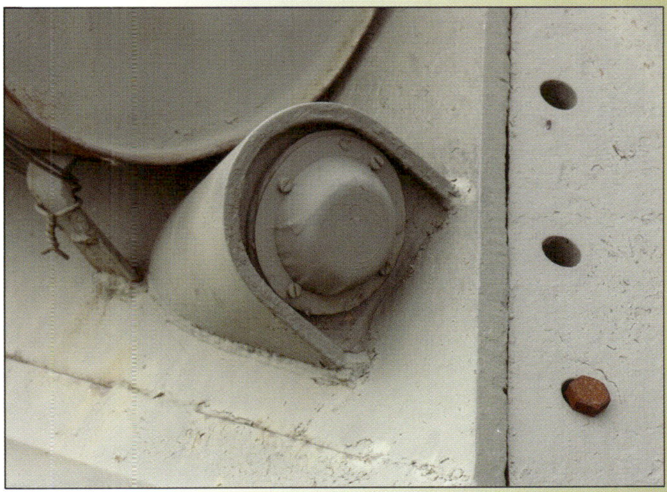

Yugoslav *Teski Tenk Vozilo A*

A Yugoslavian tank *Teski Tenk Vozilo A* preserved at the military museum in the Kalemegdan fortress in Belgrade. Note the new shape of the turret and hull armour plates. The drivetrain remained unchanged.

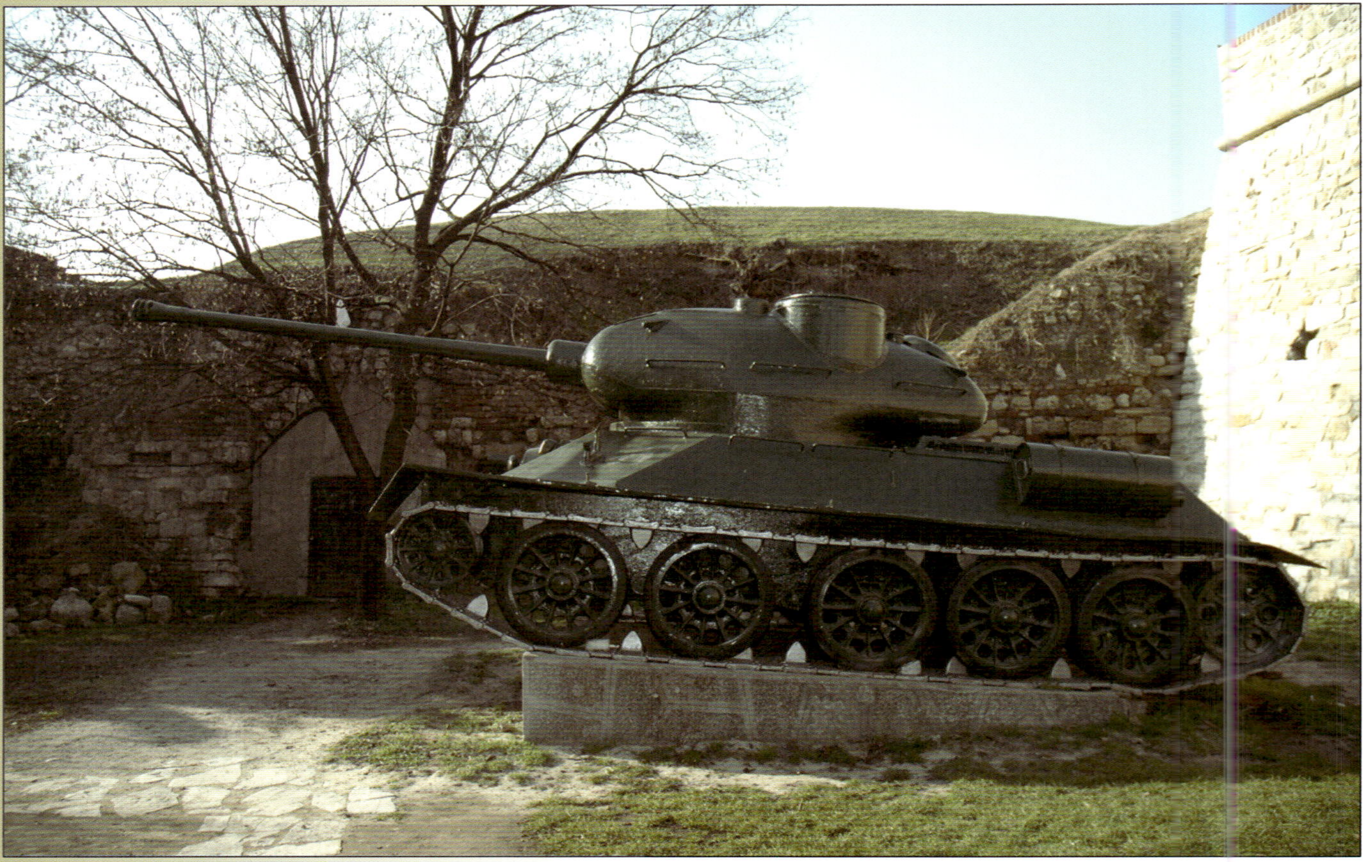

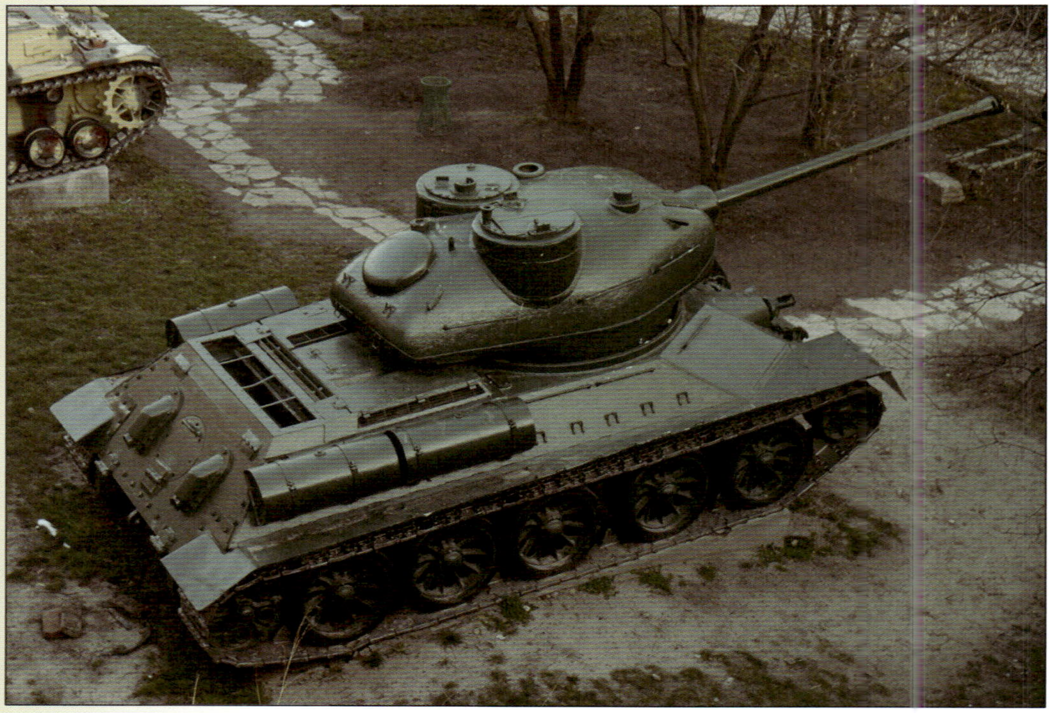

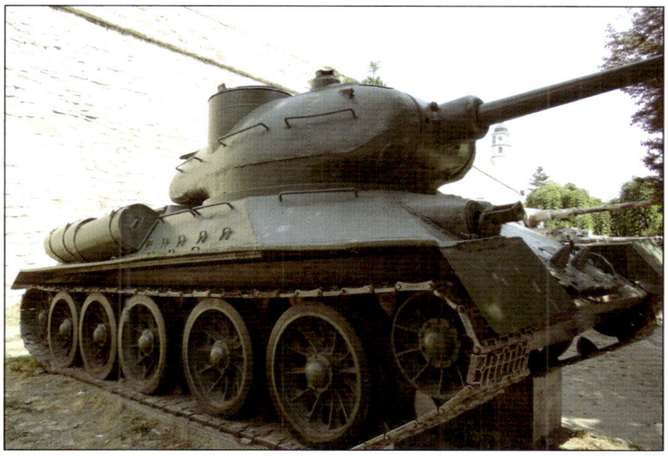
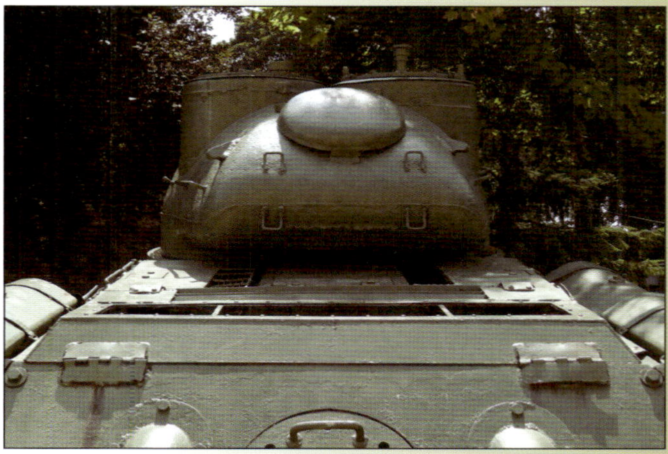
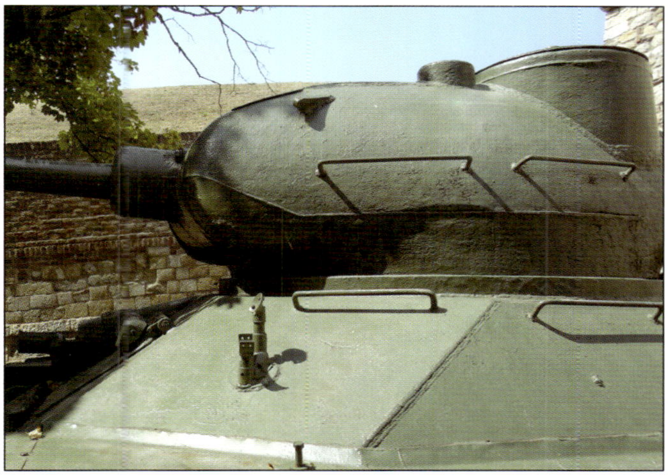
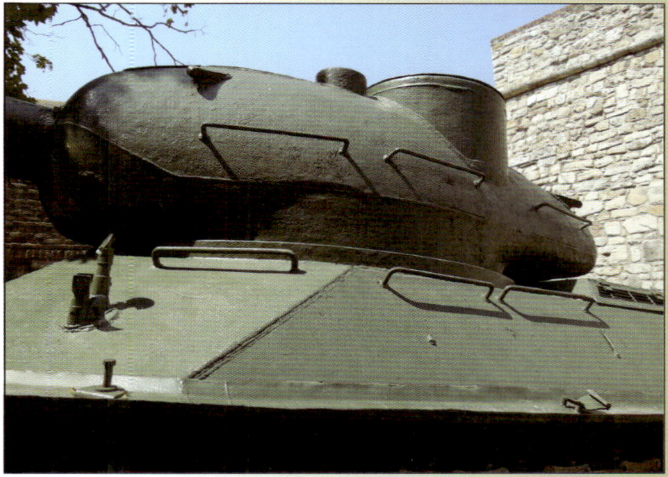
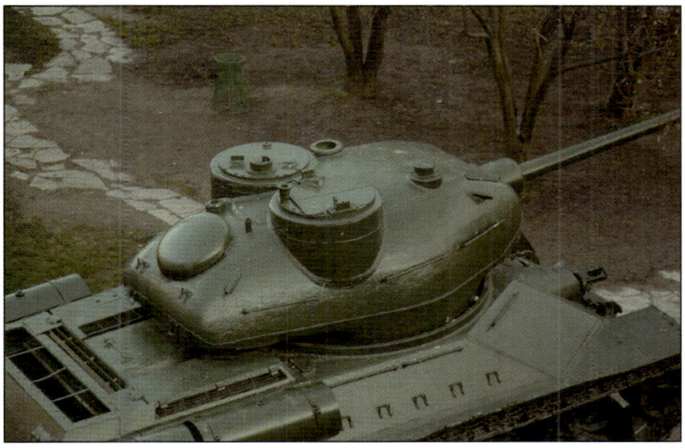
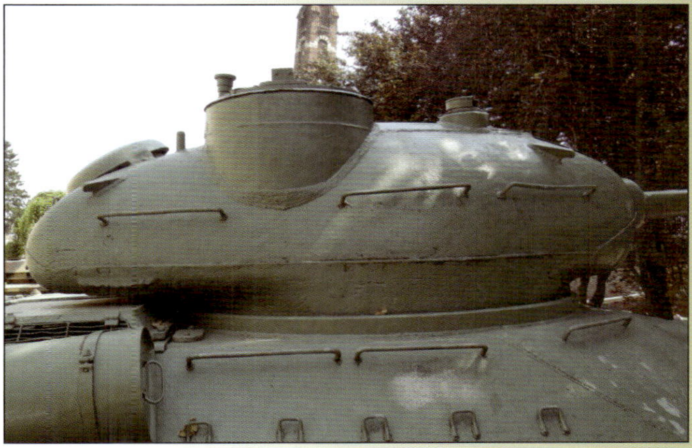
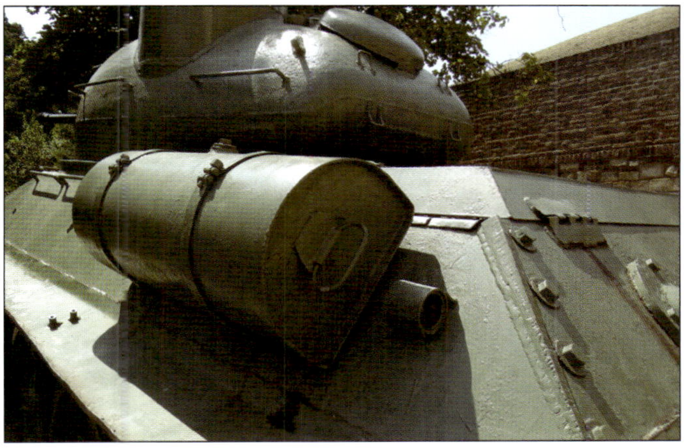
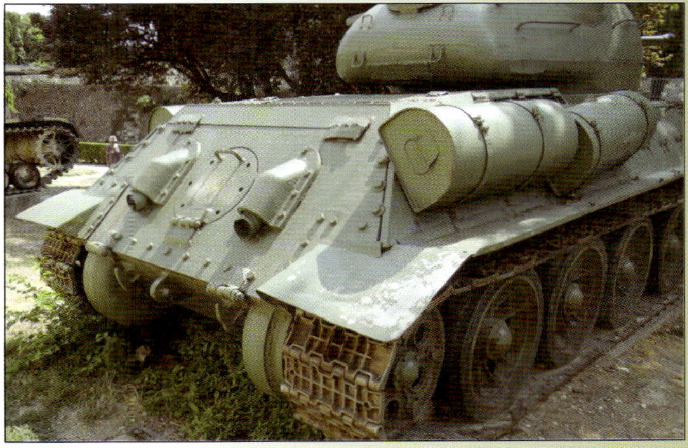

Polish T-34-85

Basic versions of Polish production T-34-85s. The photographs show tanks preserved at Armoured Weapon Museum in Poznań, Polish Arms Museum in Kołobrzeg and in private collections.

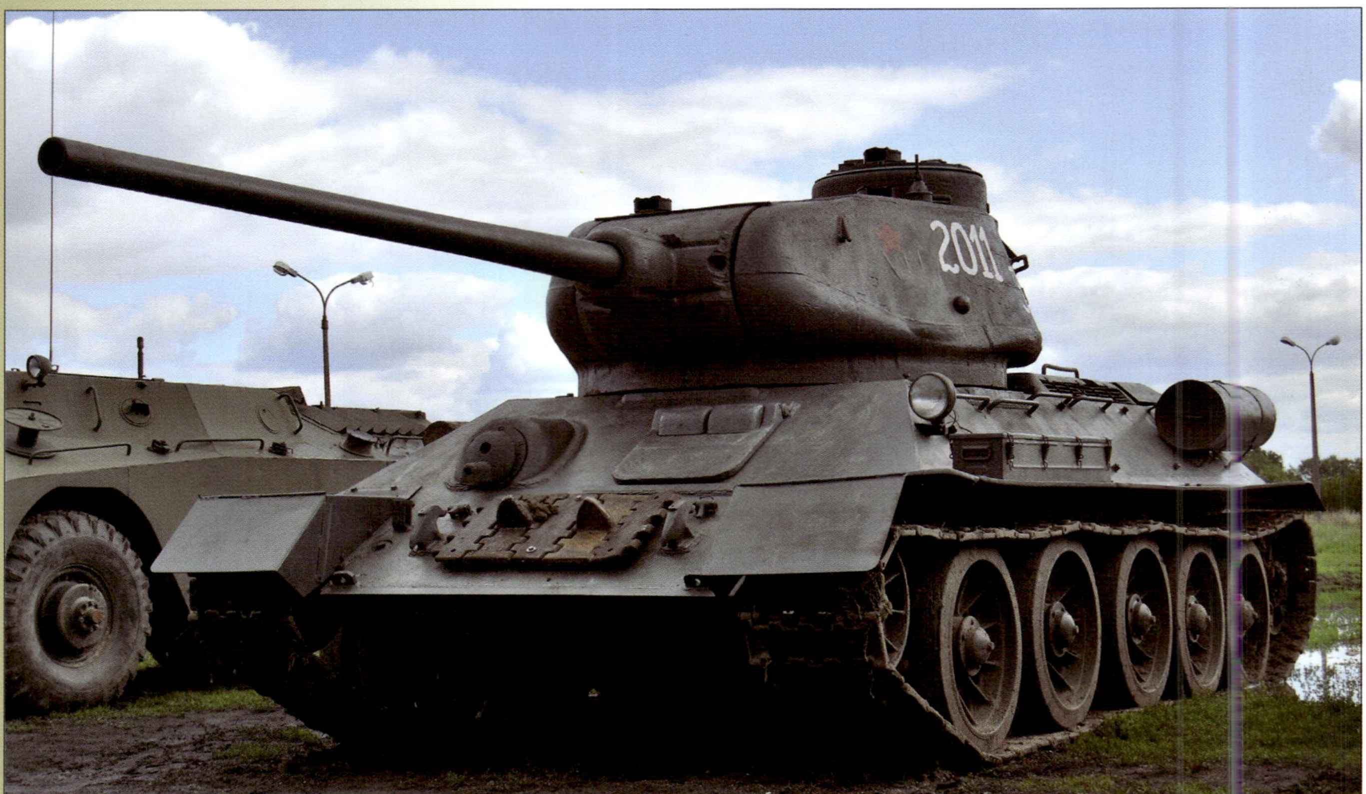

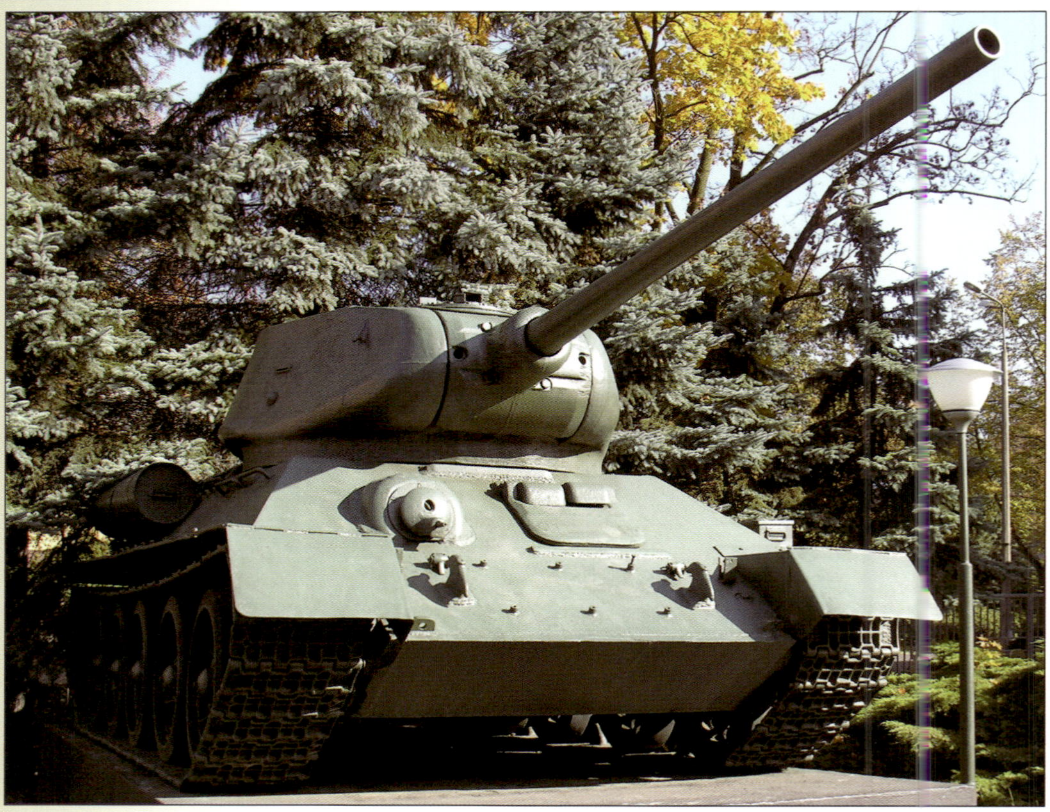

General view of a T-34-85 of Polish production.

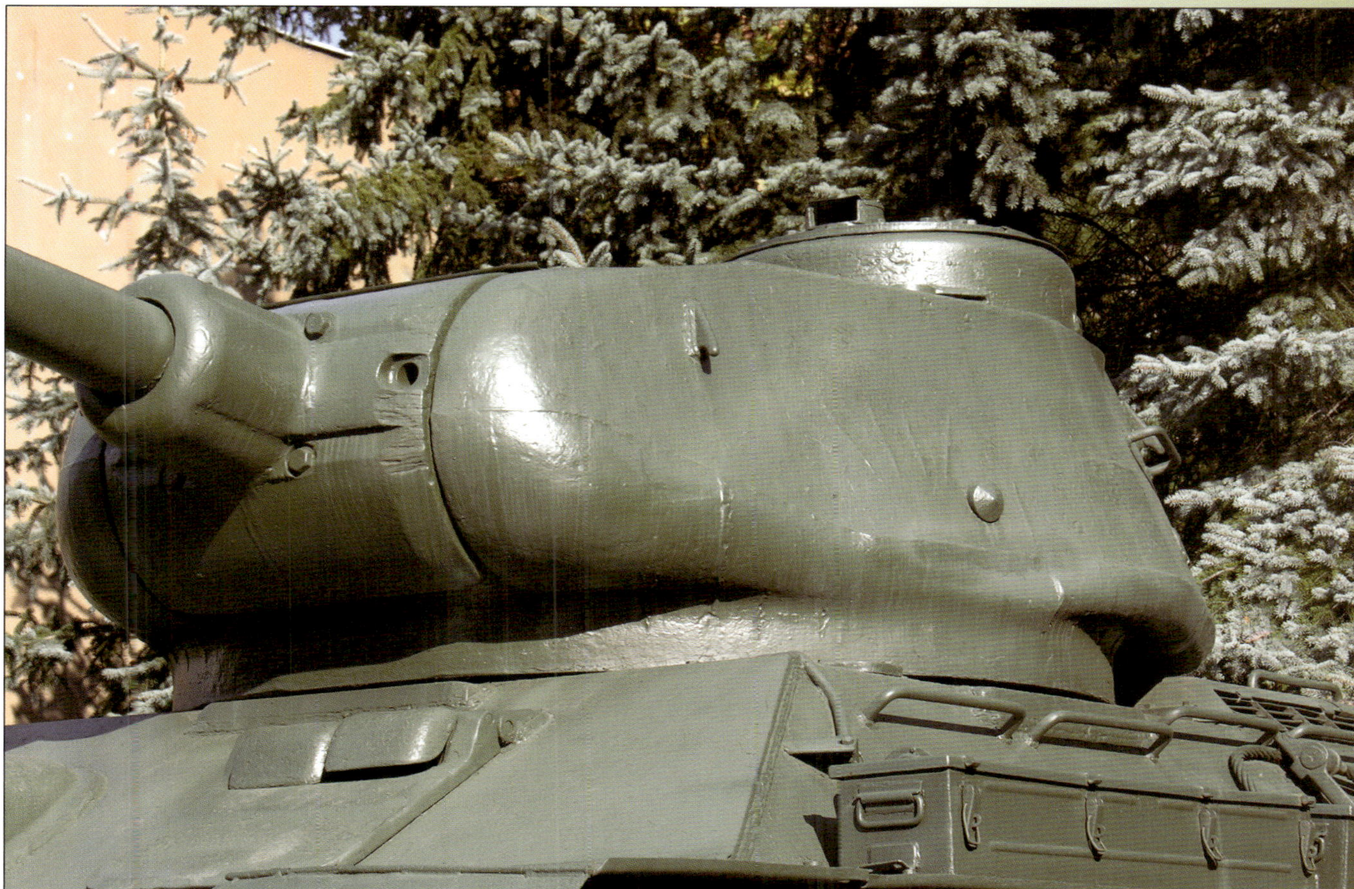

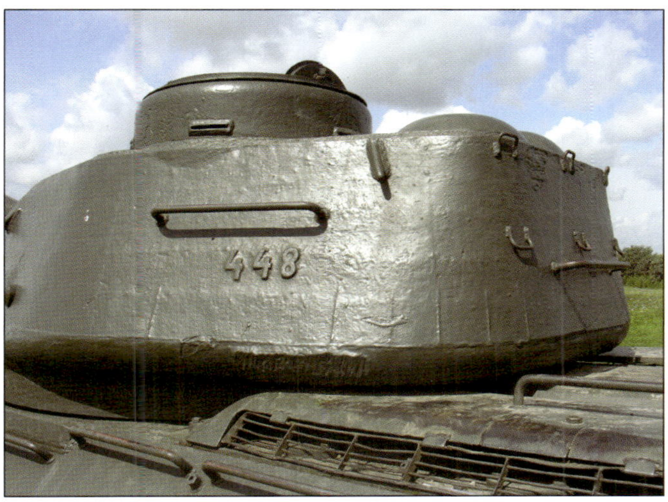

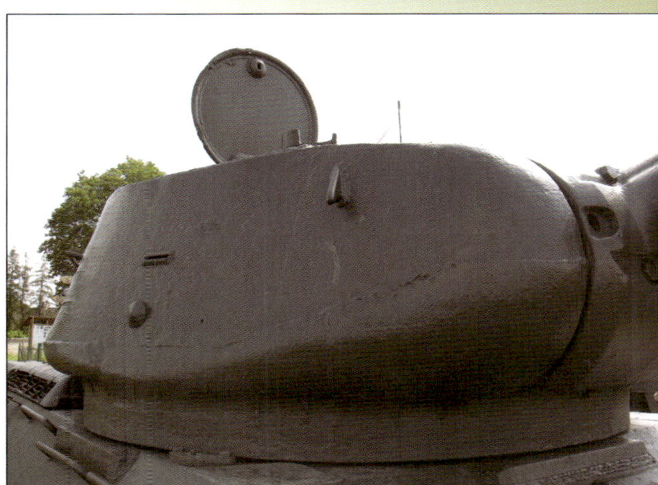

Above, three photos: Details of a turret of Polish production.

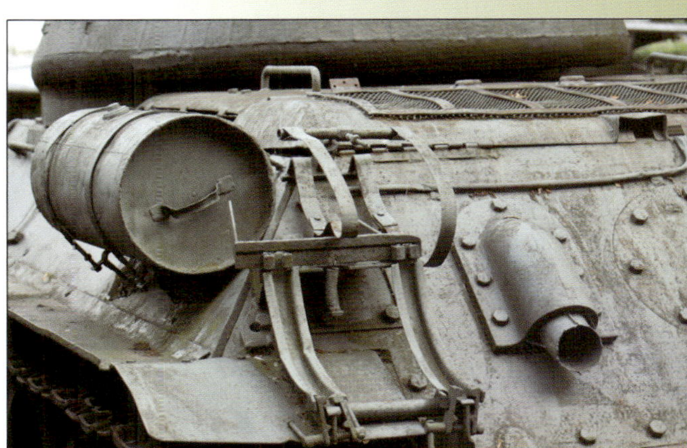

Rear section of the hull with holders for BDSh smoke canister and 200-litre fuel drum.

Tracks of a Polish T-34-85.

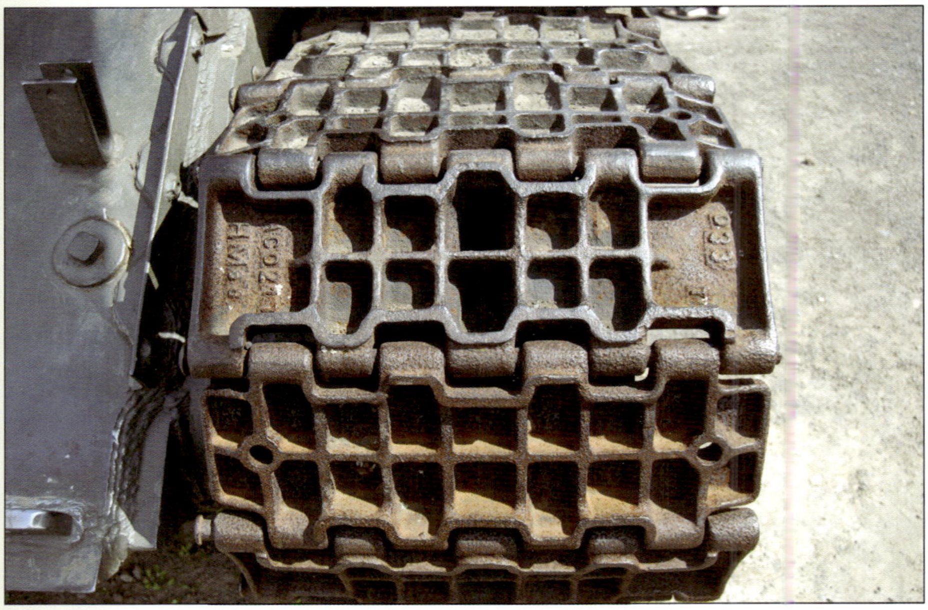

Open engine compartment hatch (transmission). Exhaust tubes with distinctive corrugated shrouds.

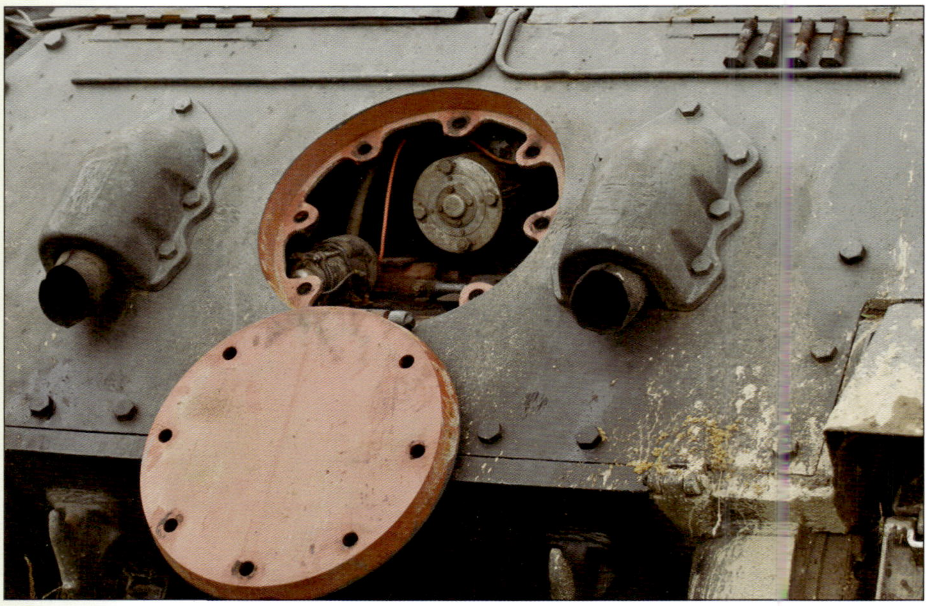

***Below:** Perforated road wheels used in most tanks of Polish production. However, some Polish T-34-85s had solid wheels (like the Czechoslovak tanks).*

***Below, right:** Idler wheel of a Polish T-34-85.*

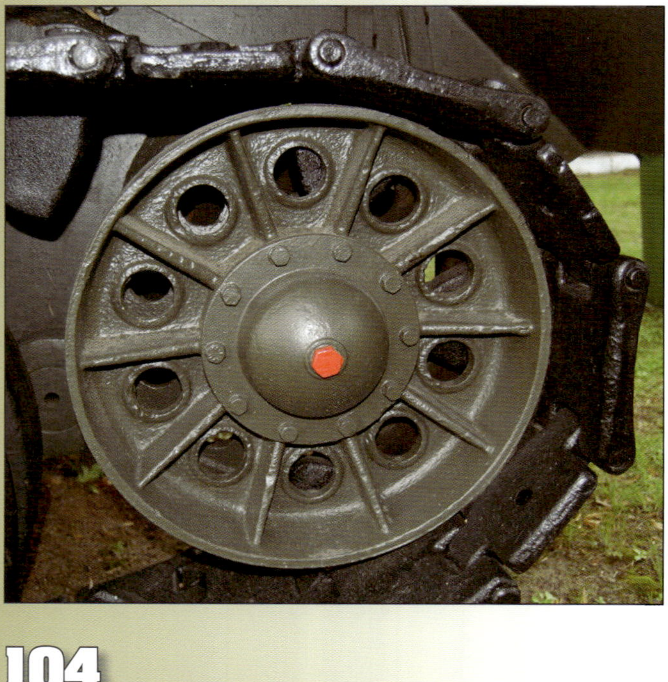

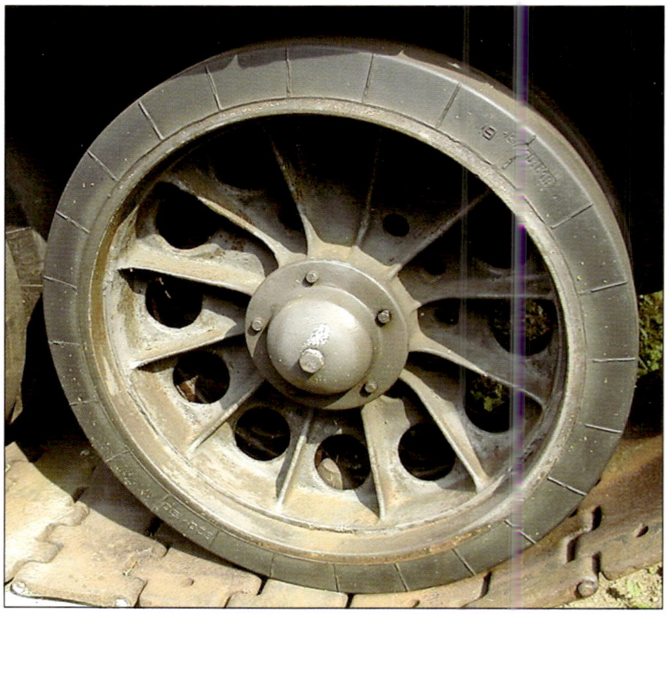

Polish T-34-85M2

Polish T-34-85M2 of Polish production, modified for crossing deep water obstacles on the bottom. The photographs show tanks preserved at museums in Bydgoszcz and Mirosławiec.

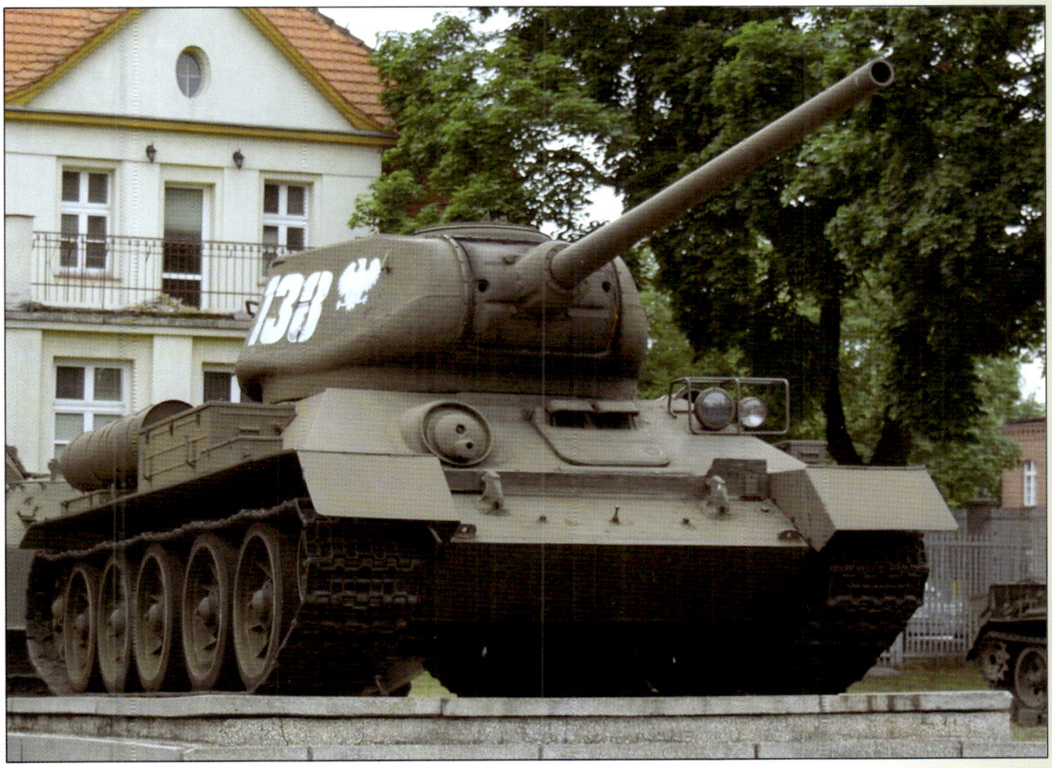

A T-34-85M2 preserved at Land Forces Museum in Bydgoszcz.

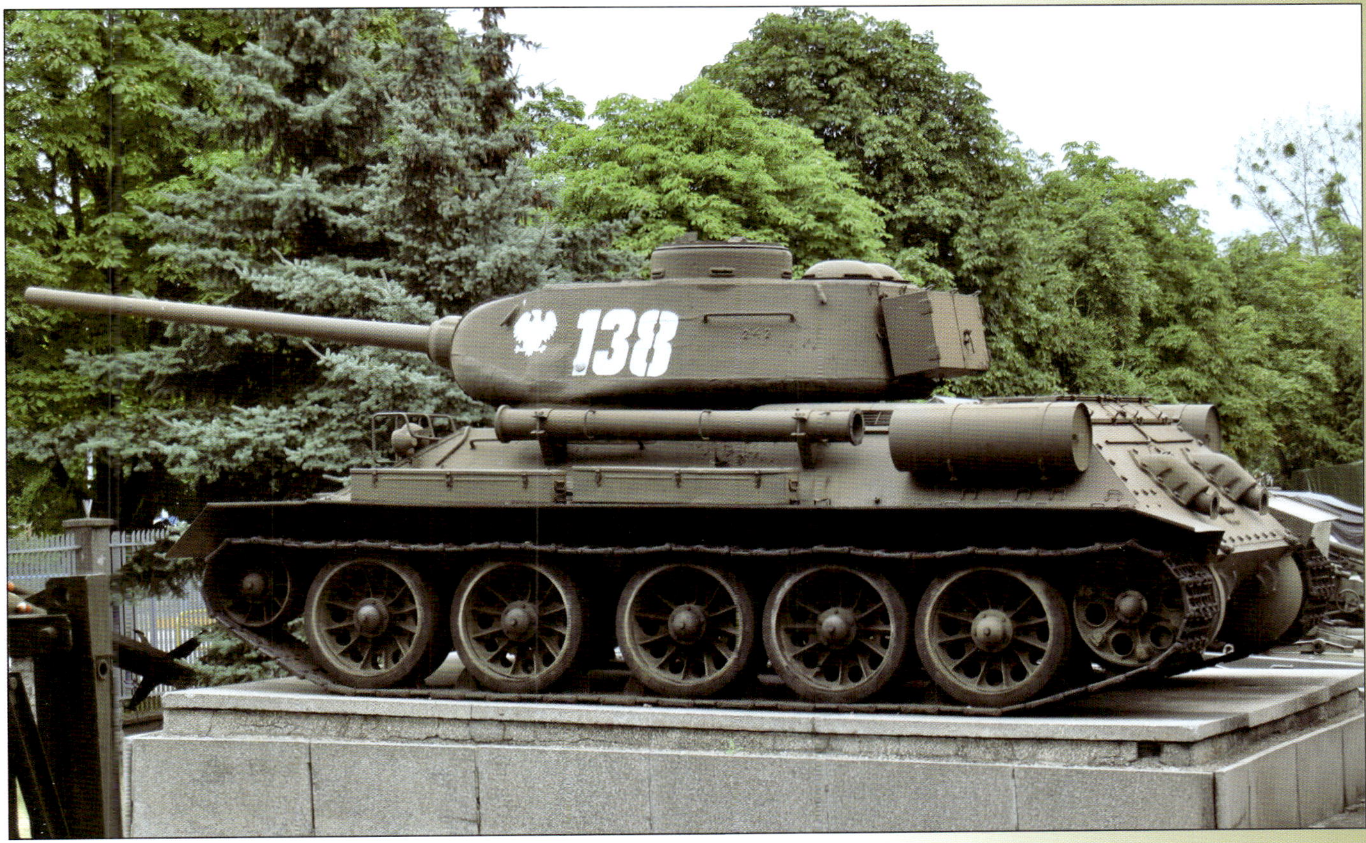

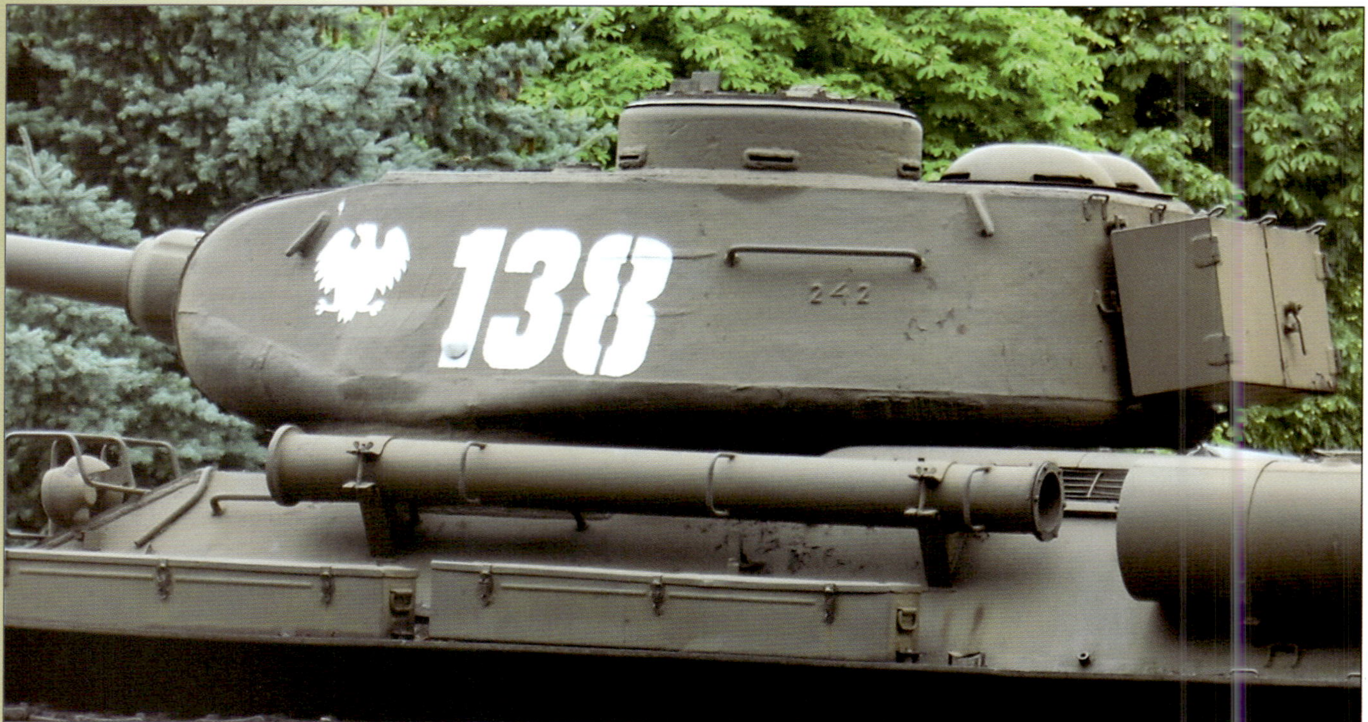

Above: Turret and middle section of the hull. The stowage box on the back of the turret and the snorkel are visible.

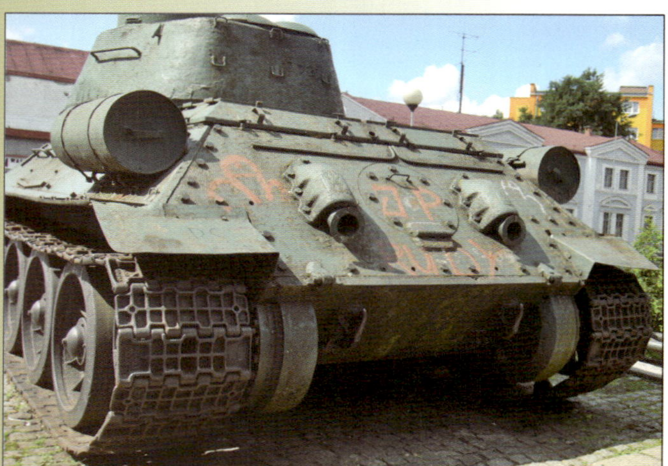

Rear section of the hull – fittings for cutoff valves on the exhaust pipes are visible.

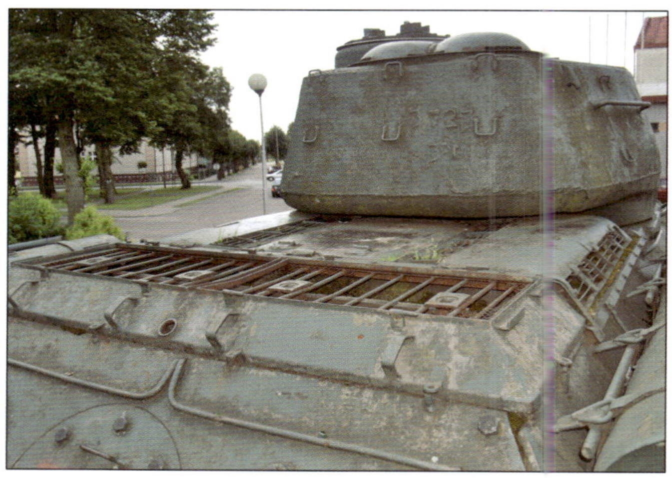

Rear section of the hull with louvres enabling sealing the engine compartment.

Forward machine gun with yoke enabling sealing.

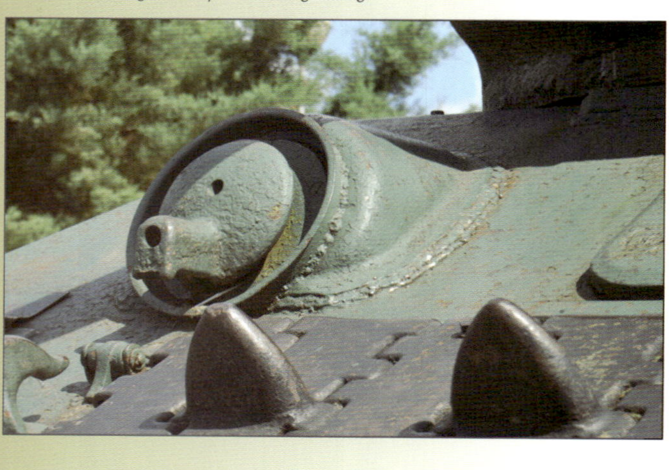

The roof of the turret with modifications enabling sealing and installation of the snorkel.

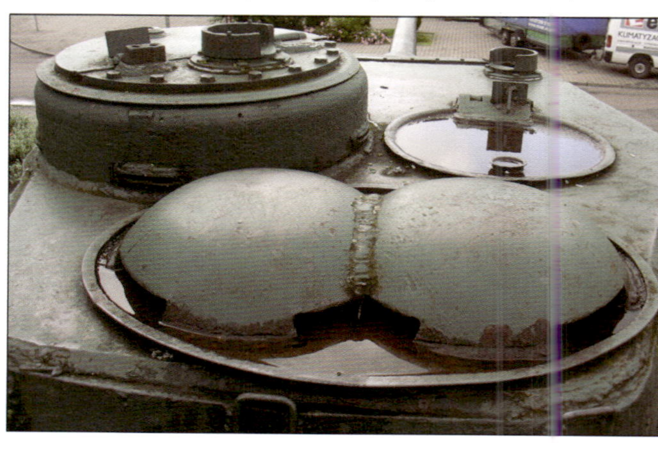

Bulgarian modernizations

The T-34-85 tanks operated by Bulgarian armoured units underwent modernization, probably in the 1960s. Although the scope of modifications was diverse, they usually consisted in addition of holders for 200-litre fuel drums on the back of the hull, installation of a stowage box on the left side of the hull and holders for BDSh smoke cannister immediately aft of it. On the right side the set of lines for fitting the unditching beam. However, most surprising were small turrets and anti-aircraft machine gun mount on the loader's hatch.

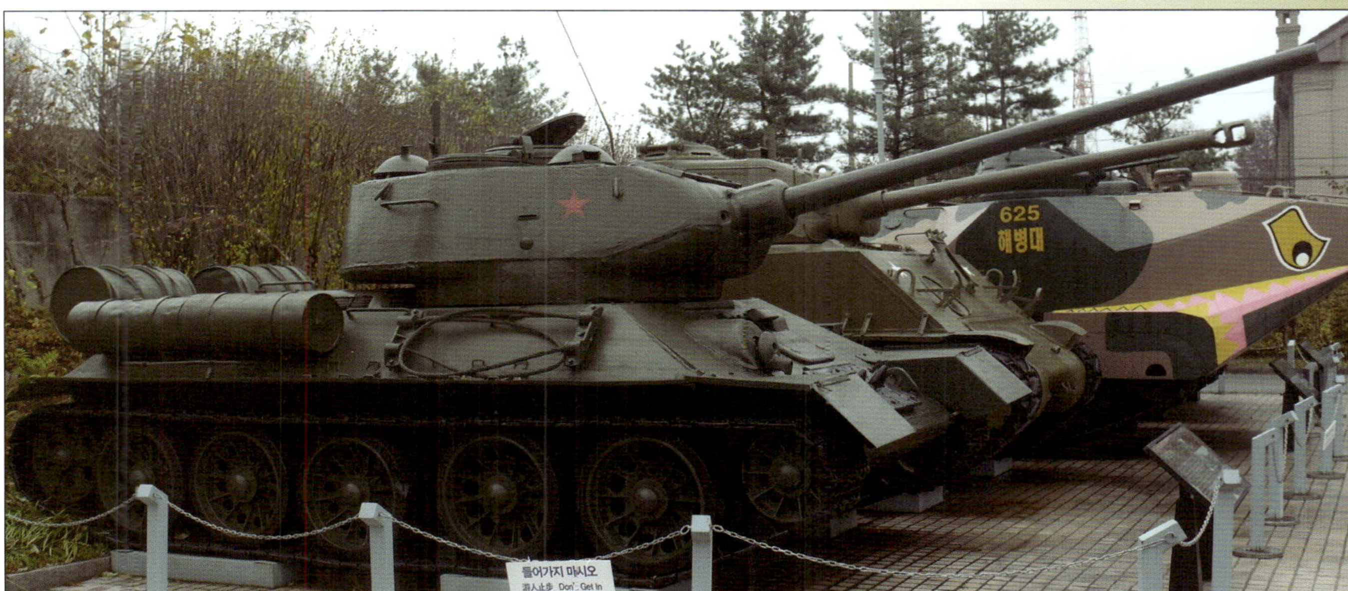

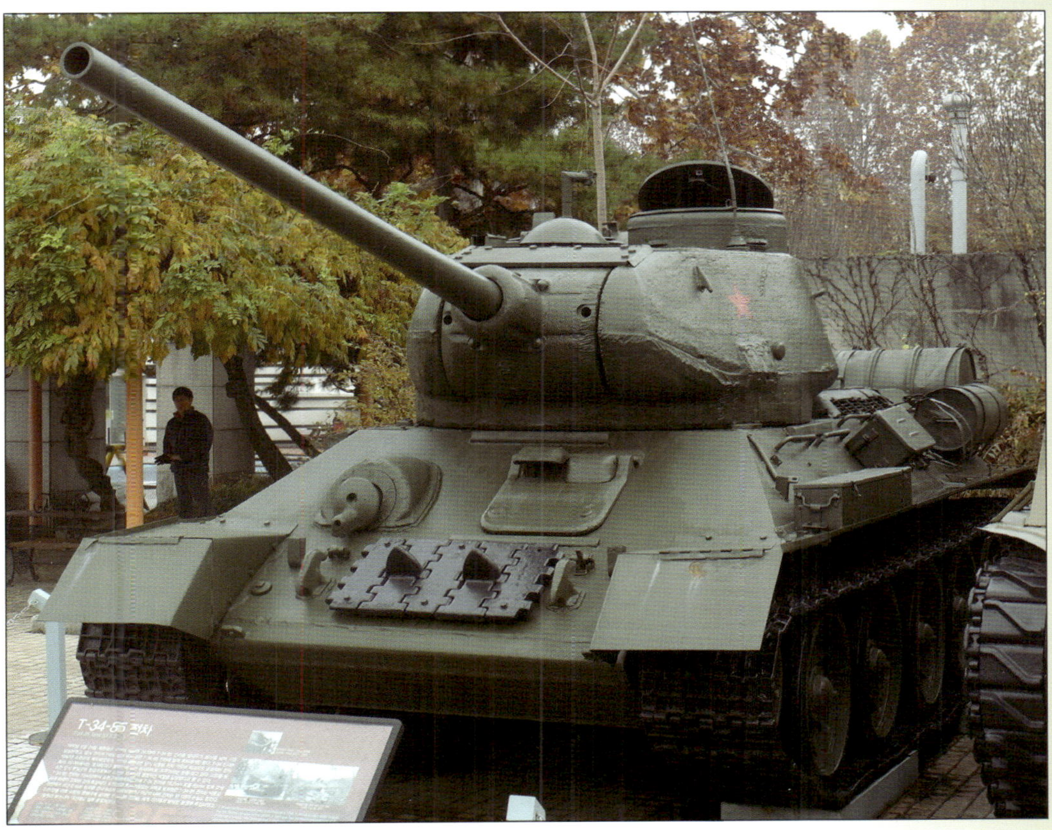

Modernized Bulgarian T-34-85 (probably of Omsk Plant No.174 post-war production).

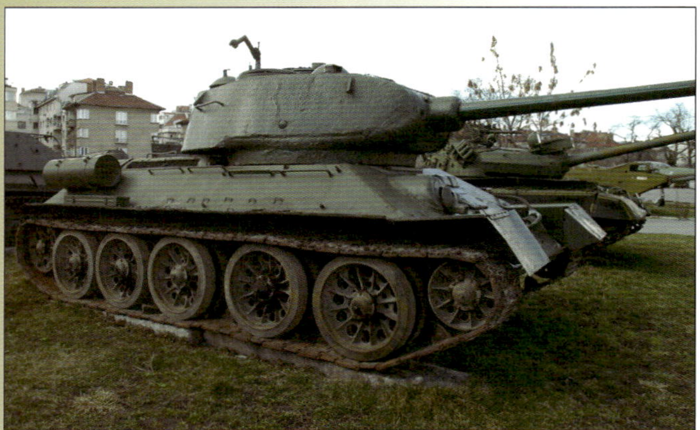

Modernized Bulgarian T-34-85 (so-called mushroom-type turret with two single ventilators of Gorki Plant No.112 production)

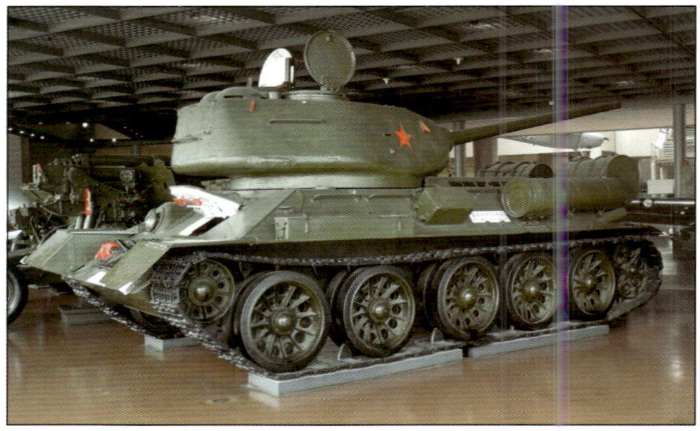

Modernized Bulgarian T-34-85 of Czechoslovak production, preserved at Korean War Memorial in Seoul.

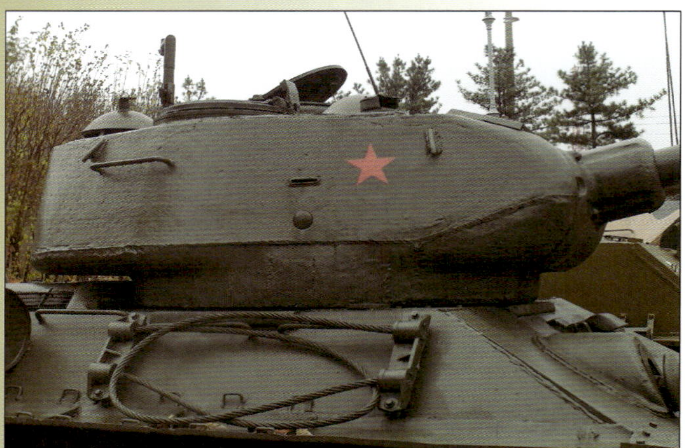

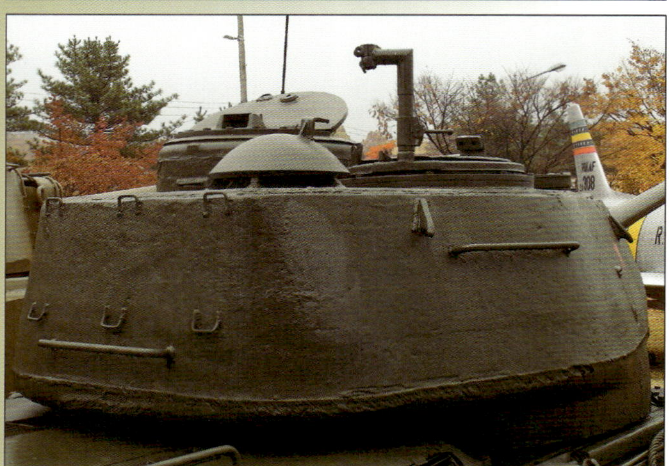

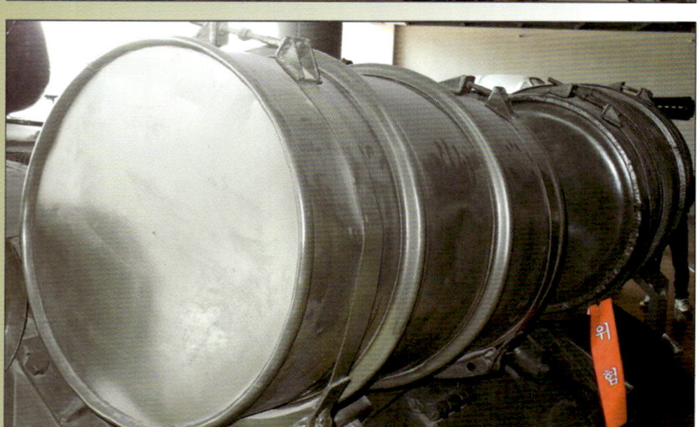

***Left, left below:** T-34-85 turret with modifications characteristic for Bulgarian tanks.*

***Below:** The turret with machine gun mount on loader's hatch.*

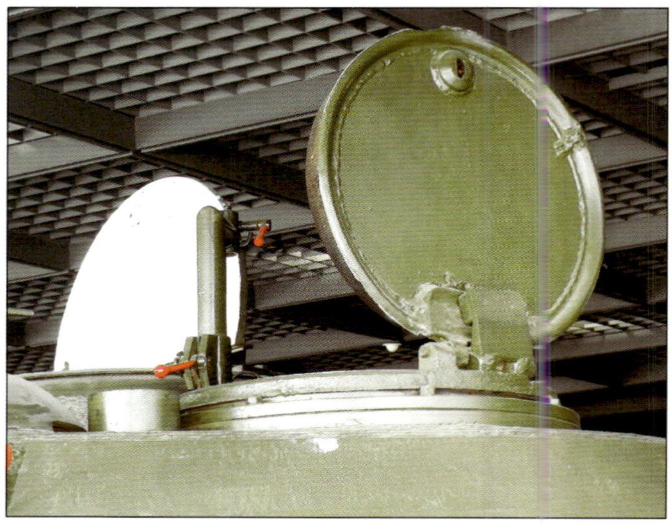

***Below, below right:** Holders for 200-litre barrels on the back of the hull.*

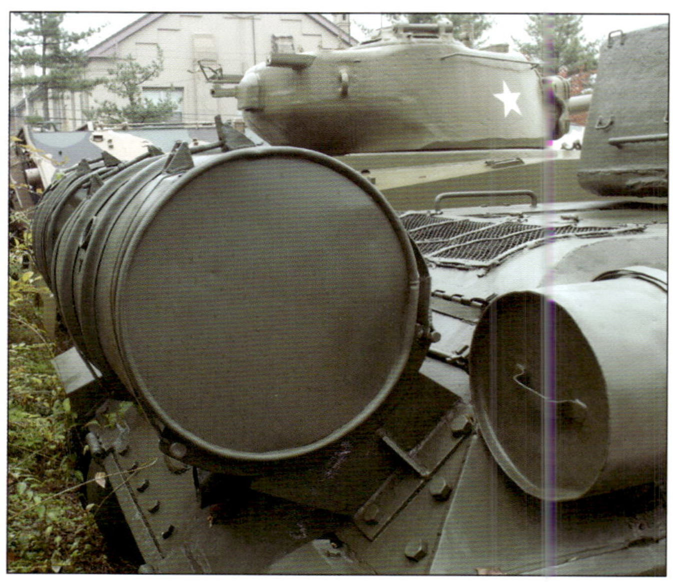

Chinese modernizations

A T-34-85 of wartime Soviet production (Plant No.174) modernized in China. The tank has new cupolas for the commander and on the loader's hatch (with machine gun mount) and modernized hinges of the rear armour plate and transmission compartment door. The tank shown in the photos had no exhaust pipes with their armoured shrouds.

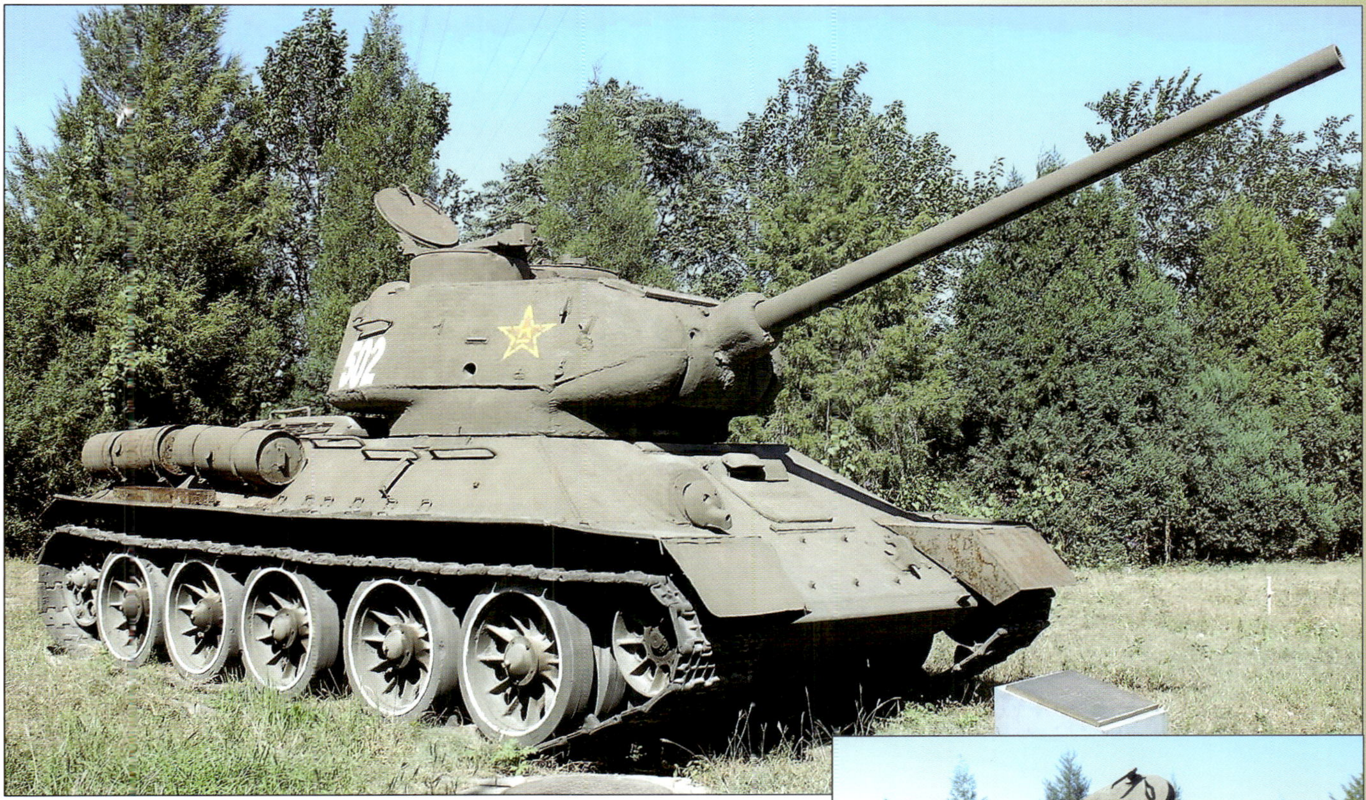

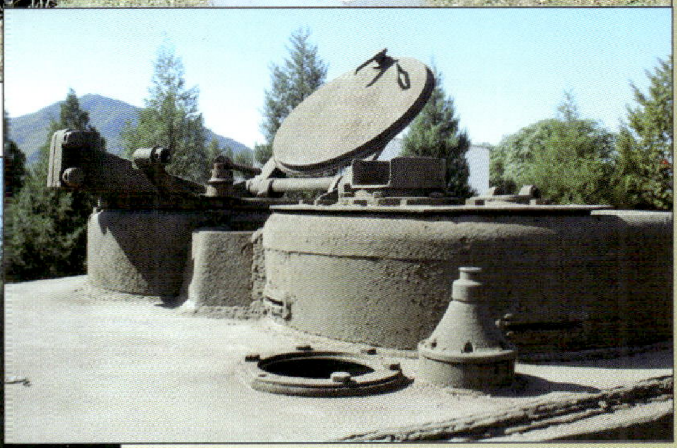

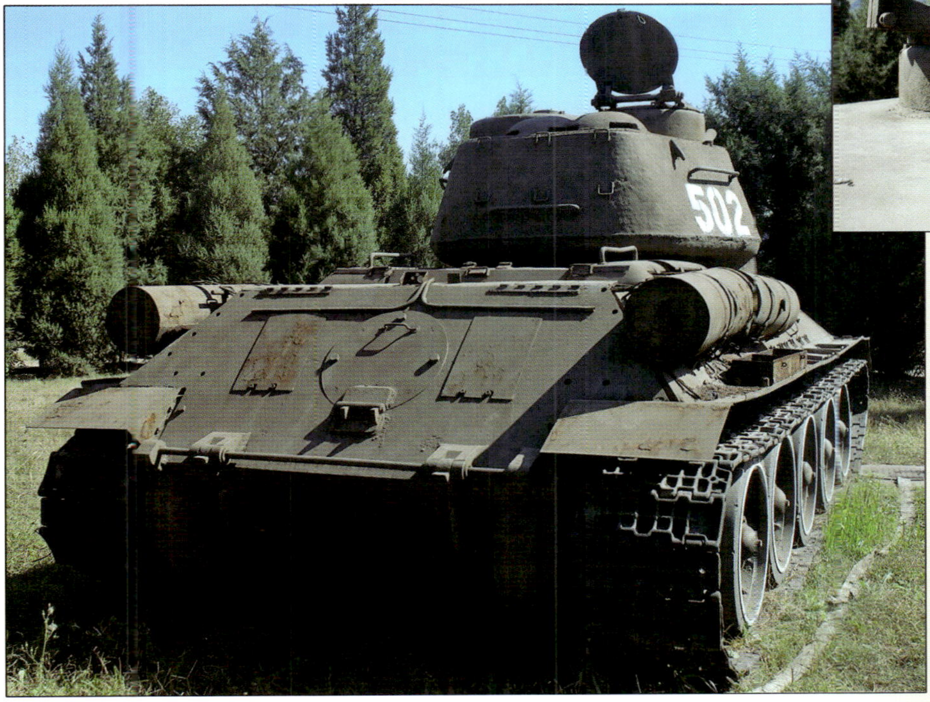

Romanian modernization

A T-34-85 of Czechoslovak production, modernized in Romania probably on the turn in 1960/70. The tank is adapted for crossing water obstacles on the bottom. It was als fitted with additional equipment, such as the toolbox on the left side of the hull and holders fo unditching beam rigging line. This tank is preserved at the military museum in Bucharest.

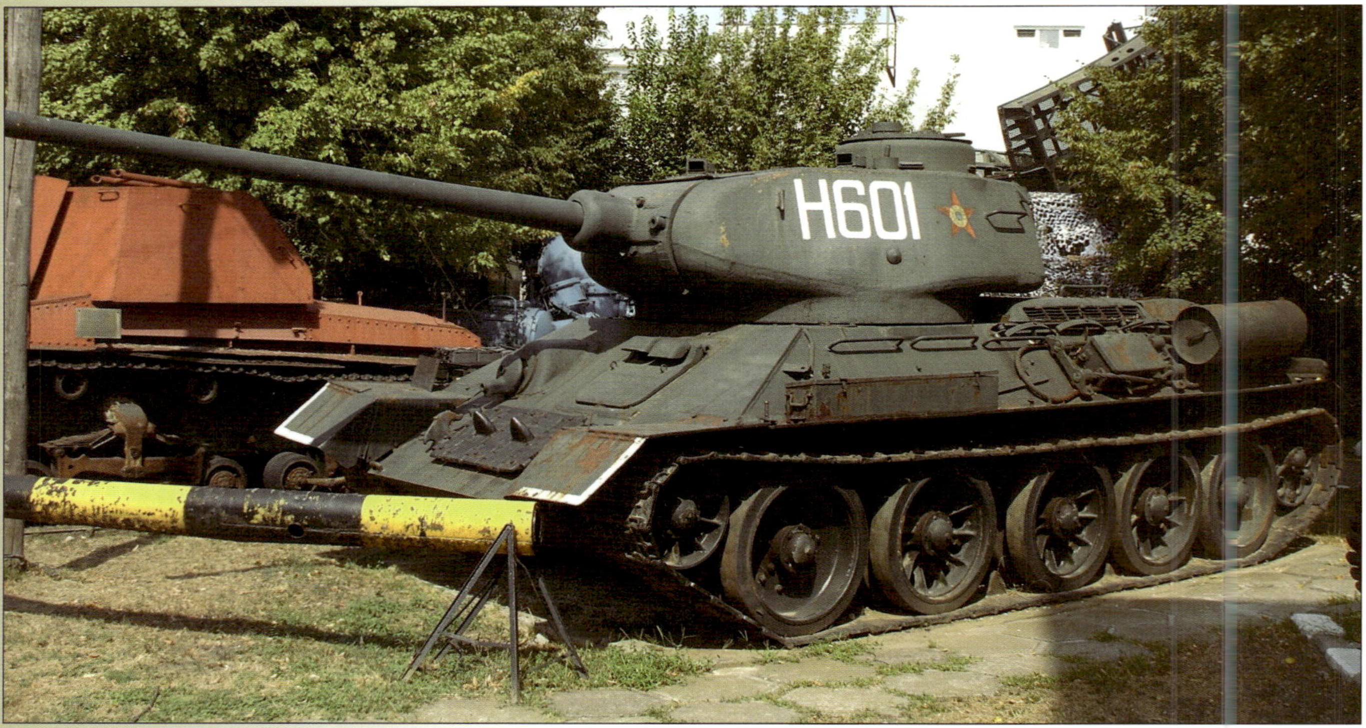

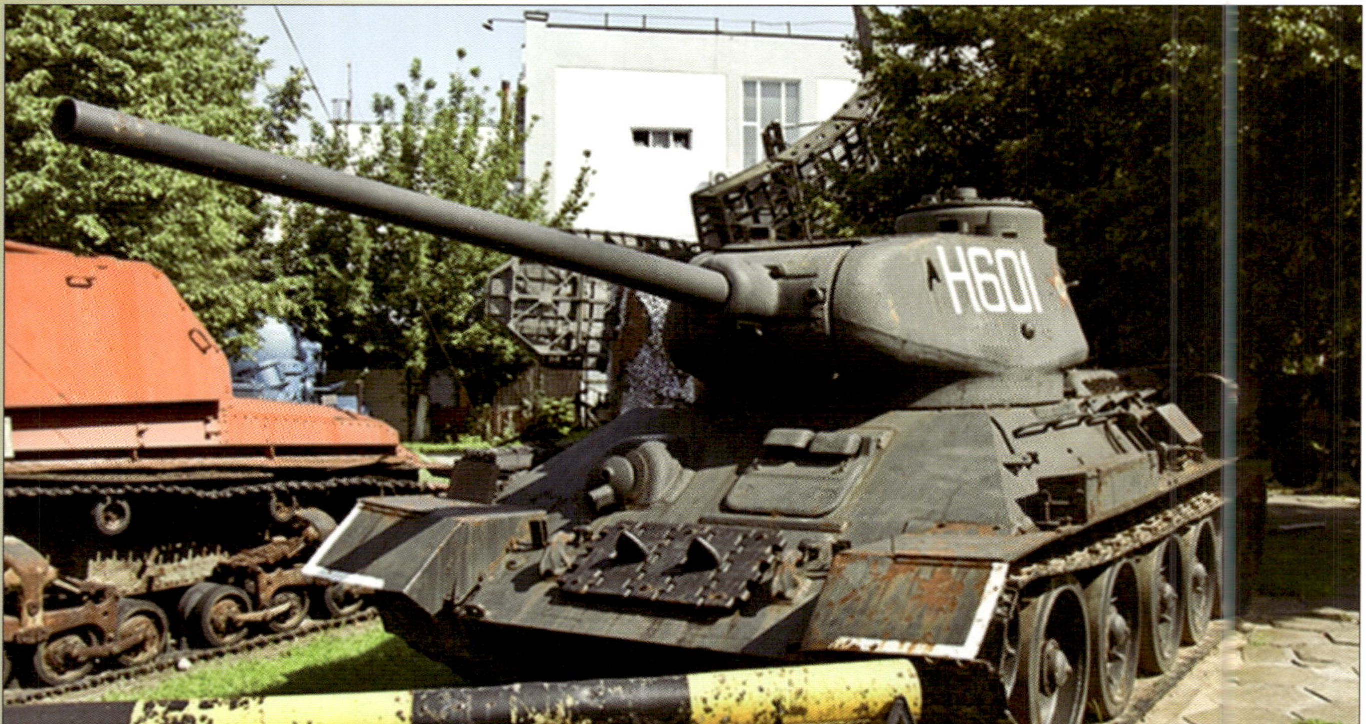

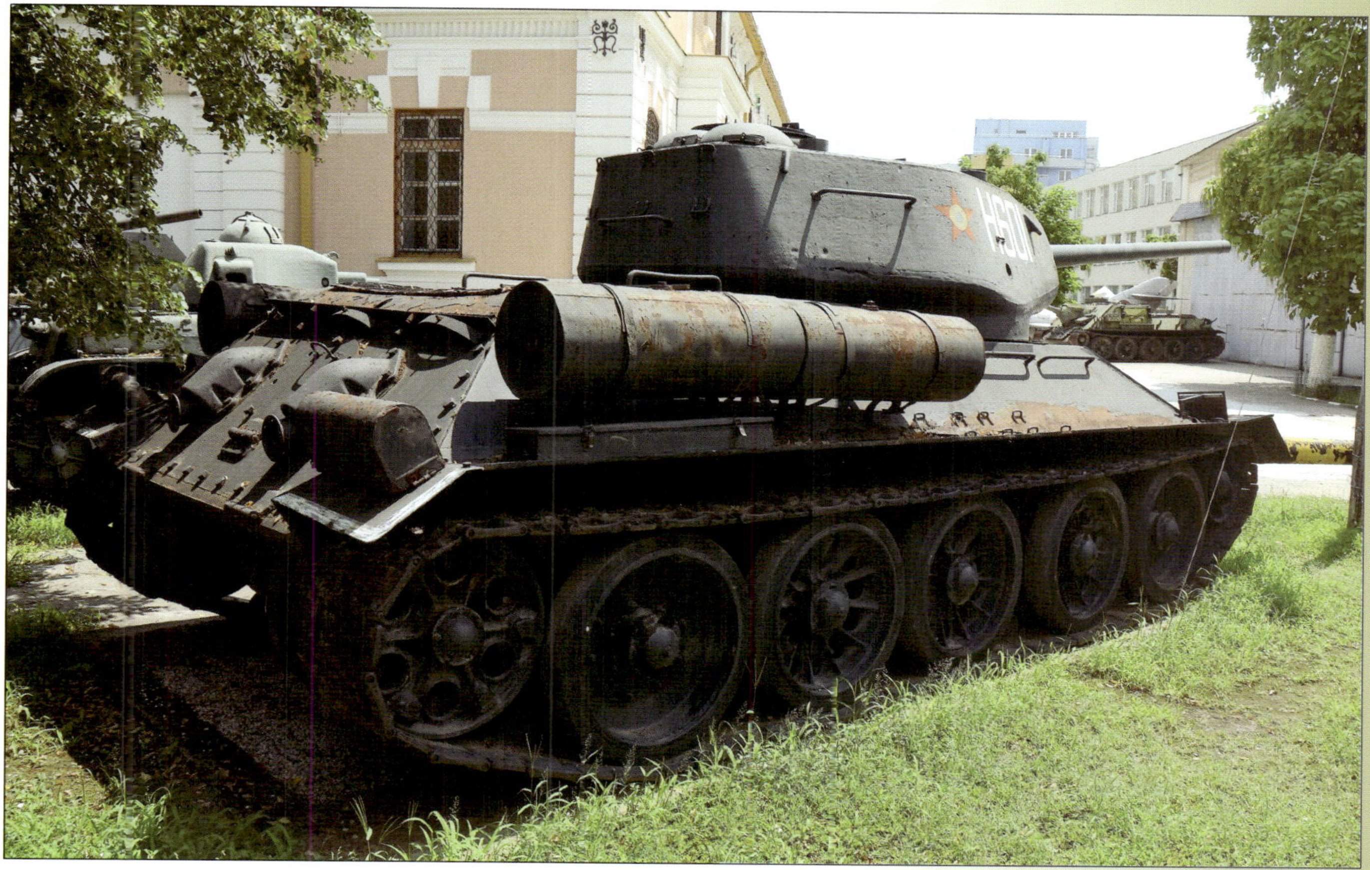
H601

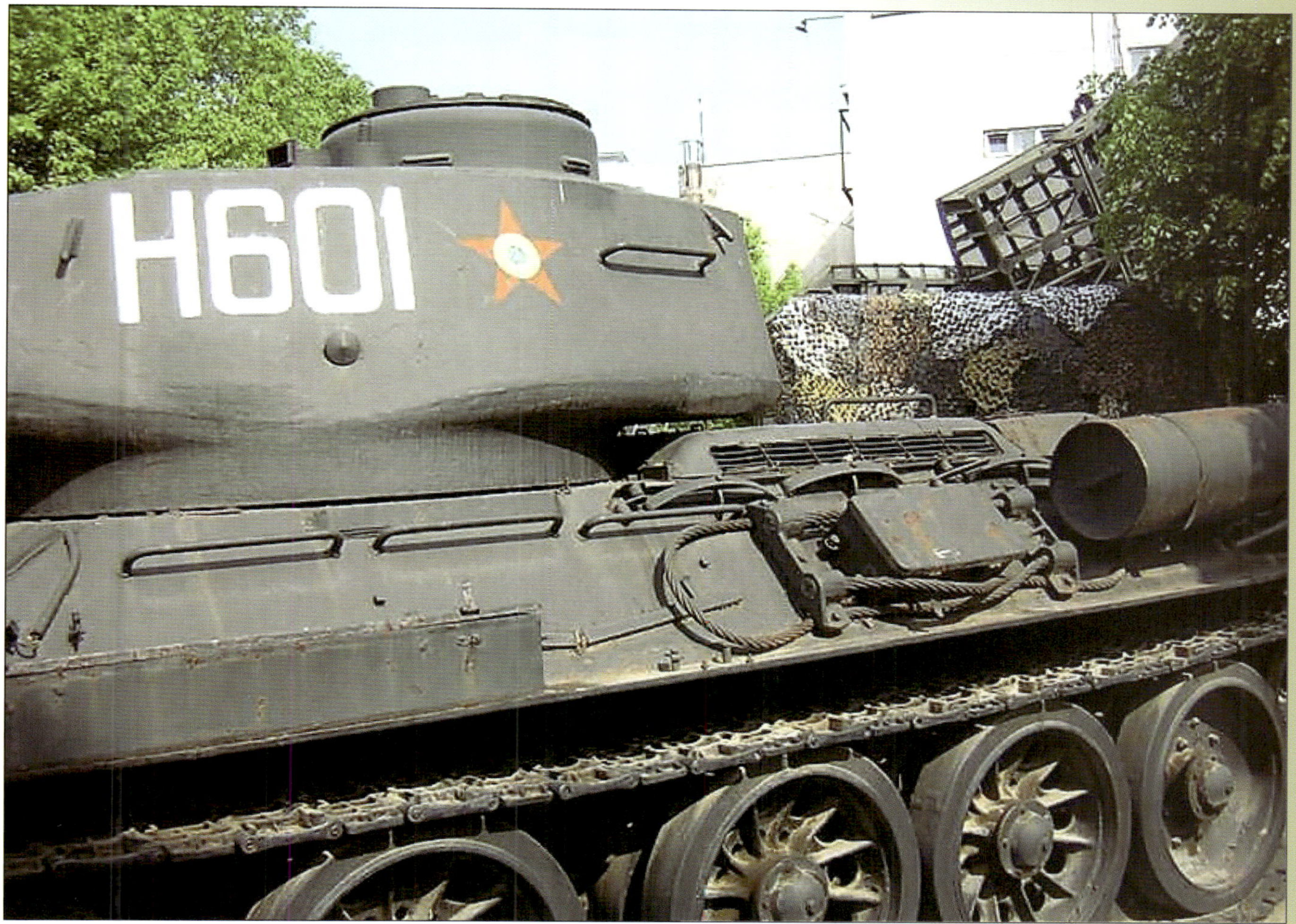
H601

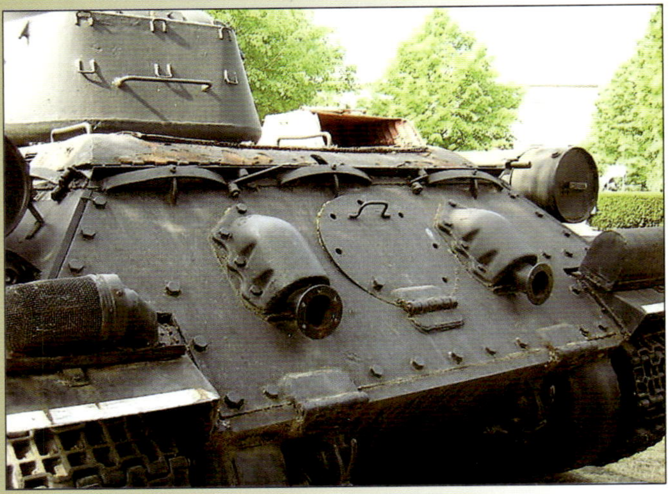
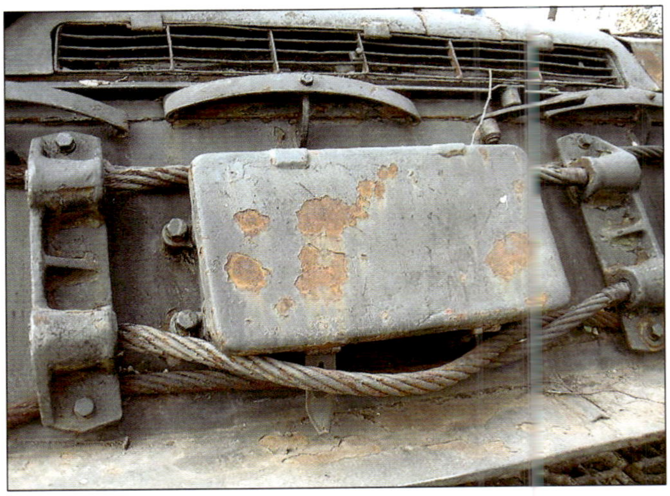
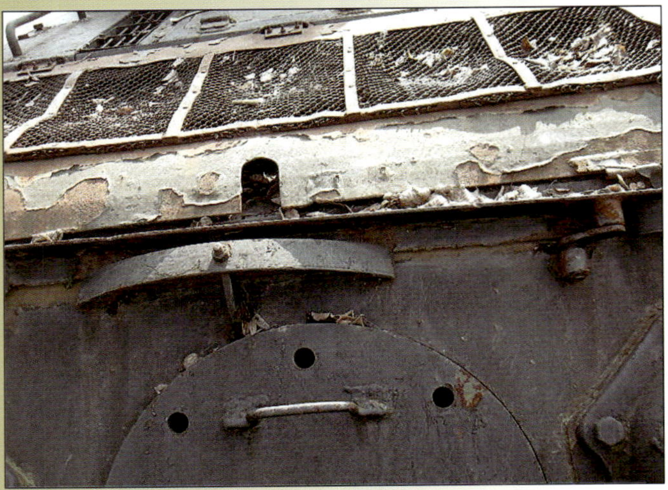
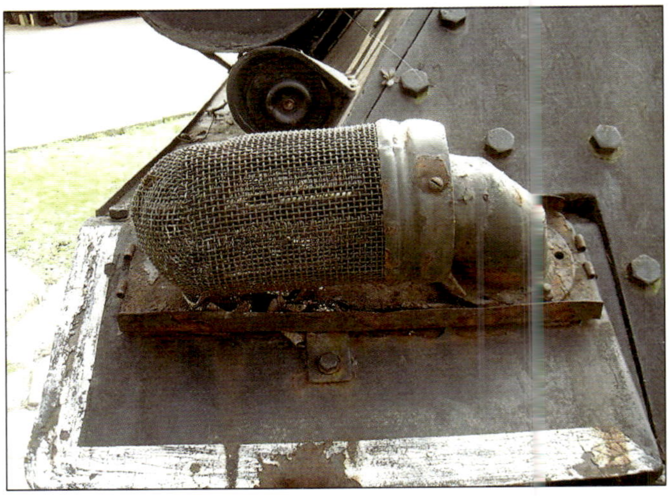
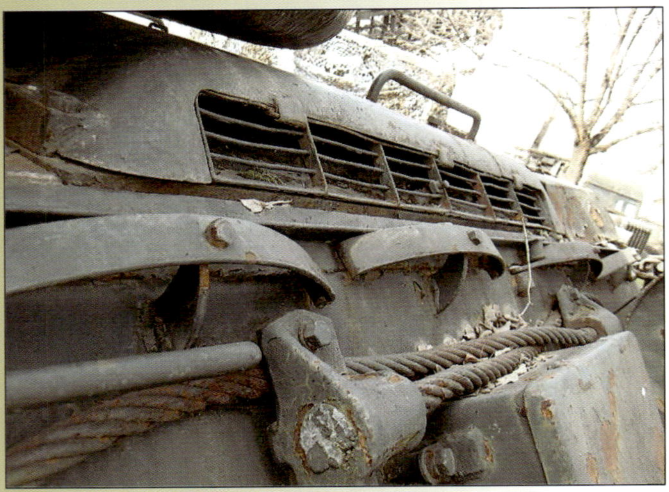
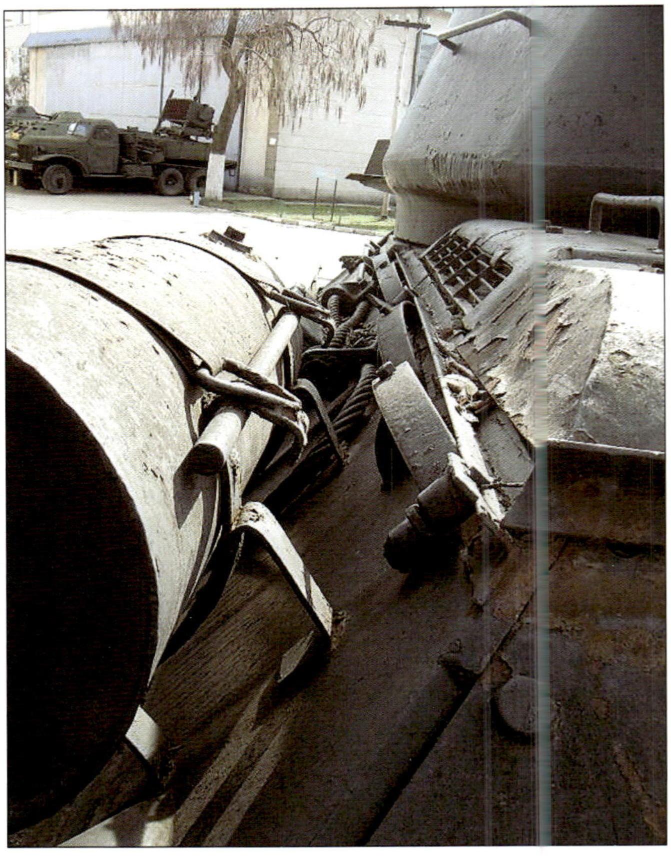

Installation for crossing water obstacles on the bottom on Romanian T-34-85.